Behavioral Interventions for Prevention and Control of Sexually Transmitted Diseases

Behavioral Interventions for Prevention and Control of Sexually Transmitted Diseases

Sevgi O. Aral, Ph.D.
John M. Douglas, Jr., M.D.
Editors

Judith A. Lipshutz, M.P.H.
Associate Editor

Division of STD Prevention
National Centers for HIV, STD, and TB Prevention
Centers for Disease Control and Prevention
Atlanta, Georgia, USA

Foreword by H. Hunter Handsfield and Edward W. Hook III

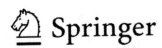 Springer

ISBN-13: 978-0-387-47863-0   e-ISBN-13: 978-0-387-48740-3

Library of Congress Control Number: 2006937338

Printed on acid-free paper.

9 8 7 6 5 4 3 2 1

springer.com

Foreword

It goes without saying that sexually transmitted diseases (STDs) are consequences of human behavior at the individual and community levels, and it stands to reason that behavioral interventions can and should contribute to STD control efforts. This is not a new idea. Throughout most of human history, the lack of effective therapy or other biomedical means of control required reliance on rudimentary behavioral strategies in attempts at prevention. Approaching the modern era, the import of behavioral assessment and intervention was emphasized by Thomas Parran, the surgeon general of the United States, in his groundbreaking road map for syphilis control, *Shadow on the Land*.[1]

However, notwithstanding Dr. Parran's insight, the dawning of the antibiotic era, soon followed by the burgeoning of microbiology, immunology, and epidemiology, ushered in an era in which markedly improved diagnosis, treatment, and understanding of the at-risk populations pushed behavior into the background. By the 1970s and early 1980s, seemingly the main solutions to control syphilis, gonorrhea, and emergent chlamydial infections were the resources and political will to apply the rapidly evolving biomedical knowledge. There was continued acknowledgment that sexual behavior, at both individual and societal levels, was fueling the rapidly rising tide of bacterial STDs, and that behavioral intervention had a potential role in prevention. However, for many generations, the public health establishment had been advising sexually active people to avoid commercial sex, to use condoms outside committed partnerships, and to seek care promptly when they developed symptoms. It was understood that many persons at risk did not follow that sage counsel, but what more could be done except to say it again? If we could not prevent people from becoming infected, at least screening, early diagnosis, and prompt treatment would make serious morbidity a thing of the past.

Then along came AIDS, growing awareness of the importance of genital herpes and sexually transmitted hepatitis, and understanding that many human papillomavirus infections are more than benign inconveniences. All of a sudden,

---

[1] Parran T. *Shadow on the Land: Syphilis*. New York: Reynal and Hitchcock; 1937.

our biomedical prevention emperor appeared thinly clothed indeed. Without curative treatment, early diagnosis of human immunodeficiency virus infection offered little obvious benefit to infected individuals. Diagnosing incurable HIV infections seemed a hollow victory, and gradually, it became apparent that screening and counseling uninfected people had little of the expected benefit in preventing transmission. Absent protective immunization, the only strategy even theoretically available to prevent accelerating transmission of the viral STDs was to understand and ultimately to influence partner selection, sex partner numbers, sexual practices, use of condoms, and the use of mind-altering substances, both at the individual level and in populations.

Thus, the emergence of AIDS and heightened appreciation of the impact of other viral STDs raised awareness that behavior matters more than theoretically. Furthermore, the forced attention on behavioral interventions prompted understanding that biomedical strategies are inherently insufficient to control any STD. Over the last twenty-five years, we have come to understand that behavior—of infected persons, of their sex partners and other persons at risk, of health care providers, of partner networks, and of entire populations—is central to success of the biomedical interventions themselves. Who visits settings where screening, diagnosis, and treatment can be implemented, and why? What factors influence persons' decisions to continue, cease, or modify their sexual behaviors in response to symptoms consistent with STD and to seek medical attention? What about compliance with therapy and follow-up? What do people do and not do to ensure that their partners are evaluated and treated, and what determines the partners' responses? What do health care providers ask or counsel their patients about risky behaviors, who do they screen, what do they understand about recommended screening criteria and treatment, and why do they use the tests and drugs they use? And, ultimately, how can we get persons at risk, those infected with STDs, their partners, and their providers to modify all these and many other behaviors to help curtail STD transmission?

Even during the heyday of biomedical prevention, a few colleagues understood what effective prevention would require, citing new models that integrated infected persons and those at risk, health care providers, social exchange, and the cultural environment. And experts historically linked to biomedical strategies began to see the light. For example, King Holmes brought a polymath's understanding to the biomedical paradigm and tirelessly promoted the importance of the behavioral sciences in STD prevention, with emphasis on the career development of social and behavioral scientists. We turned to these and other colleagues, and they opened our eyes and continue to do so.

For clinicians and public health experts, these early contributors, their peers, and their intellectual successors have provided heightened appreciation not only of the import, but also of the complexity of modifying behaviors that contribute to STD prevention and management. No longer do prevention experts consider simplistic exhortations to "just say no" or "use condoms" to be appropriate or meaningful interventions. Increasing appreciation and use of theories of behavior change, carefully crafted approaches to counseling, validated measures for evaluating behaviors, and critical assessment of intervention strategies are now increasingly embedded as crucial elements of successful STD control.

Thus, from humble beginnings dating to Dr. Parran comes this book, the first text to systematically summarize the science of behavioral interventions to prevent STDs. From theoretical underpinnings to pragmatic application, this work addresses behavioral approaches to prevention at the individual and population levels, methodologies to measure their effectiveness, and the profound policy and ethical implications. It is expected that this work not only will contribute directly to improved STD prevention, but also will stimulate further creative development of this enormously important and significant field.

H. Hunter Handsfield, M.D.
Battelle Research and University of Washington
Seattle, Washington

Edward W. Hook III, M.D.
University of Alabama at Birmingham
Birmingham, Alabama

Introduction

Sevgi O. Aral, Ph.D., Judith A. Lipshutz, M.P.H., and
John M. Douglas, Jr., M.D.

The landscape for the prevention of sexually transmitted diseases (STDs) has shifted ground over the last twenty years. A multitude of prevention trials conducted during this time along with developments in the closely related field of HIV prevention provide STD program managers and public health workers with many choices. Yet, at the same time, declining resources for STD prevention render decision making exponentially more difficult. A recent review of research on interventions for prevention of sexually transmitted infections (STIs) concluded that although many interventions were found to be effective few have been replicated, widely implemented, or carefully evaluated for effectiveness in other settings (1).

This compendium of the major behavioral interventions for prevention and control of STDs aims to provide easily accessible information on the social and behavioral parameters of STD prevention so that public health students and public health practitioners can more easily make choices in a field that has historically been and continues to be based primarily on biomedical interventions.

Choices

The decisions to be made by public health workers extend beyond the choice of interventions. Each specific intervention needs to be considered within the framework of a holistic plan that takes into account a number of factors:

- the prevalence, incidence, and distribution of infection(s);
- the epidemic potential for each infection;
- the prevalence, incidence, and distribution of risk and preventive behaviors;
- the incipient decline or increase in risk and preventive behaviors;
- the mix and coverage of interventions currently being implemented;
- costs and cost-effectiveness of available efficacious interventions;
- available resources and incipient decline or increase in such resources;
- health system parameters such as feasibility of implementation of interventions, sustainability of interventions, and feasibility of scale-up;
- estimates of achievable coverage as compared to estimates of coverage required for desirable impact;
- structures and processes that need to be put in place for quality assurance and continuous quality improvement after the implementation of the intervention.

Moreover, in light of scarce and declining resources, all choices involve difficult trade-offs.

Efficacy and Effectiveness

While at this time a considerable number of biomedical and behavioral interventions have been shown to be efficacious in randomized trials for the prevention of STDs, the effectiveness of these interventions outside the randomized trial context is often not well understood. Often, we know an intervention works if and when it is implemented correctly and consistently in a population similar to that in which it was tested, but we have limited knowledge regarding the extent to which correct and consistent implementation will occur and generalizability of the results of the intervention to other populations and other contextual situations (2). Two, by now classical, examples of efficacious practices of unknown effectiveness are abstinence and condom use. The former works in preventing the acquisition of all STIs and the latter works in decreasing the risk of acquisition for most STIs (3). However, individual people do not necessarily implement these practices correctly and consistently. Clearly, for STD prevention programs, the important factor is intervention effectiveness in the everyday context and not intervention efficacy as defined in the context of randomized controlled trials. Moreover, public health professionals lack information that would help predict the conditions under which these interventions may be effectively implemented by different subpopulations in different situations. The extent to which specific subpopulations deviate from consistent and correct implementation of an intervention and the impact of various contexts on such deviations have important implications. Such deviation on the part of subpopulations marked by low-risk behaviors and low prevalence of STIs may not carry much significance; however, even small deviation from correct and consistent implementation on the part of subpopulations marked by high-risk behaviors and/or high prevalence of STIs may contribute prominently to STI transmission. Conversely, correct and consistent implementation of an intervention for subpopulations marked by low-risk behaviors and low STI prevalence may not have much impact on population-level prevalence and incidence of STIs. Yet, correct and consistent implementation of the same intervention for subpopulations marked by high-risk behaviors and/or high prevalence and incidence of STIs may have great impact on health outcomes at the population level.

Effectiveness and Impact

The goal of STD public health interventions is to decrease the incidence and prevalence of specific STDs at the population level. In contrast to chronic disease prevention, which provides prevention benefit for the individual, infectious disease prevention interventions can be beneficial at both the individual and the population levels by preventing ongoing transmission. Yet, efficacious and even effective interventions may or may not have population-level impact depending on critical parameters that include prevalence, incidence, distribution, and epidemic potential of infection; prevalence, incidence, distribution, and incipient decline (or increase) of risk and preventive behaviors; and required *and* achieved levels of coverage of the intervention. The required level of coverage depends on the efficacy and effectiveness of the intervention under consideration as well as the networks in which the populations live. Highly efficacious/effective interventions may have population-level impact even at relatively low levels of coverage. On the other hand, interventions of relatively low efficacy may result in significant population-level impact when combined with high levels of coverage. For example, relatively low-efficacy vaccines can reduce the prevalence of infection in whole populations when full coverage is achieved (4).

Neither STIs nor risky or preventive behaviors are distributed evenly through populations. Consequently, coverage in some subpopulations is more critical to the achievement of population-level impact compared with coverage in other subpopulations. As a rule, for STD prevention and control, coverage in subpopulations marked by high-risk behaviors and high prevalence or incidence of STIs is more crucial than coverage in subpopulations marked by low-risk behaviors and low prevalence/incidence of STIs. The former have greater potential to contribute to STI spread. Often, subpopulations marked by lower behavioral and infection risk are faster in intervention uptake than those with greater behavioral and infection risks. Unfortunately, coverage in these lower risk populations generally contributes to population-level impact only in limited ways.

The concept of population-level impact associated with a specific intervention, implemented in a specific subpopulation, has been described earlier for non-infectious diseases (5). More recently, this "impact fraction" model developed for chronic conditions was adapted for STD and HIV (6). The "prevention impact model," adapted from St. Louis and Holmes (6), defines population-level impact of an intervention as

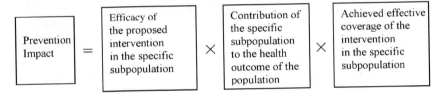

Incremental Impact and Saturation

As interventions are considered for implementation, it is important to focus on their potential "incremental" (as opposed to "absolute") impact on the health outcome of interest as well as on their potential saturation point. Interventions introduced relatively early in an epidemic in appropriately targeted populations tend to have greater impact on the prevalence and incidence of STIs than do interventions implemented later (7). Furthermore, as interventions are introduced, the incremental impact of each additional intervention can be smaller than expected due to the "saturation" effect. This pattern may be particularly relevant for behavioral interventions, since the elasticity (potential for change) of behaviors and/or the ability of the individuals to control their situation—and consequently their behaviors—may be limited. For example, most people find it difficult to abstain from sex for long periods of time. Similarly, many married women in developing countries find it difficult to use a condom against their husbands' wishes. Though public health workers encourage reduction in the number of sex partners, it is likely that most targeted persons will not find it feasible to give up a last, remaining sex partner. Similarly, once the early adopters and the easy-to-influence subpopulations have changed their behaviors, it may be particularly difficult to effect change in the behaviors of the remaining, relatively small proportion of the population (8).

This is one of the reasons why it is difficult to eliminate or eradicate adverse health outcomes after their prevalence and incidence are reduced to low levels.

Issues of saturation and diminishing, incremental impact may also be relevant for biomedical interventions. For example, the addition of an HPV 16/18 vaccine campaign may not make as large an impact on reduction of cervical cancer in a population already well covered by Pap testing as in an area with no cervical cancer prevention programs. As both biomedical and behavioral interventions are introduced and continually implemented, their incremental impact on the prevalence and incidence of STIs and their sequelae may start declining.

The Intervention Mix: Duplication, Saturation, and Synergy

At any point in time, public health programs are likely to implement a multiplicity of interventions to prevent the spread of STIs in general and of specific infections in particular. Some of these interventions target the same subpopulations, while others cover different subpopulations. When the same subpopulation is targeted by several interventions concurrently, prevention efforts may be duplicative. Similarly, when the same subpopulation is targeted by a number of interventions, concurrently or sequentially, the incremental impact of each intervention may be limited because of the saturation effect. In this context, it is important both to anticipate that diminishing marginal (or incremental) returns will occur at some point and to monitor the results of investments in interventions.

The goal of public health is to identify a package or mix of interventions with synergistic, as opposed to duplicative or opposing, effects. For example, the combination of enhanced clinical services with health promotion was key to the successful reduction of syphilis in the United States in the late 1990s (9). Another example of a multilevel intervention mix aimed at synergistic effects on increased primary prevention of STDs in adolescents is Project Connect (10). In this project, parents, health care providers, and schools are targeted simultaneously with the ultimate goal of delaying sexual debut and increasing safer sex following initiation of intercourse in middle school and high school students.

Packages of biomedical interventions coupled with behavioral interventions to magnify their effects may be particularly synergistic and effective. For example, increased screening and treatment efforts for bacterial STIs may be combined with behavioral interventions to enhance health care seeking by at-risk populations and expanded partner referral among providers.

Preventing Acquisition and Transmission of Infection

Prevention of STDs involves ensuring that uninfected persons avoid acquiring infection and that infected persons avoid transmitting their infection to susceptible sex partners. While prevention of acquisition requires that public health interventions target the very large numbers of uninfected persons, prevention of transmission allows interventions to target the smaller numbers of those who are infected. In light of limited resources, choices often need to be made about which subpopulations to target. Possible alternatives include

– infected persons with high-risk behaviors (high-frequency transmitters);
– infected persons with low-risk behaviors;

– high-risk but uninfected persons;
– low-risk, uninfected persons.

Especially for bacterial STIs, which are relatively uncommon in most populations, a focus on prevention of transmission from infected populations rather than prevention of acquisition by uninfected populations may be a more efficient and cost-effective approach to decreasing prevalence and incidence of STIs in the population. However, such an approach may run contrary to the desire of public health practitioners and public health agencies to inform and educate the general population about how to protect themselves from infections, including STIs.

Historically, STD programs have prioritized the so-called "core groups" in prevention and control efforts (11). While core groups have been defined in many different ways in the literature, all definitions include the elements of high prevalence and incidence of infection and risky behaviors. Core groups have been conceptualized as subpopulations that contribute particularly to the spread of infection in the population. Perhaps a revised approach might adopt a hierarchical ranking of subpopulations. Infected persons with high-risk behaviors that transmit infection (e.g., core groups) may be the top-priority subpopulation, followed by infected persons with low-risk transmission behaviors. Next on the hierarchy would be uninfected persons with high-risk behaviors that result in acquisition of infection followed finally by uninfected persons with low-risk acquisition behaviors. To the extent allowed by resource availability, prevention programs could attempt to cover all of the above-named subpopulations. Where resource limitations restrict coverage, the hierarchical ranking mentioned above may provide guidance for resource allocation (see Figure 1).

Hierarchy of Intervention Subpopulation Targets

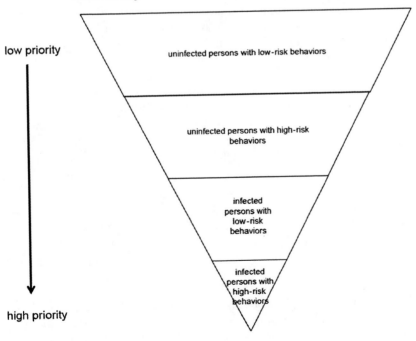

Figure 1

Intended and Unintended Consequences of Interventions

All public health interventions intend to decrease negative health outcomes in populations; however, interventions may have unintended consequences. For example, it is often suggested that the campaign to decrease the fat intake of Americans resulted in significant increases in carbohydrate intake and associated weight gain. Some argue that America's recent obesity epidemic is a direct result of the earlier low-fat prevention campaign (12,13). Similar unintended consequences can occur in STD prevention. Recent increases in bacterial STI incidence in men who have sex with men (MSM) have, in many parts of the world, been attributed not only to "prevention fatigue" associated with HIV prevention efforts but also to "disinhibition" resulting from the availability of antiretroviral therapy (14,15).

As discussed earlier, in making decisions about interventions, it is important to focus on the expected incremental, as opposed to the absolute, impact of the intervention. Similarly, in considering the potential impact of possible disinhibition associated with a specific intervention, it is important to look at the incremental (and not absolute) disinhibition. In the presence of a multiplicity of interventions for the prevention of STDs including HIV, the incremental disinhibition associated with any specific intervention is likely to be limited (15).

Cost, Cost-Efficacy, and Cost-Effectiveness

Every decision in a prevention program is associated with costs, and choosing interventions based on cost-effectiveness considerations has become an increasingly common approach to prevention. Yet, some raise serious objections to this approach. First, most cost-effectiveness analyses are based on data collected during efficacy trials, and they provide information on cost-efficacy rather than cost-effectiveness (16). Costs incurred in the context of a randomized trial may be higher (or lower) than costs incurred in the implementation of an intervention outside of the trial context (16). Second, cost-effectiveness may be given more consideration than prevention effectiveness, thereby prioritizing economic outcomes over and above health outcomes (17). Perhaps a sequential approach to decision making should prioritize interventions based first on the importance of the health outcome, second on the effectiveness of the interventions, and finally on the cost-effectiveness analysis (CEA) (not cost-efficacy) of equally effective interventions.

Multiple Epidemics; Multiple Populations

More often than not, an STI epidemic in a local area is composed of multiple epidemics in multiple subpopulations, each of which is in a different point in the epidemic trajectory (18,19). Thus, it is important for program managers to know which subpopulations are involved and whether the specific epidemic in a specific subpopulation has peaked or is just starting. Understanding the social determinants of STI epidemics, knowledge of the current social and economic context of subpopulations, and recent behavioral trends in subpopulations can help program managers analyze their current situation and predict where the next epidemic may take place. In this context, information regarding the social, cultural, economic, and behavioral factors that characterize subpopulations is important. It is such understanding that enables STD program managers to choose the most effective intervention packages and to target strategies of greatest impact. Interventions that may be most appropriate for one subpopulation may not be optimal for another.

Characteristics of STD Pathogens and Implications for Interventions

Characteristics of STDs often influence the choice of biomedical and behavioral interventions. Such characteristics include transmissibility; duration of infection; frequency and type of symptomatology; epidemiologic characteristics such as prevalence and incidence in the population as well as the partner pool; characteristics of available (and implemented) interventions; availability of a preventive vaccine and curative or suppressive antimicrobial therapy; and whether or not condoms or microbicides can reduce transmission of the particular pathogen. Recent work (20,21) suggests that some behavioral interventions may be more effective in preventing bacterial STIs, whereas others are more effective in preventing viral STIs. For example, a reduction in numbers of sex partners is more effective in reducing the incidence of gonorrhea and chlamydia (highly transmissible, curable infections), whereas a reduction in numbers of episodes of sexual intercourse with one partner is more effective in reducing the incidence of HIV (low transmissibility, incurable infection) (22). Screening—a widely used prevention intervention—is often used for relatively widespread and often asymptomatic infections such as those caused by *Chlamydia trachomatis*. In contrast, for relatively uncommon infections like syphilis, interventions such as partner management may play a relatively more important role.

Social Determinants, Future STI Trends, and Multiple Levels of Social–Behavioral Interventions

Many societal factors play a role in the determination of STI epidemiology. Such societal determinants include the demographic and socioeconomic structure of the population; the political environment and its effects on the composition of the unemployed and incarcerated populations; distribution of access to acceptable and quality health care and prevention services; social and sexual network characteristics; gender power dynamics; and sexual behaviors of different subpopulations (23). A look at these and other similar factors suggests that trends in STI incidence in the near future may create even greater challenges for STD prevention programs faced with limited and declining resources. The relatively larger size of "generation Y" portends increases in the size of sexually active age groups, and the recent increases in poverty and inequality levels suggest increased vulnerability of the population to STIs, all predictors of increased STI incidence. In this alarming context, multilevel social and behavioral interventions, ranging from the structural and policy level to couples and individual persons, constitute an important element of the STI prevention toolbox.

Volume Contents

This book is divided into five parts. The overview chapters set the stage for the intervention approaches discussed in subsequent parts. McGough and Handsfield provide a rich historical summary of STD prevention and control up to the modern AIDS era, when behavioral interventions started becoming more mainstream. St. Lawrence and Fortenberry give a comprehensive review of theories in behavioral science and intervention methods, providing the reader with a thumbnail sketch of the most important underpinnings of behavioral interventions. Given that behavioral interventions occur within what has traditionally been a biomedical field, Berman and Kamb offer a look at transmission dynamics through the lens of the Anderson–May equation, $R = bcd$ (24). They focus on two parameters that have critical interface with behavioral interventions—duration of infectivity (d) and transmissibility (b).

Following this overview, Part 2 addresses different STD intervention approaches, some related to population levels and some related to specific interventions. McCree et al. discuss behavioral interventions that specifically target couples, small groups, and communities. Moving to a larger population level and one of the newest areas of behavioral intervention research, Bloom and Cohen focus on structural-level interventions that attempt to change the context in which behaviors take place. Structures can include public and private institutions, service and educational systems, and laws and regulations. Similarly, Vega and Ghanem write about the importance of social marketing in behavior change. Social marketing campaigns for STD prevention, they contend, require not only mass communication to inform the public, but also techniques that persuade people to actually practice prevention.

The next group of chapters in Part 2 reviews more familiar STD prevention interventions. Hogben et al. focus on the classic topic of partner notification, reflecting both historical approaches and more recent innovations such as partner-delivered therapy. In the following chapter, Hogben and Schrier write about the health care system from the perspective of those who provide the care as well as those who seek it. Discussion in that chapter reflects assumed goals of public health: to increase routine prevention (e.g., yearly doctor visits) and to optimize reaction to a suspected infection. The Internet, discussed in the chapter by McFarlane and Bull, is perhaps one of the most widely discussed new intervention venues in the public health field. The authors first talk about the Internet as a risk environment, followed by the opportunities for prevention intervention that it provides. Following is the chapter on male condoms by Warner and Stone, with the latest data on condom efficacy and implications for prevention strategies. The field of vaccines for STIs is the subject of the last chapter in Part 2. While only two STI vaccines have been approved for use (HBV and HPV), both present enormous opportunities and challenges in the behavioral realm.

Part 3 shifts focus from intervention types to specific population groups. Public health practitioners have long understood that how one uses interventions must be tailored to the particular characteristics and culture of the targeted group. All population groups in Part 3 are considered at high risk for STDs. The first chapter by Ethier and Orr focuses on adolescents, the age group with highest vulnerability to STDs. The next chapter by McCree and Rompalo is about particular issues related to women, who bear the greatest burden from the sequelae of untreated STDs. The HIV/AIDS epidemic has brought to light the high-risk behaviors of MSM. The MSM population is likewise at high risk for other STDs, the topic of a chapter by Fenton and

Bloom. Leichliter et al. focus on persons who have repeat STIs. "Repeaters" have an increased risk for sequelae and may be members of a core group of people who continue to spread disease in a community. Thus, this population requires unique approaches to interventions, which are discussed in Leichliter et al.'s chapter. Williams and Kahn address the unique risks and opportunities for prevention in incarcerated populations. The authors not only review the STD burden on this population, but also discuss how the related contextual factors associated with incarceration and the effects of such imprisonment on the individual impact efforts to prevent STI transmission. Finally, the STD burden of illicit drug users and the barriers to prevention they face are addressed in the chapter by Semaan et al. Based on the limited body of available research related to STD prevention in this population, this chapter concentrates on STD prevention and control activities specific to heterosexual drug users.

To provide some insight as to how behavioral research is conducted, Part 4 is intended to help the reader understand methods. The first chapter, by McFarlane and St. Lawrence, describes several different forms of measurement and how to determine whether they are "accurate." The chapter by Gorbach and Galea outlines the main types of qualitative research approaches and how they are applied to STD prevention research. Chapel and Seechuk write about evaluation and its importance for improvement of programs. Specific examples from the STD prevention field are incorporated to demonstrate the utility of evaluation. Following is a chapter on a specific evaluation tool, cost-effectiveness analysis (CEA) by Gift and Marrazzo. The chapter introduces CEA and its limitations, followed by its important role in analyzing STD interventions. Rietmeijer and Gandelman take on the important field of research translation. They discuss the critical importance not only of understanding model behavioral interventions that work, but also of putting into practice the best methods to disseminate and adopt interventions.

The final part of the book addresses two disciplines not unique to STD prevention or public health. The first by Semaan and Leinhos is about ethical considerations in public health practice as they apply to STD prevention interventions. Key concepts in the ethics literature are described as a basis for looking at ethical issues that arise in STD prevention and control. The last chapter by Zenilman considers STD prevention-related policy and its interface with science. The topic is discussed in the context of core public health functions—assessment, assurance, policy development, and communication.

Though choices for and insights about behavioral interventions for STDs continue to grow, the chapters that follow provide a comprehensive summary of what we know to date. We hope this volume will serve as a stimulating and useful guide to the rich world of social and behavioral parameters for STD prevention.

Acknowledgment: The authors wish to thank Partricia Jackson for her outstanding support in the preparation of this manuscript.

References

1. Manhart L, Holmes KK. Randomized controlled trails of individual-level, population-level and multilevel interventions for preventing sexually transmitted infections: What has worked? *Journal of Infectious Diseases*. 2005;191: S7–S24.
2. Cates W. *HIV Prevention Research: NIH Networks, Present Status, Future Hopes*. Presented at Division of STD Prevention Seminar, Centers for Disease Control and Prevention (CDC), June 7, 2006, Atlanta, GA.
3. Steiner MJ, Warner L, Stone KM, Cates W Jr. Condoms and other barrier methods for prevention of STD/HIV infection, and pregnancy. In: Holmes KK, Sparling PF, Mardh P-A, eds. *Sexually Transmitted Diseases*, 4th ed. New York: McGraw-Hill (in press).
4. Garnett GP. Role of herd immunity in determining the effect of vaccines against sexually transmitted disease. *Journal of Infectious Diseases*. 2005;191:S97–S106.
5. Morgenstern H, Bursic ES. A method for using epidemiologic data to estimate the potential impact of an intervention on the health status of a target population. *Journal of Community Health*. 1982;7:292–309.
6. St. Louis ME, Holmes KK. Conceptual framework for STD/HIV prevention and control. In: Holmes KK, Sparling PF, Mardh P-A, et al., eds. *Sexually Transmitted Diseases*, 3rd ed. New York: McGraw-Hill; 1999;1239–1253.
7. Boily M-C, Lowndes C, Alary M. The impact of HIV epidemic phases on the effectiveness of core group intervention: Insights from mathematical models. *Sexually Transmitted Infections*. 2002;78:i78–i90.
8. Gladwell M. *The Tipping Point: How Little Things Can Make a Big Difference*. New York: Little, Brown; 2000.
9. Douglas JM, Peterman TA, Fenton KA. Syphilis among men who have sex with men: Challenges to syphilis elimination in the United States. *Sexually Transmitted Diseases*. 2005;32:S80–S83.
10. Ethier KA, DeRosa CJ, Kim DH, Afifi A, Kerndt PR. *Multi-level Correlates of Adolescent Sexual Behavior and Risk for STD*. Abstract presented at National STD Prevention Conference, May 9, 2006, Jacksonville, FL.
11. Thomas JC, Tucker MJ. The development and use of the concept of a sexually transmitted disease core. *Journal of Infectious Diseases*. 1996;174:S134–S143.
12. Atkins RC. *Dr. Atkins' New Diet Revolution: The Amazing No-hunger Weight-loss Plan that Has Helped Millions Lose Weight and Keep It Off*. New York: Avon Books; 1999.
13. Agatston A. *The South Beach Diet: The Delicious, Doctor-designed, Foolproof Plan for Fast and Healthy Weight Loss*. New York: Random House; 2003.
14. Fenton K. *Alarming Trends: Increases in STD/HIV Incidence Among MSM and Paid for Sex*. Oral presentation at the 22nd IUSTI-Europe Conference on Sexually Transmitted Infections, October 19–21, 2006, Versailles, France.
15. Aral SO. Unintended consequences of STD/HIV interventions including disinhibition. *International Journal of STD & AIDS*. 2006;17:6.
16. Pinkerton S. *Cost Effectiveness Trials in HIV Prevention Studies*. Lecture presented at the CFAR Social and Behavioral Sciences Research Network (SBSRN). First National Scientific Meeting, October 11, 2006, Philadelphia, PA.
17. Farmer PE. *Help Us Help Them Donation Presentation: Boston Health Care for the Homeless Program*. Opening Session, American Public Health Association (APHA). 134th Annual Meeting, November 5, 2006, Boston, MA.
18. Aral SO, Padian NS, Holmes KK. Advances in multilevel approaches to understanding the epidemiology and prevention of sexually transmitted infections and HIV: An overview. *Journal of Infectious Diseases*. 2005;191:S1–S6.
19. Wasserheit JN, Aral SO. The dynamic topology of sexually transmitted disease epidemics: Implications for prevention strategies. *Journal of Infectious Diseases*. 1996;174:S201–S213.

20. Garnett GP. The geographical and temporal evolution of sexually transmitted disease epidemics. *Sexually Transmitted Infections*. 2002;78:i14–i19.

21. Blanchard JF. Populations, pathogens, and epidemic phases: Closing the gap between theory and practice in the prevention of sexually transmitted diseases. *Sexually Transmitted Infections*. 2002;78:i183–i188.

22. Garnett GP. Intervention impacts dependence on socio-epidemiologic context and target groups. *International Journal of STD & AIDS*. 2006;17:6–7.

23. Aral SO. Determinants of STD epidemics: Implications for phase appropriate intervention strategies. *Sexually Transmitted Infections*. 2002;78:i1–i2.

24. Anderson RM, May RM. *Infectious Diseases of Humans: Dynamics and Control*. Oxford: Oxford University Press; 1991.

About the Editors

Sevgi O. Aral, Ph.D., is the Associate Director for Science at the Division of STD Prevention, National Centers for HIV, STD, and TB Prevention at the Centers for Disease Control and Prevention, where she is responsible for the oversight and direction of all scientific activities including the intramural and extramural research programs and science program interactions. Her work has focused on risk and preventive behaviors, gender differences, societal characteristics that influence STD and HIV rates, contextual issues, and effects of distinct types of sexual mixing on STD spread. Her research has been in both domestic and international settings, and her writings have included cross-cultural comparative analyses. Dr. Aral has served on the editorial boards of several scientific journals including *Sexually Transmitted Diseases, AIDS Education and Prevention, Sexually Transmitted Infections, AIDS,* and *American Journal of Public Health*. In addition, she is an associate editor of *Sexually Transmitted Diseases* and *Sexually Transmitted Infections*. She is the recipient of the 2006 Thomas Parran Award, which is given for lifetime achievement by the American STD Association. Dr. Aral received her Ph.D. and M.A. degrees in social psychology from Emory University and another M.A. degree in demography from the University of Pennsylvania. She completed her undergraduate training at Middle East Technical University in Turkey.

John M. Douglas, Jr., M.D., is Director of the Division of STD Prevention, National Centers for HIV, STD, and TB Prevention at the Centers for Disease Control and Prevention (CDC), where he is responsible for developing and directing CDC's national STD prevention programs as well as related behavioral, epidemiologic, surveillance, laboratory, health services, and evaluation research. Dr. Douglas brings more than 25 years of experience and leadership in the field of STD prevention to his role as Director. Prior to joining CDC in 2003, Dr. Douglas served in a combination of key management, science, and medical positions for the Denver Department of Health and Hospitals (now Denver Health). These included Director of STD Control; Director, Denver Public Health Virology Laboratory; Attending Physician in Medicine and Infectious Diseases; and Director, Denver STD Prevention Training Center. He also served on the faculty of the University of Colorado Health Sciences as Professor in the departments of Medicine and Preventive Medicine and

Biometrics. He is a significant contributor to the field of STD/HIV prevention, particularly viral STD, with over 100 scholarly articles in peer-reviewed journals and book chapters. In addition, he has served on the editorial boards of several scientific journals, including *Sexually Transmitted Diseases*. He is a member of the Infectious Disease Society of America, the American STD Association, the American Public Health Association, and the American College of Physicians. Dr. Douglas earned his B.A. degree in English, summa cum laude, from Davidson College, North Carolina, in 1974 and his M.D. degree from Harvard Medical School in 1978.

Judith A. Lipshutz, M.P.H., currently works at the Centers for Disease Control and Prevention (CDC) in the Office of the Associate Director for Science, Office of the Director, Division of STD Prevention, National Centers for HIV, STD, and TB Prevention. She serves as a central communicator to the nation's public health STD prevention community of the latest research published in peer-reviewed journals and manages the editing of major DSTDP publications. Since 1996, she has coordinated the National STD Prevention Conference, the premier domestic STD prevention meeting where scientific and programmatic leaders converge every other year. For 7 years, she served as the chief of the Communications and External Relations Office during which time she coordinated CDC's National STD Prevention Partnership as well as policy and communication efforts for the Division. Prior to coming to CDC, she spent over 11 years as the Project Director for AIDS Initiatives and the Venereal Disease Action Coalition at United Community Services in Detroit, where she initiated and oversaw the city's largest AIDS case management system. Earlier, she coordinated adolescent health services at a migrant health center in south Texas. Ms. Lipshutz received her B.A. degree from Mt. Holyoke College in 1975 and her M.P.H. degree from the University of Michigan in 1980.

Contents

Part 1 Overview Chapters: Behavioral Interventions

Part 2 Intervention Approaches

Part 4 Understanding Methods

Part 5 Ethical and Policy Issues

Contributors

Sevgi O. Aral, Ph.D.
Division of STD Prevention, National Centers for HIV, STD, and TB
Prevention, Centers for Disease Control and Prevention, Atlanta, Georgia, USA

Stuart Berman, M.D., Sc.M.
Division of STD Prevention, National Centers for HIV, STD, and TB
Prevention, Centers for Disease Control and Prevention, Atlanta, Georgia, USA

Frederick R. Bloom, R.N., Ph.D.
Division of STD Prevention, National Centers for HIV, STD, and TB
Prevention, Centers for Disease Control and Prevention, Atlanta, Georgia, USA

Devon D. Brewer, Ph.D.
Interdisciplinary Scientific Research, Seattle, Washington, USA

Sheana S. Bull, Ph.D., M.P.H.
University of Colorado Health Sciences Center, Denver, Colorado, USA

Thomas J. Chapel, M.A., M.B.A.
Office of the Director/Office of Strategy and Innovation, Centers for Disease
Control and Prevention, Atlanta, Georgia, USA

Deborah A. Cohen, M.D., M.P.H.
RAND Center for Population Health and Health Disparities, Santa Monica,
California, USA

Don C. Des Jarlais, Ph.D.
Beth Israel Medical Center and Narcotic and Drug Research Institutes,
New York, New York, USA

John M. Douglas, Jr., M.D.
Division of STD Prevention, National Centers for HIV, STD, and TB
Prevention, Centers for Disease Control and Prevention, Atlanta, Georgia, USA

Agatha Eke, Ph.D.
Division of HIV/AIDS Prevention, National Centers for HIV, STD, and TB
Prevention, Centers for Disease Control and Prevention, Atlanta, Georgia, USA

Jonathan M. Ellen, M.D.
Division of General Pediatrics and Adolescent Medicine, Johns Hopkins
University School of Medicine, Baltimore, Maryland, USA

Kathleen A. Ethier, Ph.D.
Division of STD Prevention, National Centers for HIV, STD, and TB Prevention,
Centers for Disease Control and Prevention, Atlanta, Georgia, USA

Kevin A. Fenton, M.D., Ph.D.
National Centers for HIV, STD, and TB Prevention, Centers for Disease
Control and Prevention, Atlanta, Georgia, USA

J. Dennis Fortenberry, M.D., M.S.
Indiana University School of Medicine, Indianapolis, Indiana, USA

Jerome Galea, M.S.W.
Department of Epidemiology, School of Public Health, University of
California, Los Angeles, California, USA

Alice A. Gandelman, M.P.H.
California STD/HIV Prevention Training Center, STD Control Branch,
California Department of Health Services, Oakland, California, USA

Khalil G. Ghanem, M.D.
Division of Infectious Diseases, Johns Hopkins University School of
Medicine, Baltimore, Maryland, USA

Thomas L. Gift, Ph.D.
Division of STD Prevention, National Centers for HIV, STD, and TB
Prevention, Centers for Disease Control and Prevention, Atlanta, Georgia, USA

Matthew R. Golden, M.D., M.P.H.
STD Control Program for Public Health–Seattle and King County and
Harborview Medical Center, University of Washington School of Medicine,
Seattle, Washington, USA

Pamina M. Gorbach, M.H.S., Dr.P.H.
Department of Epidemiology, School of Public Health, University of
California, Los Angeles, California, USA

Robert A. Gunn, M.D., M.P.H.
Public Health Services Division, San Diego County Health and Human
Services, San Diego, California, USA

H. Hunter Handsfield, M.D.
Battelle Centers for Public Health Research and Evaluation and University of
Washington School of Medicine, Seattle, Washington, USA

Matthew Hogben, Ph.D.
Division of STD Prevention, National Centers for HIV, STD, and TB
Prevention, Centers for Disease Control and Prevention, Atlanta, Georgia, USA

Edward W. Hook III, M.D.
University of Alabama at Birmingham School of Medicine and Jefferson
County Department of Health, Birmingham, Alabama, USA

Richard H. Kahn, M.S.
Division of Parasitic Diseases, National Center for Infectious Diseases,
Centers for Disease Control and Prevention, Atlanta, Georgia, USA

Mary L. Kamb, M.D., M.P.H.
Division of STD Prevention, National Centers for HIV, STD, and TB
Prevention, Centers for Disease Control and Prevention, Atlanta, Georgia, USA

Jami S. Leichliter, Ph.D.
Division of STD Prevention, National Centers for HIV, STD, and TB
Prevention, Centers for Disease Control and Prevention, Atlanta, Georgia, USA

Mary Leinhos, Ph.D.
National Office of Public Health Genomics, Centers for Disease Control and
Prevention, Atlanta, Georgia, USA

Nicole Liddon, Ph.D.
Division of STD Prevention, National Centers for HIV, STD, and TB
Prevention, Centers for Disease Control and Prevention, Atlanta, Georgia, USA

Judith A. Lipshutz, M.P.H.
Division of STD Prevention, National Centers for HIV, STD, and TB
Prevention, Centers for Disease Control and Prevention, Atlanta, Georgia, USA

Robert M. Malow, Ph.D., A.B.P.P.
Florida International University, Miami, Florida, USA

Jeanne Marrazzo, M.D., M.P.H.
Division of Allergy and Infectious Diseases, University of Washington
School of Medicine, Seattle, Washington, USA

Donna Hubbard McCree, Ph.D., M.P.H., R.Ph.
Division of HIV/AIDS Prevention, National Centers for HIV, STD,
and TB Prevention, Centers for Disease Control and Prevention, Atlanta,
Georgia, USA

Mary McFarlane, Ph.D.
Division of STD Prevention, National Centers for HIV, STD, and TB
Prevention, Centers for Disease Control and Prevention, Atlanta,
Georgia, USA

Laura J. McGough, Ph.D.
Department of History of Medicine, Johns Hopkins University
School of Medicine, Baltimore, Maryland, USA

Donald P. Orr, M.D.
Indiana University School of Medicine, Indianapolis, Indiana, USA

Cornelis A. Rietmeijer, M.D., Ph.D.
STD Control Program, Denver Public Health Department and University of Colorado at Denver and Health Sciences Center, Denver, Colorado, USA

Anne M. Rompalo, M.D., Sc.M.
Johns Hopkins University School of Medicine, Baltimore, Maryland, USA

Kim Seechuk, M.P.H.
Division of STD Prevention, National Centers for HIV, STD, and TB Prevention, Centers for Disease Control and Prevention, Atlanta, Georgia, USA

Salaam Semaan, Dr.P.H.
National Centers for HIV, STD, and TB Prevention, Centers for Disease Control and Prevention, Atlanta, Georgia, USA

Lydia A. Shrier, M.D., M.P.H.
Division of Adolescent/Young Adult Medicine, Children's Hospital Boston and Department of Pediatrics, Harvard Medical School, Boston, Massachusetts, USA

Lawrence R. Stanberry, M.D., M.P.H.
Sealy Center for Vaccine Development, University of Texas Medical Branch, Galveston, Texas, USA

Janet S. St. Lawrence, Ph.D.
Mississippi State University–Meridian Campus, Meridian, Mississippi, USA

Katherine M. Stone, M.D.
Atlanta, Georgia, USA

Miriam Y. Vega, Ph.D.
Latino Commission on AIDS, New York, New York, USA

Lee Warner, Ph.D., M.P.H.
Division of Reproductive Health, National Center for Chronic Disease Prevention and Health Promotion, Centers for Disease Control and Prevention, Atlanta, Georgia, USA

Samantha P. Williams, Ph.D.
Division of STD Prevention, National Centers for HIV, STD, and TB Prevention, Centers for Disease Control and Prevention, Atlanta, Georgia, USA

Jonathan M. Zenilman, M.D.
Infectious Diseases Division, Johns Hopkins University Bayview Medical Center, Baltimore, Maryland, USA

Gregory D. Zimet, Ph.D.
Indiana University Cancer Center and Medical School, Indianapolis, Indiana, USA

Part 1

Overview Chapters:
Behavioral Interventions

History of Behavioral Interventions in STD Control

Laura J. McGough, Ph.D., and H. Hunter Handsfield, M.D.

STDs comprise a wide variety of pathogens, including viruses, bacteria, fungi, and protozoa, along with an equally broad range of clinical manifestations, from mild infections localized to the genitalia to more serious diseases affecting reproductive health, the central nervous system, heart, or the immune system. The fundamental reason for placing these diverse biological agents and their sequelae under the same category of STDs is that they share a common mode of transmission—that is, a common human behavior. Given that the category of STDs is defined according to a common behavior rather than a common biological pathogen or sequela, one would expect behavioral interventions to have been at the center of historical and current strategies to prevent and control STDs. Historically, however, the opposite has been true: compared with epidemic infectious diseases such as plague and cholera, which garnered significant public health attention, STD control was relegated to private physicians and largely ignored by public health officials, except for behavioral efforts aimed largely at "marginal" groups such as prostitutes or military personnel. This chapter explains why behavioral interventions for STD control have been a relatively neglected area of public health programs.

It should be noted that the term "behavioral interventions" has come into use relatively recently (since the 1980s), while behavioral science itself is a 20th-century creation. To avoid the anachronistic practice of imposing modern categories onto the past, it is important to explain past practices within their own historical context. The categories that people in the past used to describe and explain their STD prevention and control activities often developed from fundamentally different conceptions of disease transmission, public health, and human behavior. I have retained the original language (the "pox" instead of syphilis, if that was the term commonly used) to underscore the need to understand disease control efforts in context. Similarly, depending on the context, I will refer to the historic terminology used to characterize populations, groups, behaviors, and diseases, such as prostitutes rather than commercial sex workers.

Efforts to control and treat diseases always develop out of specific historical and cultural contexts. In 19th-century Europe, for example, STD control efforts focused almost entirely on the regulation of prostitution and forced medical inspection of prostitutes. Victorian public health officials and physicians

Behavioral Interventions for Prevention and Control of Sexually Transmitted Diseases. Aral SO, Douglas JM Jr, eds. Lipshutz JA, assoc ed. New York: Springer Science+ Business Media, LLC; 2007.

regarded prostitutes as the main vectors of disease, and prostitutes' behavior as essentially unchangeable, because they were "deviant" human beings. Medical and scientific writings at the time sharply distinguished between normal and "deviant" psychology and behavior. The behavior of prostitutes' male clients, on the other hand, was not considered problematic, but a normal sexual outlet that served to protect "respectable women" from seduction. Victorian preoccupations with class and perceptions about the sexes influenced the selection of the population for health interventions: male sexual privileges were sacrosanct, whereas middle- and upper-class women were assumed to be chaste unless seduced by men. This set of assumptions left a rather narrow field for behavioral interventions, such as repressing prostitution or compelling its practitioners to obtain medical treatment, since they were "deviant" persons who could neither modify their behavior nor be trusted to seek care on their own. By showing how past STD control efforts are often the product of assumptions about disease transmission and human behavior, historical research can help present-day researchers reflect on their own (often implicit) assumptions about how and whether human behavior can change, which aspects are changeable, which populations are best able to change (and why), and through what means behavior change is best achieved.

The history of behavioral interventions in STD control provides no easy lessons for the present. Instead, it is a reminder that change in public health practice is often driven by external events, such as a new government or a war, rather than by developments within the field. The public health community can, however, prepare for and capitalize on changing circumstances in order to build more effective behavioral intervention programs. For example, the United States neglected venereal disease (VD) control after the end of World War I. After becoming Surgeon General in 1937, Thomas Parran made the reduction of syphilis morbidity his major priority. One year to the day before the bombing of Pearl Harbor and American entry into World War II, Parran and his colleagues met to develop a wartime VD control plan. Because of their planning and early meetings with military officials, they were able to change some past military practices that had been damaging to STD control, especially by suggesting public education efforts other than fear-based messages about the dangers of VD. In addition, after considerable lobbying efforts, military personnel were no longer punished for contracting VD and therefore sought rather than avoided health care.

The history of behavioral interventions in STD control shows that continuous public education about successful STD interventions is necessary, along with the development of strong relationships with public officials. Otherwise, there is enormous pressure to adopt three of the following behavioral interventions strategies, all of which (as discussed below) have limitations: 1) fear-based messages about the dangers of STDs; 2) religion-based moral approaches to STD control; and 3) efforts to control the behavior of female sex workers. Despite recent innovations in behavioral science and interventions to reduce morbidity (discussed throughout this book), public health officials need to anticipate that these historical approaches to STD control will remain popular with the wider public. These approaches dominated STD control programs from the 16th through early 20th centuries. The 20th century witnessed several important changes in behavioral intervention strategies, especially the adoption and then rejection of information-based efforts; the shift toward focusing on the behavior of health care providers rather than just the behavior of patients; and a growing concern with behavior related to surveillance, screening, and treatment, rather than with sexual behavior aimed at primary prevention. One of the principal lessons of 20th-century behavioral interventions, however, is that the behavioral component is usually an afterthought, designed to augment the efforts of control programs oriented toward surveillance and treatment. Because of the limited availability of archival material for the past 20 years, this chapter unfortunately ends in the early 1980s. It is important for future researchers to study the crucial period of the mid-1980s onwards, when the field of behavioral interventions for the control of HIV/AIDS developed and expanded rapidly. Meanwhile, however, the study of behavioral interventions prior to the 1980s yields important insights for present-day practitioners and researchers.

Early Efforts in Europe (16th to 18th Century): Morality and Hygiene

Although the history of responses to STDs can be traced to antiquity, this story will begin in the 16th century, a generation after Europeans experienced an epidemic of a new disease they called the "French disease" or the "pox," among other names. In the absence of laboratory tests, it is difficult to know whether this disease was the same as modern venereal syphilis based on highly subjective descriptions of symptoms (1). What is important for a history of behavioral interventions, however, is that, by the 1530s, physicians reached a consensus that the disease was primarily transmitted through sexual intercourse. The idea of sexual transmission was relatively new during the 16th century, an ancient Greek idea revitalized by the physician Girolamo Fracastoro (2).

Furthermore, this chapter begins with the 16th century because Europeans developed two fundamentally different, competing disease control strategies, based on different understandings of human behavior and its capacity for change—a conflict that has, in many ways, persisted to the present. By mid-16th century, the French disease or the pox was considered curable through a variety of medications: mercury, guaiacum (a wood that was ground into a powder, boiled, and then dried and used as a medication), and a variety of cures produced by popular healers (1,3,4). Despite the existence of public health offices (first in Italy and later in England) to control plague and other epidemic diseases (5), the major emphasis of STD control was treatment. All parts of Europe primarily relied on medications, sold in pharmacies or on street corners, to control the pox. Because treatment failure was acknowledged as a concern, in addition to the inconvenience and suffering associated with contracting and treating the disease, governments, churches, and physicians across Europe provided advice about prevention. Although there was considerable local variation in response, two broadly different patterns of prevention emerged during the 16th and 17th centuries: 1) the promotion of sexual hygiene for men, accompanied by a limited effort to control the behavior of female prostitutes; and 2) the promotion of religious education, especially the dangers of sins such as adultery.

The Italian city-states provide an excellent example of the former pattern. Italian physicians' advice on prevention invoked a double standard of morality that found ways for single men to enjoy sex and avoid infection, while holding women responsible for disease transmission. The celebrated University of Padua anatomist Gabriele Falloppio's lectures on the "French disease" provided a type of "behavioral intervention" for students of medicine: to clean their genitals after intercourse with a prostitute in order to avoid infection. In case cleaning alone was not sufficient, Falloppio recommended that, after coitus, men cover the penis with a bag of cloth soaked in an ointment that would prevent infection (6). Italian writers consistently displayed a sexual double standard, which allowed sexual freedom to men but demanded repentance and moral reform for women. Unmarried women who had contracted the pox and received treatment in hospitals designated for French disease patients (in contrast to wealthier women who could afford private physicians) were encouraged to repent, become nuns, and reside permanently in convents specifically devised for "fallen women" (7). Nonetheless, perhaps because of economic motives, physicians treated "guilty" patients, including prostitutes, one of whom the physician Ercole Sassonia proudly claimed to have cured so that she could continue to practice her art. As one of his colleagues explained, paid women were "worth preserving not for their own health, but primarily for the sake of their male customers" (8, p. 501).

The second approach, prevention through religion-based moral reform, is illustrated with the example of England. Physicians such as William Clowes (the Elder, d. 1604), who was influenced by Puritan thought, refrained from telling patients to wash the genitals to avoid infection. He feared that this advice would encourage illicit sexuality. The only acceptable form of prevention for Clowes was moral reform: men must avoid prostitutes and refrain from adultery. English advice focused almost exclusively on avoiding sin to prevent disease, since disease transmission was associated with sinful sexuality (6).

The differences in these two approaches can be partially explained by the underlying theological differences that developed between Roman Catholic and Protestant interpretations of Christianity. It is important not to exaggerate the differences between the two traditions, which shared a common history and common set of texts. Nonetheless, a few differences are discernible: Roman Catholics continued to emphasize the vulnerability of all human beings to sin and the subsequent importance of charitable actions, whereas certain Protestant groups viewed behavior change as nearly impossible because of predestination. According to this interpretation, some human beings could change through religious conversion; the inability of others to change, however, provided evidence of their future damnation. These differences in beliefs about human ability to change behavior led to strikingly different efforts to control the pox, with Roman Catholics emphasizing hygiene for men and repentance for women and certain Protestants focusing their efforts on the "saved" by preaching abstinence until marriage and fidelity afterwards.

In the absence of reliable annual morbidity data, it is unclear whether either approach met with success. The pox or the French disease remained major problems throughout Europe from the 16th century onward. In London, for example, approximately 20% of all hospital patients were diagnosed with the pox, while the workhouses (ostensibly charitable institutions founded on the assumption that laziness was the cause of poverty) were filled with pox patients, impoverished by disease with nowhere to turn. The pox was both the result of and a major cause of poverty in 17th- and 18th-century London, while major public health efforts focused on the plague and largely ignored the pox, regarded as a private concern for patients who could afford treatment or relegated to under-funded charities in the case of destitute patients (9). Behavior change was considered to be the domain of the churches, Protestant or Catholic; meanwhile, public health offices devoted their limited resources to the plague, while a virtual army of healers competed to fill the constant demand for cures for the pox (9).

Regulation Versus Abolition of Prostitution: 19th Century

The 19th century provides the best example of efforts to control STDs by controlling the behavior of female prostitutes. Debate raged on whether to legalize and regulate prostitution, complete with regular medical check-ups for prostitutes, or to abolish and criminalize prostitution, thereby making it difficult for clients and prostitutes alike to engage in sexual intercourse. The control of venereal diseases was virtually synonymous with the problem of prostitution from the perspective of the governments of Europe and the United States. The only behavior that mattered to public health officials was whether prostitutes regularly sought medical treatment and thereby avoided spreading infection to their male clients. Because prostitutes were regarded as an inferior class, and therefore unlikely to seek medical care, public health officials focused on regulating their behavior through legal regulation and police enforcement.

Regulation of prostitution reinforced ethnic, class, and racial prejudices, since lower-class women or nonwhite women were regarded as potential prostitutes simply because of their class and race. Laws that allowed for the detention of suspect women provided police in Europe with considerable power over women, with occasional abuses of this power through arbitrary arrest and detention. Because this period also witnessed considerable expansion of European power into Asia and Africa, including the colonization of non-European territories, Europeans took their preoccupations about venereal disease and prostitution into the territories that they ruled. In parts of Asia and Africa, the first major experience of large-scale efforts to control STDs was during the colonial period. Europeans were primarily concerned with protecting European soldiers from being infected by native prostitutes. With few if any exceptions, colonized peoples understood that VD prevention and control efforts were for the benefit of the rulers, not the ruled, and that "behavioral interventions" were directed at the colonized population, not the colonizers and their military personnel who were also likely responsible for the spread of VD.

The French took the lead in advocating legalization and regulation of prostitution rather than prohibiting it. After designing Paris's sewage system, Dr. A. Parent-Duchâtelet tackled the problem of prostitution, which he saw as fundamentally similar to the need for sewers. Following the line of reasoning that Church Fathers such as St. Augustine had provided, Parent-Duchâtelet described prostitution as an "indispensable excremental phenomenon that protects the social body from disease" (10, p. 4). Extramarital activity could be contained within the system of prostitution, but for the system to work, prostitutes had to be maintained under constant, lifelong surveillance from brothel to hospital to refuge, never allowed to return to society. Prohibition of prostitution was understood by the French authorities to be a consistent failure, so that regulation and systematic medical inspection made more sense as a means of disease control (10). Other countries, such as Italy and Russia, emulated the French system (11,12). Unfortunately, because 19th-century medical therapies were of limited efficacy, the medical inspection of prostitutes was often as dangerous to their health as it was beneficial. Russian women were rounded up and subjected to forced medical examinations in which the same speculum was used on successive women without cleaning the instrument, thereby making iatrogenic transmission possible (11).

Despite its longstanding Protestant tradition, Great Britain briefly experimented with the legalization and regulation of prostitution, because of demands made by the British army to provide a "sexual outlet" for enlisted men who were not allowed to marry. The Contagious Diseases Acts of 1864, 1866, and 1869 permitted a wide range of regulatory powers to the police to detain any woman suspected of venereal infection pending medical inspection. From the perspective of modern knowledge about, for example, the limited ability of physical examinations to detect syphilis or gonorrhea, this approach was doomed to failure as a control strategy. But the negative social consequences were drastic: Many police and other officials suspected virtually any working-class woman of possible involvement in prostitution, which meant that most or all lower-class women were subject to police harassment and detainment based on spurious grounds. Soldiers were not subject to medical inspection. Thus, the pervasive sexual double standard provoked political protests from an alliance of working-class and middle-class women, with the eventual repeal of the Contagious Diseases Acts in 1886 (13).

The British brought this system of VD regulation of women to India. In 1886, the military authorities encouraged the availability of local women for British troops, explaining that "in the regimental bazaars it is necessary to have a sufficient number of women, to care that they are sufficiently attractive, to provide them with proper houses..." (14, p. 79). Although the British Army regarded Indian women as the source of disease for its soldiers, it is likely that the reverse was as much of a problem. In fact, hospital admission rates for VD in the Native Army (composed of Indian soldiers) was one-tenth that of the British Army (14, p. 82). It is not clear whether hospital admission rates reflect differences in disease morbidity, in access to health care between English and Indian soldiers, or in lower clinical attack rates in fully or partially immune Indian soldiers. Nonetheless, from the perspective of many Indian observers, it was the behavior of white troops, not Indian women, that was a problem. The issue of prostitution and VD became part of the Indian nationalist platform when, in 1892, the eighth Indian National Congress protested state regulation of prostitution (15, p. 604). Similarly, in Shanghai, China, where the French, British, Germans, and Americans exercised political control, the regulation of Chinese prostitutes led to tensions between whites and Chinese authorities. From the European perspectives, venereal diseases were a local problem, spread from Chinese prostitutes to European soldiers; the Chinese perspective unsurprisingly was the opposite, especially in the case of syphilis, which Chinese physicians argued had not existed in China prior to European military domination (16).

The 19th-century experiment in the regulation of prostitution as the key to VD control illustrates some of the historical difficulties with this approach. Because the lower classes, racial and ethnic minorities, and women were virtually always over-represented among the population of sex workers, efforts to regulate sex workers often exacerbated social and economic inequalities that already existed in society and increased their vulnerability to disease and exploitation. Regulatory efforts therefore devolved into punitive approaches that targeted one group, sex workers, while neglecting the wider dynamics of disease transmission throughout the population. The punitive approaches also undermined disease control efforts because, fearing punishment, many patients avoided medical treatment and care.

Education for Prevention: The Age of Eugenics During the Early 20th Century

The coalition between feminists, social workers, and moral reformers that brought an end to the Contagious Diseases Acts in Great Britain endured and was reactivated in the face of the next military threat, the outbreak of the First World War. In the United States, a similar alliance between the leading social worker Jane Addams, philanthropist John D. Rockefeller, and other interested physicians and reformers founded the American Social Hygiene Association (ASHA) in 1913, which actively promoted education in order to prevent the spread of venereal diseases. The social hygiene movement brought together two groups which coexisted uneasily: moral reformers and science-based technocrats. Between these two extremes was a large middle ground of people committed to both health and sexual morality (17). The influence of the social hygiene movement on public health made this field an interesting hybrid of science and professional social reform, both fields influenced by morality and subject to internal disputes as well as external attacks. At stake was more than just a dispute about whose ideas and whose approach was more effective, but who could control resources, define the problems, and implement solutions. Because the reformers of this period had focused so heavily on prostitution and its threat of venereal disease, scientists began to distance themselves from the question of prostitution *per se* and from social and behavioral science approaches to VD control and to focus on more biological issues related to disease.

Behavior was explicitly linked to biology in the field of eugenics, still in its heyday in the early 20th century. Eugenics, a movement (defined as scientific during the time and later debunked as pseudo-science) that focused on the importance of genetic "fitness" at the individual and national level, encouraged research and education on the problem of venereal diseases. Its emphasis on "racial purity," however, undermined or even precluded any prevention efforts directed at non-whites. Although eugenics was hardly the only influence on public health research and practice during the early 20th century, it played a disproportionate role in VD prevention and treatment programs precisely because sexuality, sexual health, and reproduction were central preoccupations of the eugenics movement. Eugenics influenced how VD education programs were developed and implemented in the United States, Europe, and in European colonies in Asia and Africa (18–20).

Although eugenics influenced policies throughout the world, "moral education" as a preventive method was more common in the Anglophone countries than in continental Europe. Conflict over the best method of preventing the spread of VD produced tensions between the United States and its ally, France, where soldiers from the American Expeditionary Force (AEF) were stationed in 1917. After the American troops flocked to the local French prostitutes, who were still legally allowed to practice their trade under the system of regulation devised during the 19th century, American commanders decided to make the contraction of VD a court-martial offense. The French commanders criticized American policy on the grounds that the policy of sexual continence placed French civilian women at greater risk of rape by not providing a suitable sexual outlet for American soldiers. Of particular concern to French officials was the presence of black American soldiers, whom they (like white Americans and other Europeans) believed were not capable of sexual control and likely to rape French civilian women (17).

Condoms became widely available in the United States after a 1918 ruling by Judge Frederick Crane in the New York court of appeals that physician-prescribed birth control for the prevention of disease was neither indecent nor immoral, thereby establishing a solid legal basis for the sale of condoms. During World War I, condom sales had skyrocketed. A number of companies had entered the business in order to capture this new source of wealth. By war's end, however, condom sales had declined, leaving these companies in fierce competition. During the 1920s, condom sales moved from the "shameful" secrecy of mail-order purchases and the sanitized space of the druggist to the street: street peddlers, elevator operators, waiters, and bartenders were among the many hawking condoms to ordinary men in every walk of life. The Youngs Rubber Corporation of New York, which produced the Trojan condom, adopted a strategy that ultimately allowed the firm to beat much of the competition: to sell only at drug stores and emphasize the condom's high quality and reliability. In 1937, the Food and Drug Administration (FDA) included condoms under its jurisdiction for inspection. In order to make sure that Trojan condoms passed FDA testing, thereby living up to Trojan's advertising campaign, Youngs Rubber invested in the research and development of a machine to test condom reliability; the machine was patented in 1940. Only two condom companies (Youngs Rubber and Julius Schmid, which made the brands Ramses, Sheiks, and Trojans) passed FDA tests, thereby leaving the condom market wide open for these companies. The Schmid company's "Ramses rubbers" further benefited when the U.S. Army endorsed them in 1940, just in time for the increased demand of wartime (21).

As condom sales were expanding during the 1920s, a coalition of groups, including the United States Public Health Service (USPHS), undertook major educational efforts to warn young people about the dangers of VD. In an effort to ground the educational efforts in solid scientific research, the National Research Council established a Committee for Research in Problems of Sex specifically to examine the problem of venereal diseases, including human behavior (22). No time looked more promising for the development of behavioral interventions as a fundamental part of STD control: a major philanthropist, John D. Rockefeller, was willing to provide funding for sex behavior research and programs, while community organizations such as the YMCA and the USPHS made VD prevention and sex education their priorities. This initial postwar enthusiasm rapidly dissipated in the face of multiple conflicts: between scientists; between scientists and the American Social Hygiene Association; and between federal and local authorities over control of VD prevention activities. Furthermore, prevention efforts were undermined by the content of the messages themselves: Adolescent American boys, white and black, viewed educational posters about white men's responsibility to "lift up" inferior races with their example of moral behavior and physical fitness (23). Internationally, in European colonies in Asia and Africa, public health authorities decided not to initiate prevention and education activities since the "inferior races" were incapable of sexual control (24,25).

Still influenced by the basic Progressive Era (ca. 1890–1920) beliefs in the ability of human beings to improve society and change behavior through education and legislative reform, postwar reformers seized on sex education as an ideal instrument for the prevention of venereal disease. Between 1919 and 1924, the USPHS developed a series of slides and posters for exhibition called the "Keeping Fit" campaign, primarily fear-based representations of men and women who had sex outside of marriage as being carriers of disease. Sexuality was alluded to rather than forthrightly discussed; even depictions of anatomy were not displayed. Rather than openly discuss sexuality, the exhibit maintained discretion through the "silent lecture," that is, no lecture at all. As mentioned before, all the images were of white people, with explicit mention of the importance of avoiding venereal disease in order to maintain the strength of the (white) race. Although the campaign carefully avoided controversial images and frank discussion of sexuality, local authorities nevertheless complained that the campaign was too explicit for their constituencies, or not appropriate for their primary audiences, who might be working class or of various ethnic backgrounds. Owing to financial constraints, the program was never uniformly implemented throughout the United States, and tensions between local and federal authorities contributed to the program's demise in 1924. Education efforts were therefore sporadic and primarily founded on a moral and racial ideology of purity through sexual abstinence (23).

Research scientists were no better able to advance a thorough study of human sexual behavior and its effect on venereal disease than public health officials were able to sustain an effective sex education program. Concerned about establishing sexuality research as a legitimate field of inquiry that would be able to attract "bright young men" into the field, the Committee for Research in Problems of Sex distanced itself from direct questions about the prevention of VD. Committee members argued that research about venereal disease was too closely linked to a moral agenda promoted by ASHA. To complicate matters, Rockefeller himself had provided financial support to both ASHA and the Committee, which made researchers concerned that their work would not be accepted as scientific. Furthermore, the cutting edge of biological research at the time was physiology. At a 1921 conference to determine the research agenda, committee members agreed that the fundamental problem behind VD was the "sex impulse." Grants were therefore awarded for animal and human studies in physiology and endocrinology to gain more insight into the biology behind the "sex impulse," but not to studies dealing directly with human behavior and its relationship to VD transmission (22). American scientists deliberately excluded research on VD prevention and behavioral interventions from their agenda for the study of human sexuality.

Internationally, competition between European countries fostered a Darwinian preoccupation with the "fittest of nations," evidence of which would be high birth rates and low rates of venereal diseases. European nations failed to meet these standards, as birth rates plummeted and venereal disease continued to be common from roughly 1900 through the 1930s (19). Europeans directed their education efforts only to their own citizens, not to the "inferior" populations they had colonized. In South Africa, for example, health education was thought to be a pointless exercise for black Africans, whom doctors regarded as irresponsible regarding their own health and too "raw and ignorant" to take medications on their own (25, pp. 147–8). Across the continent, black Africans were subject to compulsory examination and treatment, while whites enjoyed voluntary services. In 1908 in Uganda, for example, the medical staff of the Royal Army Medical Corps initiated mass treatment with mercury injections because "the present state of civilization in the country does not permit any legislative measures with a view to prevention" (24, p. 101). Twenty years later, compulsory examinations of entire villages were still being carried out in rural Uganda. When a British doctor complained about the degrading and humiliating treatment of black African women, she was fired (24, p. 101). In colonial Rhodesia (now Zimbabwe), the Public Health Act of 1924 empowered authorities to examine any African and, if deemed necessary, destroy Africans' homes in order to protect whites from diseases allegedly carried by black Africans, although the rate of venereal infection in black Africans was consistently lower than in whites (26). During this period, methods of VD education, behavioral interventions and treatment were inseparable from the prevailing racial ideologies, which compromised the quality of public health efforts.

The New Deal and World War II: Comprehensive Approaches to STD Control

Although the same racial ideology continued to inform public health practices in the United States and abroad during the Second World War, the New Deal era and wartime brought about several innovations in VD control, including behavioral interventions. In the United States, Surgeon General Thomas Parran laid the groundwork for a public health approach to VD control with his book *Shadow on the Land*, published in 1937. Parran outlined a program of screening, tracing sexual contacts of infected partners, and offering treatment to those infected in order to "break the chain of infection." Parran opposed a purely moral approach to VD control, which placed the blame for infection upon patients, fueled public disregard for the patients, and undermined efforts to devote public resources to these diseases. The cost of not treating these diseases, he argued, ultimately was much higher than the costs of treating them, considering the long-term sequelae of syphilis (blindness and insanity) and the loss of worker productivity (17). At the same time, his insistence that many patients with VD were "innocent" and his desire to reduce the silence and shame surrounding VD made it difficult for him and other public health officials to confront some of the more troubling aspects of VD control, such as pediatric gonorrhea, usually the result of incest. Rather than confront the troubling problem of incest, publicly risking associating this shameful crime with VD, physicians and public health officials chose to blame toilet seats for cases of pediatric gonorrhea (27).

Parran also shifted the focus of behavioral interventions from the patient to the health care provider. Largely because of Parran's efforts, Congress passed the National Venereal Disease Control Act in May 1938, with a $15 million appropriation that enabled new clinics to open (an increase from 1,750 in July 1938 to almost 3,000 in July 1940) and provided services and medications for indigent patients of private physicians (17, pp. 143-147). This act passed partly because it was an era of large public works projects, the "New Deal," designed to lift America out of economic depression; furthermore, Parran was a long-time friend of President Roosevelt. As a result of this legislation, surveillance and treatment efforts expanded with increased screening, laboratory services, and access to medications. The major focus of behavior change efforts was to encourage and, for some populations (such as pregnant women or couples seeking marriage licenses), require syphilis screening as a routine part of health care—in other words, to "normalize" the Wasserman test for syphilis antibodies. Focusing on the behavior of health care providers, rather than only the behavior of patients, represented a major shift in public health practice.

Wartime brought a new sense of public urgency to the problem of VD control. Because historically wartime is associated with increased VD incidence and loss of military manpower due to illness, the USPHS began planning for the possibility of a VD epidemic before the United States even entered the war. On December 7, 1940, precisely one year before the bombing of Pearl Harbor, Raymond Vonderlehr, chief of the Venereal Disease Division, sent a memorandum to Thomas Parran to initiate wartime planning for VD control. Although the military adopted many of the same policies it had followed during World War I, especially the repression of prostitution, one key policy changed: Soldiers and sailors who contracted VD were no longer subject to such penalties as loss of pay. Rather than serving as a deterrent to infection, the penalties had apparently discouraged infected personnel from seeking treatment, thereby encouraging greater costs, loss of manpower, and further spread of infection, according to military medical officers and the Surgeon General (17,28). Again, the major focus of behavioral interventions was to try to encourage testing and treatment. The targets for the interventions were policies that were regarded as detrimental to patients' willingness to seek health care. Beyond the encouragement of testing and treatment, military personnel received a wide range of behavioral interventions: educational campaigns designed to provide information about VD, in addition to fear-based messages about the dangers of disease and the threats that women in particular represented; and access to prophylaxis kits, which included condoms (17).

For civilians, wartime efforts to control VD initially brought a new period of repression, especially for working-class women, but later provided the first large-scale behavioral intervention efforts. The 1941 May Act outlawed vice activities, such as prostitution and alcohol, near military installations. Like previous, historical experiences with prosecution of prostitution, the police acquired broad authority to arrest and detain "suspicious" women, which in practice often meant that working-class women were subject to arbitrary arrest and detention (17). One woman who stopped at a lunch counter near a military installation to eat by herself, for example, was regarded as suspicious, arrested and subjected to a medical examination for VD (29). In the public mind, VD control became associated with prostitution, especially because the newly opened Rapid Treatment Centers (RTCs) accepted both gonorrhea and syphilis patients directly from jails or detention centers to voluntarily serve the remainder of their sentences. With the first in March 1942 in Leesville, Louisiana,

RTCs opened throughout the country, with 30 running by September of 1943, and continued expansion to new cities and states. The largest was in Augusta, Georgia, with 470 beds. RTCs offered residential facilities for the course of treatment, which declined from six to two weeks as increasingly effective therapies became available. Public health officials were eager to use this period of treatment as a means for introducing a more comprehensive VD control program, including but not limited to arsenical therapy (and later penicillin) (28).

Penicillin therefore replaced arsenical therapy in a comprehensive residential treatment, counseling, and rehabilitation program. Interestingly, the introduction of penicillin did not alter the RTCs' approach to disease control other than to shorten the period of treatment to two weeks. RTCs offered programs that ranged from counseling from a social worker and psychiatric screening to recreational activities, job training, and even job placement. With the heavy demand for labor in wartime industries, some women were trained in skills such as riveting and metal work and offered jobs at the end of their treatment; others were trained in traditionally "female" fields such as hair dressing and sewing. These centers also provided opportunities for behavioral research, such as psychiatric research at the St. Louis center "to determine how much in this field can be offered to venereally-infected individuals with emotional and adjustment difficulties" (28). Some of the RTCs included a full-time social worker on staff, but the type and quality of services, as well as the atmosphere of each center, varied tremendously from location to location. The broad interpretation of the RTCs' mandate to prevent and control venereal diseases to include job skills training, job placement, and psychosocial support for patients developed partly because these centers often used the facilities and personnel from former New Deal social welfare programs, such as the Civilian Conservation Corps camps and the National Youth Administration. The publicity surrounding these centers focused almost entirely on the repression of prostitution, with the unfortunate consequence that the public believed that control of prostitution alone was sufficient to contain venereal diseases. "The long-term case-finding, treatment, case-holding, and prophylaxis programs that are the real heart of our effort are less dramatic and unless a special effort is made are distinctly overshadowed," Vonderlehr wrote in a memo to Parran (28).

Wartime provided the rationale for a focus on VD *per se*, while the apparatus of the New Deal programs provided public health officials with the expertise, facilities, and equipment to undertake a variety of social programs. In the aftermath of the Great Depression, social problems were often defined as the result of economic upheaval rather than personal moral failure. In this context, behavioral interventions for VD prevention and control focused upon job training and job placement, providing continuity with earlier New Deal programs. In addition to providing job skills, social workers counseled patients to accept "personal responsibility" for their health, since the availability of penicillin did not keep patients from becoming reinfected. This comprehensive, well-funded approach to VD control was the result of a unique conjunction of historical circumstances: a Surgeon General committed to VD control (Thomas Parran); strong political alliances between the USPHS and the Presidential administration; wartime concern for VD and its effect on military manpower; and the availability of trained personnel, buildings, and equipment from previous social programs that could be redirected toward the fight against

VD. This wartime allocation of resources and expertise proved difficult to sustain after the war for a variety of reasons described below.

Post-War Reappraisal: From Public to Private Health

The immediate postwar period brought no change in VD control policies and practices, since military officials acknowledged the potential danger if infected troops were allowed to return to civilian life and spread disease. As part of the process of demobilization, the Army was responsible for retaining soldiers until they were noninfectious, then lab reports were sent to state health officers to complete treatment in the demobilized soldier's state of residence. The RTCs continued to operate as well (28). In the longer term, however, interest in VD prevention and control, especially behavioral interventions, declined for two reasons. First, scientists interpreted wartime studies of the effects of behavioral interventions on VD, such as they were, as a failure. Second, with the widespread availability of penicillin, public health priorities shifted away from VD. Many clinical and public health experts confidently predicted the elimination of gonorrhea and syphilis (and many other bacterial infections) in the near future, so that further public expenditures on prevention were not warranted.

Behavioral interventions and prevention counseling during wartime had been conducted without a solid grounding in research about what worked. A 1945 training manual, for example, attempted to provide advice on human behavior in order to deftly avoid controversies over competing theories, since there was not as yet established research on which to build programs. One of the fundamental concepts of human behavior this manual taught was that "to be understood is to be helped." Counselors should take time to try to understand patients, since "it is the time and interest given rather than the particular theoretical formulation that is important" (30).

Wartime research evaluated the effects of education programs on different variables: the retention of information about VD by recipients of education programs (e.g., which type of pamphlet was more effective in imparting information) and overall morbidity (28). Public health officials and researchers assumed that information alone was sufficient to change behavior. It was an unexamined assumption, which had devastating effects on the subsequent history of prevention efforts: Prevention in general, and behavioral prevention in particular, was judged to be a failure. In assessing the result of wartime research at a conference on preventive medicine in 1954, Lt. Col. Timmerman explained that "there was no evidence that frequent VD talks or movies cut down the exposure of men to VD when overseas." Moral education also was judged not to be a solution, either, since "church membership in general was only very slightly associated with abstaining from intercourse." Certain personality types, especially borderline personalities, Timmerman concluded, were associated with VD acquisition, and persons with these personalities remained susceptible "in spite of military education, experience, or recreational opportunities" (30).

Before Alfred Kinsey created major controversy in 1948 with his publication of *Sexual Behavior in the Human Male*, his research had already influenced military policy away from prevention as early as 1946. In showing that patterns of sexual behavior were established by age 16, Kinsey's research was used by military officials to justify both their continued policy not to treat VD as a criminal offense and their decision not to focus on prevention efforts. Critics had worried that the absence of a penalty encouraged sexual promiscuity. Military leaders argued that sexual behavior was already established by the time young men enlisted, and they cited Kinsey's work in support of this claim. Although the use of Kinsey's work prevented a backlash against the decriminalization policy, it also undermined efforts to focus research and resources on prevention and behavioral interventions. If sexual patterns were already established by age 16, then the appropriate avenue of intervention was not the military or public health, but "proper home, school and church influences" (30). According to this philosophy, VD control was a fundamentally private concern.

For civilians, the story was much the same, as the government abandoned its role in providing VD treatment. Parran's successor to the post of Surgeon General, Leonard Scheele, decided to close the publicly funded RTCs in 1953 and pass the majority of treatment and care on to private physicians. Scheele presented his decision as a major victory: Research efforts and pharmaceutical production had produced penicillin and other antibiotics, thereby eliminating the need for RTCs. "Now every private physician can be an efficient venereal disease control officer, giving ambulatory treatment to patients in his office, while State and local health departments maintain the important supporting services of case finding, contact tracing, referral, treatment of many patients unable to pay for private care, and education" (31). A two-tiered system of VD treatment therefore developed in the United States: private physicians for those who could afford them; public clinics for the rest. Regarded as "cured," infectious diseases no longer represented the cutting edge of medicine, so resources moved into chronic diseases such as cancer and heart disease.

With the decline in public support for VD control, funding for behavioral interventions was all but eliminated. One of the last papers given at a 1962 "World Forum on Syphilis and Other Treponemes" was devoted to a behavioral science program at San Francisco's VD clinic, one of the only clinics in the United States to have a full-time psychiatric social worker on staff. This one worker represented a significant reduction in staffing since 1942 when the clinic employed a psychiatrist, a psychologist, and two psychiatric social workers. Because patients did not always follow through with referrals for mental health services, the San Francisco clinic found that it was useful to have a full-time mental health expert available on site. The psychiatric social worker counseled all patients under age 21, any adult patient with a problem "either personality or situational" (such as marital difficulties or alcoholism), and patients who broke "treatment rules or who otherwise has difficulty adjusting to the clinic routine" (32). This program represented virtually the only behavioral intervention in the entire country and received relatively little attention.

European countries did not follow the American pattern of shutting down public clinics, but they did shift their emphasis from prevention to treatment. In England, for example, the National Health Service was established in 1948, and VD treatment was provided free of charge. But venereal diseases, especially behavioral interventions to control VD, were no more on the radar screen in the United Kingdom or Europe than they were in the United States.

Between 1948 and the advent of AIDS was a period of "benign neglect during which there was little policy development or resource commitment, punctuated by short periods where changing epidemiological patterns or media scares stimulated political interest" (33). "Benign neglect" aptly characterizes most of the world's approach to VD control after the immediate postwar period.

Blaming the Patient: Syphilis Eradication and Noncompliant Patients, 1950s to 1970s

When the world was not ignoring the problem of STDs, as they increasingly came to be called during the 1970s, they were undertaking periodic campaigns to eradicate at least one of them, namely syphilis. Syphilis eradication campaigns had important consequences for the type of behavioral interventions that were commonly used during this period. In the United States, behavioral interventions were used to support the major efforts of the eradication campaigns, which were primarily directed towards surveillance, partner management, and treatment. Public health officials focused on the behaviors that were perceived as facilitators or barriers to disease eradication: patients' willingness to name sexual contacts; patients' cooperation with physicians' instructions, especially regarding medications (34); and the willingness of "difficult-to-reach" populations, such as male homosexuals, migrant workers, and teenagers, all regarded as reservoirs of infection, to seek health care and submit to screening.

In the United States, public health advisers, usually hired immediately after college graduation and then trained in public health practice, and nurses conducted the interviews and traced sex partners. Confidentiality was key to winning trust. Public health advisers attended "interviewing school." With a combination of classroom instruction, role playing, and feedback, public health advisers learned how to elicit information from patients, including asking about same-sex partners. Despite training in asking about same-sex partners, however, homosexual men in particular were reluctant to provide names of their partners from the 1950s through the 1970s (35–37). As one man said to the public health adviser interviewing him, "I don't mind telling you about myself, but I don't want to tell you who else is gay" (37).

The intense focus on syphilis eradication unfortunately coincided with another federal government initiative directly aimed at homosexual Americans: the "Pervert Elimination Campaign" launched by the U.S. Park Police in 1947 to crack down on gays, followed by the McCarthy-inspired Federal Loyalty Program in which approximately 1,000 persons were fired for alleged homosexuality (38). The tactics of these two separate, unrelated elimination campaigns unwittingly bore certain similarities which must have undermined gay Americans' trust in the syphilis eradication effort. To eliminate homosexuality from the federal government, vice squad officers frequented bars and clubs where homosexuals were known to congregate, interviewed co-workers and neighbors, and even compiled lists of "known" homosexuals (38). As mentioned before, public health officials tried to elicit names of contacts and, in some cities at least, maintained lists of homosexuals in order to contact them should an epidemic break out among homosexuals in that city. Public health officials perceived this relationship between homosexuals and the public health department as voluntary, but it is not clear whether gays felt the same way. At a VD seminar in Jacksonville, Florida, in 1959, for example, public health officials noted that "in Atlanta a roster of homosexuals is maintained and when an infection is found in a member of this group, word is sent out and the entire group comes in and are tested" (31). Although public health officials kept the confidentiality of their patients' names, many gays, who may have already experienced harassment from other government officials, extended their suspicion to public health officials as well. In Washington, D.C., where harassment of homosexuals reached the greatest intensity in the nation due to its large number of federal employees and location of the McCarthy hearings (38), a syphilis epidemic broke out in 1956 and continued for at least three years (31). Harassment apparently had a direct effect on gay men's willingness to seek health care.

Public health officials also had trouble reaching migrant workers and teenagers (31), who shared the same mistrust of government motives as gays did. The difficulties in reaching these "special groups" (as public health officials called them) demonstrate the limitations of the behavioral interventions being used at the time. Predicated on the idea that interviewers' techniques could be refined and developed to elicit information, interviewing methods failed to take account of the political, cultural, and economic vulnerabilities of certain groups of patients. Homosexual men and women could lose their jobs if they were identified as such. Migrant workers faced deportation. Furthermore, different branches of government were actively collecting and recording information about homosexuals and migrant workers precisely in order to fire them or deport them. It is not difficult to see why these groups had difficulty trusting another branch of government, public health, to maintain confidential information, regardless of whether they had had bad experiences with public health officials. Providing names was too big a risk to take. Behavioral interventions focused on ways of getting individuals to cooperate with government authorities, but failed to take account of the intrusive, repressive role that government played in the lives of certain populations.

Behavioral interventions scarcely appeared on the research agenda for STDs during the 1960s and 1970s. The cutting edge of scientific research during the 1970s was the microbiology of STDs, not behavioral science. Under the influence of King Holmes, who revitalized what had for several decades been a dormant field, STDs became part of the clinical specialty of infectious diseases, rather than the specialty of dermatology. This shift represented a significant change in the methods, practices and research agenda for the newly revitalized field, towards answering some of the basic questions about the microbiology of these pathogens (39).

At the same time, the success of penicillin and other antibiotics had focused attention on treatment. Patients wanted access to medications. African-American health activism after World War II, for example, focused primarily on access to treatment, especially since African Americans had largely been excluded from major government programs during the development of public health programs from 1890 to 1930. Middle-class black women organized themselves in clubs, community organizations and churches to crusade for basic public health services in black communities. Run by lay people, these efforts focused on personal hygiene, sanitation, and improvement of neighborhood water, milk, and food supplies. Although these efforts probably significantly improved health conditions and survivorship, many black Americans regarded these kinds of "behavioral interventions" and prevention activities as amateur efforts and therefore as second-class treatment, the product of government disregard for and lack of resources for black Americans while white Americans had access to physicians and medication. As a result, black health activists after the war focused on access to treatment rather than prevention and behavioral interventions (40). In many ways, however, African Americans were no different than the rest of America, focused on treatment rather than prevention.

Mistrust of syphilis prevention and treatment efforts were further undermined in 1972, when a journalist reported ethical problems with a 40-year-old continuing research study of 399 black men in Alabama, the infamous Tuskegee study. The USPHS began the study of untreated syphilis in black men in 1932 and misled the research subjects, who believed that they were receiving medical treatment for "bad blood" (a local term that referred to syphilis) when in fact researchers withheld treatment, including penicillin when it became available. When this study was made public in 1972, the public, especially blacks, expressed outrage and the study was discontinued (41). The lasting effect, however, was to further undermine public support for STD prevention and treatment programs, including for HIV/AIDS during and after the 1980s (42).

The Advent of AIDS: Behavioral Interventions at the Forefront

It took an unprecedented tragedy, the devastating AIDS epidemic that was first identified during the early 1980s, to turn attention towards behavioral interventions for the control of STDs. A fatal disease with no cure, and no effective therapy until 1996, the only way to control the epidemic was through effective prevention. Previous assumptions—that providing information about disease would change behavior, for example—were tested and evaluated systematically, as the remaining chapters in this volume describe.

The public health community had only recently turned to behavioral science to provide solutions to the burden of chronic diseases, especially cancer and cardiovascular disease, which the United States faced during the 1970s and 1980s. In 1982, for example, the leading journal *American Psychologist* devoted an entire issue to the relationship between public health and psychology (43). The majority of the articles focused on how the field of psychology could offer behavioral modification techniques, theories of learning, and communications strategies to change "health-impairing habits and life-styles," notably cigarette smoking, in addition to changing behaviors related to stress and psychosocial reactions to illness (44). Psychology's emphasis on the individual, versus public health's emphasis on the population, quickly emerged as one of the key problems in bridging these two fields. For some psychologists, however, the emphasis on the individual was one of psychology's major selling points for public health practice in an era of expanding medical costs and demands for a reduced role of government during the Reagan era. One psychologist defined the field of "behavioral health" as "an interdisciplinary field dedicated to promoting a philosophy of health that stresses *individual responsibility* in the application of behavioral and biomedical science knowledge and techniques to the *maintenance* of health and the *prevention* of illness and dysfunction by a variety of self-initiated or shared activities" (45,46, italics in original). The emphasis on individual responsibility resonated with the Republican administration's emphasis on decreasing the size of government. None of these early articles on psychology and public health discussed the potential role of behavioral science in controlling STDs. Until acquired immunodeficiency syndrome (AIDS) was acknowledged as a significant public health threat several years after its first appearance, little attention was paid to the development of effective behavioral interventions to reduce the spread of STDs. One legacy of the early 1980s' emphasis on "behavioral health" as an issue of individual responsibility and individual behavior change was an early emphasis on HIV behavioral interventions at the individual (versus community or policy) level.

This historical introduction to behavioral interventions in STD control provides a few key lessons for current practitioners. First, until the AIDS epidemic, behavioral interventions have seldom been placed at the forefront of STD control and seldom had the level of resources, research, and program planning that has been directed towards treatment and biological research. Major public health initiatives, such as the syphilis eradication programs of the 1960s, often used behavioral interventions primarily to assist interviewers find contacts and bring them into treatment, rather than to understand systematically the full spectrum of roles behavioral interventions could play to prevent and control disease.

Second, the general public has not always responded warmly to behavioral interventions. Sex education efforts often offended conservative sexual mores, but discomfort about sexuality only partially explains negative public reaction. Far more serious is the perception that prevention and behavioral interventions are a substitute for effective treatment, especially in the case of American minority groups (40), although further research is necessary to explore how widespread this perception has been during recent decades. Equally problematic is the perception that behavioral interventions are an example of government intrusion into private life. For groups whose private lives were the subject of intense public, political debate, notably gay Americans, it is hardly surprising that behavioral interventions have been regarded as one more unwanted intrusion. The future success of behavioral interventions may depend on whether the American public learns about the contributions that behavioral science and behavioral interventions can play in reducing STD and HIV acquisition and transmission—and to learn that behavioral interventions have not failed to control STDs historically, because they were virtually never tried.

References

1. Arrizabalaga J, Henderson J, French R. *The Great Pox: The French Disease in Renaissance Europe*. New Haven: Yale University Press; 1997.
2. Nutton V. The seeds of disease: an explanation of contagion and infection from the Greeks to the Renaissance. *Medical History*. 1983;27:1–34.
3. Gentilcore D. *Healers and Healing in Early Modern Italy*, Manchester: Manchester University Press; 1998.
4. Pomata G. *Contracting a Cure: Patients, Healers, and the Law in Early Modern Bologna*. Baltimore: Johns Hopkins University Press; 1998.

5. Carmichael A. Contagion theory and contagion practice in fifteenth-century Milan. *Renaissance Quarterly*. 1991; 44:213–225.
6. Schleiner W. Moral attitudes toward syphilis and its prevention in the Renaissance. *Bull. Hist. Med.* 1994;68:389–410.
7. McGough LJ. Quarantining beauty: the French disease in early modern Venice. In: Siena KP, ed. *Sins of the Flesh: Responding to Sexual Disease in Early Modern Europe*. Toronto: Centre for Reformation and Renaissance Studies; 2005.
8. Schleiner W. Infection and cure through women: Renaissance constructions of syphilis. *Journal of Medieval and Renaissance Studies*. 1994;24:499–517.
9. Siena KP. *Venereal Disease, Hospitals, and the Urban Poor: London's `Foul Wards,' 1600-1800*. Rochester: University of Rochester Press; 2004.
10. Corbin A. *Women for Hire: Prostitution and Sexuality in France after 1850* (trans. Sheridan A). Cambridge, MA: Harvard University Press; 1990.
11. Bernstein L. *Sonia's Daughters: Prostitutes and their Regulation in Imperial Russia*. Berkeley: University of California Press; 1995.
12. Gibson M. *Prostitution and the State in Italy, 1860-1915*. Columbus: Ohio State University Press; 1986.
13. Walkowitz J. *Prostitution and Victorian Society: Women, Class and the State*. New York: Cambridge University Press; 1980.
14. Kaminsky AP. Morality legislation and British troops in late nineteenth-century India. *Military Affairs*. 1979;43:78–84.
15. Levine P. Rereading the 1890s: venereal disease as "constitutional crisis" in Britain and British India. *Journal of Asian Studies*. 1996;55:585–612.
16. Hershatter G. *Dangerous Pleasures: Prostitution and Modernity in Twentieth-Century Shanghai*. Berkeley: University of California Press; 1997.
17. Brandt AM. *No Magic Bullet: A Social History of Venereal Disease in the United States since 1880*, 2nd ed. New York: Oxford University Press; 1987.
18. Gorchov L. Sexual Science and Sexual Politics: American Sex Research, 1920-1956. Ph.D. Dissertation. Baltimore: Johns Hopkins University; 2002.
19. Davidson R, Hall LA, eds. *Sex, Sin and Suffering: Venereal Disease and European Society since 1870*. New York: Routledge; 2001.
20. Haller M. *Eugenics: Hereditarian Attitudes in American Thought*. New Brunswick: Rutgers University Press; 1984.
21. Tone A. *Devices and Desires: A History of Contraceptives in America*. New York: Hill and Wang; 2001.
22. National Academies Archives, Washington, DC: Committee for Research in Problems of Sex, 1920–1965.
23. Lord A. Models of masculinity: sex education, the United States Public Health Service, and the YMCA, 1919-1924. *Journal of the History of Medicine*. 2003;58:123–152.
24. Lyons M. Medicine and morality: a review of responses to sexually transmitted diseases in Uganda in the twentieth century. In: Setel PW, Lewis M, Lyons M, eds. *Histories of Sexually Transmitted Diseases and HIV/AIDS in Sub-Saharan Africa*. Westport, CT: Greenwood Press; 1999.
25. Jochelson K. *The Colour of Disease: Syphilis and Racism in South Africa, 1880-1950*. New York: Palgrave; 2001.
26. McCulloch J. The management of venereal disease in a settler society: colonial Zimbabwe, 1900-1930. In: Setel PW, Lewis M, Lyons M, eds. *Histories of Sexually Transmitted Diseases and HIV/AIDS in Sub-Saharan Africa*. Westport, CT: Greenwood Press; 1999.
27. Sacco L. Sanitized for your protection: medical discourse and the denial of incest in the United States, 1890-1940. *Journal of Women's History*. 2000;14: 80–104.
28. National Archives, College Park, MD, Record Group 90.

29. Hegarty M. Patriots, prostitutes, patriotutes: the mobilization and control of female sexuality in the U.S. during World War II. Ph.D. Dissertation. Columbus: Ohio State University; 1998.

30. National Archives, College Park, MD, Record Group 112.

31. National Archives, Southeast Region, East Point, GA, Record Group 442.

32. Angell M. A behavioral science action program in a venereal disease clinic. In: *Proceedings of World Forum on Syphilis and Other Treponematoses*. Atlanta: Communicable Disease Center, Venereal Disease Branch; 1964.

33. Evans D. Sexually transmitted disease policy in the English National Health Service, 1948-2000: continuity and social change. In: Davidson R, Hall LA, eds. *Sex, Sin and Suffering: Venereal Disease and European Society since 1870*. New York: Routledge; 2001:237–252.

34. Greene JA. Therapeutic infidelities: `noncompliance' enters the medical literature, 1955-1975. *Social History of Medicine*. 2004;17:327–343.

35. Spencer J. Personal Interview: February 22, 2005, Atlanta, GA and February 24, 2005, Gainesville, GA.

36. Martich, F. Personal Interview: February 10, 2005, Atlanta, GA.

37. Naehr, J. Personal Interview: January 18, 2005, Atlanta, GA.

38. Johnson DK. *The Lavender Scare: The Cold War Persecution of Gays and Lesbians in the Federal Government*. Chicago: University of Chicago Press; 2004.

39. Aral SO and Douglas JM. Personal Interviews: March 25, 2005, Atlanta, GA.

40. Smith S. *Sick and Tired of Being Sick and Tired: Black Women's Health Activism in America, 1890-1950*. Philadelphia: University of Pennsylvania Press; 1995.

41. Jones JH. *Bad Blood: The Tuskegee Syphilis Experiment*, 2nd ed., New York: Free Press; 1993.

42. Gamble VN. Under the shadow of Tuskegee: African Americans and health care. *American Journal of Public Health*. 1997;87:1773–1778.

43. DeLeon PH, Pallak MS. Public health and psychology: an important, expanding interaction. *American Psychologist*. 1982;37:934–935.

44. Singer JE, Krantz DS. Perspectives on the interface between psychology and public health. *American Psychologist*. 1982;37:955–960.

45. Matarazzo JD. Behavioral health's challenge to academic, scientific, and professional psychology. *American Psychology*. 1982;37:1–14.

46. Matarazzo JD. (1980). Behavioral health and behavioral medicine: frontiers for a new health psychology. *American Psychology*. 1980;35:807–817.

2

Behavioral Interventions for STDs: Theoretical Models and Intervention Methods

Janet S. St. Lawrence, Ph.D., and J. Dennis Fortenberry, Ph.D, M.D., M.S.

Adverse health consequences from sexual behavior, such as infections with STDs, are conservatively estimated to be at least threefold higher in the United States than in any other developed country (1). This disparity in disease prevalence and the serious personal, social, and financial consequences of sexually transmitted infections are generating a growing body of literature that describes the development, implementation, and evaluation of behavioral interventions addressing STD/HIV prevention. These interventions are designed to inform, change attitudes and perceptions, modify social norms, promote sexual health and reduce risky behaviors, transform social contexts, and alter policies that are facilitators or barriers to healthy behaviors. However, a careful review of the literature reveals that exhortations to intervene and recommendations for interventions far outnumber credible interventions that have been subjected to a thorough statistical evaluation demonstrating their effectiveness.

Up to the present, interventions for STD/HIV prevention have been implemented primarily at the individual, small-group, and community-levels, with varying degrees of population coverage associated with these efforts (2). A source of confusion for many consumers of this research is that not all of these intervention efforts are correctly labeled as "behavioral" interventions. Intervention strategies that are described in the literature can range from atheoretical to theoretical; from straightforward information provision to complex multi-method, multi-component programs; from minimally to rigorously evaluated; and from individual to multilevel programs. Some may be grounded in beliefs about how things should work in the real world; others are empirically grounded in evidence about how things actually happen. The objective of this chapter, then, is to describe and evaluate theoretical approaches to behavior change; to review the basic structure of behavioral interventions; and to summarize interventions conducted at various individual, group, and community levels.

What Is a Behavioral Theory and How Can It Be Used?

A theory is a systematic way of describing events and behaviors. It incorporates a set of concepts, definitions, and hypotheses that explain or predict behaviors by examining the relationships between variables. Theories are, by

Behavioral Interventions for Prevention and Control of Sexually Transmitted Diseases. Aral SO, Douglas JM Jr, eds. Lipshutz JA, assoc ed. New York: Springer Science+ Business Media, LLC; 2007.

nature, abstract. Most of the theories that are applied to health promotion were originally developed to explain other topics and were later adapted to explain health behaviors. Many of the theories to be described in the sections that follow have not been rigorously evaluated; therefore they constitute theoretical frameworks for understanding and predicting behavior that await empirical verification.

Given the unproven nature of most theoretical models, why then do behavioral scientists use them in developing and evaluating an intervention? Theoretical models provide a logical framework for designing, measuring, and evaluating behavioral interventions. They enable the program developer or evaluator to consider what they are planning within a larger context, applying relevant theoretical models to develop tailored programs and measurement of the effectiveness of those programs. Thus, behavioral theories provide us with a roadmap for studying a health problem, explaining the relationships between behaviors (including the social and physical contexts surrounding them), and specifying the measurement that will provide useful outcome evaluations from an intervention.

In other words, our theories provide a way of organizing the reasons why people do or do not engage in specific behaviors, helping to identify what we need to know before we develop a health promotion program, and suggesting what we need to monitor and measure in order to know whether our intervention manages to change the intended outcomes. Simply put, a large body of literature underscores the reality that interventions based on a theoretical model are far more likely to succeed than programs delivered without the benefit of a theoretical model.

Two different types of theories will be described in this chapter. Some theories are explanatory, describing the reasons why a problem arises. These theories are used to identify variables that contribute to a problem that can potentially be changed to alleviate the problem. Other theories focus on behavior change. These latter theories are most often used to guide the development of interventions and their evaluation. Their focus is on extracting the interventions methods and messages thereby providing a framework for program evaluation.

What Is a Behavioral Intervention?

Two approaches characterize the structure of behavioral interventions. The first approach is to define *a priori* the components to be incorporated into a behavioral intervention. The second method is extrapolated from research syntheses and meta-analyses of effective behavioral interventions. This latter strategy extracts the cross-cutting characteristics of effective interventions. When these two methods are contrasted, the convergence between them demonstrates remarkably consistent agreement between their conclusions.

A priori definitions of behavioral interventions are characterized by 1) a specified theoretical model; 2) intervention using evidence-based methods of behavior change; 3) rigorous outcome evaluation; 4) sound research designs; and 5) measurement of multiple domains such as cognitions (e.g., knowledge, attitudes, perceptions, self-efficacy beliefs, readiness for change), behavioral skills (e.g., correct condom application skill, social competencies to refuse unwanted sex), or biological variables representing a direct outcome of the behavior in question (e.g., STD diagnosis or a pregnancy test).

Post hoc research syntheses and meta-analyses examine cross-cutting characteristics of effective behavioral interventions and provide remarkably congruent support for the above definition. Cross-cutting characteristics of effective behavioral interventions are that they 1) have a clear focus on reducing sexual risk; 2) are based on sound theoretical models; 3) deliver interventions of sufficient magnitude and duration; 4) utilize a variety of evidence-based intervention methods; 5) personalize the information to the participants; 6) provide specific and accurate information; 7) provide participants with skill training and with opportunities to practice these newly acquired skills; 8) reinforce clear messages that strengthen values and norms that favor safety; 9) are tailored to the community and cultural norms of the participants; 10) make an effort to include the target group in program planning; 11) have clear goals and objectives; and 12) systematically document their results relative to the goals using sound research designs and rigorous evaluation (3–6).

Integrating Behavioral Interventions and Public Health

Research summaries consistently document the effectiveness of behavioral interventions in changing risky behaviors of specific groups, including drug users (7), adolescents (8), heterosexual adults (9), and men who have sex with other men (10). With such strong support for the efficacy of behavioral interventions, integration of the fields of behavioral science and public health presents a high priority.

However, continuing challenges have limited the integration of behavioral sciences and public health. Behavioral sciences have had a greater influence on research and demonstration activities than on the continuing services of public health departments (11). Behavioral interventions are often rooted in theoretical models that are familiar to the behavioral scientists, but are not as well known by public health practitioners. If these models are applied in a faulty manner, the desired outcomes may not be attained, as was the case in several intervention reports (12–15). Such failures may widen the gap between behavioral science and public health practice (16). For example, when Flowers et al. (15) and Elford et al. (14) attempted to replicate an intervention that had consistently demonstrated risky behavior reductions of 30% in communities of men who have sex with men, they incorporated only one of the nine core elements from the model. As a result, unlike the programs that incorporated all—or even most—of those core components, their interventions yielded no behavior changes. Therefore, careful analysis of the situation is necessary to estimate how piecemeal adaptation of theory-based interventions could have undesired consequences (11).

Given the importance behavioral scientists attribute to their theoretical models, let us next examine what these models are, as well as their comparative strengths and shortcomings. Although there is no theoretical model specifically developed to explain sexual behavior, a number of existing theoretical models have been adapted and extended to STD/HIV research.

Theoretical Models Applied to STD/HIV Interventions

Seven conceptual "families" of theoretical models appear in the STD and HIV intervention literatures. These conceptual domains include 1) psycho-educational approaches that stress information provision; 2) cognitive theories that emphasize internal decision-making processes; 3) behavioral models based on the principles derived from learning theories; 4) theories of motivation and emotional arousal; 5) social marketing and social influence theories; 6) a stage theory, the transtheoretical model; and 7) blended theories that integrate more than one of these domains into a single model, such as the Information-Motivation-Behavior model.

Psycho-Educational Theories Stressing Information Provision

Education and information provision continue to be prominent public health responses to STD/HIV. Information provision programs generally have three goals: 1) providing accurate information to recipients; 2) influencing attitudes and behaviors so that the recipients will translate knowledge into behavior change; and 3) reducing the number of infections (17). Psycho-educational interventions often accomplish the first of these three goals, but they are usually insufficient to attain the last two goals.

A number of studies illustrate the limitations of information-based interventions. For example, Brandt et al. (18) found that the quality and accuracy of printed educational materials varies widely. When they evaluated 21 printed educational materials about human papillomavirus (HPV), most were found to be "not suitable" or "barely adequate"; information was inconsistent from one pamphlet to another; and the content was sometimes highly inaccurate. In addition, the language in most of materials required a reading comprehension level that exceeded the literacy of a large proportion of the U.S. population.

In many public health and medical settings, information provision is often the only available intervention. The limitations of this approach are illustrated by a study of women who were tested and found to be positive for HPV infection. All of the women were counseled about their HPV infection. However, follow-up interviews showed that fewer than half recalled ever hearing of HPV or having been told that they had HPV infection (19).

Information provision may accomplish some important public health objectives. For example, the national educational campaign initiated in 1988 by former Surgeon General C. Everett Koop in response to HIV and AIDS was a key effort to quickly educate the U.S. population about an emerging epidemic. At a time when misconceptions about AIDS were prevalent, an educational brochure was mailed by the U.S. Public Health Service to every household in the United States. This monumental task, accompanied by substantial advocacy by the Surgeon General, contributed to a substantial reorientation of public awareness of HIV/AIDS (20).

Cognitive Theories Applied to STD/HIV Prevention

Cognitive theoretical models emphasize the relationship between cognitive processes (attitudes, values, perceptions, intentions, and beliefs) and behavior, and these models view cognition as the proximal determinant of sexual behaviors. Each cognitive theory shares in common the assumption that cognitions are causal, predisposing factors that explain sexual behaviors. These theoretical approaches are widely applied, with varying success, as explanatory models in the STD/HIV behavioral intervention literature.

The Health Belief Model

The Health Belief Model (HBM) hypothesizes that cognitive mediators such as 1) perceived vulnerability to a health threat; 2) perceived severity of the threat; 3) beliefs in the effectiveness of taking precautionary action; 4) perceived costs of implementing that action; and 5) the presence of environmental cues that interact to produce behavior change. Additionally, the model indicates that the perceived efficacy of behavior change is subsequently balanced against perceived social, physical, and psychological barriers to implementing the behavior. Finally, the model states that specific, identifiable cues are necessary to trigger the decision-making process (21,22).

A large body of literature has examined the utility of HBM in explaining STD/HIV risk behavior (23). Some studies have found that perceptions of susceptibility, severity, and benefits are significant predictors of sexual behavior, while others have found little or no relationship (17). In many instances, predictors specified by HBM accounted for only a modest amount, that is, 15% to 20% of the behavioral variance (24). An important limitation of HBM from a public health perspective is that it does not explain how perceptions of risk originate, nor does the model describe how health beliefs develop or persist over time (25,26). In addition, the theoretical perspective that beliefs necessarily precede behavior is not substantiated by contemporary research, which suggests that many health beliefs are a consequence rather than a precursor of behavior.

Theory of Reasoned Action

The Theory of Reasoned Action (TRA) postulates that an individual's attitudes, beliefs, perceptions about peers' attitudes, and the extent to which the individual values the peer group's approval all interact to form an intention to behave in a specific fashion (27,28). This specific intention is the proximal determinant of a specified behavior. Although similar to other cognitive theories in viewing behavior as an outcome of beliefs, addition of social norms as contributing factors and emphasis on behavioral intentions differentiate the TRA from the other cognitive theories. TRA has been widely used in survey research to explain the observed correlations between attitudes and precautionary behavior or intentions to engage in safer behavior in the future (29).

An important limitation of TRA is the assumption that sexual risk and protective behaviors result from a conscious decision-making process. However, substantial recent research suggests that many behaviors in sexual situations are motivated at least in part by affect and emotion rather than by the deliberative evaluations. Other research raises questions about the strength of the intentions–behavior relationship, which may differ across behaviors and populations (30). The limitations described in the previous section for the HBM also apply to the TRA, including the modest behavioral variance explained by the theory, the unclear origins of the cognitive progenitors of intentions, and the implicit directionality in the model that could just as easily be reversed with equal plausibility. Finally, while the model explains relationships between variables and suggests where to intervene, it offers no specific guidance regarding how to implement intervention strategies that might produce changes in these observed relationships. The model can also be criticized for leading to truncated measurement when it is applied in several intervention studies for STD/HIV prevention (31). Despite these limitations, the TRA is a popular framework in the intervention literature.

Theory of Planned Behavior

Icek Azjen later modified the TRA (32). This modified theory became known as the Theory of Planned Behavior (TBP). The TPB differs from the TRA in that it added one additional construct to the original model-perceived behavioral control. Perceived behavioral control is a person's belief that it is possible to control a given behavior. Azjen added this construct to account for situations in which people's behavior or behavioral intentions are influenced by things that they believe are beyond their ability to control. The model argues that people will be more successful in performing a behavior if they believe that they have a high degree of control over whether or not they engage in the behavior. Like the TRA, this theory emphasizes the relationships between behavior and cognitions such as beliefs, attitudes, and intentions. Like the TRA, it assumes that behavioral intention is the most important determinant of behavior and that behavioral intentions, in term, result from a person's attitudes toward performing a behavior and by beliefs about whether the individuals who are important to the person would approve or disapprove of the behavior. Both of these models largely ignore factors such a culture or the surrounding environmental context, assuming that they do not add further explanatory benefit to the models' explanations of the likelihood that a person will behave in a particular manner. Like the TRA, the TPB describes a causal chain of beliefs, attitudes, perceptions of controllability, and intentions that are believed to drive behavior.

Decision-Making Theory

Decision-making models, similar to HBM and TRA, are based on the assumption that people make rational choices about sexual risk and protection, expecting their choices to produce positive outcomes (33–35). As applied to STD/HIV prevention, these models offer an explanatory framework for how decisions should be made, then examine differences between decisions that increase risk and those that maximize safety. Several aspects of the model call into question whether it should be used to explain sexual behavior. The model does not reconcile the decisional balance from the immediate gratification offered by risky behaviors such as sexual intercourse or drug use and the delayed and uncertain long term negative consequences of a decision not to engage in these actions. As suggested previously, emotions may be more important than rational choice in decisions about sexual behavior. Finally, many decades of evidence show that immediate gratification usually overwhelms alternatives requiring delay of gratification (36).

Theories Based on the Principles of Learning

Learning theories are widely applied to behavioral interventions for STD/HIV prevention. Behavioral interventions based on learning theory often focus on identification of cues to risky behavior and on teaching new skills intended to reduce infection risk. Theoretical models based upon learning theories are often misunderstood to a greater extent than other theoretical models.

Operant Learning Theory

Unlike the cognitive theories, operant learning theory relies on measurable behaviors and identification of stimulus cues and reinforcers to explain the acquisition, performance, and maintenance of behaviors (37). Operant learning-based approaches concentrate on three components: 1) specifying the behavior; 2) identifying current consequences of the behavior (reinforcers) that operate (hence the term "operant") to strengthen or maintain the behavior; and 3) identifying discriminative stimuli in the environment that serve as cues and "trigger" the behavior. Behavior change strategies that derive from operant learning theory include managing the consequences of behavior (reinforcement, punishment, and extinction), shaping, counter conditioning, and stimulus control. The key construct in operant approaches is the concept of reinforcements that follow a behavior and affect whether or not the behavior is repeated in the future. Positive reinforcements (often described as "rewards") increase a person's likelihood of repeating the behavior in the future. Negative reinforcement also increases future performance of a behavior because it eliminates some continual negative condition (e.g., giving in to pressures to have sex without a condom). Reinforcements can be internal or external. Internal rewards are things that people do to reward themselves, while external rewards are provided by others. Behavior change strategies using reinforcement always are designed to increase the incidence of behaviors.

By contrast, there are also strategies that are designed to reduce or suppress behaviors. These are referred to as punishing consequences or extinction. Punishment is the application of a negative consequence perceived as being decidedly unpleasant by the recipient. Punishment is often misapplied; although it can successfully suppress a behavior for some period of time, it does not eliminate it and the behavior typically recurs. Elimination is achieved through a carefully designed process called extinction that identifies and then systematically removes the reinforcers that give rise to or maintain the behavior.

Shaping is the process of changing discrete steps along a sequence of behaviors by interrupting the sequence and replacing behaviors in the chain that led to risky behavior in the past with alternatives that do not lead to the same end point. For example, there are many behaviors in a linked chain of occurrences between leaving one's place of work and arriving home. When the commute involves passing a location where unsafe sex has taken place repeatedly, the chain of events can be altered by designing a different route between the office and home that is not associated with any cues to embark on the chain of behaviors (events) that have led to the unsafe sexual occurrences in the past.

Counter conditioning involves substituting an incompatible alternative to the problematic behavior. For example, someone who is easily led by others to engage in risky behavior may benefit from assertiveness training. In that case, the counter conditioning would replace passive response patterns with assertive responses. If negative mood stages are associated with risky behavior, learning when and how to use positive self-statements may effectively counter this chain of behaviors.

Stimulus control refers to avoiding or countering stimuli that elicited the problem behaviors in the past, restructuring one's personal environment, avoiding cues that previously "triggered" high-risk behavior, and using gradual fading techniques, if necessary, to make the transition from maladaptive to adaptive behavior (38). The example given above about changing a route between work and home to avoid locations associated with unsafe sex also addresses stimulus control, since changing the route also avoids the "stimulus" of seeing (and responding to) the location where such acts took place, for example, a "massage parlor" along the way where sexual behaviors are included in the establishment's services.

Clinicians use operant approaches extensively in interventions for other health concerns such as smoking cessation, weight control, and medication adherence (39–41). Operant approaches are designed to change the chain of past behavior that culminated in risk; to provide participants with new behavioral skills that they can employ in the future; to modify the stimulus cues in the environment that were associated with risky behaviors; to replace past behavior patterns; and to change the reinforcers that make it more likely that a past risky behavior will be repeated in the future. Usually, operant learning theory is embedded into the behavior change methods included in intervention programs based on the social learning theories described below.

Social Learning and Self-Efficacy Theory

Social learning theory (SL) and its later derivative, social cognitive theory (SCT), are popular models in the intervention literature. Social learning theory adds to operant approaches by explaining that new behaviors also are acquired by observational learning: watching others, noting consequences, then imitating the observed skills that led to positive consequences (42). More recently, Bandura expanded social learning theory to incorporate the concept of self efficacy -confidence in one's ability to successfully implement changes (43). This modified theory is called SCT. In reality, these terms are often used interchangeably although they refer to two distinct conceptual stages in the development of Bandura's theory. In its newer form, SCT specifies three main components that affect the likelihood that a person will change a health-related behavior: a) self-efficacy, b) goals, and c) outcome expectancies. In other words, if a person is confident about his or her ability to make a successful change (self-efficacy), he or she can change behaviors even if faced with barriers. If one does not believe that one has such control, one may not be motivated to act or may not persist when faced with resistance. However, the importance of changing self-efficacy as a critical step for promoting STD/HIV risk reduction has not been conclusively demonstrated.

SL and SCT are the most frequently used and most robust theoretical models for successful behavioral interventions. In practice, behavioral interventions that employ learning theories also attend to information provision and to cognitive processing. Thus, the learning theories, in reality, are additive to the earlier models rather than stand-alone explanations.

The Becoming a Responsible Teen (BART) intervention is one example from a large number of behavioral interventions based on the learning theories (17). Initially, the intervention provided its participants with information and education about STDs and HIV. In the next step, the intervention addressed motivation by attending to values, beliefs, handling peer pressure, and mobilizing positive attitudes toward change. Most of the intervention was devoted to modeling and practice of the skills that would be needed to act effectively on decisions to reduce risk taking. The skill training addressed technical competencies such as correct condom application and correct needle cleaning. Training in social competencies such as refusing sex or drug initiations, partner negotiation, sharing information with peers and family members, and condom purchases were also practiced. Finally, the intervention also attended to cognitive skills such as risk appraisal, problem solving, self-management of mood states, coping skills, and self-reinforcement for engaging in desired behavior.

Evaluation of the intervention showed that young people who had not reached their sexual debut were less likely to initiate sexual activity in the following year than were young persons who did not participate in BART. Only 11% of the abstinent BART participants became sexually active in the following year; in comparison, nearly 33% of the abstinent young persons who did not receive the BART program became sexually active. The intervention was also effective in changing the risk behavior of young persons who were already sexually active. Sexually active boys reduced the number of their sex partners, discontinued unprotected anal intercourse entirely, and sustained condom use over time. Sexually active BART girls reduced their number of sex partners, as well as the frequency of unprotected vaginal, oral, and anal intercourse. Thus, there were clear and measurable positive changes, and these changes endured for the following year.

Theories of Motivation and Emotional Arousal

Theories grounded in motivation and arousal were generally developed to explain health-risk and health-protective behaviors, at least partially to amplify the motivational aspects with the cognitive theories introduced earlier. Among the theories within this category are 1) the Fear-Drive model (44); 2) the Dual Process Model (45); and 3) Protection Motivation Theory (46,47).

The Fear-Drive and the Dual Process Models

The Fear-Drive Model states that fear generates a subjective discomfort that motivates some action to reduce the unpleasant emotional state. The Dual Process Model extended the Fear-Drive Model one step further so as to regard fear as an effective motivator when it is paired with a health threat. In addition, the Dual Process Model recognizes that fear-generated behaviors may be irrational and may fail to effectively alleviate the threat. Instead of alleviating the threat, fear leads to maladaptive strategies that reduce the unpleasant emotional state while leaving the risk-producing behavior intact. Denial is one such example of an emotional coping strategy that can be behaviorally maladaptive because it minimizes the likelihood that an individual will take any effective action to reduce risk. The Dual Process Model adds learned helplessness as its explanation for failure to react to a perceived threat. Learned helplessness refers to the generation of feelings of helplessness by intense fear, leading to reduced likelihood of constructive courses of action.

Fear-Drive and Dual-Process Models are rarely used as a basis for behavioral interventions to prevent STD/HIV. Contemporary studies suggest that differential power (based on gender or economic reasons) is a more important source of inhibition of self-protective behaviors.

Protection Motivation Theory

Protection Motivation Theory (PMT) (47) is a hybrid theory that combines cognition and emotional arousal into a single framework. This theory posits that concern in response to a health threat initiates a generalized coping appraisal that, in turn, generates coping responses that may be either adaptive or maladaptive. The particular coping responses that people ultimately choose depend on their perceptions and beliefs regarding available options and on their ability to enact those options. In this way, PMT encompasses many of the concepts that appear in the cognitive theoretical models.

PMT starts with recognition of a potential threat to which an individual can respond in either an adaptive or a maladaptive fashion. The response is mediated by a balance between "threat appraisal" and "coping appraisal." Threat appraisal is the balance between anticipated rewards associated with the behavior and the perceived severity of and personal vulnerability to the threat. The rewards can be extrinsic (related to social, peer, or parental influences) or intrinsic (associated with the person's personality traits and physical feelings of pleasure). The coping appraisal process is mediated by balancing the behavioral efficacy of an action (perceived likelihood that the action will reduce the threat) and perceived belief that the person can complete the adaptive response) with the response cost (barriers or inconvenience) of the possible protective behaviors. PMT expands theories of motivation and emotional arousal by also incorporating attention to the dynamic cognitive process in making a decision about behavior change.

PMT is not one of the theories at the forefront of intervention research, but it is applied as an explanatory theory in studies examining the factors associated with risky and protective behavior (24). As is true for the cognitive models, this model's constructs may be statistically significant in studies assessing the model's "fit" as an explanatory framework, but all of the measured variables taken together account for only modest amounts of the total variance. In the Li et al. study (24) cited above, for example, all of the constructs of PMT accounted for only 17% of the total variance in risky sexual behaviors, similar to the small amount of variance explained by the cognitive theories.

The Limits of Emotional Arousal as Stimulus for Behavior Change

The emotional arousal models share an emphasis on health messages designed to arouse fear as the starting point needed to motivate action. Obviously, the degree of arousal is critical since too much fear may generate despair instead of motivating action. Therefore, practitioners who rely on such models believe that interventions must 1) induce a level of anxiety that motivates sustained precautionary behavior; 2) assist people to maintain their psychological equilibrium in the face of this anxiety; and 3) contain the anxiety below a debilitating threshold level (48).

In practice, fear-inducing messages can be memorable (49), but their effectiveness in motivating precautionary behavior is questionable. Moreover, an unanticipated increase in denial associated with anxiety induction can have inadvertent undesirable consequences when it results in increases, rather than decreases, in health-harming behaviors. Thus, emotional arousal theories present an implicit conundrum when they are applied to STD/HIV prevention. On one hand, individuals at risk need to initiate safer behavior if they are to preserve their health. Yet, if they are recipients of fear arousal and do not use denial as their coping strategy, they may be vulnerable to high levels of anxiety. The alternative is to react with denial, thereby undermining the likelihood they will initiate any effective behavior changes (50). In the context of STDs and HIV, denial is never functional because even infrequent risky activity can confer exceedingly high risk (48,51).

Sadly, despite extensive evidence that scare tactics are inadvisable, such programs continue to be implemented. As recently as 2005, a small-print media campaign relying on fear tactics was underway in San Francisco in response to syphilis outbreaks in men having sex with men (MSM) who used crystal methamphetamine. The "Meth = Death" campaign materials, in addition to their verbal emotional appeal, also featured a male whose head is in the process of morphing into a skull, graphically illustrating the campaign's fear arousal approach. The San Francisco Department of Public Health, which sponsored the "Meth = Death" campaign, monitored requests for the "Meth = Death" print materials as well as requests for a factual informational brochure that took a harm-reduction approach to methamphetamine use titled, "A Few Things to Know About Speed." Physicians requested both types of materials, but more often requested the "Meth = Death" materials. In stark contrast, outreach workers and organizations in the gay community requested only the harm-reduction brochure, never asking for the fear induction materials associated with the "Meth = Death" campaign (52). This disconnect between this campaign and its target community may reflect a lack of understanding of the target community on the part of the health department or unfamiliarity with more effective intervention methods, but it also suggests that community input early in the campaign's development may have been able to prevent such a misguided effort.

Social Influence Theories

Intervention programs based on the social influence theories typically attempt to reach a critical mass of people at the community or population level with information, motivation, and skills to alter the social norms that either regulate or support behavior (53). Social marketing theories and diffusion of innovation theory generally provide the conceptual underpinnings of such programs.

Social Marketing

Social marketing approaches are based on commercial marketing philosophies adapted for health promotion. Such strategies reflect implicit belief that the knowledge, beliefs, attitudes, and needs of the target groups—the "consumers" of information—are the most important determinants of effective prevention. Embedded in the social context of the targeted "consumer," social marketing attempts to offer recipients personal benefits they will value, in language that is familiar, and at a "price" (not necessarily monetary) that they are willing to pay in order to achieve a meaningful goal (54). Silvestre et al. (55, p. 223) defined social marketing as "the design, implementation, and control of programs seeking to increase the acceptability of a social idea or practice in a target group." Public health programs have relied on social marketing concepts for decades and are now adapting these concepts to STD/HIV prevention.

STOP AIDS (56) was the first major AIDS prevention intervention that used social marketing. STOP AIDS began in San Francisco and capitalized on community mobilization by using members of the local gay community to provide risk-reduction information to other gay men. The developers modeled the program on home-marketing methods that were then used to sell housewares and personal care products. Epidemiological evidence suggests that STOP AIDS initiated dramatic behavior changes in homosexual men in San Francisco and later in other urban centers, but there are no program evaluation data that can extricate the STOP AIDS contribution from other factors that may have been taking place at the same time unrelated to the campaign. Later, Miller et al. (57) replicated and evaluated the STOP AIDS program in southern California and found significant post-discussion changes on all measures. However, there was no longitudinal measurement to assess the extent to which the program changed actual behavior or, if so, whether the results were enduring.

Diffusion of Innovation Theory

A theoretical model that has proven useful in explaining how new behavioral trends become established in communities is Diffusion of Innovation theory (DOI) (16). This approach has more recently come to be known as the "popular opinion leader" (POL) approach when it is applied to changing sexual behaviors that pose STD/HIV risk within communities. Opinion leaders are the people within social groups who are respected or popular; individuals whom others naturally observe and imitate. DOI suggests that new innovations are most effective when a critical mass of opinion leaders, usually 15% of the total population, adopt and endorse the innovation.

POL uses ethnographic methods to systematically identify the popular and socially influential individuals within the target population. These individuals are then recruited and trained in how to communicate risk-reduction messages to their peers during everyday conversations. The core elements of the POL model that must be incorporated into an intervention include (58):

1. Intervention directed to an identifiable target population in well-defined community venues where the population size can be estimated and where social interactions take place;
2. Ethnographic techniques to identify segments within the target population and the popular persons within each segment who are well-liked and trusted by others;
3. Enlisting 15% of the POLs into the intervention;
4. Teaching the POLs skills for initiating risk-reduction conversations with friends and acquaintances during everyday conversations and to use themselves as an example;
5. Training POLs to use the characteristics of effective behavior change messages that address risk-related attitudes, norms, intentions, and self-efficacy. In their conversations, the POLs endorse the benefits of safer behavior and use themselves as examples of for practical steps that can be used to implement changes;
6. Intervention that takes place weekly in sessions that use instruction, facilitator modeling, and extensive role play practice to help the POLs refine their skills and gain confidence about delivering the messages to others. Intervention groups are small enough to allow for extensive practice for all of the POLs;
7. POLs who set specific goals for the number of risk-reduction conversations they will initiate with friends and acquaintances between the weekly sessions;
8. Review of the POLs experiences delivering the messages followed by discussion and reinforcement in subsequent sessions. Successful conversations provide modeling to other participants; difficult conversations are addressed with problem-solving strategies to apply in a future interaction; and
9. Logos, symbols, or other stimulus cues that are made available as conversation starters between the POLs and others in their social or sexual networks.

Applied to sexual behavior, this model was first evaluated in an experimentally tested community-level intervention in clubs frequented by gay men in three small cities (59,60). Bartenders in the clubs identified socially influential men from each of the customer subgroups who patronized the bar. These men were then recruited to participate in four weekly group training sessions. Three months after the intervention and at two 6-month intervals thereafter, the surveys were repeated to detect whether the intervention produced changes in the risk behavior of gay men in each city. These population-wide surveys revealed consistent and substantial reductions in the proportion of gay men who engaged in risky behavior following the intervention in each city, ranging from 19% to 30% reductions in risk behavior from baseline levels in the proportion of men who engaged in unprotected anal intercourse. Because these changes followed the stepwise introduction of the intervention in each city, it was clear that the POL intervention was responsible for these reductions. Three years later, the surveys were again repeated and clearly documented that these changes were enduring; even lower levels of risk behavior were present in all three cities three years after the intervention (61).

Transtheoretical Model (Stages of Change)

The Transtheoretical Model (TTM) has two distinct characteristics (62). First, it defines five distinctive stages through which people cycle in making behavior changes. As a result, it is often called the "Stages of Change" theory. Second, it explicitly identifies intervention methods linked with each stage. According to the model, if a given treatment is mismatched to the person's stage of readiness for change, it is likely to be ineffective. Thus, the hallmark of interventions based on TTM is assessing the person's readiness, or stage of change, and then tailoring the intervention accordingly (63). Briefly, the five stages are:

1. *Precontemplation*, the stage at which there is no intention to change behavior in the foreseeable future. Friends and family may be aware of the problem and may even apply pressure to change. Resistance to recognizing a problem is the defining characteristic of precontemplation. People in the precontemplation stage can be responsive to consciousness-raising techniques such as observations, confrontations, and interpretations.
2. *Contemplation* is the stage at which people become aware that a problem exists but are not committed to taking action. They may weigh the pros and cons of continuing or changing the behavior, counterbalancing their past positive experiences with the behavior against the time, energy, and loss they believe they will experience if they change the problematic behavior. Individuals who say they are considering changing a behavior within the next six months would be classified in the contemplation stage. In this stage, dramatic relief techniques that raise positive emotions about the benefits of change and clarify negative emotions that could be lowered by change can be effective. If the problem behavior is central to their self-identify, this reevaluation may require altering their definitions of themselves. During this process, the person may also reevaluate how his or her behavior is affecting others. Such a reevaluation might involve, for example, a man redefining himself as being a responsible person who is going to protect others by engaging in safer sex.
3. *Preparation* is the time when people begin making small steps toward action. People in this stage make some tentative reductions in their behavior and indicate that they clearly plan to change, but have not yet committed themselves

to take actions even though they "intend" to do so within the very near future. Change methods that are well matched to this stage include initiating counter conditioning and stimulus control to begin altering their behavior or to avoid situations in which risky behavior has commonly occurred in the past. In this stage, they move into a greater commitment to avoid the risks that characterized their past behavior.

4. *Action* is the stage in which people initiate overt changes in their behavior and environment. This is the point at which efforts to change become visible to others. People are classified in this stage if they have successfully modified the problem behavior for a period of time ranging from one day to six months. Successful action entails having and using the requisite skills to make changes, accompanied by effective use of counter conditioning and stimulus control in order to modify the stimuli that frequently trigger a relapse. During this stage, social support and helping relationships can buoy behavior change efforts. An example of a stimulus control step might be a decision to always carry condoms as a reminder to practice safer sex and to ensure they are "on hand" if needed.

5. *Maintenance* is the stage when people consolidate the gains from the action stage and concentrate on preventing relapses into unsafe behavior. This stage represents a continuation, not an absence, of change. The hallmarks of this stage are stabilization of the behavior change and avoiding relapses. This stage is present from six months after successful change and it lasts indefinitely. For some behaviors, maintenance may need to last a lifetime. Successful maintenance builds on all the change strategies that helped the person get to this point. In addition, very specific preparation and planning to anticipate situations that will arise when relapse is more likely and to identify or develop specific alternate ways of dealing with those situations become important interventions in preserving maintenance.

Information, Motivation, Behavior (IMB) Model

The IMB model (64) is a parsimonious and practical model that has become widely applied. In brief, the model states that AIDS risk-reduction interventions need to provide people with information about AIDS transmission and prevention, incorporate strategies that increase motivation to reduce AIDS risk, and train people in behavioral skills that will be needed to enact the specific behaviors required for successful risk reduction. The model has been applied to both primary prevention campaigns (for those who are uninfected to prevent disease acquisition) and to secondary prevention interventions (for those who are already infected to prevent both transmission and acquisition or reacquisition).

The IMB model was proposed following a thorough review of the AIDS risk-reduction literature that identified intervention characteristics favoring risk-reduction behavioral changes (64). The reviewers consistently found that interventions with evidence of effectiveness were all characterized as providing AIDS risk-reduction information, motivation, and behavioral skills. Information regarding the means of transmission and information about specific methods of preventing infection are regarded as necessary prerequisites of risk-reducing behavior. Motivation to change risky behavior affects whether one acts on the overt knowledge regarding transmission and prevention. Finally, having the necessary behavioral skills to perform the specific preventive behaviors is a critical determinant of whether even a knowledgeable, highly motivated person will be able to change his or her behavior. This model, in many respects, integrates educational, cognitive, and behavioral theories into a coherent whole.

The IMB theory explicitly describes the process of intervention development beginning with elicitation research to identify the population's existing level of knowledge, factors that determine their motivation for change, and their existing prevention behavioral skills. Then, on this basis of this population-specific information, the next steps are to create appropriate and evidence-based interventions that address the elicitation findings to produce changes in knowledge, motivation, and behavioral skills leading to preventive behavior. Finally, this model stresses the need to implement methodologically sound evaluation research to determine whether the intervention has produced short-term changes in these multiple indicators (knowledge, motivation, and behavioral skills) and then to assess to what extent those changes resulted in long-term risk-reduction behavior changes.

Summary

During the review for this chapter, several themes emerged from the intervention literature. First, although the need for theoretically driven interventions has been stressed for many years (65,66), most interventions have been based on an informal blend of logic and practical experience. Even 25 years into the AIDS epidemic, published interventions based on formal theoretical conceptualizations of any kind are exceedingly few. Second, although investigators have stressed the importance of tailoring interventions to specifically meet the needs of target groups for decades (67), descriptions of formal elicitation research to identify group-appropriate intervention tactics are rare. When elicitation research is present, the intervention's effectiveness appears to increase. Regrettably, the number of such interventions that were preceded by an elicitation phase is exceedingly small (68–70). Third, although many authors allude to the need for interventions that focus on the informational, motivational, and behavioral skills needed for change (65,64,67,70,71), such a broad focus is uncommon in the intervention literature. When interventions do stress all three components, their effect is enhanced (57,72–75). Finally, many authors stress the need for systematic evaluation research to monitor the effectiveness of interventions (64,65,70,71,75), but even of these interventions that have been evaluated, there are often limitations with respect to their experimental design and control groups, reliance only on self-report measures, high subject self-selection bias, unacceptably high attrition, multiple confounded interventions, and failure to assess the intervention's effect on mediating factors that presumably affect intervention uptake. These methodological limitations make the attribution of changes to an intervention or to specific components within interventions virtually impossible in many cases. It also appeared that the more broad-based the intervention (vs. narrowly focused interventions) the more serious the methodological problems became.

The most defensible uses of the existing theories at present are in the organization that they provide for measurement and for identifying determinants that need to be addressed by an intervention. Relatively few of these theoretical models provide any concrete guidance regarding the strategies that will produce the desired changes. Questions are also raised as to whether the specific theory is critical or whether the benefit is in having any overarching model that guides development of the measurement plan and intervention strategies. When St. Lawrence and her colleagues (76) specifically tested interventions based on three different theoretical models against one another and compared them with a control comparison condition, all three theoretically grounded interventions produced comparable changes in behavior, perhaps because although the rationales differed, the intervention procedures associated with each of these models were very similar. These interventions, conducted with low-income inner city women, also found that change was greater for women when they were entering new relationships than for women who remained in an ongoing relationship, suggesting that the existing intervention models may not be entirely adequate for women whose primary risk derives from a partner's behavior and not from their own behaviors.

Levels for Intervention Delivery

Just as there are different theoretical models that can inform the development of an intervention, behavioral interventions also differ markedly in their population coverage and in the intensity (in terms of cost, staff, or training) that is required for their delivery. Interventions may be implemented at a variety of "levels": societal, population, community, schools, small groups, dyads, or individuals. Figure 1 illustrates differences between some of the intervention approaches discussed in this chapter and their comparative intensity and coverage. Several chapters in this volume review the potential levels for intervention delivery in depth and they will be addressed only briefly in this chapter.

Structural, Legal, and Policy-Level Interventions

Societal interventions are those that affect an entire population, typically through either a policy or legal mandate. Governments frequently enact laws and impose regulations to promote the public's health by discouraging unhealthy behaviors and promoting healthy behaviors. In addition to direct appeals through public education and law, government also can influence individual choices by taxation and spending priorities, as well as by penalizing

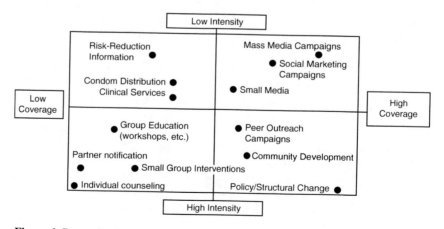

Figure 1 Prevention interventions: population coverage and delivery intensity.

harmful activities by imposing civil and criminal penalties. Despite the magnitude, costs, and scope of governmental efforts to promote health, few such initiatives have been subjected to rigorous evaluation. Nor is the process of creating such policy-level changes efficient or clearly delineated. The foremost examples are in the decline in deaths owing to heart disease over the past 40 years, significant reductions in the rate of cigarette smoking, and dramatic decreases in the rate of motor vehicle crash deaths per million miles driven (77). Each of these changes resulted from government mandates, legal imperatives, and selective application of taxation.

The process by which behavioral scientists can help translate scientific findings into public health policy formation is not well understood. Typically, so many variables affect behavior that it is extraordinarily difficult to demonstrate a causal relationship between the policy and the health effect (78,79).

In some instances, changes in laws have unintended, but beneficial, health effects. Chesson and colleagues (80) examined the relationship between changes in alcohol consumption and STD incidence rates in the 50 United States and the District of Columbia. From 1983 to 1998, they found that reductions in alcohol consumption (usually as a consequence of increases in alcohol taxes) were significantly associated with decreases in gonorrhea and syphilis rates. Each 1% decrease in per capita alcohol consumption was paralleled by decreases of 0.4% to 0.7% in reported gonorrhea incidence and 1.8% to 3.6% in reported syphilis incidence. The findings suggest that increases in alcohol tax could potentially reduce alcohol consumption, thereby reducing the burden of STDs.

Media Interventions

Population-level interventions are often characterized by using media interventions as the preferred delivery medium. The best of these media interventions are informed by social marketing principles, with the goal of delivering the right message to the largest number of people. The limitations of that approach have already been discussed in the earlier section on psycho-educational theory (see "Psycho-educational Theories Stressing Information Provision").

Effective health communication campaigns are characterized by use of a variety of mass communication channels, making sure that the audience is exposed to the message, and providing a clear and specific action for the people to take. Effective campaigns are usually based in formative research such as focus groups to develop the messages and inform the campaign's strategy. Many of the better-designed interventions include other social marketing strategies such as market segmentation, channel analysis, and message pretesting (81). They also link media strategies with community programs, thus reinforcing the media message and providing local support for the desired behavior changes (82).

One media campaign based on social marketing principles evaluated the effect of a brief community-level condom social marketing campaign in a high syphilis prevalence region of the United States (83). The campaign's development was preceded by qualitative research phase and community engagement activities to identify what the messages should be and then to pretest media materials. Radio and small-print media, retail distribution of condoms, and community outreach workers all promoted a novel condom brand during a 12-week social marketing campaign. Post-intervention evaluation showed that almost 80% of residents interviewed in the targeted community reported exposure to the intervention, but almost no one in the comparison area did so. In the community where the campaign was implemented, condom use with main and casual partners increased, while no changes were reported in the comparison community. Of considerable importance, residents in the intervention community reported a 20% decrease in the number of sex partners, changes that did not occur in the comparison community. The results suggest that community-based and theoretically driven social marketing campaigns can, in even a brief intervention, produce measurable outcomes in areas of high STD prevalence in the United States.

Community-Level Interventions

Community-level interventions may be "community level" or "community-based," and these terms are not interchangeable. Community-level approaches target an entire community or a population segment within the community. Community-level interventions are at the heart of many public health approaches (84). Interventions that are conducted in partnership with communities, rather than being applied from outside the communities, are more likely to enlist the community in addressing health issues and to yield behavior changes. This latter approach is considered to be community-based. Public health approaches more often rely on involving selected individuals from communities in program planning (85), an approach that falls short of the true partnerships needed to fully engage communities with an active voice in problem definition, data collection, intervention delivery, and the subsequent application of the results to address the community's concerns. In addition, community-level participation and buy-in are likely to produce more sustainable interventions by leaving an infrastructure in place after the research ends. Earlier in this chapter, several community-level interventions were described in sections 2.5 and 2.6.

School-Based Interventions

School-based prevention programs have been viewed as a desirable way to prevent young people from adopting risky behaviors, even as early as elementary school (3,86). Many studies of young people of different ages and from different locales indicate that most youth initiate sexual activity while they are of school age, whether or not they are in school (87) and numerous reviews and studies confirm that effective interventions that are delivered prior to sexual debut can prevent later STDs (3,69,88,). Finally, schools are an accepted venue for many interventions, given that their purpose is to equip young people with education for life. They have a defined location; they are sustained within the community; their hours and operations are well known; they already have established mechanisms for introducing new programs and accessing students; and their target population's size is known. In addition, schools are linked into the larger community through families and other community organizations, potentially enhancing local ownership of intervention programs.

Social and Sexual Network Interventions

Social network analysis identified the ties between people and how the structure of these ties affects the spread of disease within and between social groups. While research on sexual networks can be complex, this approach is providing unique insights into the spread of STDs that traditional epidemiological and behavioral approaches may not capture. To date, most of the research has focused on understanding the structure of and relationships between networks, illustrating how different network types affect the distribution of STDs, and generating information on which network-based interventions could be developed (89). Relatively few intervention studies to date have been reported that target networks, but this is a promising approach for the future. Amirhanian et al. (90) provided a practical blueprint explaining how to 1) access high-risk networks in a community; 2) identify and enumerate the membership of these networks; 3) identify the key persons within each network; and 4) establish the levels of risky behavior within the networks. To date, most network interventions have targeted the networks of drug injectors who share needles (91,92). Cottler et al. (93) showed that interventions delivered by peers within social networks of out-of-treatment drug abusers reduced their injection-related risk behavior. Trotter et al. (92) demonstrated that when HIV risk-reduction counseling for intravenous drug users (IDUs) is provided to all members of social networks, risk-reduction outcomes are greater. Training peer leaders within drug using networks to be HIV behavior change agents has also produced injection risk reduction within injectors' risk networks (91,94). Broadhead et al. (95) estimated that the cost of reaching drug users through a social network approach is only one-thirtieth the cost of reaching drug users through traditional community outreach programs. One example of a network intervention applied to changing sexual behavior was reported by Kincaid (96). Kincaid compared the effectiveness of different strategies to promote the adoption of contraceptives by married women in Bangladesh. He found that peer-delivered social network-based intervention produced significantly greater adoption of contraceptives than did discussions led by fieldworkers from family planning settings. Taken together, these findings offer promising support for the potential usefulness of network-delivered interventions.

Small-Group Interventions

Small-group interventions involve the delivery of an intervention to cohorts of 6 to 18 participants and have been the most common intervention format in the United States. Large numbers of studies attest to the effectiveness of sound behavioral interventions when provided to small groups (68,72,97–99). The largest of these small-group intervention studies was the National Multisite HIV Prevention Trial, sponsored by the National Institute of Mental Health. In this randomized controlled HIV prevention behavioral intervention trial, 3706 high-risk adults from 37 clinics across the United States were randomly assigned to attend either a seven-session intervention of 14 hours or a single-session educational program (100). During a 12-month follow-up period, the participants from the more intensive skills training intervention reported significantly fewer unprotected sex acts and higher levels of condom use.

Kalichman et al. (68) used the small-group format to deliver an intervention for persons living with HIV/AIDS. The results of this randomized controlled trial showed that a behavioral intervention grounded in social cognitive theory reduced unprotected sexual behavior of both men and women living with HIV infection, with the greatest reductions in HIV transmission risk behavior taking place with non-HIV seropositive sex partners. The intervention was developed and the content identified in consultation with a community advisory group using elicitation research. Their effective five-session group intervention focused on enhancing motivation through self-reflection and developing coping efficacy skills for HIV disclosure decision-making, active listening, assertiveness skills, and problem solving for disclosure and transmission risk-reduction behaviors. The intervention components were tailored for gender and sexual orientation. Integrated skills practice sessions used coached role-plays developed from elicitation and films. The intervention was proven to be effective within a community service delivery setting and could be adapted for use by HIV-related service organizations, delivered within support groups or in health department settings.

Interventions for Dyads

STD transmission takes place during a dyadic interaction; therefore dyad interventions would seem to be a logical level for intervention delivery. Evidence that women who participate in interventions are less likely to initiate condom use within an ongoing relationship than when they enter into a new relationship (76) also suggests that dyads, rather than individuals or unconnected individual people within small groups, would be a fruitful intervention focus. Although we were unable to locate any dyadic interventions in the existing literature, this is another potential approach that warrants further attention.

Individual Counseling Interventions

Individual-level interventions are provided one-by-one to persons at risk or who have contracted an STD. Individual-level interventions are common in the literature, along with small-group interventions. One notable example is a large intervention study (101) that was conducted with 5700 heterosexual patients from five inner-city STD clinics. Patients were randomly assigned to one of three individual-level interventions coupled with HIV testing: 1) standard clinic practice; 2) STD/HIV prevention counseling with two 20-minute sessions intended to increase risk perception and negotiating a behavior change step; and 3) enhanced counseling consisting of four theory-based interactive sessions. The first 20-minute session took place during the initial clinic visit and was identical in all three interventions. The next three sessions in the third experimental condition were approximately one hour in length. All interventions focused on promoting consistent condom use with all sex partners as their outcome goal. After three months, self-reported frequencies of consistent condom use were significantly higher for the second and third arms than for those who received standard practice messages. After six months, more participants in the standard practice group developed new STDs (10.4%) than in the enhanced (7.2%) or intensive counseling (7.4%) conditions. This trend was similar both for men and women in all five participating sites.

In another individual-level intervention study, Belcher et al. (102) employed motivational enhancement interviewing techniques combined with skills training for high-risk women who used drugs and traded sex for drugs. In the study, women were randomized to receive either a one-on-one single session of two hours with motivational enhancement and skills training or to an AIDS education-only comparison condition of the same duration. Results demonstrated the potential promise of even brief, well designed, individual-level behavior interventions when they focus on building motivation and skills. Women in the experimental condition increased their self-reported frequency of condom use by 44%, while women in the education-only condition increased to a much lesser degree, changes that were sustained through a three-month follow-up assessment.

Multilevel Interventions

Achieving our health promotion goals will require more than a single intervention that teaches people skills and providing them with information. It will require efforts to change organizational behavior, social norms, as well as the physical and social environments within communities. Ideally, it also requires policy changes that support health. Thus, the optimal health promotion effort would address health issues across a spectrum by using a range of different strategies and operating at multiple, rather than single, levels. Given the substantial heterogeneity of determinants of STD/HIV-relevant health outcomes, it is not realistic to expect that a single intervention addressing only one determinant delivered only once will ever be sufficient to eliminate STDs or even to produce substantial sustained reductions. A multilevel approach intervening at multiple levels of influence, including the individual, interpersonal, institutional, familial, community, and policy levels over a sustained duration is rare, but is more realistic if long-term changes are to be produced and sustained. Fortunately, there is a small number of intervention reports that attest to the benefits of taking a multilevel approach for intervention delivery (77,103–107). This multilevel approach recognizes that sustained positive health outcomes will be the result of interplay between individual, familial, school, and larger social contexts that influence health risks. However, interventions targeting STD/HIV health behavior change have a tradition of focusing first on individual- or group-level factors such as increasing knowledge, motivating positive attitudes, or transmitting skills relevant to implementing behavior changes, and such interventions have only rarely taken a multilevel approach.

The obvious advantage of a multilevel intervention is that by linking interventions at multiple levels, consistent intervention messages, support, and maintenance can culminate in a positive synergy over time. Relatively few multilevel interventions are to be found in the literature, but those that are cited in the previous paragraph all suggest that health behavior changes are supported and reinforced well after such multilevel interventions have concluded. Some of the most extensive multilevel efforts have been in tobacco prevention, but in any area of health behavior, coordinated, multilevel interventions may offer the greatest promise to accomplish public health goals.

The Seattle Social Development Project (SSDP) (104–106), for example, provides an excellent example of how a well-designed multilevel program that was provided to elementary school children, their teachers, and their parents can yield measurable benefits even two decades later. This multilevel intervention involved 1) training teachers in proactive classroom management, interactive teaching, and cooperative learning; 2) training parents in child management and skills to support their child's educational development; and 3) providing the children with cognitive and social skills training. Although the SSDP did not address specific health risks, its effects on behavior and health were far-reaching. A decade later, participants in the SSDP showed evidence of delaying the onset of sexual activity, decreasing unprotected sexual intercourse after sexual debut, and had fewer STDS and unplanned pregnancies (106). Even 20 years later, the intervention still demonstrated beneficial effects, still lowering the sexual risk behaviors of SSDP participants, underscoring the value of early intervention as well multilevel approaches (105).

Another example of a multilevel program that intervened with schools, parents, and young people was the Safer Choices project (108). This project included a school-based curriculum, staff development, peer resources within the schools, parent and parent-surrogate educational programs, and active school-community linkages. Evaluation of the program demonstrated its effectiveness in reducing recent unprotected intercourse.

What Behaviors Should Be Changed?

Considerable discussion has addressed the selection of appropriate outcome goals for behavioral interventions. For the most part, these debates cluster into two types: 1) deeply held and heartfelt opinions as to whether behavioral interventions should strive to obtain complete cessation of risk behavior versus a harm-reduction approach that promotes risk reduction; and 2) academic debates over measurement, research designs, and theoretical frameworks.

Abstinence Versus "Safer Sex" Interventions?

Contentious debate characterizes a deep division between those who argue that abstinence until marriage should be the only acceptable goal of interventions and those who argue that a range of options need to be available, especially given the STD and sexual behavior statistics for the United States. Where the debate begins, however, is with regard to the best strategies for prevention.

Comprehensive sexuality intervention programs typically provide information, encourage abstinence, promote condom use for those who are sexually active, encourage fewer sex partners, and transmit sexual communication skills. The evidence is clear that comprehensive sexuality interventions do not accelerate sexual debut (109) and do reduce unwanted pregnancy rates (110). These multi-spectrum programs decrease the likelihood of unprotected sexual intercourse at the time of sexual debut (3,4,111) and reduce the sexual risk behavior that contribute to STDs and HIV (69,106,112,113). Such programs not only decrease high-risk sexual behaviors, but they also increase the number of adolescents who abstain from sex (69,113). Sexually active youth who participate in these programs increase condom acquisition and use (114–117) and are more likely to use condoms when they have sex for the first time (118,119). Taken together, there is a considerable body of evidence that comprehensive sexual risk-reduction interventions that address *both* abstinence and condom use produce reductions in risky sexual behavior and delays in the onset of intercourse (4,69,113,120,121). It is also reassuring that the majority of parents support comprehensive programs for their children (122).

There are few published scientific studies evaluating the efficacy of abstinence-only and abstinence-until-marriage programs (123,124) and these studies tend to be quite limited since most lack random assignment to programs and enroll a very homogeneous sample, making behavior change difficult to measure and the results impossible to generalize with reliability. Overall, the evidence is not encouraging. Several published studies evaluating abstinence-only programs have failed to document any reduction in sexual behavior (125–127). Virginity pledges, abstinence-only programs, and abstinence-until-marriage programs have been shown to have the unintended consequence of increasing the likelihood that adolescents have unprotected intercourse at the time of their first intercourse (128–130) and virginity pledgers who contract an STD are less likely to realize they are infected (130). No long-term randomized controlled studies have shown these programs to be effective, especially for sexually experienced adolescents (126,128,131, 132), although several evaluations of abstinence-only programs are currently underway. Thus, such programs may not be the most defensible strategy for reducing STDs in youth and young adults. Abstinence-until-marriage programs have also been criticized for their insensitivity to gay, lesbian, and transgendered youth and young adults who are precluded by law from marrying in most jurisdictions; therefore, they cannot achieve abstinence until marriage.

Cessation Versus Harm Reduction: The Needle Exchange Controversy

Injection drug use is associated with one third of the AIDS cases and one half of all hepatitis C cases in the United States (133). As a result, interventions have been conducted to change drug use behaviors as well as sexual behaviors. Numerous studies have shown unequivocally that needle exchange programs (NEPs) and pharmacy sales of sterile syringes are effective in reducing transmission of both diseases. The evidence supporting positive outcomes from NEPs is overwhelming. There are more than a million injection drug users in the United States (134) who are estimated to inject approximately 1000 times a year (135). Only a fraction of drug users who seek substance-abuse treatment are able to be served by existing treatment programs (136). Studies have clearly documented that injection-related risk behavior is associated with restricted syringe access (95,137,138). Other studies clearly document that needle exchange programs are associated with reductions in needle reuse, syringe sharing, and other indirect sharing of paraphernalia (139–142), and that regular use of needle exchange programs is associated with less drug-related HIV risk behavior and lower rates of seroconversion (143), reduced incident hepatitis C infection (144), and that the incidence of HIV in IDUs who use NEPs is less than one third of the HIV incidence in IDUs who do not use NEPs (145). Further, IDUs who use needle exchange programs exhibit reductions in the mean average number of injections per syringe as well as reductions in the number of injections per day (141), and participation in NEPs is associated with improved access to health care and drug treatment (146). Such programs are clearly cost effective (147–150) and neither result in increased use of illicit drugs nor encourage first-time drug use (140). The available evidence also confirms that if sterile syringes are available, injection drug users will obtain them (151,152), and access to sterile injection equipment through pharmacies has been associated with reduced rates of both needle sharing and HIV transmission (153).

The Measurement Debate

Self-reported behaviors have often been the primary outcome measure from behavioral prevention studies. One reservation about self-report is whether study participants provide truthful or accurate information in response to sensitive questions about sexual or drug use behaviors. Some argue that one can have confidence only in self-reported data when there are biological outcome measures that corroborate self-reported behavior change (2). Although most intervention researchers would agree that disease incidence offers strong confirmatory support, this can be difficult when there is a low incidence in such diseases as HIV in the population under study. STDs have been recommended as surrogate markers for HIV, despite the lack of a true empirical relationship between specific STDs and HIV. However, the relationship between the incidence and prevalence of a given STD and HIV incidence is equally as complex as the relationship between self-reported behaviors and HIV incidence (154).

Because of self-reported data, two psychometric aspects of such data have been of concern: their reliability and their validity. Reliability confirms that the instrument is free of random error, and validity demonstrates whether the instrument measures what we think it is measuring. People may bias self-reported information either because the person does not accurately remember his or her behavior during the period under question or because the person does not accurately report behavior that is recalled. A large volume of literature has addressed these questions and found that, in general, people provide truthful information if they are 1) assured that their information will be anonymous; 2) provided with motivating instruction that stresses the importance of their information; 3) not required to report the information face-to-face; and 4) able to confirm that their answers are truthful (154).

Given truthful responding, the accuracy of the information that is provided will be dependent on the length of the recall period, the question format, and individual differences (i.e., recall may be less accurate for those who engage in the behavior with high frequency). Most of the research suggests that moderate recall intervals are preferable to those that are short or lengthy (155,156). Recall can also be affected by the respondents' education or age, the data collection methods being used, and demand characteristics of the situation. However, the research suggests that only a small percentage of persons provide inaccurate responses when the conditions listed in the preceding paragraph is present (154).

A panel constituted by the National Institute of Mental Health (NIMH) examined the issue of self-report and biological data as outcome variables and prepared a National Institutes of Health Policy Statement based on its conclusions (154). This report noted that there are many reasons why biologic data may not be congruent with self-reported information. The report concluded that the failure to find a linear relationship between self-report and incident STDs cannot be taken as an indication of dishonesty or inaccuracy. In fact, that panel concluded that when appropriate assessment conditions are established, well-designed questions result in reliable and valid self-reported information about sensitive behaviors.

Are Behavioral Interventions Cost Effective?

The relatively modest resources for public health efforts need to be carefully allocated if they are to have the greatest benefit for public health. Often, this necessitates weighing alternative intervention and measurement strategies and prioritizing those that are expected to yield the greatest benefit at the lowest cost. Cost-effectiveness analyses (CEAs) are needed to help public health officials and community leaders establish priorities and assess the utility of different interventions. CEA is an umbrella term covering a variety of analyses that compare alternative interventions, often using measures such as the potential years of life gained, infections averted, or quality-adjusted life years to assess the tradeoffs between interventions. CEA therefore yields a ratio that expresses the value of an intervention relative to its cost. The cost effectiveness of behavioral interventions has been the subject of several recent empirical investigations, primarily after the public and private costs of managing HIV and AIDS became evident to policy-makers and raised questions about the cost-effectiveness of other approaches (97). The CEAs that have appeared in the literature indicate that a preventive public health approach to the AIDS epidemic based on social and behavioral science would be cost-effective, saving thousands of dollars for each HIV infection averted. In an analysis of one of the POL intervention studies conducted by Kelly et al. (157) on urban women in the United States, for example, Holtgrave and Kelly (158) concluded that the cost-utility ratio of the POL intervention was at a level generally regarded to be very cost effective. Taken together, the available literature indicated that behavioral interventions are both cost saving and cost effective (159–162).

Moving Interventions from Research to Service Delivery

Dissemination of new diagnostic tests and treatments in health care average 15 to 17 years (163). Consider the record of uptake into clinical practice of newer, more specific and sensitive laboratory tests for chlamydia and gonorrhea. More than a decade after they were shown to offer improved sensitivity and specificity, less than 3% of practicing clinicians reported that they were using the newer and more sensitive tests (164).

If dissemination of new diagnostic tests and clinical treatments seems unreasonably long, dissemination of behavioral interventions is even more uncertain in the absence of the intensive marketing that characterizes the pharmaceutical and diagnostics industries. The best developed dissemination efforts for behavioral interventions were organized by the Centers for Disease Control and Prevention (CDC). Although limited in both their scope and their duration, these were model efforts attempting to get sound interventions into the hands of community organizations and agencies that provide programs on a local level. In the first instance, the Division of Adolescent and School Health (DASH) at the CDC sponsored programs for youth with evidence of effectiveness and no evidence of untoward consequences. Potential candidates for DASH's dissemination effort were identified by program staff from the literature. Independent panels, one of scientists and another of program end users, then reviewed and rated the interventions, using rigorous criteria. A small number of programs was subsequently selected for their "Programs that Work" designation. Program materials were prepared by education contractors, and then trainers from state Departments of Education were funded to attend a centralized "train the trainer" program. The trainers' attendance at the initial training was supported by CDC in exchange for their commitment to train others within their states to deliver the programs after they returned home. In this way, DASH made a concerted effort to move sound research programs into broad use in a timely manner. The "Programs that Work" effort was a commendatory and model effort, but the effort was abruptly discontinued in response to intensive conservative political pressures. The second model effort was initiated by the Division of HIV Prevention (DHAP), also within CDC, when DHAP initiated a program called "Interventions in a Box" to disseminate effective interventions for adults. The selected interventions were packaged in a "box" that contained training videos, an intervention manual, and intervention handouts. As of 2005, 13 programs had been packaged, and almost 3000 people had participated in the sponsored training programs using these materials. Finally, the NIMH is currently supporting a large international trial of the popular opinion leader intervention in five countries. This well-funded and carefully controlled experimental trial is likely to yield exciting information, but it leaves the issue of how to accomplish widespread dissemination of effective programs largely unresolved.

Ethical Considerations About Behavioral Interventions

Unanticipated and detrimental behavioral outcomes have accidentally resulted from some biomedical interventions. For example, one problematic consequence of successful antiretroviral treatment and the subsequent advertising campaigns that reframed AIDS as a "chronic manageable disease" is that some people resumed risky behavior as their HIV viral load decreased, believing either that they were no longer infectious or that HIV's severity had been lessened. Ven and colleagues (165) reported that 40% of gay men whose viral load became undetectable as a result of treatment with antiretroviral drugs resumed engaging in unprotected anal intercourse. Such resumptions of risky behavior following improved health, restoration of higher energy levels, and beliefs that they could no longer transmit HIV to sex partners have been widely reported and are unquestionably problematic. In behavioral interventions, questions about the possibility of adverse outcomes are usually based on 1) uncertainty whether the usual participant incentive payments may be coercive or create opportunities for continued risk behavior and 2) whether the intervention itself produces untoward effects by increasing risky behaviors, as it appears was the case for pharmacological treatments such as Viagra and antiretroviral medications.

Effect of Incentive Payments on Risk Behaviors

Research studies going back a quarter of a century consistently confirm that ethical concerns about incentives for participants are unwarranted (166). Clearly, the size of incentive payments has a positive effect on participants' retention in longitudinal research; however, there is no evidence that incentive payments increase risky behavior. For example, when cash or voucher incentives of varying amounts were paid to active drug abusers, neither the mode nor the magnitude of payment had any significant effect on rates of drug use or on participants' perceptions of coercion (167). Consistent with other studies on contingency management (168), higher incentive payments produce higher retention in research studies, a serious concern in maintaining the validity and generalizability of the research results (167,169), but incentive payments have not been shown to introduce any deleterious consequences.

Are There Adverse Behavioral Outcomes from Behavioral Interventions?

Concerns are often voiced as to whether behavioral interventions give rise to undesirable outcomes. For example, critics express their concern that safer sex interventions or condom distribution may promote an increase of sexual behaviors or earlier sexual debut. Despite an extensive literature review covering a quarter of a century of intervention science, we were unable to locate any evidence of such untoward outcomes.

Summary and Future Directions

You cannot defend the truth with lies.

A.S. Byatt, Whistling Women

The main purpose of this chapter is to offer perspectives about the essentials of public health interventions that are necessary to prevent STD in those who are uninfected, and about the limits of adverse sequelae of infections that do occur. Our goal was to provide for nonspecialists an interdisciplinary blueprint about the architecture of behavioral interventions. We believe there are four general principles that may be distilled from the details that were presented.

First, we encourage readers to carefully consider the goals of public health behavioral intervention efforts to reduce STI morbidity. An effective public health intervention may achieve at best modest health improvements, often with an investment of substantial effort and resources. Such interventions may yield only minor behavior change but still may be associated with substantial public health benefit. Consider, for example, the likely benefit of a net reduction of the caloric equivalent of one bag of potato chips each month on rates of adult obesity. The efforts to achieve such a goal would likely require coordinated efforts of manufacturers to produce a less-fattening chip, and from communities, retailers, advertisers, and public health teams to encourage reduced consumption. Many individuals would not adhere to such a change, and some might paradoxically increase potato chip consumption. It is unlikely that efforts to completely eliminate chips would be successful. Yet, important public health gains still could result. However, interventions to change sexual risk behavior appear to be held to higher standards. This may be because many public health approaches to STI (sexually transmitted infection) control traditionally involve reinforcement of strong social controls on sexuality. This artificial standard for STI interventions leads to substantial policy mischief when, for example, sexual abstinence as an individual behavior is confused with sexual abstinence as a public health intervention. For individuals, abstinence is 100% effective for STI prevention because an individual person cannot simultaneously be abstinent and nonabstinent. At a population level, however, some individuals will fail to be abstinent. Failure to consider abstinence from a public health perspective leads to policies grounded in false assumptions about efficacy. This belief has led to an increasingly widespread practice of withholding information about effective approaches to prevention (170,171). Such systematic withholding of information raises a number of moral and ethical concerns.

Second, readers should consider the place of behavioral interventions within the larger contexts of a society. Our society, like all societies, is a dynamic entity. Larger societal developments such as economic expansion or contraction, shifts in the demography of poverty, or changes in attitudes about family formation will all have effects on the design, implementation, and success of a given intervention. Readers should also remember that the population of people "at risk" for STIs is neither homogenous nor static. This means that various components of a population become sexually active as they age from adolescence into adulthood. Not only are the prevention needs of younger people different from those of older folks, but prevention needs change as cohorts age. Thus, with age, a cohort's sexual health needs (including the need for disease prevention) also change. One of the challenges yet to be met by intervention science is creation of interventions that match the diversity and developmental dynamism of a diverse population.

Third, readers are encouraged to consider interventions within the context of future biomedical innovations. Phrases such as "until we have a vaccine or a cure, we must rely on behavioral interventions to reduce rates of sexually transmitted infections" reverberate through public and professional discourse about STIs. These phrases are quaintly optimistic in their faith in technological solutions to public health problems. Yet, these phrases emphasize a pessimistic, even fatalistic, sense that behavioral interventions are little better than nothing at all. In considering the various types of technological solutions to the various epidemics of STI—drugs, vaccines, microbicides, improved condoms—the various ways people must incorporate these advances into their sexual lives remains the gist of public health science and practice about prevention. For example, consider the implications for STI prevention of a vaccine to prevent genital HPV infections. Preliminary data suggest that such a vaccine will be highly effective for prevention of the most common HPV types associated with cervical and other genital cancers. However, other common STIs are not prevented by this vaccine. A new generation of interventions will be required to help people differentiate vaccine-prevented STIs from those to which susceptibility remains. This is but one example of several imminent challenges to STI prevention practice.

Fourth, readers are encouraged to consider the fundamentals of science presented in this chapter. It should be obvious that effective behavior change is not a simple product of education and exhortation. Many in public health seem to feel that a sufficient intervention is defined by some posters and pamphlets, a rhetorical question such as "you don't want to get an STI, do you?" and an admonition to change. Data reviewed in this chapter should make the limitations of this approach quite clear. These data also suggest some alternative means by which public health personnel and institutions can help people understand and target specific behaviors, identify appropriate target behaviors, and acquire skills to achieve those targets. This, of course, is the essence of public health prevention practice.

References

1. Ebrahim SH, McKenna MT, Marks JS. Sexual behaviour: related adverse health burden in the United States. *Sexually Transmitted Infections.* 2005;81:38–40.
2. Manhart LE, Holmes KK. Randomized controlled trials of individual-level, population-level, and multilevel interventions for preventing sexually transmitted infections. What has worked. *Journal of Infectious Diseases.* 2005; 191:S7–S24.

3. Kirby D. School based interventions to prevent unprotected sex and HIV among adolescents. In: Peterson JL, DiClemente RJ, eds. *Handbook of HIV Prevention*. New York, NY: Kluwer/Plenum Publishers; 2000:103–107.
4. Kirby D. *Emerging Answers: Research Findings on Programs to Reduce Teen Pregnancy*. National Campaign to Prevent Teen pregnancy, 2001.
5. Nation M, Crusto C, Wandersman A, et al. What works in prevention: principles of effective prevention programs. *American Psychologist*. 2003;56:449–456.
6. St. Lawrence JS. *What Works in Prevention: Principles of Effective Programs*. Symposium presented at the International Union for the Study of Sexually Transmitted Infections (IUSSTI). Punta del Este, Uruguay; December 2003.
7. Semaan S, Des Jarlais D, Sogoglow E, et al. A meta-analysis of the effect of HIV prevention interventions on the sex behaviors of drug users in the United States. *Journal of Acquired Immune Deficiency Syndromes and Human Retrovirology*. 2002;30:S73–S93.
8. Robin L, Dittus P, Whitaker D, et al. Behavioral interventions to reduce incidence of HIV, STD, and pregnancy among adolescents: a decade in review. *Journal of Adolescent Health*. 2004;34:3–26.
9. Neumann MS, Johnson WD, Semaan S, et al. Review and meta-analysis of HIV prevention intervention research for heterosexual adult populations in the United States. *Journal of Acquired Immune Deficiency Syndromes and Human Retrovirology*. 2002;34:S106–S117.
10. Johnson WD, Hedges LV, Ramirez G, et al. HIV prevention research for men who have sex with men: a systematic review and meta-analysis. *Journal of Acquired Immune Deficiency Syndromes and Human Retrovirology*. 2002;4:S118–S129.
11. Leviton LC. Integrating psychology and public health: challenges and opportunities. *American Psychologist*. 1996;51:42–51.
12. COMMIT Research Group. Community intervention trial for smoking cessation (COMMIT): 1. Cohort results from a four year community intervention. *American Journal of Public Health*. 1995;85:183–192.
13. COMMIT Research Group. Community intervention trial for smoking cessation (COMMIT): II. Changes in adult cigarette smoking prevalence. *American Journal of Public Health*. 1995;85:193–200.
14. Elford J, Bolding G, Sherr L. Peer education has no significant impact on HIV risk behaviours among gay men in London. *AIDS*. 2002;15:535–538.
15. Flowers P, Hart GJ, Williamson IM, Frankis JS, Der GJ. Does peer-led sexual health promotion have a community level effect amongst gay men in Scotland? *International Journal of STD & AIDS*. 2002;13:102–108.
16. Rogers EM. *Diffusion of Innovation*. New York, NY: Free Press; 1983.
17. St. Lawrence JS, Brasfield T, Jefferson K, Alleyne E. Theoretical models applied to AIDS prevention. In: Goreczny A, ed. *Handbook of Health and Rehabilitative Psychology*. New York, NY: Plenum Publishing Company; 1995:555–582.
18. Brandt HM, McCree DH, Lindsey LL, Sharpe PA. *A formal evaluation of existing printed HPV educational materials*. Presented at the annual meeting of the American Public Health Association. Washington, DC; 2003.
19. Sharpe PA, Brandt HM, McCree DH. (2005). Knowledge and beliefs about abnormal Pap test results and HPV among women with high-risk HPV: results from in-depth interviews. *Women and Health*. 2005;42:107–133.
20. AIDS brochure launched despite doubts. *Nature*. 1988;333:87.
21. Becker HM. The Health Belief Model and personal health behavior. *Health Education Monographs*. 1974;2:236–473.
22. Janz N, Becker HM. The Health Belief Model: a decade later. *Health Education Quarterly*. 1984;11:1–47.
23. Brown LK, DiClemente RJ, Reynolds LA. HIV prevention for adolescents: utility of the Health Belief Model. *AIDS Education and Prevention*. 1991;3:50–59.

24. Li X, Fang X, Lin D, et al. HIV/STD risk behaviors and perceptions among rural-to-urban migrants in China. *AIDS Education and Prevention*. 2004;16:536–558.

25. Cleary PD, Rogers TF, Singer E, et al. Health education about AIDS among seropositive blood donors. *Health Education Quarterly*. 1986;13:317–319.

26. Prochaska TR, Albrecht G, Levy A, Sugrue N, Kim, JH. Determinants of self-perceived risk for AIDS. *Journal of Health and Social Behavior*. 1990;31: 384–395.

27. Fishbein M, Azjen I. *Belief, Attitude, Intention, and Behavior: An Introduction to Theory and Research*. Reading, MA: Addison-Wesley; 1975.

28. Fishbein M, Middlestadt SE. Using the Theory of Reasoned Action as a framework for understanding and changing AIDS related behaviors. In: Mays VM, Albee GW, Schneider SF, eds. *Primary Prevention of AIDS: Psychological Approaches*. Newbury Park: Sage Publications; 1989:93–110.

29. Jemmott LS, Jemmott JB. Applying the theory of reasoned action to AIDS risk behavior: condom use among black women. *Nursing Research*. 1991;30:228–234.

30. Sheeran P, Orbell S. Do intentions predict condom use? Meta-analysis and examination of six moderator variables. *British Journal of Social Psychology*. 1998;37:231–250.

31. Schnell DJ, Galavotti C, Fishbein M, Chan DK, The AIDS Community Demonstration Projects. Measuring the adoption of consistent use of condoms using the stages of change model. *Public Health Reports*. 1996;111:59–68.

32. Azjen I. Perceive behavioral control, self-efficacy, locus of control, and the theory of planned behavior. *Journal of Applied Social Psychology*. 2002;32:665–683.

33. Fischhoff B. Making decisions about AIDS. In: Mays VM, Albee GW, Schneider SF, eds. *Primary Prevention of AIDS: Psychological Approaches*. Newbury Park: Sage Publications; 1989:168–206.

34. Lebow RN, Stein J. Beyond deterrence. *Journal of Social Issues*. 1987;43:5–72.

35. Eddy DM. Probabilistic reasoning in clinic medicine: problems and opportunities. In: Kahneman D, Slovic P, Tversky A, eds. *Judgment under Uncertainty: Heuristics and Biases*. New York: Cambridge University Press; 1980:46–53.

36. Mischel W, Ebbeson EB. Attention to delay of gratification. *Journal of Personality and Social Psychology*. 1970;16:329–337.

37. Ferster CB, Skinner BF. *Schedules of Reinforcement*. New York: Appleton-Century-Crofts, Inc.; 1957.

38. Kelly JA, St. Lawrence JS. *The AIDS Health Crisis: Psychological and Social Interventions*. New York: Plenum; 1988.

39. Brownell KD. Obesity: Understanding and treating a serious, prevalent, and refractory disorder. *Journal of Consulting and Clinical Psychology*. 1982;50:820–840.

40. Chesney M. Behavior modification and health enhancement. In: JD Matarrazo, SM Weiss, JA Herd, NE Miller, SM Weiss, eds. *Biobehavioral Health: A Handbook of Health Enhancement and Disease Prevention*. New York: Wiley; 1984:658–663.

41. Prechacek TF. Modification of smoking behavior. In: Krasnegor N, ed. *The Biobehavioral Aspects of Smoking*. National Institute on Drug Abuse Research Monograph 26. Rockville, MD: US Department of Health, Education, and Welfare; 1979. Available at: http://www.nida.nih.gov/pdf/monographs/26.pdf.

42. Bandura AA. *Social Learning Theory*. Englewood Cliffs, NJ: Prentice-Hall; 1977.

43. Bandura AA. Perceived self efficacy in the exercise of control over AIDS infection. In: Mays VM, Albee GW, Schneider SF, eds. *Primary Prevention of AIDS: Psychological Approaches*. Newbury Park: Sage Publications; 1989:128–141.

44. Leventhal H, Safer MA, Panagis DM. The impact of communication on self-regulation of health beliefs, decisions, and behavior. *Health Education Quarterly*. 1983;10:3–31.

45. Leventhal H, Zimmerman R, Gutmann M. Compliance: A self-regulation perspective. In: Gentry WD, ed. *Handbook of Behavioral Medicine.* New York: Guilford; 1984:369–436.
46. Maddox J, Rogers R. Protection motivation and self-efficacy: a revised theory of fear appeals and attitude change. *Journal of Experimental Social Psychology.* 1983;19:469–479.
47. Rogers R. Cognitive and physiological processes and attitude change: a revised theory of protection motivation. In: Cacioppo JT, Petty RE, eds. *Social Psychophysiology: A Sourcebook.* Guilford Press, New York, NY; 1983: 53–176.
48. Bauman IJ, Siegel K. Misperception among gay men of the risk for AIDS associated with their sexual behavior. *Journal of Applied Social Psychology.* 1987;17:329–350.
49. Rhodes F, Wolitski RJ. Perceived effectiveness of fear appeals in AIDS education: relationship to ethnicity, gender, age, and group membership. *AIDS Education & Prevention.* 1990;2:1–11.
50. Lazarua AA. *The Practice of Multimodal Therapy.* New York: McGraw-Hill; 1981.
51. St. Lawrence JS, Hood HV, Brasfield TL, Kelly JA. Differences in gay men's AIDS risk knowledge and behavior patterns in high and low AIDS prevalence cities. *Public Health Reports.* 1989;391–395.
52. Mitchell SJ, Klausner JD. *Methamphetamine & STDs Including HIV Infection: A Local Public Health Department Responds.* Seminar presented to the National Center on HIV, STD, & TB Prevention, Centers for Disease Control & Prevention. Atlanta, GA; February 9, 2005.
53. Miller HG, Turner CF, Moses IE, eds. *AIDS: The Second Decade.* Washington, DC: National Academy Press; 1990.
54. MacDonald G, Schneider A. *The Importance of Social Marketing Techniques in Creating Effective Medical Campaigns.* Paper presented to the VII International Conference on AIDS, Florence, Italy; 1991.
55. Silvestre A, Lyster DW, Rinaldo CR, Kingsley IA, Forrester R, Huggins J. Marketing strategies for recruiting gay men into AIDS research and education projects. *Journal of Community Health.* 1986;11:222–231.
56. Puckett SB, Bye LL. *The Stop-AIDS Project: An Interpersonal AIDS Prevention Plan.* Report to the San Francisco AIDS Foundation, San Francisco; 1987.
57. Miller T, Booraem C, Flowers J, Iverson A. Changes in knowledge, attitudes, and behavior as a result of a community-based AIDS prevention program. *AIDS Education & Prevention.* 1990;2:12–25.
58. Kelly JA. Popular opinion leaders and HIV prevention peer education: Resolving discrepant findings, and implications for the development of effective community programmes. *AIDS Care.* 2004;16:139–150.
59. Kelly JA, St. Lawrence JS, Diaz YE, et al. HIV risk behavior reduction following intervention with key opinion leaders of a population: an experimental community-level analysis. *American Journal of Public Health.* 1991;81:168–171.
60. Kelly JA, St. Lawrence JS, Stevenson LY, et al. Producing population wide reductions in HIV risk behavior among small-city gay men: Results of an experimental field trial in three cities. *American Journal of Public Health.* 1992; 82:1483–1489.
61. St. Lawrence JS, Brasfield TL, Diaz YE, Jefferson KW, Reynolds M, Leonard M. Longitudinal follow-up from a community AIDS/HIV risk reduction intervention training popular peers as change agents: population risk behavior three years later. *American Journal of Public Health.* 1994;84:2027–2028.
62. Prochaska JO, DiClemente CC, Norcross JC. In search of how people change: application to addictive behaviors. *American Psychology.* 1992;47:1102–1114.

63. Prochaska JO, Redding CA, Harlow LL, Rossi JS, Velicer WF. The transtheoretical model of change and HIV prevention: a review. *Health Education Quarterly*. 1994;21:471–485.
64. Fisher JD, Fisher WA. Changing AIDS risk behavior. *Psychological Bulletin*. 1992;111:455–474.
65. Coates T. Strategies for modifying sexual behavior for primary and secondary prevention of HIV disease. *Journal of Consulting and Clinical Psychology*. 1990;58:37–49.
66. Leviton LC. Theoretical foundations of AIDS prevention programs. In: Valdiserri RO, ed. *Preventing AIDS: The Design of Effective Programs*. New Brunswick, NJ: Rutgers University; 1989:42–90.
67. McKusick L, Conant M, Coates TJ. The AIDS epidemic: a model for developing intervention strategies for reducing high risk behavior in gay men. *Sexually Transmitted Diseases*. 1985;12:229–234.
68. Kalichman SC, Rompa D, Cage M. Group intervention to reduce HIV transmission risk behavior among persons living with HIV/AIDS. *Behavior Modification*. 2005;29:256–285.
69. St. Lawrence JS, Brasfield TL, Jefferson KW, Alleyne E, O'Bannon RE, Shirley A. Cognitive-behavioral intervention to reduce African-American adolescents' risk for HIV infection. *Journal of Consulting and Clinical Psychology*. 1995;63:221–237.
70. Winett RA, Altman DG, King DG. Conceptual and strategic foundations for effective media campaigns for preventing the spread of HIV infection. *Evaluation and Program Planning*. 1990;13:91–104.
71. Flora JA, Thoresen CE. Reducing the risk of AIDS in adolescents. *American Psychologist*. 1988;43:965–970.
72. Kelly JA, St. Lawrence JS, Hood HV, Brasfield TL. Behavioral intervention to reduce AIDS risk activities. *Journal of Consulting and Clinical Psychology*. 1989;57:60–67.
73. Kelly JA, St. Lawrence JS, Betts R, Brasfield TL, Hood HV. A skills training group intervention model to assist persons in reducing risk behaviors for HIV infection. *AIDS Prevention & Education*. 1990;2:24–35.
74. Rotheram-Borus MJ, Koopman C, Haignere C, Davies M. Reducing HIV sexual risk behaviors among runaway adolescents. *Journal of the American Medical Association*. 1991;266:123–127.
75. Valdiserri RO, Lyter DW, Leviton LC, Callahan CM, Kingsley LA, Rinaldo CR AIDS prevention in homosexual and bisexual men: results of a randomized trial evaluating two risk reduction interventions. *AIDS*. 1989;3:21–26.
76. St. Lawrence JS, Wilson T, Eldridge G, Brasfield T, O'Bannon R. Evaluation of community-based intervention to reduce low income African-American women's risk of sexually transmitted diseases: a randomized controlled trail of three theoretical models. *American Journal of Community Psychology*. 2001;29:937–964.
77. Institute of Medicine. *Promoting Health Intervention Strategies fro Social and Behavioral Research*. Washington, DC: National Academy Press; 2000.
78. Flay BR, Cook TD. Evaluation of mass media prevention campaigns. In: Rice RE, Atkins CK, eds. *Public Communication Campaigns*. Newbury Park, CA: Sage Publications; 1990.
79. Gostin LA. Legal and public policy interventions to advance the population's health. In: Institute of Medicine. *Promoting Health: Intervention Strategies from Social and Behavioral Research*. Washington, DC: National Academy Press; 2000:340–416.
80. Chesson HW, Harrison P, Stall R. Changes in alcohol consumption and in sexually transmitted disease incidence rates in the United States: 1983–1998. *Journal of Studies on Alcohol*. 2003;64:623–630.

81. Lefebvre C, Flora J. Social marketing and public health intervention. *Health Education Quarterly*. 1988;15:299–315.

82. Wallace L, DeJong W. Mass media and public health. In: US Department of Health and Human Services. *The Effects of Mass Media on the Use and Abuse of Alcohol*. Bethesda, MD: National Institutes of Health; 1995:253–268.

83. St. Lawrence JS. Social marketing to increase condom acceptance and use in a high syphilis morbidity community. *Manuscript under editorial review*. 2007.

84. Coyle RT. *Theory: A Guide for Health Promotion Practice*. Washington, DC: US Department of Health and Human Services, National Institutes of Health; 2005.

85. Sorenson G, Emmons K, Hunt M, Johnson D. Implications of the results of community intervention trials. *Annual Review of Public Health*. 1998;19:379–416.

86. Finger B, Lapertina M, Pribla M, James-Traore T. *Intervention Strategies that Work for Youth: Summary of yhe FOCUS on Young Adults End of Program Report*. Arlington, VA: Family Health Interventional, YouthNet Program; 2002.

87. World Health Organization (WHO). *School Health Education to Prevent AIDS and Sexually Transmitted Diseases*. Geneva: WHO; 1992. WHO AIDS Series.

88. Grunseit A, Kippax S, Aggleton P, Baldo M, Slutkin G. Sexuality education and young people's sexual behavior: a review of studies. *Journal of Adolescent Research*. 1997;12:421–453.

89. Doherty IA, Padian NS, Cameron M, Aral SO. Determinants and consequences of sexual networks as they affect the spread of sexually transmitted infections. *Journal of Infectious Diseases*. 2005;191:S42–S54.

90. Amirhanian YA, Kelly JA, McAuliffe TI. Identifying, recruiting, and assessing social networks at high risk for HIV/AIDS: methodology, practice, and a case study in St. Petersburg, Russia. *AIDS Care*. 2005;17:58–75.

91. Latkin C, Mandell W, Vlahov D, Oziemkowska M, Celentano D. People and places: behavioral settings and personal network characteristics as correlates of needle sharing. *Journal of Acquired Immune Deficiency Syndromes and Human Retrovirology*. 1996;13:273–280.

92. Trotter RT II, Bowen AM, Potter JM Jr. Network models for HIV outreach and prevention programs for drug users. *NIDA Research Monograph*. 1995;151: 144–180.

93. Cottler LB, Compton WM, Ben Abdallah A, et al. Peer-delivered interventions reduce HIV risk behaviors among out-of-treatment drug abusers. *Public Health Reports*. 1998;113(suppl 1):31–41.

94. Latkin C, Glass GE, Duncan T. Using geographic information systems to assess spatial patterns of drug use, selection bias and attrition among a sample of injection drug users. *Drug and Alcohol Dependence*. 1998;50:167–175.

95. Broadhead RS, van Julst Y, Heckathorn DD. The impact of a needle exchange's closure. *Public Health Reports*. 1999;114:439–447.

96. Kincaid DL. Social networks, ideation, and contraceptive behavior in Bangladesh: a longitudinal analysis. *Social Science and Medicine*. 2000;50:215–231.

97. Belcher L, St. Lawrence JS. Women and HIV. In: Sherr L, St. Lawrence JS, eds. *Women, Health, and the Mind*. London: John Wiley & Sons; 2000:205–326.

98. Exner T, Seal D, Ehrhardt A. A review of HIV interventions for at-risk women. *AIDS & Behavior*. 1997;1:93–124.

99. Ickovics J, Yoshikawa J. Preventive interventions to reduce heterosexual HIV risk for women: current perspectives, future directions. *AIDS*. 1998;12(Suppl. A):197–208.

100. National Institute of Mental Health. The NIMH Multisite HIV Prevention Trial: reducing sexual HIV risk behavior. *Science*. 1998;280:1889–1894.

101. Kamb M, Fishbein M, Douglas J, et al. HIV/STD prevention counseling reduces high risk behaviors and sexually transmitted diseases: results from a multicenter randomized controlled trial (Project RESPECT). *Journal of the American Medical Association*. 1998;280:1161–1167.

102. Belcher L, Kalichman S, Topping M, et al. A randomized trial of a brief HIV risk reduction counseling intervention for women. *Journal of Consulting and Clinical Psychology*. 1998;66:856–861.

103. Emmons KM. Behavioral and social science contributions to the health of adults in the United States. In: Institute of Medicine. *Promoting Health: Intervention Strategies from Social and Behavioral Research*. Washington, DC: National Academy Press; 2000:254–321.

104. Hawkins JD, Catalona RF, Kosterman R, Abbot R, Hill KG. Preventing adolescent health risk behaviors by strengthening protection during childhood. *Archives of Pediatric Adolescent Medicine*. 1999;153:438–447.

105. Lonczak HA, Abbott ES, Hawkins JD, Kosherman R, Catalnno RF. Effects of the Seattle Social Development Project on sexual behavior, pregnancy, birth, and sexually transmitted disease outcomes by age 21 years. *Archives of Pediatric Adolescent Medicine*. 2002;156:438–447.

106. O'Donnell J, Hawkins JD, Catalano RF, Abbott RD, Day LE. Preventing school failure, drug use, and delinquency among low income children: long term intervention in elementary schools. *American Journal of Orthopsychiatry*. 1995;65:87–100.

107. Perry CL. Preadolescent and adolescent influences on health. In: Institute of Medicine, *Promoting Health: Intervention Strategies from Social and Behavioral Research*. Washington, DC: National Academy Press; 2000:217–253.

108. Coyle K, Basen-Enquist K, Kirby D. Short term impact of Safer Choices: a multi-component school based HIV, other STD, and pregnancy prevention program. *Journal of School Health*. 1999;69:181–188.

109. Blake SM. Condom availability programs in Massachusetts high schools: relationships with condom use and sexual behavior. *American Journal of Public Health*. 2003;3:955–962.

110. Centers for Disease Control and Prevention. *HIV/STD/TB Prevention News Update*. May 11, 2004. Available at: http://listmanager.aspensys.com/read/messages?id=32247

111. Main DS, Iverson DC, McGolin J, et al. Preventing HIV infection among adolescents: evaluation of a school-based education program. *Preventive Medicine*. 1994;23:409–417.

112. Centers for Disease Control and Prevention. *Compendium of HIV Prevention Interventions with Evidence of Effectiveness from CDC's HIV/AIDS Prevention Research Synthesis Project* November 1999 (Revised on August 31, 2001). Available at http://www.cdc.gov/hiv/pubs/hivcompendium/hivcompendium.htm

113. St. Lawrence JS, Crosby RA, Brasfield TL, O'Bannon RE. Reducing HIV/STD risk behavior of substance-dependent adolescents: a randomized controlled trial. *Journal of Consulting and Clinical Psychology*. 2002;40:1010–1021.

114. Harper GW, Robinson WL. Pathways to risk among inner city African American adolescent females: the influence of gang membership. *American Journal of Community Psychology*. 1999;27:383–404.

115. Jemmott JB, Jemmott LS. HIV behavioral interventions for adolescents in community settings. In: Peterson JL, DiClemente RJ, eds. *Handbook of HIV Prevention*. New York, NY: Kluwer Academics/Plenum Publishers; 2000:103–127.

116. Lightfoot M, Rotherm-Borus MJ. Interventions for high risk youth. In: Peterson JL, DiClemente RJ, eds. *Handbook of HIV Prevention*. New York, NY: Kluwer Academics/Plenum Publishers; 2000:129–145.

117. Peterson JS, DiClemente RJ, eds. *Handbook of HIV Prevention*. New York, NY: Kluwer Academics/Plenum Publishers; 2000.

118. Rosenfeld A, Myer L, Merson M. *The HIV/AIDS pandemic: The Case for Prevention*. Menlo Park, CA: Henry J. Kaiser Family Foundation; 2001.

119. Low-Beer D, Stoneburner S. *In Search of the Magic Bullet: Evaluating and Replicating Prevention Programs*. Menlo Park, CA: Henry J. Kaiser Family Foundation; 2001.

120. Collins C, Alagiri P, Summers T, Morin SF. *Abstinence Only vs. Comprehensive Sex Education: What Are the Arguments? What Is the Evidence?* San Francisco: University of California at San Francisco; March 1992. AIDS Research Institute, Policy Monograph Series.

121. Pedlow CT, Carey MP. *Developmentally Appropriate Features of HIV Risk Reduction Interventions for Adolescents.* Paper presented to the National HIV Prevention Conference. Atlanta, GA; August 13, 2001.

122. Henry J. Kaiser Family Foundation. *Sex Education in America: A View from Inside the Nation's Classrooms.* 2000. Available at: http://www.kff.org/youthhivstds/3048-index.cfm. Accessed February 18, 2005.

123. Thomas MH. Abstinence based programs for prevention of adolescent pregnancies: a review. *Journal of Adolescent Health.* 2000;26:5–17.

124. Denny G, Young M, Rausch S, Spear C. An evaluation of an abstinence education curriculum series: sex can wait. *American Journal of Behavior.* 2002;26:366–377.

125. Christopher FS, Roosa MW. An evaluation of an adolescent pregnancy prevention program: is "just say no" enough? *Family Relations.* 1990;39:68–72.

126. Kirby D, Korbi M, Barth RP, Cagampang HH. The impact of the Postponing Sexual Involvement curriculum among youth in California. *Family Planning Perspectives.* 1997;29:100–108.

127. Roosa MW, Christopher FS. Evaluation of an abstinence only adolescent pregnancy prevention program: a replication. *Family Relations.* 1990;39:363–367.

128. Bearman P, Bruckner H. Promising the future: virginity pledges and first intercourse. *American Journal of Sociology.* 2001;106:859–912.

129. Bearman PS, Bruckner H. *The relationship between virginity pledges in adolescence and STD acquisition in young adulthood.* Paper presented at the 2004 National STD Conference. Philadelphia, PA; March 9, 2004. Available at http://www.cdc.gov/stdconference/2004/PlenMiniPlen/Bearman.pps.

130. Bruckner H, Bearman P. After the promise: the STD consequences of adolescent virginity pledges. *Journal of Adolescent Health.* 2005;36:271–278.

131. Jemmott JB, Jemmott LS, Fong GT. Abstinence and safer sex HIV risk reduction interventions for African American adolescents: a randomized controlled trial. *Journal of the American Medical Association.* 1998;279:1529–1536.

132. Zimmerman R. *Why Haven't Abstinence Programs Worked.* Presented at the annual meeting of the American Public Health Association. Philadelphia, PA; December 12, 2005.

133. Centers for Disease Control and Prevention. *HIV/AIDS Surveillance Report, 2003* (Vol. 15). Atlanta: US Department of Health and Human Services, Centers for Disease Control and Prevention; 2004. Also available at: http://www.cdc.gov/hiv/stats/hasrlink.htm.

134. Aceijas C, Stimson GV, Hickman M, Rhodes T. Global overview of injecting drug use and HIV infection among injecting drug use. *AIDS.* 2004;18:2295–2303.

135. Lurie P, Jones TS, Foley, J. A sterile syringe for every drug user injection: how many injections take place annually and how might pharmacists contribute to syringe distribution. *Journal of Acquired Immune Deficiency Syndromes and Human Retrovirology.* 1998;18(suppl):S45–S51.

136. Centers for Disease Control and Prevention. Policy Issues and Challenges in Substance Abuse Treatment. *Prevention among Injection Drug Users Fact Sheet Series.* February 2002. Available at http://www.cdc.gov/idu/facts/Policy.htm.

137. Gostin LO, Lazzarini Z., Jones TS, Flaherty K. Prevention of HIV/AIDS and other blood-borne diseases among injection drug users: a national survey on the regulation of syringes and needles. *Journal of the American Medical Association.* 1997;277:53–62.

138. Rich JD, Dickinson B, Liu K. Strict syringe laws in Rhode Island are associated with high rates of reusing syringes and HIV risks among injection drug users.

Journal of Acquired Immune Deficiency Syndromes and Human Retrovirology. 1998;18(suppl):S140.

139. Hagan J, Thiede H. Changes in injection risk behavior associated with participation in the Seattle needle exchange program. *Journal of Urban Health.* 2000;77:369–382.

140. Vlahov D, Junge B. The role of needle exchange programs in HIV prevention. *Public Health Report.* 1998;113:75–80.

141. Vlahov D, Junge B, Brookmeyer R, et al. Reductions in high risk drug use behaviors among participants in the Baltimore needle exchange program. *Journal of Acquired Immune Deficiency Syndromes and Human Retrovirology.* 1997;16:400–406.

142. Blumenthal RN, Kral AH, Gee L, Erringer EA, Edlin B. The effect of syringe exchange use on high risk injection drug users: a cohort study. *AIDS.* 2000;14:605–611.

143. Des Jarlais DC, Marmor M, Paone D, et al. HIV incidence among injecting drug users in New York City syringe exchange programs. *Lancet.* 1996;348:987–991.

144. Taylor A, Goldberg D, Hutchinson S, et al. Prevalence of hepatitis C virus infection among injecting drug users in Glasgow 1990–1996: are current harm reduction strategies working? *Journal of Injections.* 2000;40:176–183.

145. Des Jarlais DC. Research, politics and needle exchange. *American Journal of Public Health.* 2000;90:1392–1394.

146. Strathdee SA, Celentano DD, Shah N, et al. Needle exchange attendance and health care utilization promote entry into detoxification. *Journal of Urban Health.* 1999;76:448–460.

147. Gold M, Safni A, Melligan P, Millson P. Needle exchange programs: an economic evaluation of a local experience. *Canadian Medical Association Journal.* 1998;157:255–262.

148. Holtgrave D, Pinkerton SD. Updates of cost of illness and quality of life estimates for use in economic evaluations of HIV prevention programs. *Journal of Acquired Immune Deficiency Syndromes and Human Retrovirology.* 1997;16:54–62.

149. Holtgrave D, Pinkerton SD, Jones TS, Lurie P, Vlahov D. Cost and cost effectiveness of increasing access to sterile syringes and needles as an HIV prevention intervention in the United States. *Journal of Acquired Immune Deficiency Syndromes and Human Retrovirology.* 1998;18(suppl):S133–S138.

150. Jacobs P, Calder P, Taylor M, Houston, S, Saunders LD, Alvert T. Cost effectiveness of Streetwork's needle exchange program of Edmonton. *Canadian Journal of Public Health.* 1999;90:168–171.

151. Junge B, Vlahov D, Riley E, Huettner S, Brown M, Beilenson P. Pharmacy access to sterile syringes for injecting drug users: attitudes of participants in a syringe exchange program. *Journal of the American Pharmaceutical Association.* 1999;39:17–22.

152. Heimer R, Khoshnood K, Biggs D, Guydish J, Junge B. Syringe use and reuse: effects of needle exchange programs in three cities. *Journal of Acquired Immune Deficiency Syndromes and Human Retrovirology.* 1998;18(suppl):S37–S44.

153. Cotton-Oldenburg NU, Car P, DeBoer JM, Colison EK, Novotny G. Impact of pharmacy-based syringe access on injection practices among injecting drug users in Minnesota, 1998 to 1999. *Journal of Acquired Immune Deficiency Syndromes and Human Retrovirology.* 2001;27:183–192.

154. Pequegnat W, Fishbein M, Celentano D, et al. NIMH/APPC Workgroup on behavioral and biological outcomes in HIV/STD prevention studies: a position statement. *Sexually Transmitted Diseases.* 2000;27:127–132.

155. Kauth MR, St. Lawrence JS, Kelly JA. Reliability of retrospective assessments of sexual risk behavior: a comparison of biweekly, three-month, and twelve-month self-reports. *AIDS Education & Prevention.* 1991;3:207–215.

156. McFarlane M, St. Lawrence JS. Adolescents' recall of sexual behavior: Consistency of self-report and the effect of variations in recall duration. *Journal of Adolescent Health*. 1999;25:199–206.

157. Kelly JA, Somlai AM, Benetsch EG, et al. Distance communication transfer of HIV prevention interventions to service providers. *Science*. 2004;305:1953–1955.

158. Holtgrave D, Kelly JA. Preventing HIV/AIDS among high risk urban women: the cost effectiveness of a behavioral group intervention. *American Journal of Public Health*. 1997;86:1442–1445.

159. Kumaranayake L, Vickerman P, Walker D, et al. The cost effectiveness of HIV preventive measures among injecting drug users in Svetlogorsk, Belarus. *Addiction*. 2004;12:1565–1576.

160. Pinkerton SD, Holtgrave DR, Jemmott JB. Economic evaluation of HIV risk reduction intervention in African-American male adolescents. *Journal of Acquired Immune Deficiency Syndromes & Human Retrovirology*. 2000;25:1634–172.

161. Pinkerton SD, Johnston-Masotti AP, Holtgrave DR, Farnham PG. Using cost effectiveness league tables to compare interventions to prevent sexual transmission of HIV. *AIDS*. 2001;15:917–928.

162. Pinkerton SD, Holtgrave DR, DiFranceisco MA, Stevenson LY, Kelly JA. Cost effectiveness of a community level HIV risk reduction intervention. *American Journal of Public Health*. 1998;88:1239–1242.

163. Institute of Medicine. *Crossing the Quality Chasm: A New Health System for the 21st Century*. Washington, DC: National Academy Press; 2001.

164. St. Lawrence JS, Montano DA, Kasprzyk D, Phillips WR, Armstrong K, Leichliter J. National survey of US physicians' STD screening, testing, case reporting, clinical and partner notification practices. *American Journal of Public Health*. 2002;92:1784–1788.

165. Ven PV, Mao LA, Fogarty AA, et al. Undetectable viral load is associated with sexual risk taking in HIV serodiscordant gay couples in Sydney. *AIDS*. 2005;19:179–184.

166. St. Lawrence JS. Efficacy of a money deposit contingency on clinical outpatients' attendance and participation in assertive training. *Journal of Behavior Therapy and Experimental Psychiatry*. 1981;12:237–240.

167. Festinger DS, Marlowe DB, Croft JR, et al. Do research payments precipitate drug use or coerce participation? *Drug and Alcohol Dependence*. 2005;11:11–18.

168. Higgins D, Galavotti C, O'Reilly K, et al. Evidence for the effects of HIV antibody counseling and testing on HIV risk behavior. *Journal of the American Medical Association*. 1991;266:2419–2429.

169. Kasprzyk D, Montano DE, St. Lawrence JS, Phillips WR. The effect of variations in mode of delivery and monetary incentive on physicians' responses to a mailed survey assessing STD practice patterns. *Evaluation and the Health Professions*. 2001;24:3–17.

170. DeLamanter J. *Values Trump Data: The Bush Administration's Approach to Sexual Science*. Paper presented at the annual meeting of the American Public Health Association. Philadelphia, PA; December 12, 2005.

171. Kerry J. *Keynote address*. Presented to the annual meeting of the American Public Health Association. Philadelphia, PA; December 10, 2005.

3

Biomedical Interventions

Stuart Berman, M.D., Sc.M., and Mary L. Kamb, M.D., M.P.H.

Biomedical interventions for STD are not new. In fact, the 19th century discoveries related to syphilis in large part presaged the biomedical model of intervention. Three major discoveries at the dawn of the 20th century set the stage for subsequent medical advances: the identification of *Treponema pallidum* as organism responsible for syphilis; a complement fixation blood test that could diagnose the presence of the organism; and the identification by Paul Ehrlich of an arsenical, salvarsan (though not the magic bullet hoped for), that could kill the organism (1). Subsequently, the availability of penicillin and the publication of Surgeon General Thomas Parran's "Shadow on the Land" contributed to the national effort to control syphilis transmission, supported by the National Venereal Disease Control Act (1938), the model for modern public health interventions based on the biomedical model. However, as this book demonstrates, the array of available interventions aimed at preventing and controlling sexually transmitted infections (STIs) now include many other non-medical approaches. Nevertheless, in many ways biomedical interventions are still the critical mainstay of prevention, and new biomedical approaches are constantly being evaluated and added to the armamentarium.

In considering biomedical interventions, we have found that the Anderson-May equation, $R = bcd$, serves as a useful framework (2). In this construct, R, the reproductive number, is the average number of secondary cases associated with an index case; b is the measure of transmissibility, given exposure; c is the average number of susceptibles exposed during the period of infectivity; and d is the average period of infectivity. Although biomedical interventions may affect any of these transmission parameters, two of these, d—duration of infectivity, and b—transmissibility, are most directly affected and are the focus of this chapter. Some aspects of c are addressed by biomedical interventions (e.g., vaccines); however, this parameter is primarily affected by sexual behaviors that are addressed elsewhere in this book.

Reducing d—Duration of Infectivity

Reducing duration of infection (i.e., affecting d) is the most obvious and historically most common means by which biomedical interventions reduce transmission. Case identification and prescribed antibiotic treatment of STD

Behavioral Interventions for Prevention and Control of Sexually Transmitted Diseases.
Aral SO, Douglas JM Jr, eds. Lipshutz JA, assoc ed. New York: Springer Science+Business Media, LLC; 2007.

infection clears infection and renders the index case noninfectious—achieving "prevention" by reducing the period of infectivity, and thus reducing prevalence. Although case identification and treatment is the biomedical intervention that probably comes to mind first, there are a variety of other biomedical approaches that can reduce duration of infectivity. STD screening of asymptomatic populations can identify unrecognized infections and allow treatment of cases that would otherwise have been missed. "Mass treatment" of an entire at-risk population—regardless of symptoms or behavioral risks—is a strategy that aims to reduce STD prevalence in the entire community. In addition to prescribed treatment approaches, nonprescribed approaches such as traditional therapies and folk remedies have been used to attempt to reduce symptoms and eliminate disease (and thereby infectivity).

The various approaches and contexts by which biomedical interventions affect d are addressed here primarily for the curable STDs targeted by national control programs, typically for syphilis, gonorrhea, and chlamydia. However, some therapeutic approaches aimed at viral STDs such as herpes simplex virus (HSV) and human immunodeficiency virus (HIV) may also affect duration of infectivity, and these are commented on as relevant.

Case Identification and Prescribed Antibiotic Treatment

There are few more established, fundamental biomedical interventions than the antibiotic treatment of infectious disease. In fact, the landmark paper in 1944 promoting use of penicillin to treat syphilis (a disease that was already a public health priority) and gonorrhea was among the first published applications of the drug (3,4). The availability of this powerful and effective antibiotic therapy was a revolutionary advance that changed medical management of STDs and other communicable diseases forever, as antibiotic treatment not only prevented adverse consequences in the individual, but also affected disease transmission, incidence, and prevalence.

Gonorrhea

Classically, antibiotic treatment was primarily provided to those persons presenting with symptoms; in terms of gonorrhea, male urethritis was the typical presenting complaint, and was one of first demonstrated uses for penicillin (5). The treatment was highly effective—symptoms were relieved and in addition, infection was cured; the reduction in infectivity could be clearly demonstrated by microbiologic culture. In fact, treatment of gonococcal urethritis with an appropriate antibiotic has been demonstrated to eliminate infectivity in a matter of hours (6). Treatment for gonorrhea has been observed to be so effective that some experts recommend that only therapies with greater than 95% efficacy would meet an acceptable standard of care (7). However, maintaining that rate of efficacy has been challenging since *N. gonorrhoeae* has proved quite nimble at acquiring antimicrobial resistance (8). In fact, evolving antibiotic resistance over time has resulted in substantial changes in the antibiotic regimens recommended for treatment of gonorrhea. As resistance emerged to penicillin and tetracycline, these drugs were no longer sufficiently effective, and have ceased to be recommended in most national STD guidelines (9). Currently, as an increasing percentage of *N. gonorrhoeae* strains have demonstrated resistance to quinolone antibiotics, this class of drug treatment is also becoming less relevant even in the United States. As of 2005, resistance has reached high enough levels in certain settings or subpopulations that quinolone use for gonorrhea is no longer recommended in several western states including Hawaii and California, or among men who have sex with men regardless of location (10,11). In such situations, cephalosporins are the primary treatment recommended for gonorrhea, and although clinical failures have been reported and low levels of resistance to some cephalosporin preparations have been observed (12), resistance has not as yet been documented to ceftriaxone. If widespread antimicrobial resistance to ceftriaxone were to develop, gonorrhea treatment options would be severely limited (13).

Although antibiotic treatment of gonorrhea has been observed to be highly effective at the individual level, the broader public health benefit of treating symptomatic disease—primarily males who present with urethritis—is less obvious. The community trial conducted in Mwanza, Tanzania, during the early 1990s found that increased access to and quality of symptomatic STD treatment was associated with a 49% reduction in prevalence of male symptomatic urethritis compared with control communities, although prevalence of gonorrhea among women attending antenatal clinics in the treatment and control communities did not differ (14). Furthermore, evidence from mathematical models has demonstrated the importance of providing prompt treatment to men and women with symptoms (15). Given reports of increasing delays in obtaining services in genitourinary medicine clinics in Britain, modelers evaluated the public health impact of such compromise. The models indicated that when disease incidence is elevated, if access is limited a "vicious" cycle can be set in motion, whereby "inadequate treatment capacity leads to many untreated infections, generating further high incidence and high demand and thus maintaining the inadequacy of services" (15). Additionally, other data support the concept that compromises in treatment efficacy can also have population-level public health impact, as at least one gonorrhea outbreak was attributed to prevalence of antibiotic resistant gonorrhea (16).

How effective is case identification and treatment of gonorrhea in controlling disease prevalence? In the United States, rates of gonorrhea disease did not decline dramatically until three years after a national gonorrhea control program, with broadly applied culture-based screening for gonorrhea among women, was launched in 1972 (17). Rates of gonorrhea continued to decline over the next 25 years, although the relative contributions of behavior change, partner notification, and screening are unknown (Fig. 1). However, some experts estimated that the gonorrhea prevention program—which relies primarily on antibiotic treatment—had shortened duration of gonorrhea infectivity by 70% (18).

Syphilis

Assessing the role of case identification and treatment regarding prevention of syphilis transmission is somewhat more challenging than for gonorrhea. As is the case for gonorrhea, studies that document the effectiveness of penicillin are historic—before the era of randomized trials. But, additionally, evidence of antimicrobial efficacy is challenging to gather since the causative agent of syphilis, *Treponema pallidum,* cannot be readily cultured (19), and thus outcome measures of efficacy have not been based on assessing microbiologic cure as is done for treatment of gonorrhea. Instead, assessments of efficacy have relied upon the imperfect approach of following serologic titers (20). Despite

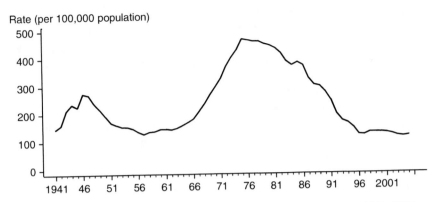

Rate (per 100,000 population)

Figure 1 Rates reported for gonorrhea, prevalence in the United States, 1941–2004.

the difficulties in accurately assessing treatment efficacy for a disease with such an unpredictable course, and one that can result in complications years later following long periods of latency, clinical experience is consistent in suggesting that antibiotic treatment for syphilis has been highly effective (21).

Another area of contrast between syphilis and gonorrhea is that treatment recommendations for syphilis have been remarkably consistent since 1944. Penicillin was quickly adopted as the treatment of choice for syphilis when early studies demonstrated that the antibiotic was rapidly treponemicidal (22). (The arsenic-derived drug salvarsan also killed the treponeme but had many side effects associated with it. Interestingly, Alexander Fleming was one of the few physicians administering salvarsan; that experience encouraged him to search for other antimicrobials, leading to discovery of penicillin (23)). In fact, after longer-acting penicillin formulations were available in the 1950s, there have been minimal changes in drug treatment schedules for syphilis (21). *T. pallidum* has remained exquisitely sensitive to penicillin, and resistant strains have never been identified. This may be related to fact that the *T. pallidum* genome is quite limited (24); the organism has very few genes and a very limited metabolic repertoire (19,25). However, strains of the organism that demonstrate antibiotic resistance to azithromycin have been identified (26), and such resistance can compromise effectiveness of a drug (27) whose efficacy otherwise appears comparable to that of benzathine penicillin (28).

As noted, from the earliest clinical studies it was apparent that acute lesions of syphilis resolved promptly after penicillin treatment (5). Since the lesions of early syphilis are very infectious, effective treatment should theoretically shorten duration of infectivity. However, the lesions associated with early syphilis are also self-limited and of short duration, and this, coupled with the lower infectiousness of later stage syphilis, has limited the impact of treatment (outside or early syphilis) on disease transmission. Importantly, early treatment also prevents the development of subsequent stages or relapses of syphilis, when individuals may become infectious again. Therefore, the earlier in the course of syphilis that treatment is provided, the greater is the reduction in duration of infectivity and the greater the prevention benefit (29). In sum, reduction in duration of infectivity is greatest—and the contribution to prevention greatest—when syphilis is treated in primary stage (29).

The contribution of syphilis treatment to prevention would seem to vary by gender and perhaps by sexual orientation. Females with syphilis are less likely to be diagnosed with primary stage lesions than heterosexual males (30), probably because the primary chancre is classically painless and may go unnoticed, or the primary lesion may occur on the cervix where it is not easily observed without a speculum examination. Similarly, it is assumed that the occurrence of rectal and pharyngeal lesions among men who have sex with men (MSM) are less likely to be noticed than penile lesions (31) and thus MSM are less likely to present with primary stage lesions than are heterosexual males. (Note: such gender differences also exist with regard to treatment of gonorrhea and chlamydia; males are more likely to present with incident, symptomatic infection, whereas infections among women, are more likely to be diagnosed by screening.)

Some evidence indicates that providing primarily symptomatic treatment for syphilis (manifested as genital ulcer disease) could have a population effect, shown by the Mwanza community trial of enhanced syndromic case management discussed earlier(14). In this study, in which the symptomatic treatment provided to those with genital ulcers included penicillin, syphilis seroprevalence was 29% lower in the intervention communities than in the comparison communities. Prevalence of active syphilis was also 38% lower in the intervention than in the comparison communities, although differences did not achieve statistical significance at $p < 0.05$. In that trial, no differences in syphilis prevalence were observed among pregnant women receiving antenatal care in the intervention and control communities (14).

Historically, however, treatment for syphilis was not provided primarily to reduce acute symptomatology or even reduce transmission; the primary objective was to prevent the long term complications (32). Soon after the U.S. national program to control syphilis was established in 1938, rapid treatment centers were set up to screen and identify infected individuals; this occurred even prior to penicillin availability. With a national program already in place, provision of penicillin treatment began to be implemented broadly, and treatment was not limited to just those seeking symptomatic care.

Although the population-level impact of the syphilis control program was quite effective, it is difficult to tease out how much of this was related to penicillin treatment as opposed to other control strategies. As noted earlier, penicillin treatment was initiated in 1944 as part of a national STD control program that already included syphilis screening. By 1956, reported incidence of primary and secondary syphilis in the United States had fallen to 3.9 per 100,000 from a rate of 70.9 a decade earlier (Fig. 2) (33). As the national program evolved, aggressive locating and treatment of exposed sexual partners was emphasized in the 1950s, and has continued to the present. The limitations of antibiotic treatment alone began to be observed as syphilis has become less common in the general population, and more concentrated in "core groups" (subpopulations with high STI prevalence and high rates of partner change). At the turn of the 21st century, after achieving historic low syphilis prevalences, Sweden, Canada, the United Kingdom, and the United States have all begun to see a resurgence in disease rates (34–37).

Chlamydia

Chlamydia is the third bacterial STD for which there is a national control program in the United States, and that program's structure is similar to that of the

Cases (in thousands)

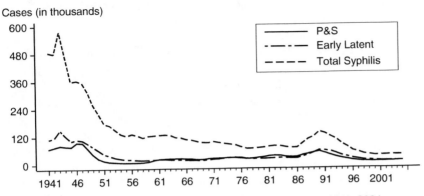

Figure 2 Rates reported syphilis, prevalence in the United States, 1941–2004.

national gonorrhea control program. Historically, men presented to care for treatment of symptomatic urethritis; when this was caused by something other than gonorrhea, it was termed non-gonococcal urethritis (NGU). Typical studies found that *C. trachomatis* caused 30–50% of NGU in heterosexual males (38). However, the purpose of NGU treatment was to provide symptomatic relief; specific etiologic diagnoses were rarely made, and evidence of microbiologic cure following treatment typically was not available. Subsequently, clinical studies have demonstrated that the antibiotics used to provide symptomatic relief for NGU—typically a week's course of tetracycline—were effective treatment for chlamydia infection, eradicating the organism in over 95% of cases among males, and over 90% among females in trials of up to 21 days of follow-up (39). Clinical entities, such as mucopurulent cervicitis, were identified which were regarded as manifestations of chlamydia infection among women corresponding to NGU (40); such entities warranted antimicrobial treatment for chlamydia. Until the availability of azithromycin, treatment involved multiple-day regimens (41). However, although a single-dose regimen is associated with greater adherence, there is thus far little evidence supporting enhanced treatment effectiveness of this approach compared with multiple dose regimens (42,43).

It is not yet clear whether or not antibiotic treatment efficacy for chlamydia is compromised by antimicrobial resistance. Some anecdotal evidence supports the existence of clinically relevant antimicrobial resistance; however, substantial uncertainty exists about the relevance of such evidence, and the appropriateness of the methodologies used for assessing resistance (44). Treatment efficacy has become an issue, however. As data have accumulated from follow-up evaluations of women treated for chlamydia, it is apparent that approximately 5–10% of women "successfully" treated for chlamydia (i.e., women who have negative chlamydia tests at approximately one month after treatment) test positive for chlamydia some months later (45,46). Such infections have typically been assumed to result from exposure to an infected partner (reinfection); however, prevalence frequently seems unassociated with such exposure (46,47), suggesting biologic persistence. Subclinical persistence is a characteristic of the organism (48), independent of any formal antimicrobial resistance.

Antibiotic treatment, which effectively cleared chlamydia infection, was clearly associated with decreased transmission on an individual level, especially in light of evidence that duration of chlamydia infection is quite long (probably over a year in women) (49). However, there are little available data to assess the population impact of treatment of symptomatic chlamydia infection. Effective symptomatic treatment for male urethritis, whether gonococcal or non-gonococcal, was standard care and widely available for years prior to the implementation of a national chlamydia prevention program. Nevertheless, prior to program implementation, chlamydia prevalence among young women in clinical settings was typically 10% or more (50,51), suggesting that symptomatic treatment had limited effect on community prevalence (Fig. 3). Supporting this, the Mwanza, Tanzania, community trial found little impact on prevalence of chlamydia among pregnant women, although, as noted earlier, prevalence of symptomatic urethritis among males was lower in intervention communities (14).

The impact of the U.S. national program on chlamydia transmission has become increasingly difficult to determine. In 1988, the beginning of the national infertility prevention program was launched and was subsequently implemented across the United States; it focused primarily on screening among young women. Screening programs were first implemented extensively in the Pacific northwestern states (Washington, Idaho, Alaska, and Oregon), and were observed to have apparently a substantial prevention effect as, from 1988 to 1994, prevalence among 15–24-year-old women declined from 15.1% to 5.7% (34,51) in those states. Similar declines were noted in other regions as their screening programs were implemented (50). However, neither national nor regional chlamydia prevalence has continued to decline over time, and prevalence may have in fact been increasing in some locales. Other countries (52) have also experienced increases in rates of chlamydia despite ongoing program activities. It is possible that limited screening coverage (52,53) or limited treatment of partners (54) explain some of the waning declines in chlamydia rates. Other mechanisms have also been hypothesized. Brunham (55) postulates that existing chlamydia control activities resulted in shortened duration of infection, which interfered with development of the immunologic protection that has been observed with repeated chlamydia infections. This would increase the number of susceptibles, permitting increases in incidence and re-infection rates. This is a complicated scenario, and is still only conjecture. Of note, this hypothesis would not apply to gonorrhea, since there is little evidence that gonococcal infection is associated with any subsequent immunologic protection.

Viral STDs

The role of treatment as an STD prevention strategy by means of reducing infectivity is also relevant for the viral STDs. For example, antiviral therapies have been shown to be associated with a 20-fold decrease in genital shedding of HSV-2 compared with placebo, and measured by culture (relative risk = 0.05) (56). Consistent with this finding, Corey demonstrated that, among discordant couples, provision of acyclovir (500 mg/day) to symptomatic partners was associated with a 48% reduction in HSV-2 incidence compared with placebo among the uninfected partners (57). Such an approach has obvious benefit on the individual level; however, it is as yet unclear whether sufficient numbers of HSV-2 infected individuals will utilize the approach to produce a population-level impact.

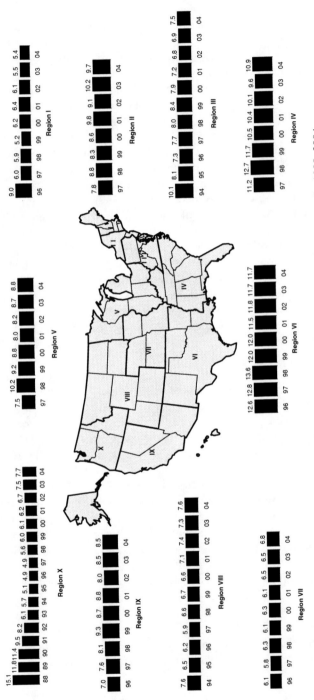

Figure 3 Chlamydia prevalence, 15–24-year-old females, family planning clinics, by HHS region, U.S., 1988–2004.

Direct evidence that antiviral treatment of HIV can reduce infectivity and HIV transmission is lacking. However, antiretroviral therapy has been shown to be very effective in reducing HIV viral load—an important finding for HIV prevention, since, as demonstrated by studies from Rakai, Uganda, risk of HIV transmission has been directly related to HIV viral load (58). Moreover, antiretroviral therapy has been associated with reductions in HIV concentration in semen, although few such studies have evaluated genital shedding among women receiving such treatment (59,60). On the other hand, mathematical modeling suggests that the population-level benefit provided by reducing infectivity can be countered by modest increases in risk-taking behavior—so called "disinhibition" (61,62). Unfortunately such increased risk-taking has already been observed among MSM in many wealthier nations, and this has been in large part attributed to the availability of highly active antiretroviral therapies (HAART) (31,63,64). In sum, the role of antiviral agents such as HAART as an HIV prevention strategy is still unclear, and is an area of active research.

In some situations there is evidence that antiretroviral therapy (ART) may reduce the probability of HIV transmission. Considerable evidence demonstrates that ART prevents mother-to-child HIV transmission (65,66). In addition, an early case-control study conducted among persons who had occupational, percutaneous HIV exposure suggested that post-exposure prophylaxis (PEP) reduced HIV acquisition through that route; PEP has also been promoted for sexual HIV exposure (CDC Guidelines). There is speculation that pre-exposure prophylaxis (PrEP) for sexual exposure may also reduce likelihood of HIV acquisition; this is currently being evaluated in studies assessing the utility of tenofovir in reducing HIV acquisition (discussed in more detail under *b*) (67).

In summary, case identification and antibiotic treatment has been demonstrated to effectively prevent transmission of the three common curable STDs, gonorrhea, syphilis, and chlamydia, most certainly at the individual level. Increasing evidence also suggests antiviral therapies may reduce duration of infectiousness for viral STDs including HSV and possibly HIV (although the mechanism of action may be aimed at transmissibility rather than duration). However, the population effects of case identification and treatment in the absence of broader control programs (i.e., including other interventions discussed in this book) are much less obvious, particularly for diseases that are largely asymptomatic. Interestingly, at this point, none of the three national prevention programs currently implemented in the United States appear to be sustaining ongoing decreases in disease rates. In fact, for the chlamydia prevention program, this point has been reached while the disease is still quite widespread in the general population (34,68). Gonorrhea and syphilis are more concentrated in core groups and subpopulations (34), and may be more amenable to focused approaches (69). Sustaining reductions in chlamydia transmission after a control program is established is, as discussed, an important challenge, and there is uncertainty about how to proceed; just what accounts for "rebound" in prevalence is not clear (70).

Screening and Treatment to Reduce *d*

As is clear from the above discussion, case identification and treatment of those with symptomatic infection with chlamydia, gonorrhea, or syphilis has limited public health impact. However, population level effects on transmission have been observed when such treatment has been part of a broad disease control approach. Since infection with the above bacterial STDs is frequently asymptomatic, many if not most infections would not be treated unless identified by screening. In fact, screening is a critical component of the national chlamydia and gonorrhea control programs in the United States as currently implemented, although this is no longer true for syphilis. (Note: Viral STDs are also frequently asymptomatic. However, although HIV is targeted by a national control program, HIV screening and case finding is performed primarily to address issues of personal wellbeing, rather than to reduce duration of infectivity.)

Treatment based on screening asymptomatic individuals requires having a suitable diagnostic capacity. As discussed earlier, a complement fixation test for syphilis (i.e., the Wasserman test) was available since 1906, well before the national program was initiated or penicillin was available. The national gonorrhea control program, launched in 1972, with an extensive screening component among women, was feasible only after the discovery in 1962 of Thayer-Martin media for culturing *N. gonorrhoeae* (71). Similarly, the infertility prevention program, which focuses on screening women for chlamydia, was made possible by the availability in the 1980s of suitable commercial tests for chlamydia (17). In addition to availability, suitable STD screening tests must have acceptable performance characteristics (i.e., sensitivity and specificity) (72). Appropriately accurate tests are now available for syphilis, as for the other bacterial STDs targeted by national programs (73). However, after the national syphilis program was launched, there had been widespread use of the Wasserman test despite performance limitations; although some have estimated that as many as 25% of Wasserman test positives were false positives, between 1937 and 1940, 31% of Chicago residents received such tests (1,74).

The contribution of screening and treatment to disease control seems most clear for gonorrhea, in light of the dramatic decrease in incidence that the United States and other countries experienced following wide implementation of screening. The issues now facing the gonorrhea control program involve how to best use the diagnostic tools that are available, given that the disease is now quite rare in the general population and given performance limitations of tests used for gonorrhea screening. The situation regarding the chlamydia program is different. As noted earlier, the impact that screening has on chlamydia transmission is not clear. Although chlamydia prevention has emphasized screening among sexually active women 25 years of age or younger, it may be that the strategy should be altered. For example, the role that screening asymptomatic males for chlamydia (or for gonorrhea) should play in prevention is still not known. The question is not whether asymptomatic infection in males plays role in disease transmission but rather, given an environment of limited resources, if and when resources should be directed to male screening rather than to other options such as expanding screening to older women, or supporting increased efforts to facilitate partner treatment (75).

For syphilis, the role of screening as a prevention modality has changed substantially over the years. Screening among general clinic populations is no longer recommended, nor is premarital testing or routine testing of hospital patients. As the disease has become less common, and more likely to involve core group populations, screening is recommended primarily for high-risk populations such those entering detention, commercial sex workers, and risk-taking MSM (76,77). (Screening among all antenatal women is still recommended because its cost-effectiveness against congenital syphilis has been demonstrated even when prevalence is exceedingly low) (78,79). The role screening now plays in control of the disease is also uncertain, even though syphilis seropositivity is rather prevalent in certain settings (i.e., MSM in STD clinics; women in detention) (34). Yet, some locales, a substantial proportion of cases of early syphilis have been identified by screening at detention facilities (80).

Screening for these three bacterial STDs has typically been venue or facility based, in large part because of the somewhat invasive nature of testing, along with the handling requirements that some specimens had required. However, more recently with new technological developments, testing for chlamydia and gonorrhea can be performed on urine specimens from either males or females or even on self-collected vaginal swabs (72,81). Furthermore, the specimens are sufficiently stable to be sent via the mail (82,83). With such advances, screening for those entities can be performed in a wide variety of contexts and settings, since clinics and clinical examinations are no longer required. This has allowed school-based screening, screening of street-accessed youth, home collection, and screening implemented via internet contact (84). Such technologies allow public health practitioners to rethink the usual approach to disease control. Some believe that such approaches allow "in field" targeting of core-group members (85). Such approaches would seem to be most appropriate for STDs such as gonorrhea and syphilis which are concentrated in core groups. Clearly, such an approach benefits those infected individuals and their partners who are diagnosed and treated. However, as yet there is little evidence of the public health value of such an approach, and little agreement about the role of such strategies in a comprehensive disease control program. This is true for both gonorrhea and syphilis, since the contribution that outreach screening for syphilis would make towards community disease prevention also remains questionable. The yield of outreach screening for syphilis, even among high risk populations, has been found to be quite low, with few (e.g., prevalence lower than 1% among those tested) untreated cases of early syphilis identified (86). Thus, the contribution that rapid, point-of-care treponemal tests would offer for syphilis control is unknown. However, it should be noted that such tests, which are available in many parts of the world but not in the United States, provide an important opportunity to improve prevention of congenital syphilis, facilitating screening and treatment among pregnant women in developing countries (73).

Rescreening (Persons Diagnosed with an STD)

There is a growing recognition that individuals found to have an STD either by screening or by clinical presentation are at increased risk of for future infection. The data, indicating a risk among women for recurrent or persistent chlamydial infection of approximately 10% at four months, prompted a CDC recommendation to rescreen women with chlamydial infection three to four months after treatment (77). With additional data, it is becoming clear that increased risk of repeated or recurrent infection is not confined to women, and applies not only to chlamydia (47,87,88). CDC treatment guidelines in 2006 recommend that clinicians consider STI rescreening in other populations (i.e., men, and men and women with gonorrhea).

Mass Antibiotic Treatment

The purpose of treatment has primarily been for improvement of personal health, and secondarily for population-level prevention, even though improved public health was an objective with the first National Venereal Disease Control Act (1938) in the time of Thomas Parran. Mass treatment, on the other hand, is a strategy whose purpose is explicitly for its population level effect. However, the effects of mass treatment on STD prevalence seem to be mixed. Mass treatment that addressed multiple STDs in the general population was provided in a community trial conducted in Rakai, Uganda, in an attempt to reduce HIV transmission. Antibiotic treatment was provided on a community basis every 10 months for three rounds, with control communities receiving a placebo every 10 months. The approach was not found to be effective in its primary goal of reducing HIV transmission; however, at follow-up, prevalence of active syphilis was 20% lower and trichomoniasis was 41% lower in the intervention group (89). No significant decreases in prevalence were found for gonorrhea or chlamydia, however, prevalences were low and sample sizes were small for these infections. Among pregnant women, prevalences of trichomoniasis, bacterial vaginosis, gonorrhea, and chlamydia were 30–70% lower in the intervention group, with all differences statistically significant (14). Although mass treatment may be effective for reducing specific STDs in the individual, its ambivalent population effects suggest little likelihood of its being widely implemented for the purpose of STD control.

The use of mass treatment may be more feasible for targeting high-risk populations, such as commercial sex workers. In an effort to curtail a syphilis outbreak in Vancouver, BC, public health officials provided single doses of azithromycin (1.8 g) to commercial sex workers, injection drug users, and their accessible partners within a defined area. Rates of syphilis declined initially but then rebounded to a higher level within several months. Findings from mathematical modeling supported the hypothesis that, although acute infection was being treated, treatment increased the number of susceptible high-risk individuals, who were then re-exposed to infectious syphilis (90). Canadian public health officials cautioned against such implementation in the absence of thorough understanding of the size of the population at risk, and of infection prevalence in the relevant network structures.

On the other hand, mass penicillin treatment appeared effective in California when used among sex workers and migrant workers, initiated because partner notification was not productive (91). Similarly, in Indonesia, the long-standing practice of providing routine penicillin injections (i.e., benzathine penicillin (1.2 mU) every two weeks) to sex workers was associated with a reported decrease in prevalence of active syphilis from 50% to 10% in those women (92). Furthermore, in South Africa, periodic presumptive treatment provided to commercial sex workers who worked in villages adjacent to gold mines (1 g azithromycin) was associated with a decrease in prevalence of gonorrhea or chlamydia among the miners from 10.9% to 6.2% over nine months; prevalence of genital ulcer disease also decreased among the miners from 5.8% to 1.3% (93).

Thus, for population level approaches, mass treatment may be useful to reduce prevalence of STDs, but existing data suggest that effective approaches must be targeted (e.g., most typically to commercial sex workers) and sustained.

Nonprescribed Treatment Approaches to Shorten *d*

In addition to prescribed therapies, a variety of over-the-counter treatments and traditional or folk remedies have been used to treat STIs and other reproductive tract infections (RTIs). Although relatively unstudied, nonprescribed treatment approaches are widely practiced, and may even be the most common first line approach used to deal with symptomatic RTIs.

Vaginal Douching

Vaginal douching—the use of a liquid solution to wash out the vaginal cavity–is a particularly commonly used nonprescribed treatment that seems to be at least partially aimed at reducing infectivity. Although the practice has been described to be primarily adopted for reasons of hygiene or contraception, many women report douching to prevent or treat infection or at least remove harmful organisms (94,95). Vaginal douching is practiced by women all over world, although appears to be more prevalent in some cultures than others (96). In developing world settings, douching has been reported as common among low-income or rural women who may be unable to bathe regularly, and also among sex workers who may be self-treating RTIs (97,98). In the United States, douching is reportedly most prevalent among African-American women and perhaps older age cohorts (99). However, it is quite commonly practiced among younger women, including those from a broad range of ethnic, cultural and socioeconomic backgrounds, to "treat infections" (94,100). U.S. research studies have also reported that women who douche tend to be more likely to have STI risk factors, including a history of prior STI (94). Taken together, these findings suggest that at least some women may douche to treat infections or symptoms associated with infections, rather than for cleanliness or hygiene only.

There is very little evidence that vaginal douching is effective at treating RTIs, and, in fact, some evidence suggests that douching may even predispose women to develop certain infections such as bacterial vaginosis and *Chlamydia trachomatis*, or STI sequelae such as pelvic inflammatory disease or tubal infertility (96,97,99,101,102). Douching practices seem to be able to be influenced fairly readily. Several investigators have noted douching practices are swayed by recommendations from mothers, peers, and health care providers (100,103). Douching has also been observed to be influenced by marketing strategies including television and internet advertisements (96,99).

In addition to attempts at destroying pathogens that would reduce *d*, douching solutions may be used to reduce vaginal pH or affect vaginal flora in ways that make the vaginal environment less susceptible to STDs or other RTIs. This application of douching solutions is directed at *b* or transmissibility (or susceptibility) and is discussed in more detail in the next section.

Reducing *b*—Transmission Efficiency

The transmissibility of STI pathogens is dependent on host resistance and susceptibility factors, which are determined by intrinsic defenses and by adaptive immunity (104). Intrinsic characteristics such as gender and age affect anatomical structures, formation of epithelial surfaces and presence and concentration of endogenous sex steroids. Biomedical interventions affecting *b* generally influence the host's environment in some way that blocks or inactivates sexually transmitted pathogens before they are able to invade the genital mucosa. Some examples of this are mechanical barriers such as the male latex condom, the female condom, and other devices that protect the female cervix (e.g., female condom, diaphragm, or cervical cap). Male circumcision has been postulated as a type of physical barrier, as the keratinized epidermis resulting from circumcision appears to be less susceptible to acquiring (and possibly transmitting) pathogens. In addition, an assortment of chemical barriers have been proposed that attempt to protect against STI transmission through various mechanisms aimed at inactivating pathogens at the genital mucosal surface where infection is likely to occur. Chemical barriers primarily refer to microbicides for topical intravaginal (or possibly rectal) use. Several microbicidal candidates have been developed and are undergoing safety or efficacy trials, and an even larger number of potential candidates are under development (105,106). In addition to commercial pharmaceutical products, various traditional or folk remedies draw on commonly available household products in an attempt to reduce vaginal pH or affect vaginal flora and, thus, STI acquisition.

This section provides a general overview of host and environmental factors associated with b, followed by descriptions of the major biomedical interventions affecting STI susceptibility or transmissibility. Susceptibility to STIs may also be influenced by social or cultural factors that play a role in how effectively biomedical interventions are implemented. Since these considerations are covered in other chapters of this book, they are mentioned here only when particularly relevant to a specific biomedical intervention (Table 1).

Host Characteristics Affecting b

Mucosal surfaces of the male and female genital and anal tracts are believed to be the primary entry sites for many sexually transmitted pathogens.

Table 1 Biomedical interventions against STDs.

Intervention type and target
Targeting d—duration of infectivity
Case identification and prescribed antibiotic treatment
Screening among asymptomatic individuals
Mass antibiotic treatment (including periodic presumptive treatment)
Non-prescribed treatments (including traditional or folk therapies)
Targeting b—transmission efficiency
Mechanical barriers
Male condom (latex, polyurethane, natural membrane)
Female condom (polyurethane)
Cervical barriers (diaphragm, cervical cap, sponge, shield)
Chemical barriers (microbicides, including pharmaceutical and non-pharmaceutical products)
Male circumcision
Targeting c—the average number of susceptibles
STI vaccines (HBV, HPV)

Table 2 Portals of entry and exit for STD pathogens.

Disease/Agent	Urethra	Cervix	Vagina	Vulva/Penis	Anus/Rectum
Gonorrhea	✓	✓			✓
Chlamydia	✓	✓			✓
Trichomonas	✓	✓	✓		
HIV	✓	✓	✓		✓
HBV	✓	✓	✓		✓
Syphilis	✓	✓	✓	✓	✓
Chancroid	✓	✓	✓	✓	✓
HSV	✓	✓	✓	✓	✓
HPV	✓	✓	✓	✓	✓

Adapted from: Stone KM. HIV, other STDs, and barriers. In: Mauck CK et al., eds. *Barrier Contraceptives: Current Status and Future Prospects.* New York, NY: Wiley-Liss, Inc: 1994:207.

Although the exact sites of entry for every STI are not exactly known, for several infections (and particularly gonorrhea and chlamydia) the cells most susceptible are the columnar epithelia of uterine cervix in women and the male urethra in men. However, HPV and trichomonas can also attach to squamous epithelial surfaces, *T. pallidum* (the bacterium causing syphilis) appears to infect both squamous and columnar epithelium, and HIV appears to infect mucosal Langerhans' cells that are present throughout the male and female genital tracts (107) (Table 2).

Transmission of STIs concentrated in semen, such as gonorrhea, chlamydia, HBV, and particularly HIV, has been observed to be more efficient from men to women than women to men (108–110). Increasing evidence supports that herpes simplex virus (HSV) is also more efficiently transmitted from men to women (111). Reasons for differential transmission of STIs among genders has been postulated by some to be related to the larger surface area and more susceptible vaginal mucosa in women, or perhaps because the cervix is more easily infected than the male urethra (110). The abundance of Langerhans' cells, an HIV target cell, in the female lower genital tract compared with circumcised males may help explain differential HIV transmission. It has also been observed that relatively little differential transmission exists between genders for the pathogens causing syphilis and chancroid. This suggests that other factors unrelated to *b* also play a role in STI susceptibility, such as more extended contact post-sexual exposure for women when STI pathogens remain in the vagina deposited in semen, thus enhancing *d* (duration) (110).

Environmental and Other External Factors Affecting *b*

For women, susceptibility to STIs may be enhanced by changes in the vaginal microenvironment. Studies in humans and animal models have identified that the vaginal flora is a "dynamic and closely interrelated system" and that disturbances in this vaginal microenvironment have the potential to affect STI susceptibility (112). Early laboratory investigations indicated an inverse relationship between the concentration of lactobacilli and other bacteria, particularly anaerobes, during menarche, pregnancy, postpartum, menopause, and postoperatively (112). In 1983, Paavonen (112) reported that during these periods, decreased concentrations of aerobic bacteria were observed while anaerobic bacteria remained constant, and hypothesized that such disturbances to the vaginal microbial flora had potential impact on STI susceptibility. Subsequent clinical studies appear to have borne this out (113–116).

Animal and human research suggests that, through hormonal influences, the normal vaginal flora is colonized with lactobacilli that help the vagina maintain a low pH that inhibits invading pathogens. Some H_2O_2-producing lactobacillus strains may also have direct bactericidal effects (113). Several clinical studies have linked the loss of vaginal flora with an increased risk for HIV and other STI (115,117). In particular, studies of sex workers have found that women with low or absent lactobacilli have higher risk for HIV and other STI (116,118).

A woman's vaginal pH undergoes continual physiologic changes from birth to menopause which appears to affect susceptibility to STI. The changes are greatly related to variations in endogenous steroid hormones, but also to other factors such as sexual practices (e.g., use of drying agents or douching solutions), sexual frequency, type of sexual activity, systemic diseases, and concurrent vaginal infections such as candidiasis, trichomoniasis, and bacterial vaginosis, which are all associated with higher vaginal pH. Use of some systemic agents (e.g., hormonal contraceptives) and topical intravaginal therapies also affect the vaginal microenvironment (119–121) and thus may affect susceptibility to STDs.

Mechanical Barriers that Reduce *b*

Several mechanical barriers have been developed, primarily as contraceptive methods, which also protect against certain STIs. These include male condoms, female condoms and devices that cover the uterine cervix such as the diaphragms, cervical caps and sponges.

Male Condoms

Of all barriers, the male latex condom is the oldest, best studied and (at least to date) most effective in preventing STD acquisition or transmission. An in-depth discussion of the male latex condom is provided in Chapter 10, and so is addressed only briefly here.

The male latex condom is designed to cover the penile glans and shaft, thus protecting the male anatomical areas most susceptible to acquiring or transmitting certain STI. Laboratory studies have demonstrated that latex bars passage against even the smallest sexually transmitted pathogen (122). However, *in vivo* studies indicate that condom efficacy against specific STIs varies based on the transmission route of the pathogen. If used correctly, the male latex condom can be quite effective in preventing those sexually transmitted infections that are transmitted to or from the penile urethra such as gonorrhea, chlamydia, trichomoniasis, HBV, and HIV (123–125). The data on condom effectiveness against HIV transmission are particularly compelling (126,127). More recent studies suggest male latex condoms can also reduce transmission of those STIs that may be transmitted through skin-to-skin contact, such as genital herpes (128,129) and HPV (130). In addition, several clinical studies support that male condoms reduce the risk of syphilis and genital ulcer disease in settings where the ulcers were primarily related to chancroid or syphilis (131,132). Although no published research has specifically addressed condom effectiveness against chancroid, the fragility of this bacterium, as well as limited detection methods (at least in the past), have made such studies difficult.

Male condoms can also be made of materials other than latex. Natural membrane condoms, also known as "natural skin" or "lambskin," contain pores large enough to permit the passage of viruses, including small viruses such as HBV and phage X174 as well as larger HIV and HSV, and thus are not believed to offer the same level of protection as latex condoms (122). Other synthetic condoms (usually polyurethane) have *in vitro* efficacy similar to latex condoms, and although relatively few clinical investigations have specifically studied synthetic (nonlatex) condoms, existing information suggests their effectiveness in protecting against STI is probably similar to latex condoms (133). Some advantages of the synthetic condoms are their lack of odor and color and their ability to be used with oil-based lubricants (which dissolve latex). They are also resistant to deterioration when stored over time (122).

Female Condoms

Over the past 15 years, considerable effort has focused on developing effective female barrier methods that women might be able to use as an alternative to male condoms for protection against HIV and other STI. In response to this effort, a female condom was developed, intended to be used during sex (like the male condom) but under control of the woman. The product has been available since 1992 and since that time has been marketed around the world under various names.

The FC female condom (formerly Reality) is a loose-fitting, prelubricated polyurethane pouch or sheath that entirely lines the vagina from labia to cervix (Fig. 4). Each end of the pouch contains a firm, flexible ring. The free-floating inner ring is inserted to fit around the uterine cervix and to hold the female condom in place, while the larger outer ring remains outside the vulva and holds the opening of the pouch open and acts as a guide during penetration. The female condom has one distinct advantage over the male

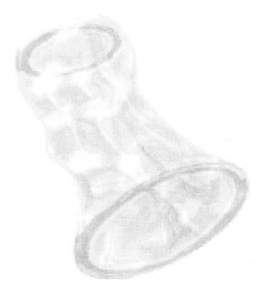

Figure 4 Female condom.

condom in that it can be introduced before sex and can be used for multiple coital acts.

As was discussed with the male synthetic condom, laboratory data support that polyurethane effectively protects against STI, and *in vitro* studies evaluating the female condom have also demonstrated its impermeability to HIV and other viruses (134). Relatively few clinical epidemiologic studies have assessed the effectiveness of the female condom against STI pathogens; however, existing data have been consistent in supporting that the device's effectiveness is probably similar to that of male condoms (135). Three randomized controlled trials ranging in from 500 to 1800 users each found the female condom to be as effective as the male condom against chlamydia, gonorrhea, and trichomonas. In addition, a small prospective cohort study assessing trichomonas reinfection found none over 45 days among compliant female condom users compared with 14% reinfection among nonusers, and 14.7% in "noncompliant" condom users (135). This study's findings of inconsistent use suggest the product may be unacceptable or difficult to insert for some users. In fact, the female condom is a somewhat bulky device. However, numerous small studies from around the world have demonstrated reasonable acceptability of the female condom, and particularly strong acceptance has been reported among many high-risk women such as commercial sex workers (136) and STD clinic patients (137).

A disadvantage of the female condom its relatively high cost (U.S. $0.88 to $1.20) compared with the male latex condom (which costs only pennies). However, given the durability of polyurethane, the condoms appear to be able to be safely reused after cleaning. In 2002, the World Health Organization convened a consultation to examine this issue, and concluded that reuse was not ideal, but with careful attention to disinfection (e.g., 1:20 dilution of household bleach), washing, drying and relubrication after each use the polyurethane condom could probably be safely reused (138). Subsequent evaluations have suggested that the female condom can be reused up to five times with an acceptable level of safety, although noted that excessive or rough handling can damage the condom (139). Nevertheless, neither the manufacturer nor the World Health Organization supports or recommends reuse.

Although not developed for this purpose, some users have adapted the female condom for anal sex by removing the inside cervical ring. Relatively little data have been published regarding safety or effectiveness of this practice, although it has been widely promoted on Internet sites. A large prevention trial among men who have sex with men (MSM) found about half of the participants had heard about use of the female condom for anal sex, and 6% reported such use of the condom during the preceding six months (140). A small San Francisco study that interviewed MSM found about half of men reported preferring the female condom over the male condom for anal sex, although some men reported it to be difficult to insert and occasionally painful (141). In a crossover study among a small number of HIV-seroconcordant monogamous male couples, men reported more frequent condom slippage, pain, discomfort, and rectal bleeding with the female condom than with male latex condoms, and frequently reported pain or discomfort and rectal bleeding (142), suggesting use of the condom for anal sex may not be without risk.

Two additional types of female condom are commercially available, although thus far no data exist on their effectiveness in preventing STIs. The Reddy female condom (V-Amour Women's Condom) is a latex pouch with a firm, flexible outer ring resembling the FC female condom, but with a soft polyurethane sponge that holds the condom in place inside the vagina. The Natural Sensation Panty Condom is made of a thin synthetic material (thinner than latex) that is worn like a woman's panty with a built-in condom (143).

Cervical Barriers

Diaphragms, cervical caps, and cervical shields are all soft latex or silicone devices that cover the uterine cervix and are promoted to be used in conjunction with spermicides. Cervical sponges are polyurethane foam barriers containing spermicide as part of the device. Although initially developed as contraceptive methods, increasing interest in cervical barrier methods for protection against HIV and other STDs (particularly when used with microbicides) has led to renewed research in these devices. Advantages to diaphragms, caps, and shields are that they are reusable, can be inserted up to 6 hours before, and left in place for up to 24 hours after intercourse (thus offering protection for multiple coital acts) and they can be used without a partner's knowledge (122,143). Currently, three sponges and about a dozen silicone or latex cervical barrier devices are being marketed, and at least nine of these cervical barrier devices have been formally approved by U.S. or European regulatory authorities (143).

The diaphragm is a shallow latex or silicone cup with a flexible rim that is folded for insertion, covering the cervix and held in place by the posterior fornix of the vagina, the pubic arch, and the vaginal walls. The shallow dome of the diaphragm is meant to be coated with spermicide (or microbicide). Smaller and firmer than a diaphragm, the cervical cap is a thimble-shaped latex or silicone device designed to adhere to the cervix by suction. Although generally observed to be more difficult to insert and remove than the diaphragm, many users find cervical caps more convenient because they can be left in place longer, up to 48 to 72 hours (143). The Lea's Shield is a silicone cup similar to the diaphragm but with an air valve, and a loop to aid in removal. Three cervical sponges are available for contraceptive use, although none are licensed in the United States (the Today Sponge was removed from the U.S. market in 1995) (143).

Designed to be used with spermicides or microbicides rather than alone, cervical barrier methods can be effective contraceptives if used consistently and correctly with every act of intercourse (143). Their efficacy against STIs is less well documented. A 2005 review identified 10 published studies evaluating diaphragm efficacy against STD (135). All were observational studies and thus subject to limitations of those designs (135,144). For example, diaphragm users and nonusers may have varied on their STI risk in ways that could not be adjusted for in the risk comparisons. The studies also assessed only current method use rather than ever use. Control groups varied, making comparisons between studies difficult. Furthermore, in several studies, the concurrent use of nonoxonyl-9 (N-9) containing spermicidal gel with the diaphragm may have influenced STI prevention effectiveness as N-9 has *in vitro* efficacy against several STIs, including HIV, syphilis, gonorrhea, chancroid, and HSV (122). It is interesting to note that all 10 existing evaluations supported some STI prevention effectiveness of diaphragms (144). Three cross-sectional studies suggested 60–75% prevention efficacy against chlamydia, gonorrhea, or both. Seven case-control studies suggested similar efficacy against gonorrhea, chlamydia, pelvic inflammatory disease, tubal infertility, and cervical cancer and its precursors. One large prospective cohort study demonstrated a substantial, highly significant preventive effect against cervical cancer in diaphragm users compared with nonusers. Most of the studies were older, and none were large enough to address a protective effect against HIV, thus there are no data documenting any benefit of the diaphragm against the virus (144).

Other cervical barriers are less well studied. The vaginal contraceptive sponge appears to provide some protection against cervical infections such as gonorrhea (145); however, it contains N-9 as its principal spermicide, which has proved to be problematic (discussed below under "Chemical Barriers"). As is the case with the diaphragm, none of the other cervical barrier methods have documented protection against HIV.

Because none of the cervical barrier methods cover the vaginal epithelium, it is assumed that these methods will not protect against STIs as effectively as the female condom. However, as noted earlier, the cervix is highly susceptible to certain STIs (including HIV), and the protective benefits of cervical barriers may turn out to be substantial, particularly if introduction of the diaphragm allows women to increase the proportion of protected sex acts and does not reduce their use of latex condoms or other prevention interventions. At least one study of men and women attending a family planning clinic in Harare, Zimbabwe found that introducing the diaphragm increased protected sex acts overall and did not reduce use of the male latex condom, although female condom use was observed to decline (146).

With increasing focus on female-controlled methods to prevent HIV, the use of cervical barrier methods along with microbicides has become a topic of renewed interest in HIV prevention research. Currently, there are randomized controlled trials underway in at least five African settings evaluating the effectiveness of the diaphragm plus a microbicidal agent against HIV or STI (discussed in more detail in the next section).

Chemical Barriers that Reduce b—Pharmaceutical Agents

Microbicides are chemical substances developed for topical use inside the vagina to protect against HIV and other STI through a range of possible mechanisms. Some are detergents or acids that would kill or inactivate STI microbes, some enhance or reinforce the vagina's own natural defenses against pathogens, some simply coat the vagina or cervix to prevent infections, and others block HIV or other viral entry into susceptible vaginal, cervical, or rectal target cells (105,143). Although it would be primarily targeted at preventing HIV, an ideal microbicide has been described as one that would also protect against other STIs, protect the vaginal as well as rectal mucosa, be resistant to temperature variations and durable enough to transport easily, and help protect men as well as women (145). Some researchers also suggest an ideal microbicide should have contraceptive efficacy; however, this might also be a negative factor if women desired pregnancy but also desired HIV and STD protection. Practically speaking, an effective microbicide must at least be acceptable to users, effective against HIV, and ideally would have more than one mechanism of HIV protection (147).

Candidate agents studied thus far have used a variety of formulations including gels, creams, foams, and films that have been used alone or in combination with a cervical barrier method. More than 60 agents have been identified to have *in vitro* activity against HIV, and by 2006 at least 18 of these have advanced to some type of clinical testing. These have included detergent-type barriers that cause viral envelope disruption (e.g., N-9, ACIDFORM), poly-meric broad entry or viral fusion inhibitors (e.g., Emmelle, PRO 2000, Carraguard, Ushercell), herbal extracts (e.g., Praneem), Lactobacillus suppositories, acidifying gels (e.g., BufferGel), HIV target cell inhibitors (e.g., RANTES), and viral replication inhibitors (e.g., Tenofovir) (105,106,148,149). Thus far, no microbicide has been found safe and effective at preventing HIV or other STI; however, several efficacy studies are currently underway and results from most of these will not be available for 3 to 10 years.

Ongoing microbicide studies have helped clarify several issues fundamental to HIV prevention, including realization of the critical importance of product safety. A very promising early candidate agent, N-9, was a long-used active ingredient of many over-the-counter spermicides, and is still used in small dosages for many lubricated condoms. *In vitro* studies have demonstrated N-9's ability to disrupt cell membranes, particularly bacterial membranes and the HIV envelope (148). However, five subsequent clinical trials evaluating various N-9 formulations (including N-9 preparations alone as a gel or a film, with lubricated condoms, and with a contraceptive sponge) failed to demonstrate an *in vivo* protective effect against HIV. More concerning, with frequent use or higher dosages, N-9 was observed to be associated with local mucosal inflam-mation and micro-ulcerations of the vaginal and cervical epithelia, thus perhaps increasing the host's susceptibility to HIV or other infections (150,151). Although the rectal use of N-9 has not been specifically studied, the rectal epithelium is more fragile than vaginal epithelium and richer in HIV CD4 receptor cells. Given the potential for mucosal inflammation and disruption, many health experts particularly advise against the use of lubricants containing N-9 during anal intercourse.

Several challenges have slowed the design and development of microbicidal agents (135,148). Product formulation and delivery has proved to be compli-cated, requiring acceptable application methods, dosage, and volume, as well as good coverage of the vaginal area and minimal systemic effects. It has been particularly challenging to provide formulations with sufficiently high dosages to offer protection for multiple hours, or multiple sexual acts, yet not cause local inflammation or mucosal disruption (135). Development of formulations that can be safely used rectally has also proven difficult, but important as increasing data indicates that a substantial minority of heterosexual women, and most homosexual men, engage in anal intercourse. Additionally, most of the development of new microbicidal agents has been done by small biotech-nology companies without substantial funding. Profit margins are of ongoing concern, particularly as the principal market for microbicides is perceived to be women with limited incomes.

The field of microbicidal research has been embroiled in a number of methodological, ethical, and political controversies over the past decade. Although laboratory-based methods exist that assess toxicity and provide surrogates for anticipated efficacy, the lack of a fully adequate animal model for determining clinical efficacy of microbicides or well-validated surrogate markers that correlate with clinical findings remains a problem. Without these, HIV seroconversion must be evaluated as an endpoint, requiring enrollment of thousands of HIV-uninfected, high-risk women who must be followed for many years. International ethical standards require that condoms are available to participants assigned to both active and placebo arms. This has resulted in a situation in which microbicide efficacy trials actually assess the marginal effectiveness of the microbicide above and beyond condom use—increasing the numbers of participants needed and adding complexity and expense over a traditional "placebo only" control group. Substantial controversy exists about the proper choice of control groups for efficacy studies. In 2004, the U.S. Food and Drug Administration required that initial microbicide effectiveness trials should include, in addition to the treatment arm, both a placebo (blinded) control arm and "condom only" (nonblinded) control arm, arguing that further clarification was needed on whether the placebo gel increased HIV risk or resulted in less condom use. Investigators have been mixed in their support for this strategy, which adds even greater numbers, complexity, length, and expense to already difficult trials (152–154). Development of a placebo that lacks antimicrobial effectiveness has been a further challenge (135). Ensuring that HIV status of participants and nonparticipants is kept confidential is another obstacle that must be carefully addressed in each setting. Additionally, although many observers believe it is most efficient to test a microbicide in developing nations where HIV incidence is higher and costs lower, local public sentiment has sometimes risen against conducting controlled trials in developing world settings. A tenofovir trial in Cambodia was halted because of local public and governmental concern about the agent's potential to harm participating women; this situation has been reported to indicate need for an international consensus on research ethics, study design, and oversight (155).

Additional challenges for microbicidal research loom in the future, such as the possibility that general resistance can develop to entire classes of drugs, and the persistent concern that microbicide development might discourage successful condom promotion efforts. As noted, sufficient funding is an ongoing concern. Although U.S. governmental funding for microbicidal research has more than tripled since 1997, few private companies, and none of the larger pharmaceutical companies, are involved in this research. Despite all this, researchers working in the area are remarkably optimistic that at least one safe and effective agent against STIs or HIV will be available within the next few years (Alliance for Microbicide Development) (148). However, the lack of effective agents thus far has been somewhat discouraging.

Male Circumcision

Increasing evidence indicates that male circumcision (the surgical removal of the foreskin of the penis) can protect men from acquiring certain sexually transmitted infections, particularly HIV (156–160). Circumcision also appears to be highly protective against squamous cell carcinoma of the penis, which is believed to be primarily caused by carcinogenic subtypes of HPV (156). Several mechanisms by which circumcision might protect against HIV or other STI risk, or both, have been postulated (156,157). One hypothesis is that the keratinized skin resulting from circumcision may serve as a physical barrier to bacteria and viruses and be less susceptible to scratches, tears, and abrasions that might provide portals of entry for pathogens during sexual intercourse. The prepuce in uncircumcised men is presumed to be especially vulnerable to traumatic lesions during intercourse, and thus more susceptible to sexually transmitted pathogens such as HIV and possibly syphilis, chancroid and genital herpes. Another hypothesis is that circumcision may act by reducing presence of HIV target cells, as the Langerhans' cells are abundant in the epithelial foreskin but unusual in the penile urethra (107). A third hypothesis relates to the possibility that circumcision reduces STD co-factor effects, thus reducing likelihood of HIV acquisition. It has been theorized that the intact foreskin may serve as a reservoir for bacteria or viruses, and thus perhaps increasing contact time (or "duration" of exposure) to the viruses or bacteria (156,157).

Over the past 15 years, a number of studies from around the world, including multiple cross-sectional and at least three cohort studies among adult, heterosexual males (158,159,161), have found lack of circumcision associated with significant 1.5- to 3-fold increased risk of HIV acquisition . In addition, a 1993 cross-sectional study of homosexual men found lack of circumcision to be associated with a two-fold risk of prevalent HIV infection (162); and a 1995–1997 cohort of MSM found uncircumcised men were twice as likely as circumcised men to develop new HIV infection (140). Despite remarkable consistency in results, the likelihood that important confounding factors (e.g., condom use, sexual behavior, ethnicity) could also account for the association, and could not be well controlled, led some to be skeptical about the potential effectiveness of circumcision as an HIV prevention strategy (156).

Recently, three randomized controlled clinical trials studying the effect of circumcision in adult, heterosexual males on HIV acquisition were conducted in South Africa (163), Uganda (164), and Kenya (165). In early 2006, the interim analysis of the South African study found differences between intervention groups were sufficient to warrant recommendation that the trial be stopped early. The intent-to-treat analysis found elective circumcision of 18–24-year-old adult males was associated with a 60% reduction in new HIV infection over the 18-month follow-up period (163). No serious adverse outcomes were observed, although some cross-over occurred (about 7 % of men assigned to each arm chose the alternative intervention during the study period). In late 2006, the trials in Uganda and Kenya were also stopped early because interim analyses indicated significant outcome differences. Both trials found approximately 50% reductions in HIV incidence among men assigned to receive circumcision. Further results (including the impact of male circumcision on other STDs, or on HIV acquisition among female partners of circumcized males) are not yet available. The consistency of the results of these rigorously conducted trials from three different African settings supports that circumcision can reduce an individual male's risk for HIV fairly substantially. The implications of the trials are being widely discussed, particularly regarding next programmatic steps to be taken.

Although based primarily on observational studies or clinical data, considerable data indicate that circumcision may protect against other STIs, particularly chancroid, syphilis, and gonorrhea. Several studies, including two cohort studies, have found genital ulcer disease associated with bacterial STDs (primarily chancroid and syphilis) to be associated with intact foreskin (166,167). Gonorrhea has also been associated with lack of circumcision in some studies, including at least one cohort study (160), although other studies have found no association. The link between circumcision and genital herpes infection is still unclear: cross-sectional, case-control, and at least three cohort studies have attempted to assess the association between circumcision and genital herpes infection, with some suggesting an association and others no association. The relationship of male circumcision and HSV is a specific area of study in the ongoing trials, and thus more information on this should be available in the near future. Anecdotally, clinicians have long noted that chancroid, a major cause of genital ulcer disease in the past, rarely occurs in circumcised men. In addition, circumcision has been associated with reductions in genital ulcer disease and has been documented in areas where chancroid was the predominant cause of ulcers (132). However, the effect of male circumcision on chancroid or other STDs other than the ones described here is not well documented in the published literature.

Some evidence suggests that circumcised men infected with HIV or other STIs may be less likely to transmit infections to their female partners than uncircumcised men. Ecologically, cervical cancer, which, like penile cancer, is mediated by sexually transmitted HPV, has been observed to be remarkably unusual among Israeli women compared with other women; and Jewish women living in New York City have similar low cervical cancer incidence as Israeli women (168). Further support for this notion comes from a pooled analysis of data from seven case-control studies assessing risk for cervical cancer and that included male partner data. This study found women who reported circumcised male partners had a lower risk of cervical cancer than women with uncircumcised partners; the difference in risk was most notable among women whose partners had a history of multiple partners (169). This same research group later assessed pooled data on 305 adult heterosexual couples who enrolled in five case-control studies assessing risk for invasive cervical cancer and found women with circumcised partners had approximately one-fifth the risk of seropositivity for *C. trachomatis* compared with women with uncircumcised partners (odds ratio = 0.18; 95% confidence interval, 0.05, 0.58) (170). In contrast, no significant differences associated with circumcision were found for *C. pneumonia*, a chlamydial infection that is not sexually transmitted (170). More recent though not yet published data, out of the Rakai community trial, suggested significantly lower incidence of HIV and bacterial vaginosis among female partners of circumcised men compared with partners of uncircumcised men; similar but nonsignificant results were observed for HSV-2 and HPV infections (171). Although these data are intriguing in their suggestion that male circumcision may reduce transmission of some STDs to female partners, other factors may also account for the observed findings. Whether and to what extent circumcision among infected males might reduce transmission of HIV or other STI to male partners through anal sex remains unstudied.

Although the recent trial results at least suggest that male circumcision may provide substantial protection against HIV acquisition for individuals at risk, the population effects of circumcision on HIV, particularly in industrialized nations such as the United States and Europe, are unclear. This is particularly the case because of varying HIV transmission modes globally. In most sub-Saharan African nations HIV and other STI prevalences are relatively high, and heterosexual sexual transmission is the most common mode of disease spread. But most new HIV infections in Europe, Australia, and the United States are related to injection drug use or to male-to-male transmission. As noted earlier, the possibility of a protective effect of circumcision on male partners practicing anal sex is undocumented. Also, should ongoing trials bear out the protective benefits of circumcision against HIV observed in the

South African trial, some scientists have warned that benefits could be attenuated by behavioral disinhibition or (i.e., risk compensation) if newly circumcised men believed they were fully protected from HIV and thus practiced riskier sex (i.e., less condom use, and therefore more unprotected sex acts) (172).

Nonprescribed Treatments Affecting *b*

Clinicians, researchers, and patients themselves have experimented with a variety of nonpharmaceutical treatments to provide contraception as well as protection against STI acquisition (105). For some time, a few clinical experts have recommended that women use a vinegar douche as a sort of post-exposure prophylaxis after rape or other unprotected sexual exposure, both to protect against pregnancy and to lower vaginal pH and thus inactivate HIV (173,174). Men have been advised to wipe their penis with lemon or lime juice or vinegar directly after intercourse to inactivate HIV or other viruses before they have a chance to infect (175). Some researchers have reported on the *in vitro* virucidal effects of lemon and lime juice, noting that a pH of 4 has been demonstrated to inactivate HIV and kill other STD in culture, including HSV-2, *N. gonorrhoeae*, *T. pallidum*, and *C. trachomatis* (175). A few cross-sectional studies of women using intravaginal solutions of vinegar, lemon or lime juice, or carbonated soft drinks have suggested acceptability of such solutions (105). Nigerian researchers have reported on the spermicidal and pH-lowering effects of several carbonated solutions, including water, colas, and lemonade (176). A 2005 study of sexually active Nigerian women found more than 60% of sex workers were frequent users of these products, believing them to protected against both pregnancy and STDs (177). Phase 1 clinical trials of the acceptability and safety of intravaginal lime juice have been recently initiated; however, some experts warn that until such studies are completed lemon or lime juice should not be recommended for general use (105). This opinion is supported by recently published data on another "natural" and inexpensive topical microbicide candidate, zinc salt solutions, which were touted as a potential agent against herpes simplex virus type 2. However, animal studies indicated that at the therapeutic concentrations needed to protect against HSV-2, the salt solutions were associated with vaginal epithelial sloughing severe enough that it might increase susceptibility to secondary infections (178).

In some regions of the United States, douching with carbonated beverages, primarily colas, has been reportedly practiced as a folk remedy against pregnancy, STIs, and other RTIs (100). U.S. researchers have also reported on the use of other household products as douching solutions, many of them quite caustic (96,99,100,113,114). In one cross-sectional study of adolescent girls, the teens reported using such douching solutions as commercially available baking soda, Betadine, Pine-sol, and Lysol, among other products (100). Most household solutions are entirely untested (and potentially harmful) as STI prevention methods.

In addition to douching solutions, other nonpharmaceutical intravaginal agents have been used to avert STI. Application of various dairy products (e.g., yogurt) containing *Lactobacillus acidophilus* has long been recommended by some practitioners as a mechanism to restore or maintain vaginal flora and health, particular aimed at preventing bacterial vaginosis or urinary tract infection (105,179,180). A recent Cochrane search posted on the Internet found six small, randomized trials evaluating treatment of bacterial infections, four assessing treatment of active disease (bacterial vaginosis) and two aimed at preventing recurrence of urinary tract infections (181). The results of these small trials were mixed. Three of the four treatment studies suggested some objective improvement of vaginitis with intravaginal use of either lyophilized *Lactobacillus acidophilus* or yogurt versus a control intervention, at least in short-term follow-up, whereas the remaining trial found women with vaginitis assigned to intravaginal application of fermented milk fared more poorly than women treated with metronidazole. Of the two prevention trials, one suggested a 50% reduction in recurrence of urinary tract infection in women assigned to use *Lactobacillus* suppositories compared with women using sterilized skimmed milk; the other trial of twice weekly doses of two lactobacilli species versus placebo found no significant differences in infection rates among the two groups of women (181). The evidence-based research group summarizing these data reported that the existing trials do no constitute sufficient evidence to recommend using yogurt or *Lactobacillus* to cure vaginal infections. The authors suggested there may be some effect in ameliorating symptoms of bacterial vaginosis, but no evidence of any beneficial effect on suppressing urinary tract infections (181). A capsule containing an H_2O_2-producing *Lactobacillus* strain has been developed for intravaginal use, and safety and efficacy studies are being conducted in animal models (182).

Despite a certain attractiveness associated with using "natural" products to reduce STI risk, numerous reports documented a range of risks associated with use of intravaginal substances (96,99,100,113,114), such as inflammation or trauma to the cervical mucosa caused by the solution itself (see earlier discussion on zinc salt solutions), or through abrasions caused by the applicator, through alteration of the vagina's natural protective mechanisms and flora, or even through direct introduction of pathogens (105,114). Although promoted as STI and pregnancy prevention methods, vaginal douching has been linked to several long-term adverse reproductive and gynecologic outcomes including chronic bacterial vaginosis, preterm and low-birth-weight infants, endometritis, pelvic inflammatory disease, chlamydial infection, tubal pregnancy, higher rates of HIV acquisition and cervical cancer (99,113). Given this, many experts have advised against douching with solutions of any type (98,183–185). In addition, some investigators hypothesize that promotion of such widely available nonprescription substances as STI protective mechanisms could encourage behavioral "disinhibition"—providing a false sense of security that might lead women to abandon other more effective prevention strategies, such as condoms (105).

Reducing *c*—The Average Number of Susceptible Hosts

Although most interventions aimed at *c* are related to reducing number of sex partners, and thus affect primarily behavioral rather than biomedical parameters, immunity, whether adaptive or vaccine-related, can also affect the average number of susceptibles in a given population. At least two examples of adaptive immunity exist for curable STIs, observed with syphilis and with *C. trachomatis*. (55). However, it is the incurable, virally mediated STIs (particularly HIV) that have most illuminated our understanding of relevant cellular and humoral responses. In addition, over the past 25 years, a growing number of vaccines have been developed that confer immunity against specific STIs. (Note: one can regard vaccines as reducing c to the extent that complete individual protection is afforded, since vaccination would truly reduce the number of susceptibles in the population.) Plasma-derived (and later recombinant) vaccines against HBV have been used since 1980 (186). More recently, effective vaccines protecting against carcinogenic subtypes of HPV have been developed (187,188). Preventive vaccines against genital herpes infection are being clinically evaluated. Vaccines against gonorrhea, chlamydia, cytomegalovirus (CMV), and HIV-1 are continually under development. In this section we discuss biomedical interventions that affect c, including acquired immunity in STD and a brief discussion of currently available vaccines. Vaccines against STDs are discussed in much greater length in Chapter 11.

Acquired Immunity

Growing information about a host's adaptive immunity to various STIs has helped researchers to develop new biomedical interventions or applications against these pathogens; this is particularly the case for HIV. In addition, the acquired immunity afforded by effective vaccines, although still relatively uncommon for STDs, is perhaps the most exciting application of biomedical interventions as vaccines can have beneficial effects at both the individual and population levels.

Adaptive Immunity

It is often assumed that curable STIs provoke little or no immunity; however, as noted in the discussions on d, a few examples may occur. One is the complex immunity observed with syphilis in which ongoing infection appears to produce immunity to reinfection. A second example occurs with *Chlamydia trachomatis*, in which re-exposure leads to less frequent reinfection over time (perhaps related to acquiring a balance between antigen specific interferon (IFN)-γ and interleukin (IL)-10 responses producing lymphocytes) (55). Although certain protozoal infections, such as *E. histolytica* and Giardia have characteristics suggesting adaptive immunity (189), these are uncommon STIs. Prior infection with *T. vaginalis*, the most common sexually transmitted protozoa, does not seem to protect against repeated infection (190).

For viral STIs, cell-mediated and humoral immune mechanisms appear to play important roles in controlling infection (e.g., for HSV and cytomegalovirus). Effective immune responses to HPV infection appear to be complex and type specific. In the case of HIV, reduced host susceptibility has been linked to acquired immunity through the roles of protective cytotoxic T-lymphocytes and host genetic variation (e.g., specific HLA class I alleles) (191). Susceptibility to HIV has also been related to differences in humoral responses at mucosal surfaces (191,192). New work in the fields of genetics and genomics will likely yield additional breakthroughs in the next few years that further enhance understanding of STI immunity, which may in turn lead to new and more effective biomedical interventions.

STI Vaccines

Among the most exciting biomedical interventions aimed at STI prevention and control over the past quarter century are breakthroughs in vaccine development for HBV and HPV, both common viral STIs that result in a substantial source of morbidity and mortality globally. Hepatitis B vaccines provide protection against development of viral hepatitis by stimulating production of neutralizing antibodies against HBV (anti-HBs). The early randomized clinical trials evaluating HBV vaccine efficacy were conducted among MSM. Efficacy trials found vaccine reduced new HBV infections by 90 to 95% (193,194), and results also suggested some degree of postexposure protection (195). The hepatitis B vaccine's effectiveness and safety have been rigorously documented: 95% of children and 90% of adults receiving the full three-dose series develop protective antibodies (193). In the United States, HBV vaccine is currently recommended as part of the early childhood vaccination package, and vaccination rates among children aged 1 to 9 years have increased substantially over the past 10 years (now approaching 90%) (CDC). More recently the plasma-derived vaccines used in the past have been largely replaced by recombinant vaccines, which are safe, also have a protective efficacy in the 90 to 95% range, and are less costly.

A quadrivalent vaccine against HPV, which includes the subtypes associated with most cervical cancers (i.e., types 16, 18) and genital warts (i.e., types 6, 11), was licensed in the United States in 2006 and appears highly effective and safe; results suggest these HPV vaccines have the potential to significantly reduce cervical cancer and its precursors in the future (187,188,196). In terms of widespread vaccine dissemination, the issue about which groups to vaccinate for greatest benefit has been considered. Ideally, HPV vaccines would be administered to the general population prior to the initiation of sexual activities, suggesting administration to those 10–12 years of age. If this is the case, education programs aimed at supporting widespread vaccine acceptance by both patients and providers will be important in determining uptake of the new vaccines (197).

Unintended Consequences of Biomedical Interventions

Biologic interventions may result in an almost limitless array of unintended consequences, many of them negative. Adverse outcomes range from fairly minor problems, such as self-limited side effects of prescribed antibiotic therapies, to much graver outcomes, such as disfigurement, chronic pain, high cost, and even death in rare instances. This section focuses on some of the more common consequences, particularly those that are often misunderstood or involve population rather than individual level concerns.

Case Identification and Prescribed Antibiotic Treatment

Prescribed antibiotic treatment is associated with a number of obvious unintended consequences. Most adverse outcomes, such as nausea, diarrhea, or vaginal yeast infections associated with certain antibiotics, are primarily annoying. However, side effects to antimicrobials can be consequential, as demonstrated by the severe lipodystrophies associated with certain protease inhibitors used in HIV management. Such side effects can have significant consequences on quality of life. Several antibiotics are associated with rare but severe allergic reactions which can be life threatening. Of note, antimicrobial resistance to gonorrhea or other bacterial STIs is seldom a consequence of STI treatment, but is an increasingly problematic consequence of widespread use of antibiotics for other (non-STI) conditions.

Screening

The most important unintended consequence of STI screening in asymptomatic populations is the occurrence of false positive tests, particularly problematic in low-prevalence settings (198,199). Adverse outcomes associated with any positive STD test can include anxiety, additional health care and resource utilization, negative impacts on sexual relations (e.g., accusations of infidelity), and stigma that may be severe and profound; these are particularly problematic if the test was false positive. Stigma is an important issue with any sexually transmitted infection, but in the case of HIV can have powerful implications. Histories of abandonment and much worse have occurred after notification of positive HIV test results, some of which were later determined to be negative.

Barrier Methods

Mechanical barriers such as the male and female condoms and cervical barriers are generally fairly safe. The male latex condom is easy to use, widely available and inexpensive. However, many men report decreased sensitivity and sensation, and 1–3% of people have allergic reactions to latex that make condom use impractical for them. Male condoms have some other issues: they must be in place before sex, and a new condom must be used for each sex act. If used incorrectly, condoms can break or slip off (200). Latex condoms deteriorate with use of oil-based lubricants or oil-based vaginal yeast medications such as butoconazole, miconazole and terconazole (123).

As is the case with the male latex condom, relatively few adverse effects have been reported on use of the female condom in women. However, some use issues exist although different from those associated with the male condom. Penile displacement outside the loose-fitting pouch has been reported to occur, and the device may be difficult to insert and cause more noise than other products (122). However, because the FC female condom is made of polyurethane, oil-based lubricants may be safely used.

Most currently available cervical barrier methods have relatively few safety risks. However, toxic shock syndrome (TSS), a rare but sometimes fatal syndrome caused by *Staphylococcus aureus*, has been linked to prolonged use of a now discontinued cervical sponge and may also be associated with the diaphragm (201). Although some observational studies have found urinary tract infections (UTIs) associated with diaphragm use, others have not and variable study methods have hampered meaningful comparisons (143).

Chemical Barriers

With the exception of N-9, few vaginal microbicides are currently marketed. The spermicide nonoxynol-9 has been more consistently correlated with urinary tract infections. In addition, as noted earlier, higher or more frequent doses of N-9 have been associated with localized cervical micro-ulcerations that may increase risk of STI and HIV acquisition (145,150,151,202).

"Condom migration"—movement by women away from condoms toward less effective devices or products, is an issue of considerable concern to microbicide researchers (135), but it could also pertain to other, noncondom barrier methods. Many health experts are concerned that vulnerable women may choose easier to apply but less effective prevention methods over more effective methods, thereby actually increasing their STI and HIV risk (203). Some data suggest that, at least for microbicides, the availability of additional products may change the type of protective method used but does not reduce the proportion of protected sex acts (135,203). Modeling data also indicate that condom migration should not lead to a greater proportion of unprotected sex acts unless condom use is at very low levels (<70% or acts) and microbicide use is lower than 50% for sex acts when no condom use occurred (203). However, further population-based research in this area would be helpful.

Circumcision
A variety of serious complications and potential risks to circumcision have been reported. The prevalence of complications due to the procedure appears to be fairly rare, but some data are available from case series of infant circumcisions in developed countries and reports from the recently published South Africa trial (which reported no serious adverse outcomes) (163). Among infants, the two largest series estimate complication rates ranging from 0.2% to 0.6%, with the most frequent complications reported as bleeding, infection, wound separation, and poor cosmetic outcome (204,205). Serious complications are unusual, but the procedure is associated with adverse outcomes such as meatal stenosis, urethral fistula, penile necrosis, unintended amputation of the glans, and, very rarely, death (156,157). Clinicians around the world are quite mixed in their support for this practice, and discussions often seem more related to ambient sociocultural norms than scientific data. Currently, the American Academy of Pediatrics neither advises for nor against infant circumcision (204).

Some health educators worry that if circumcision is found to be highly effective, men who opt for the procedure may experience "behavioral disinhibition"—a compensatory increase in risky sex behaviors in response to perceptions of safety conferred by the procedure. This phenomenon has been previously invoked in a variety of areas and is sometimes referred to by psychologists as "risk compensation" or "risk homeostasis" (206). In the arena of STDs and sexual behavior, STDs have been observed to be increasing in younger gay men over the past several years in the United States and Europe, believed to be related to the availability of highly effective antiretroviral therapies for treating HIV. A type of behavioral disinhibition has been observed in long-time condom users: it has been demonstrated that people tend to have more or riskier sex partners when they use condoms than when they do not (207). Economists have also recognized the phenomenon in other areas affecting health such as seat belt use (i.e., people seem to drive more recklessly while wearing seat belts), noting "circus performers take more chances when practicing with nets" (208).

Vaccines
Conventional vaccines have some drawbacks (186). On the individual level, a small but significant proportion of the population does not adequately respond to the vaccines and rarely, adverse vaccine-associated events have been reported. On the population level, if large numbers of persons remain unvaccinated, a community-level prevention effect may not be achieved, despite individual level protection. In addition, as is the case with circumcision, some people are concerned that vaccines against certain STDs may result in behavioral disinhibition (e.g., a vaccine against an STD, such as HPV, may lead people to have more unprotected sex, and thus be at greater risk for other STDs). Likelihood of disinhibition has been cited as an ethical concern in HIV

vaccine efficacy studies, both for current study participants and for future populations if a vaccine were found to be safe but only partially effective. It has been feared that vaccine study participants may perceive that they are protected against HIV and therefore take more risks than they would have had they not participated in the study. Recent follow-up data of participants in such a trial suggest that, although risk taking was substantial, trial participants were not necessarily more risky than nonparticipants (209). On the other hand, models evaluating the potential impact of widespread implementation of a partially effective HIV vaccine have indicated that behavioral disinhibition could profoundly affect impact of the vaccine (210). As vaccine recipients are likely to constitute a large proportion of the total population, any substantial increase in risk behaviors could result in a rising HIV incidence, abolishing all benefits of vaccination (210). Behavioral inhibition will continue to be an important element of STD vaccine research, and it appears likely that behavioral prevention efforts to promote safe sex will continue to be critical to the public health benefits of new vaccines.

Summary

Brunham notes that "a distinctive characteristic of infectious disease epidemiology (as opposed to the epidemiology of chronic diseases) is that incidence depends on prevalence, and therefore case detection and treatment is a major approach in bacterial STI prevention efforts. In short, "treatment is prevention" (104). The history of biomedical interventions aimed at reducing STI certainly bears this out, since the treatment and screening interventions that were first used early in the 20th century and which address d, duration, remain the backbone of most national STD programs. In the latter part of the 20th century, biomedical interventions aimed at b began to become an important part of STD prevention and research. These interventions include barrier methods for women as well as men, microbicides (although these largely remain in the research realm), and possibly the role of male circumcision in preventing HIV and other STI. STD vaccines are biomedical interventions aimed at c, and thus far include vaccines against HBV and HPV. Vaccines hold great promise to be the most consequential biomedical interventions against STDs in the future.

Although biomedical interventions certainly play an enormous role in STD control and prevention, they shouldn't be provided without attention to the behavioral issues discussed in some of the other chapters of this book. Behavioral research can help us address how, in what circumstances, and when biomedical interventions can be used most effectively. For example, a fundamental understanding of patient and provider attitudes, perceptions, and acceptability of the various biomedical interventions is critical for their effective application. This is true whether we are considering STD screening programs, promoting barrier methods to high risk populations, proposing circumcision strategies, or promoting vaccines. Similarly, behavioral disinhibition could undermine any beneficial effect of a biomedical intervention against STD. Concerns that behavioral disinhibition will mitigate the public health benefits of biomedical interventions such as cervical barrier methods, vaginal microbicides, male circumcision, and HIV vaccine are being voiced even before the primary trials determining efficacy of these strategies have been completed. Such concerns have led to debates about appropriate study designs and even the ethics of specific study criteria, and these in turn have led researchers to reconsider the best ways of studying the efficacy of these interventions.

Educating practitioners and the public about the limitations as well as the strengths of biomedical interventions, and promoting interventions in ways that ensure the greatest public health benefit depends on a foundation of solid behavioral research. Until the unlikely discovery of the elusive "magic bullet" against STD, effective STD prevention and control programs must continue to depend on the complementary use of behavioral and biomedical interventions.

References

1. Brandt AM, Jones DS. Historic perspectives on sexually transmitted diseases: challenges for prevention and control. In: Holmes KK, Sparling PF, Mardh PA, et al., eds. *Sexually Transmitted Diseases*. 3rd ed. New York: McGraw-Hill; 1999:15–21.
2. May RM, Anderson RM. Transmission dynamics of HIV infection. *Nature*. 1987;326:137–142.
3. Mahoney JF, Arnold RC, Sterner BL, Harris A, Zwally MR. Penicillin treatment of early syphilis: II. *JAMA*. 1944;126:63–67.
4. Mahoney JF, Ferguson C, Bucholtz M, Van Slyke CJ. The use of penicillin sodium in the treatment of sulfonamide-resistant gonorrhea in man. *Am J Syph Gonor & Ven Dis*. 1943;27:525–528.
5. Arnold HL. Penicillin and early syphilis. *JAMA*. 1984;251:2011–2012.
6. Haizlip J, Isbey SF, Hamilton HA, et al. Time required for elimination of Neisseria gonorrhoeae from the urogenital tract in men with symptomatic urethritis: comparison of oral and intramuscular single-dose therapy. *Sex Transm Dis*. 1995;22:145–148.
7. Handsfield HH, McCutchan JA, Corey L, Ronald AR. Evaluation of new anti-infective drugs for the treatment of uncomplicated gonorrhea in adults and adolescents. Infectious Diseases Society of America and the Food and Drug Administration. *Clin Infect Dis*. 1992;15(suppl 1):S123–S130.
8. Hook EW, III, Holmes KK. Gonococcal infections. *Ann Intern Med*. 1985;102:229–243.
9. Rice RJ, Thompson SE. Treatment of uncomplicated infections due to *Neisseria gonorrhoeae*. A review of clinical efficacy and in vitro susceptibility studies from 1982 through 1985. *JAMA*. 1986;255:1739–1746.
10. Increases in fluoroquinolone-resistant *Neisseria gonorrhoeae* among men who have sex with men—United States, 2003, and revised recommendations for gonorrhea treatment, 2004. *MMWR*. 2004;53:335–338.
11. Antibiotic resistant gonorrhea. 2006. 2-20-2006. Ref Type: Internet Communication.
12. Muratani T, Akasaka S, Kobayashi T, et al. Outbreak of cefozopran (penicillin, oral cephems, and aztreonam)-resistant *Neisseria gonorrhoeae* in Japan. *Antimicrob Agents Chemother*. 2001;45:3603–3606.
13. Tapsall JW. What management is there for gonorrhea in the postquinolone era? *Sex Transm Dis*. 2006;33:8–10.
14. Grosskurth H, Gray R, Hayes R, Mabey D, Wawer M. Control of sexually transmitted diseases for HIV-1 prevention: understanding the implications of the Mwanza and Rakai trials. *Lancet*. 2000;355:1981–1987.
15. White PJ, Ward H, Cassell JA, Mercer CH, Garnett GP. Vicious and virtuous circles in the dynamics of infectious disease and the provision of health care: gonorrhea in Britain as an example. *J Infect Dis*. 2005;192:824–836.

16. Faruki H, Kohmescher RN, McKinney WP, Sparling PF. A community-based outbreak of infection with penicillin-resistant *Neisseria gonorrhoeae* not producing penicillinase (chromosomally mediated resistance). *N Engl J Med.* 1985;313:607–611.
17. Wasserheit JN, Aral SO. The dynamic topology of sexually transmitted disease epidemics: implications for prevention strategies. *J Infect Dis.* 1996;174(suppl 2):S201–S213.
18. Brunham RC, Plummer FA. A general model of sexually transmitted disease epidemiology and its implications for control. *Med Clin North Am.* 1990;74:1339–1352.
19. Radolf JD, Steiner B, Shevchenko D. *Treponema pallidum:* doing a remarkable job with what it's got. *Trends Microbiol.* 1999;7:7–9.
20. Zenker PN, Rolfs RT. Treatment of syphilis, 1989. *Rev Infect Dis.* 1990;12(suppl 6):S590–S609.
21. Rolfs RT. Treatment of syphilis, 1993. *Clin Infect Dis.* 1995;20(suppl 1):S23–S38.
22. Parkes R, Renton A, Meheus A, Laukamm-Josten U. Review of current evidence and comparison of guidelines for effective syphilis treatment in Europe. *Int J STD AIDS.* 2004;15:73–88.
23. People and discoveries: Alexander Fleming 1881–1995. Available at: http://www.pbs.org/wgbh/aso/databank/entries/bmflem.html Accessed September 8, 2006.
24. Fraser CM, Norris SJ, Weinstock GM et al. Complete genome sequence of *Treponema pallidum,* the syphilis spirochete. *Science.* 1998;281:375–388.
25. Pennisi E. Genome reveals wiles and weak points of syphilis. *Science.* 1998;281:324–325.
26. Lukehart SA, Godornes C, Molini BJ, et al. Macrolide resistance in *Treponema pallidum* in the United States and Ireland. *N Engl J Med.* 2004;351:154–158.
27. Azithromycin treatment failures in syphilis infections—San Francisco, California, 2002–2003. *MMWR Morb Mortal Wkly Rep.* 2004;53:197–198.
28. Riedner G, Rusizoka M, Todd J, et al. Single-dose azithromycin versus penicillin G benzathine for the treatment of early syphilis. *N Engl J Med.* 2005;353:1236–1244.
29. Kahn RH, Peterman TA, Arno J, Coursey EJ, Berman SM. Identifying likely syphilis transmitters: implications for control and evaluation. *Sex Transm Dis.* 2006;33:630–635.
30. Musher DM. Early syphilis. In: Holmes KK, Sparling PF, Mardh PA, et al., eds. *Sexually Transmitted Diseases*, 3rd ed. 1999:479–485.
31. Marcus U, Bremer V, Hamouda O, et al. Understanding recent increases in the incidence of sexually transmitted infections in men having sex with men: changes in risk behavior from risk avoidance to risk reduction. *Sex Transm Dis.* 2006;33:11–17.
32. Cates W Jr, Rothenberg RB, Blount JH. Public health measures for syphilis control. In: Hook EW, III, Lukehart SA, eds. *Syphilis*. Cambridge, MA: Blackwell Scientific; 1994.
33. Garnett GP, Brunham RC. Magic bullets need accurate guns—syphilis eradication, elimination, and control. *Microbes Infect.* 1999;1:395–404.
34. Centers for Disease Control and Prevention. *Sexually Transmitted Disease Surveillance, 2004*. Atlanta, GA: U.S. Department of Health and Human Services; 2005.
35. Simms I, Fenton KA, Ashton M, et al. The reemergence of syphilis in the United Kingdom: the new epidemic phases. *Sex Transm Dis.* 2005;32:220–226.
36. Karlsson A, Hejdeman B, Pernetun T, Sandstrom E. [HIV, gonorrhea, chlamydia and syphilis are increasing among homosexual men]. *Lakartidningen.* 2001;98:1793–1795.

37. Wong T, Singh A, Mann J, Hansen L, McMahon S. Gender differences in bacterial STIs in Canada. *BMC Womens Health*. 2004;(4 suppl 1):S26.
38. Stamm WE. *Chlamydia trachomatis* infections of the adult. In: Holmes KK, Sparling PF, Mardh PA, et al., eds. *Sexually Transmitted Diseases*, 3rd ed. New York: McGraw-Hill; 1999:407–422.
39. Toomey KE, Barnes RC. Treatment of *Chlamydia trachomatis* genital infection. *Rev Infect Dis*. 1990;12(suppl 6):S645–S655.
40. Brunham RC, Paavonen J, Stevens CE, et al. Mucopurulent cervicitis—the ignored counterpart in women of urethritis in men. *N Engl J Med*. 1984;311:1–6.
41. 1989 Sexually Transmitted diseases treatment guidelines. *MMWR Morb Mortal Wkly Rep*. 1989;38(suppl 8):1–43.
42. Hillis SD, Coles FB, Litchfield B, et al. Doxycycline and azithromycin for prevention of chlamydial persistence or recurrence one month after treatment in women. A use-effectiveness study in public health settings. *Sex Transm Dis*. 1998;25:5–11.
43. Handsfield HH, Stamm WE. Treating chlamydial infection: compliance versus cost. *Sex Transm Dis*. 1998;25:12–13.
44. Wang SA, Papp JR, Stamm WE, Peeling RW, Martin DH, Holmes KK. Evaluation of antimicrobial resistance and treatment failures for *Chlamydia trachomatis*: a meeting report. *J Infect Dis*. 2005;191:917–923.
45. Whittington WL, Kent C, Kissinger P, et al. Determinants of persistent and recurrent *Chlamydia trachomatis* infection in young women: results of a multicenter cohort study. *Sex Transm Dis*. 2001;28:117–123.
46. Schillinger JA, Kissinger P, Calvet H, et al. Patient-delivered partner treatment with azithromycin to prevent repeated *Chlamydia trachomatis* infection among women: a randomized, controlled trial. *Sex Transm Dis*. 2003;30:49–56.
47. Golden MR, Whittington WL, Handsfield HH, et al. Effect of expedited treatment of sex partners on recurrent or persistent gonorrhea or chlamydial infection. *N Engl J Med*. 2005;352:676–685.
48. Stamm WE. *Chlamydia trachomatis*—the persistent pathogen: Thomas Parran Award Lecture. *Sex Transm Dis*. 2001;28:684–689.
49. McCormack WM, Alpert S, McComb DE, Nichols RL, Semine DZ, Zinner SH. Fifteen-month follow-up study of women infected with *Chlamydia trachomatis*. *N Engl J Med*. 1979;300:123–125.
50. Addiss DG, Vaughn ML, Ludka D, Pfister J, Davis JP. Decreased prevalence of *Chlamydia trachomatis* infection associated with a selective screening program in family planning clinics in Wisconsin. *Sex Transm Dis*. 1993;20:28–35.
51. Mosure DJ, Berman S, Fine D, DeLisle S, Cates W, Jr., Boring JR, III. Genital chlamydia infections in sexually active female adolescents: do we really need to screen everyone? *J Adolesc Health*. 1997;20:6–13.
52. Low N, Harbord RM, Egger M, Sterne JA, Herrmann B. Screening for chlamydia. *Lancet*. 2005;365:1539.
53. Centers for Disease Control and Prevention. Chlamydia screening among sexually active young female enrollees of health plans—United States, 1999–2001. *MMWR*. 2004;53:983–985.
54. Centers for Disease Control and Prevention. Expedited partner therapy in the management of sexually transmitted diseases. 2006. Atlanta, GA: US Department of Health and Human Services. 2-20-2006. Ref Type: Report
55. Brunham RC, Pourbohloul B, Mak S, White R, Rekart ML. The unexpected impact of a *Chlamydia trachomatis* infection control program on susceptibility to reinfection. *J Infect Dis*. 2005;192:1836–1844.
56. Gupta R, Wald A, Krantz E, et al. Valacyclovir and acyclovir for suppression of shedding of herpes simplex virus in the genital tract. *J Infect Dis*. 2004;190:1374–1381.

57. Corey L, Wald A, Patel R, et al. Once-daily valacyclovir to reduce the risk of transmission of genital herpes. *N Engl J Med.* 2004;350:11–20.
58. Quinn TC, Wawer MJ, Sewankambo N, et al. Viral load and heterosexual transmission of human immunodeficiency virus type 1. Rakai Project Study Group.[comment]. *New England Journal of Medicine.* 2000;342:921–929.
59. Vernazza PL, Troiani L, Flepp MJ, et al. Potent antiretroviral treatment of HIV-infection results in suppression of the seminal shedding of HIV. The Swiss HIV Cohort Study. *AIDS.* 2000;14:117–121.
60. Hosseinipour M, Cohen MS, Vernazza PL, Kashuba AD. Can antiretroviral therapy be used to prevent sexual transmission of human immunodeficiency virus type 1? *Clin Infect Dis.* 2002;34:1391–1395.
61. Blower S. Calculating the consequences: HAART and risky sex. *AIDS.* 2001;15:1309–1310.
62. Law MG, Prestage G, Grulich A, Van d, V, Kippax S. Modelling the effect of combination antiretroviral treatments on HIV incidence. *AIDS.* 2001;15:1287–1294.
63. Douglas JM, Jr., Peterman TA, Fenton KA. Syphilis among men who have sex with men: challenges to syphilis elimination in the United States. *Sex Transm Dis.* 2005;32:S80–S83.
64. Wohlfeiler D, Potterat JJ. Using gay men's sexual networks to reduce sexually transmitted disease (STD)/human immunodeficiency virus (HIV) transmission. *Sex Transm Dis.* 2005;32:S48–S52.
65. Connor EM, Mofenson LM. Zidovudine for the reduction of perinatal human immunodeficiency virus transmission: pediatric AIDS Clinical Trials Group Protocol 076–results and treatment recommendations. *Pediatr Infect Dis J.* 1995;14:536–541.
66. Connor EM, Sperling RS, Gelber R, et al. Reduction of maternal-infant transmission of human immunodeficiency virus type 1 with zidovudine treatment. Pediatric AIDS Clinical Trials Group Protocol 076 Study Group. *N Engl J Med.* 1994;331:1173–1180.
67. Celum CL, Robinson NJ, Cohen MS. Potential effect of HIV type 1 antiretroviral and herpes simplex virus type 2 antiviral therapy on transmission and acquisition of HIV type 1 infection. *J Infect Dis.* 2005;191(suppl 1):S107–S114.
68. Miller WC, Ford CA, Morris M, et al. Prevalence of chlamydial and gonococcal infections among young adults in the United States. *JAMA.* 2004;291:2229–2236.
69. Turner KM, Garnett GP, Ghani AC, Sterne JA, Low N. Investigating ethnic inequalities in the incidence of sexually transmitted infections: mathematical modelling study. *Sex Transm Infect.* 2004;80:379–385.
70. Fine, D, Mosure, D. J., Dicker, L. W., and Berman, S. Increasing chlamydia positivity among women attending region X family planning clinics, 1997–2004: is NAAT testing the reason? *ISSTDR.* 2005.
71. Thayer JD, Martin JE, Jr. A selective medium for the cultivation of *N. gonorrhoeae* and *N. meningitis. Public Health Rep.* 1964;79:49–57.
72. Johnson RE, Newhall WJ, Papp JR, et al. Screening tests to detect *Chlamydia trachomatis* and *Neisseria gonorrhoeae* infections–2002. *MMWR Recomm Rep.* 2002;51:1–38.
73. Peeling RW, Ye H. Diagnostic tools for preventing and managing maternal and congenital syphilis: an overview. *Bull World Health Organ.* 2004;82:439–446.
74. Brandt AM. *No Magic Bullet.* New York: Oxford University Press; 1985.
75. Kretzschmar M, Welte R, van den HA, Postma MJ. Comparative model-based analysis of screening programs for *Chlamydia trachomatis* infections. *Am J Epidemiol.* 2001;153:90–101.
76. Calonge N. Screening for syphilis infection: recommendation statement. *Ann Fam Med.* 2004;2:362–365.
77. Sexually transmitted diseases treatment guidelines 2002. Centers for Disease Control and Prevention. *MMWR Recomm Rep.* 2002;51:1–78.

78. Stray-Pedersen B. Economic evaluation of maternal screening to prevent congenital syphilis. *Sex Transm Dis*. 1983;10:167–172.
79. Garland SM, Kelly VN. Is antenatal screening for syphilis worth while? *Med J Aust*. 1989;151:368,370,372.
80. Kahn RH, Voigt RF, Swint E, Weinstock H. Early syphilis in the United States identified in corrections facilities, 1999–2002. *Sex Transm Dis*. 2004;31:360–364.
81. Schachter J, Chernesky MA, Willis DE, et al. Vaginal swabs are the specimens of choice when screening for *Chlamydia trachomatis* and *Neisseria gonorrhoeae*: results from a multicenter evaluation of the APTIMA assays for both infections. *Sex Transm Dis*. 2005;32:725–728.
82. Andersen B, Ostergaard L, Sorensen H, et al. Diagnosis of urogenital *Chlamydia trachomatis* infections by home-obtained, mailed samples: do we need a telephone hotline for information and advice? *Scand J Infect Dis*. 2002;34:262–266.
83. Sparks R, Helmers JR, Handsfield HH, et al. Rescreening for gonorrhea and chlamydial infection through the mail: a randomized trial. *Sex Transm Dis*. 2004;31:113–116.
84. Gaydos A, Barnes M, Dwyer K, Rizzo-Price P, Wood BJ, Flemming T, Hogan T. Can the internet be used to facilitate screening for *Chlamydia trachomatis* by reaching non-clinic populations. ISSTDR. 2005.
    Ref Type: Conference Proceeding
85. Rietmeijer CA, Yamaguchi KJ, Ortiz CG, et al. Feasibility and yield of screening urine for *Chlamydia trachomatis* by polymerase chain reaction among high-risk male youth in field-based and other nonclinic settings. A new strategy for sexually transmitted disease control. *Sex Transm Dis*. 1997;24:429–435.
86. Ciesielski C, Kahn RH, Taylor M, Gallagher K, Prescott LJ, Arrowsmith S. Control of syphilis outbreaks in men who have sex with men: the role of screening in nonmedical settings. *Sex Transm Dis*. 2005;32:S37–S42.
87. Kissinger P, Mohammed H, Richardson-Alston G, et al. Patient-delivered partner treatment for male urethritis: a randomized, controlled trial. *Clin Infect Dis*. 2005;41:623–629.
88. Peterman TA, Tian LH, Metcalf CA, et al. High incidence of new sexually transmitted infections in the year following a sexually transmitted infection: a case for rescreening. *Ann Intern Med*. 2006;145:564–572.
89. Wawer MJ, Sewankambo NK, Serwadda D, et al. Control of sexually transmitted diseases for AIDS prevention in Uganda: a randomised community trial. Rakai Project Study Group [comment]. *Lancet*. 1999;353:525–535.
90. Rekart ML, Patrick DM, Chakraborty B, et al. Targeted mass treatment for syphilis with oral azithromycin. *Lancet*. 2003;361:313–314.
91. Jaffe HW, Rice DT, Voigt R, Fowler J, St John RK. Selective mass treatment in a venereal disease control program. *Am J Public Health*. 1979;69:1181–1182.
92. Joesoef MR, Valleroy LA, Kuntjoro TM, et al. Risk profile of female sex workers who participate in a routine penicillin prophylaxis programme in Surabaya, Indonesia. *Int J STD AIDS*. 1998;9:756–760.
93. Steen R, Vuylsteke B, DeCoito T, et al. Evidence of declining STD prevalence in a South African mining community following a core-group intervention. *Sex Transm Dis*. 2000;27:1–8.
94. Rosenberg MJ, Phillips RS, Holmes MD. Vaginal douching, who and why? *J Reprod Med*. 1991;36:753–758.
95. Foch BJ, McDaniel ND, Chacko MR. Racial differences in vaginal douching knowledge; attitude; and practices among sexually active adolescents. *J Pediatr Adolesc Gynecol*. 2001;13:29–33.
96. Martino JL, Vermund SH. Vaginal douching: evidence for risks or benefits to women's health. *Epidemiol Rev*. 2002;24:109–124.
97. Reed BD, Ford K, Wirawan DN. The Bali STD/AIDS study: association between vaginal hygiene practices and STDs among sex workers. *Sex Transm Dis*. 2001;77:46–52.

96 Stuart Berman and Mary L. Kamb

98. Joesoef MR, Sumampouw H, Linnan M, Schmid S, Idajadi A, St. Louis ME. Douching and sexually transmitted diseases in pregnant women in Surabaya, Indonesia. *Am J Obstet Gynecol.* 1996;174:115–119.
99. Cottrell BH. Vaginal douching. *J Obstet Gynecol Neonatal Nurs.* 2003;32:12–18.
100. Oh MK, Merchant JS, Brown P. Douching behavior in high-risk adolescents. What do they use, when and why do they douche? *J Pediatr Adolesc Gynecol.* 2002;15:83–88.
101. Scholes D, Stergachis A, Ichikawa LE, Heidrich FE, Holmes KK, Stamm WE. Vaginal douching as a risk factor for cervical *Chlamydia trachomatis* infection. *Obstet Gynecol.* 1998;91:993–997.
102. Scholes D, Daling JR, Stergachis A, Weiss NS, Wang SP, Grayston JT. Vaginal douching as a risk factor for acute pelvic inflammatory disease. *Obstet Gynecol.* 1993;81:601–606.
103. Martino JL, Youngpairoj S, Vermund SH. Vaginal douching: personal practices and public policies. *J Womens Health (Larchmt).* 2004;13:1048–1065.
104. Brunham RC. Parran Award Lecture: insights into the epidemiology of sexually transmitted diseases from Ro = betacD. *Sex Transm Dis.* 2005;32:722–724.
105. Holmes W. Investigating widely available substances as vaginal microbicides. *Sex Health.* 2004;1:73–79.
106. Alliance for Microbicide Development. 2006. 5-31-2006.
Ref Type: Internet Communication
107. Cohen MS, Anderson DJ. Genitourinary mucosal defences. In: Holmes KK, et al., eds. *Sexually Transmitted Diseases,* 3rd ed. New York: McGraw Hill; 1999:173–180.
108. Peterman TA, Stoneburner RL, Allen JR, Jaffe HW, Curran JW. Risk of human immunodeficiency virus transmission from heterosexual adults with transfusion-associated infections. *JAMA.* 1988;259:55–58.
109. Padian NS, Shiboski SC, Glass SO, Vittinghoff E. Heterosexual transmission of human immunodeficiency virus (HIV) in northern California: results from a ten-year study. *Am J Epidemiol.* 1997;146:350–357.
110. Bolan G, Ehrhardt AA, Wasserheit JN. Gender perspectives and STDs. In: Holmes KK, et al., eds. *Sexually Transmitted Diseases,* 3rd ed. New York: McGraw Hill; 1999:121–122.
111. Sacks SL, Griffiths PD, Corey L, et al. HSV-2 transmission. *Antiviral Res.* 2004;63(suppl 1):S27–S35.
112. Paavonen J. Physiology and ecology of the vagina. *Scand J Infect Dis Suppl.* 1983;40:31–35.
113. Hillier SL. Normal vaginal flora. In: Holmes KK, et al., eds. *Sexually Transmitted Diseases,* 3rd ed. New York: McGraw Hill; 1999:191–203.
114. Hillier SL. The vaginal microbial ecosystem and resistance to HIV. *AIDS Res Hum Retroviruses.* 1998;14(suppl 1):S17–S21.
115. Mardh PA. The vaginal ecosystem. *Am J Obstet Gynecol.* 1991;165:1163–1168.
116. Martin HL, Richardson BA, Nyange PM, et al. Vaginal lactobacilli, microbial flora, and risk of human immunodeficiency virus type 1 and sexually transmitted disease acquisition. *J Infect Dis.* 1999;180:1863–1868.
117. Hillier SL. The vaginal microbial ecosystem and resistance to HIV. [Review] [27 refs]. *AIDS Research & Human Retroviruses.* 1998;14(suppl 1):S17–S21.
118. Hillier SL. The vaginal microbial ecosystem and resistance to HIV. *AIDS Research & Human Retroviruses.* 1998;14(suppl 1):S17–S21.
119. Melis GB, Ibba MT, Steri B, Kotsonis P, Matta V, Paoletti AM. Role of pH as a regulator of vaginal physiological environment. *Minerva Ginecol.* 2000;52:111–121.
120. Denenberg R. HIV and the vaginal ecosystem. *GMHC Treat Issues.* 1997;11:8–10.
121. Hillier SL. The vaginal microbial ecosystem and resistance to HIV. [Review] [27 refs]. *AIDS Research & Human Retroviruses.* 1998;14(suppl 1):S17–S21.

122. Stone KM. Barrier methods for the prevention of sexually transmitted diseases. In: Holmes KK, ed. *Sexually Transmitted Diseases*, 3rd ed. New York: McGraw Hill; 1999:1307–1321.

123. Stone KM. HIV, other STDs, and barriers. In: Mauck CK, ed. *Barrier Contraceptives: Current Status and Future Prospects*. New York: Wiley-Liss; 1994.

124. Warner L, Stone KM, Macaluso M, Buehler JW, Austin HD. Condom use and risk of gonorrhea and chlamydia: a systematic review of design and measurement factors assessed in epidemiologic studies. *Sex Transm Dis*. 2006;33:36–51.

125. Warner DL, Hatcher RA, Steiner M. Condoms. In: Hatcher RA, Trussell J, Stewart FH, eds. *Contraceptive Technology*. 18th ed. New York: Ardent Media; 2004.

126. Pinkerton SD, Abramson PR. Effectiveness of condoms in preventing HIV transmission. *Soc Sci Med*. 1997;44:1303–1312.

127. Weller S, Davis K. Condom effectiveness in reducing heterosexual HIV transmission. *Cochrane Database Syst Rev*. 2001;CD003255.

128. Wald A, Langenberg AG, Link K, et al. Effect of condoms on reducing the transmission of herpes simplex virus type 2 from men to women. *JAMA*. 2001;285:3100–3106.

129. Holmes KK, Levine R, Weaver M. Effectiveness of condoms in preventing sexually transmitted infections. *Bull World Health Organ*. 2004;82:454–461.

130. Manhart LE, Koutsky LA. Do condoms prevent genital HPV infection, external genital warts, or cervical neoplasia? A meta-analysis. *Sex Transm Dis*. 2002;29:725–735.

131. Zenilman JM, Weisman CS, Rompalo AM, et al. Condom use to prevent incident STDs: the validity of self-reported condom use. *Sex Transm Dis*. 1995;22:15–21.

132. Jessamine PG, Plummer FA, Ndinya Achola JO, et al. Human immunodeficiency virus, genital ulcers and the male foreskin: synergism in HIV-1 transmission. *Scand J Infect Dis Suppl*. 1990;69:181–186.

133. Potter WD, De Villemeur M. Clinical breakage, slippage and acceptability of a new commercial polyurethane condom: a randomized, controlled study. *Contraception*. 2003;69:39–45.

134. Drew WL, Blair M, Miner RC, Conant M. Evaluation of the virus permeability of a new condom for women. *Sex Transm Dis*. 1990;17:110–112.

135. Minnis AM, Padian NS. Effectiveness of female controlled barrier methods in preventing sexually transmitted infections and HIV: current evidence and future research directions. *Sex Transm Infect*. 2005;81:193–200.

136. Elias C, Coggins C. Acceptability research on female-controlled barrier methods to prevent heterosexual transmission of HIV: Where have we been? Where are we going? *J Womens Health Gend Based Med*. 2001;10:163–173.

137. Artz L, Macaluso M, Brill I, et al. Effectiveness of an intervention promoting the female condom to patients at sexually transmitted disease clinics. *Am J Public Health*. 2000;90:237–244.

138. World Health Organization. The safety and feasibility of female condom reuse: report of a WHO consultation. January 28–29, 2002, 1–18. 2002. Geneva, World Health Organization. Ref Type: Report.

139. Potter B, Gerofi J, Pope M, Farley T. Structural integrity of the polyurethane female condom after multiple cycles of disinfection, washing, drying and relubrication. *Contraception*. 2003;67:65–72.

140. Buchbinder SP, Vittinghoff E, Heagerty PJ, et al. Sexual risk, nitrite inhalant use, and lack of circumcision associated with HIV seroconversion in men who have sex with men in the United States. *J Acquir Immune Defic Syndr*. 2005;39:82–89.

141. Gibson S, McFarland W, Wohlfeiler D, et al. Experiences of 100 men who have sex with men using the Reality condom for anal sex. *AIDS Educ Prev*. 1999;1:65–71.

142. Renzi C, Tabet SR, Stucky JA, et al. Safety and acceptability of the Reality condom for anal sex among men who have sex with men. *AIDS*. 2003;17:727–731.
143. Ellertson C, Burnes M. Reexamining the role of cervical barrier devices. *Outlook*. 2003;20:1–8.
144. Moench TR, Chipato T, Padian NS. Preventing disease by protecting the cervix: the unexplor4ed promise of internal vaginal barrier devices. *AIDS*. 2001;15:1595–1602.
145. Kreiss J, Ngugi E, Holmes K, et al. Efficacy of nonoxynol 9 contraceptive sponge use in preventing heterosexual acquisition of HIV in Nairobi prostitutes. *JAMA*. 1992;168:477–482.
146. Posner SF, van der SA, Kang MS, Padian N, Chipato T. Introducing Diaphragms into the mix: what happens to male condom use patterns? *AIDS Behav*. 2005;1–7.
147. D'Cruz OJ, Uckum FM. Clinical development of microbicides for the prevention of HIV infection. *Curr Pharm Des*. 2004;10:315–336.
148. Dhawan D, Maher KH. Microbicides to prevent HIV transmission: overcoming obstacles to chemical barrier protection. *Journal of Infectious Diseases*. 2006;193:36–44.
149. Keller MJ, Zerhouni-Layachi B, Cheshenko N, et al. PRO 2000 gel inhibits HIV and herpes simplex virus infection following vaginal application: a double-blind placebo-controlled trial. *Journal of Infectious Diseases*. 2006;193:27–35.
150. Wilkinson D, Ramjee G, Tholandi M, Rutherford G. Nonoxynol-9 for preventing vaginal acquisition of HIV infection by women from men. *Cochrane Database Syst Rev*. 2002;CD003936.
151. Wilkinson D, Tholandi M, Ramjee G, Rutherfold GW. Nonoxynol-9 spermicide for prevention of vaginally acquired HIV and other sexually transmitted infections: systematic review and meta-analysis of randomised controlled trials including more than 5000 women. *Lancet Infect Dis*. 2002;2:613–617.
152. Stein Z, Susser M. The design of prophylactic trials for HIV: the case of microbicides. *Epidemiology*. 2003;14:80–83.
153. Coplan PM, Mitchnick M, Rosenberg ZF. Regulatory challenges in microbicide development. *Science*. 2004;304:1911–1912.
154. Padian N. Commentary: The design of prophylactic trials for HIV. *Epidemiology*. 2003;14:83–84.
155. Ahmad K. Trial of antiretroviral for HIV prevention on hold. *Lancet Infect Dis*. 2004;4:597.
156. Moses S, Bailey RC, Ronald AR. Male circumcision: assessment of health benefits and risks. *Sex Transm Infect*. 1998;74:368–373.
157. Bailey RC, Plummer FA, Moses S. Male circumcision and HIV prevention: current knowledge and future research directions. *Lancet Infect Dis*. 2001;1:223–231.
158. Cameron DW, Simonsen JN, D'Costa LJ, et al. Female to male transmission of human immunodeficiency virus type 1: risk factors for seroconversion in men. *Lancet*. 1989;2:403–407.
159. Mehendale SM, Shepherd ME, Divekar AD, et al. Evidence for high prevalence & rapid transmission of HIV among individuals attending STD clinics in Pune, India. *Indian J Med Res*. 1996;104:327–335.
160. Diseker RA, III, Peterman TA, Kamb ML, et al. Circumcision and STD in the United States: cross sectional and cohort analyses. *Sex Transm Infect*. 2000;76:474–479.
161. Gray RH, Kiwanuka N, Quinn TC, et al. Male circumcision and HIV acquisition and transmission: cohort studies in Rakai, Uganda. Rakai Project Team. *AIDS*. 2000;14:2371–2381.
162. Kreiss JK, Hopkins SG. The association between circumcision status and human immunodeficiency virus infection among homosexual men. *J Infect Dis*. 1993;168:1404–1408.

163. Auvert B, Taljaard D, Lagarde E, Sobngwi-Tambekou J, Sitta R, Puren A. Randomized, controlled intervention trial of male circumcision for reduction of HIV infection risk: the ANRS 1265 Trial. *PLoS Med*. 2005;2:e298.

164. U.S. National Institutes of Health. Trial of male circumcision: HIV, sexually transmitted disease (STD) and behavioral effects in men, women and the community. National Institutes of Health. 2006. Ref Type: Electronic Citation.

165. U.S. National Institutes of Health. Male circumcision and HIV rates in Kenya. National Institutes of Health. 2006. Ref Type: Electronic Citation.

166. Lavreys L, Rakwar JP, Thompson ML, et al. Effect of circumcision on incidence of human immunodeficiency virus type 1 and other sexually transmitted diseases: a prospective cohort study of trucking company employees in Kenya. *J Infect Dis*. 1999;180:330–336.

167. Todd J, Munguti K, Grosskurth H, et al. Risk factors for active syphilis and TPHA seroconversion in a rural African population. *Sex Transm Infect*. 2001;77:37–45.

168. Persaud V. Geographical pathology of cancer of the uterine cervix. *Trop Geogr Med*. 1977;29:335–345.

169. Castellsague X, Bosch FX, Munoz N, et al. Male circumcision, penile human papillomavirus infection, and cervical cancer in female partners. *N Engl J Med*. 2002;346:1105–1112.

170. Castellsague X, Peeling RW, Franceschi S, et al. *Chlamydia trachomatis* infection in female partners of circumcised and uncircumcised adult men. *Am J Epidemiol*. 2005;162:907–916.

171. Reynolds S, et al. Circumcision and the risks of female HIV and STD acquisition in Rakai, Uganda. 13th Conference on Retroviruses and Opportunistic Infections, Denver, Colorado, February 8, 2006. Ref Type: Conference Proceeding.

172. Siegfried N. Does male circumcision prevent HIV infection? *PLoS Med*. 2005;2:e393.

173. Foster IM, Bartlett J. Anti-HIV substances for rape victims. *JAMA*. 1989;261:3407.

174. Bartlett JG, Finkbeiner AK. *The guide to living with HIV infection. Developed at Johns Hopkins AIDS Clinic*. Baltimore: Johns Hopkins University Press; 1993.

175. Short RV. New ways of preventing HIV infection: thinking simply, simply thinking. *Phil Trans R Soc B*. 2006;1–10.

176. Oyelola OO, Ayangade SO, Amole F. In vitro inhibition of sperm motility by some local mineral water drinks. *Contraception*. 1987;36:435–440.

177. Imade GE, Sagay AS, Onwuliri VA, et al. Use of lemon or lime juice douches in women in Jos, Nigeria. *Sex Health*. 2005;2:237–239.

178. Bourne N, Stegall R, Montano R, Meador M, Stanberry LR, Millagan GN. Efficacy and toxicity of zinc salts as candidate topical microbicides against vaginal herpes simplex virus type 2 infection. *Antimicrob Agents Chemother*. 2005;49:1181–1183.

179. Neri A, Sabah G, Samra Z. Bacterial vaginosis in pregnancy treated with yoghurt. *Obstet Gynecol Scand*. 1993;72:17–19.

180. Epigee Women's Health website encouraging use of yoghurt for vaginal infection. Epigee Women's Health. 2006. Ref Type: Electronic Citation.

181. Moore A, McQuay H, Muir Gray JA. Bandolier: evidence based health care. *Bandolier: Evidence based thinking about health care*. 1999;60:2–4. Accessible at: http://www.jr2.ox.ac.uk/bandolier/band60/b60-3.html.

182. Patton DL, Cosgrove Sweeney YT, Antonio MA, Rabe LK, Hillier SL. Lactobacillus crispatus capsules: single-use safety study in the Macaca nemestrina model. *Sex Transm Dis*. 2003;30:568–570.

183. Holzman C, Leventhal JM, Qui H, et al. Factors linked to bacterial vaginosis in nonpregnant women. *Am J Public Health*. 2001;91:1664–1670.

184. Ness RB, Hillier SL, Richter HE, et al. Douching in relation to bacterial vaginosis, lactobacilli, and facultative bacteria in the vagina. *Obstet Gynecol.* 2002;2002:765.

185. Ness RB, Soper DE, Holley RL, et al. Douching and endometritis: results from the PID evaluation and clinical health (PEACH) survey. *Sex Transm Dis.* 2001;28:240–245.

186. Kao JH, Chen DS. Global control of hepatitis B virus infection. *Lancet Infect Dis.* 2002;2:395–403.

187. Koutsky LA, Ault KA, Wheeler CM, et al. A controlled trial of a human papillomavirus type 16 vaccine. *N Engl J Med.* 2002;347:1645–1651.

188. Harper DM, Franco EL, Wheeler C, et al. Efficacy of a bivalent L1 virus-like particle vaccine in prevention of infection with human papillomavirus types 16 and 18 in young women: a randomised controlled trial. *Lancet.* 2004;364:1757–1765.

189. Guerrant RL, Sears CL, Ravdin JI. Intestinal protozoa: *Giardia lamblia, Entamoeba Histolytica,* Cryptosporidium and new emerging protozoal infections. In: KK Holmes, et al., eds. *Sexually Transmitted Diseases.* 3rd ed. McGraw-Hill; 1999:613–614.

190. Krieger JN, Alderete JF. *Trichomonas vaginalis* and trichomoniasis. In: Holmes KK, ed. *Sexually Transmitted Diseases,* 3rd ed. McGraw-Hill; 1999:590–591.

191. Telenti A, Ioannidis JPA. Susceptibility to HIV infection—disentangling host genetics and host behavior. *Journal of Infectious Diseases.* 2006;193:4–6.

192. Mazzoli S, Trabattoni D, Lo CS, et al. HIV-specific mucosal and cellular immunity in HIV-seronegative partners of HIV-seropositive individuals. *Nat Med.* 1997;3:1250–1257.

193. Hadler SC, Francis DP, Maynard JE, et al. Long-term immunogenicity and efficacy of hepatitis B vaccine in homosexual men. *N Engl J Med.* 1986;315:209–214.

194. Szmuness W, et al. Hepatitis B vaccine: demonstration of efficacy in a controlled clinical trial in a high-risk population in the United States. *N Engl J Med.* 1980;3030:833.

195. Francis DP, Hadler SC, Thompson SE, et al. The prevention of hepatitis B with vaccine. Report of the centers for disease control multi-center efficacy trial among homosexual men. *Ann Intern Med.* 1982;97:362–366.

196. Villa LL, Costa RL, Petta CA, et al. Prophylactic quadrivalent human papillomavirus (types 6, 11, 16, and 18) L1 virus-like particle vaccine in young women: a randomised double-blind placebo-controlled multicentre phase II efficacy trial. *Lancet Oncol.* 2005;6:271–278.

197. Kahn JA, Zimet GD, Bernstein DI, et al. Pediatricians' intention to administer human papillomavirus vaccine: the role of practice characteristics, knowledge, and attitudes. *J Adolesc Health.* 2005;37:502–510.

198. Zenilman JM, Miller WC, Gaydos C, Rogers SM, Turner CF. LCR testing for gonorrhoea and chlamydia in population surveys and other screenings of low prevalence populations: coping with decreased positive predictive value. *Sex Transm Dis.* 2003;79:94–97.

199. Grimes DA, Schulz KF. Uses and abuses of screening tests. *Lancet.* 2002;359:881–884.

200. Trussell J, Warner DL, Hatcher RA. Condom slippage and breakage rates. *Fam Plann Perspect.* 1992;24:20–23.

201. Broom CV. Epidemiology of toxic shock syndrome in the United States: overview. *Review of Infectious Diseases.* 1989;11:S14–S21.

202. WHO/CONRAD technical consultation on nonoxynol-9, World Health Organization, Geneva, 9-10 October 2001: summary report. *Reprod Health Matters.* 2002;10:175–181.

203. Foss AM, Vicerman PT, Heise L, et al. Shifts in condom use following microbicide introduction: should we be concerned? *AIDS.* 2003;17:1227–1237.

204. American Academy of Pediatrics: Report of the Task Force on Circumcision. *Pediatrics.* 1989;84:388–391.
205. Neonatal circumcision revisited. Fetus and Newborn Committee, Canadian Paediatric Society. *CMAJ.* 1996;154:769–780.
206. MacCoun RJ. Toward a psychology of harm reduction. *American Psychologist.* 1998;53:1199–1208.
207. Peterman TA, Lin LS, Newman DR, et al. Does measured behavior reflect STD risk? An analysis of data from a randomized controlled behavioral intervention study. Project RESPECT Study Group. *Sex Transm Dis.* 2000;28:446–451.
208. Hemenway D. *Prices and Choices: Microeconomic Vignettes,* 2nd ed. Cambridge, MA:Ballinger; 1988.
209. Bartholow BN, et al. HIV sexual risk behavior over 36 months of follow-up in the world's first HIV vaccine efficacy trial. *J Acquir Immune Defic Syndr.* 2005;39:90–101.
210. Gray RH, Li X, Wawer MJ, et al. Stochastic simulation of the impact of anti-retroviral therapy and HIV vaccines on HIV transmission; Rakai, Uganda. *AIDS.* 2003;17:1941–1951.

Part 2

Intervention Approaches

Dyadic, Small Group, and Community-Level Behavioral Interventions for STD/HIV Prevention

Donna Hubbard McCree, Ph.D., M.P.H., R.P.h, Agatha Eke, Ph.D., and Samantha P. Williams, Ph.D.

STD/HIV prevention efforts, including education, information, and counseling, have frequently been used to motivate individuals to reduce their risk behaviors. Many of these prevention approaches are drawn from theories that link risk behavior to individual psychological processes such as cognition, beliefs, attitudes, self-efficacy, and perception of risk (1). Although these approaches can help individuals initiate risk-reduction steps and make short-term changes in their risk behaviors, most individual beliefs, attitudes, and, ultimately, behaviors are influenced by the larger environmental and community contexts within which they reside (2). Therefore, long-lasting maintenance of protective behaviors is likely only when peer group social norms, relationships, the environment, and public health policies support personal behavior change effort (2,3). Thus, prevention may also target the community, or special groups of individuals at higher risk for, or more vulnerable to STD/HIV (4). This chapter will focus on and provide examples of STD/HIV interventions that target couples, small groups, and communities.

Utilization of the "Group" Format to Facilitate Behavioral Change

A classic definition of a "group" is a collection of 3–15 interdependent members with a common goal and who meet face-to-face, or in such a way as to develop personal relationships with one another. The group should have perceived boundaries and regular interaction (5). Although this definition has stood the test of time in group communication literature, it does not describe the structure of small groups that have been constructed for empirical purposes. In the intervention modality, group members may not have had prior relationships, and the group interactions may not lead to interpersonal connections. According to Bormann (6), an aggregation does not become a small group until the participants have communicated enough to form a structure and impression of one another. Ideally, the structure and impressions of a group develop over time through norms that may evolve shared experiences and behaviors so that it becomes difficult to distinguish between group members and nonmembers. In this respect, the definition of group may best fit larger

Behavioral Interventions for Prevention and Control of Sexually Transmitted Diseases. Aral SO, Douglas JM Jr, eds. Lipshutz JA, assoc ed. New York: Springer Science+ Business Media, LLC; 2007.

group structures such as communities, or natural groups that were formed prior to empirical engagement.

The purpose of the "group" format for behavior change interventions is to 1) disseminate information to a number of people in a similar manner, and 2) to utilize the social interactions among them to both enhance the likelihood of acquiring new information and skills and facilitate behavioral change. The group format for behavioral interventions enables the group members to learn with and from each other in a "safe" environment. Establishment of a "safe" environment is particularly important for the types of behavioral interventions most often implemented for STD/HIV prevention, especially when sexuality-related topics are discussed.

Group level interventions can be utilized in a variety of settings such as health departments, community-based organizations, private health care settings such as a physician's office, and nontraditional venues such as a community center or apartment complex. However, the specific type of group intervention format may vary depending on the intervention targets (to whom), facilitators (by whom), purpose (why), timing (when), and location (where).

In STD/HIV prevention interventions, efforts are made to assemble groups with members who have similar backgrounds and/or risk profiles and who are gathered together in the same place or at the same time (7). The basic assumption behind STD/HIV prevention interventions that target groups is that some individuals require interventions specifically tailored for their circumstances in order to adopt or change to healthy behaviors (7). The intent of group-level interventions is to assist individuals in learning and applying skills that will reduce a risk behavior or address a factor that influences behavior. The three types of interventions that will be discussed in this chapter are dyadic, small-group, and community-level interventions. Dyadic interventions are those that target couples, irrespective of gender. This particular format is most closely related to a counseling modality and has been more recently used in interventions that target HIV discordant and concordant partners (8). Small-group interventions are those that target more than two individuals meeting together for an identified purpose (9), and have been used most often to attempt to efficiently disseminate and train same-gender groups to adopt and engage in self-protective sexual behaviors (10). Community-level interventions are those that target pre-existing groups that have established but not explicit norms, rituals, and histories such as organizations and neighborhoods. The aim of community-level interventions is to induce widespread and durable behavior change throughout the target population (11–13). Community-level interventions may require the most immediate and long-term time investment out of the three intervention formats. This is due to both the broader audience focus and the difficulty of affecting norms via individual-level efforts. Proximity and social exchange between the intervention targets and facilitators increases the chances that dyadic and small-group interventions will identify and transform risk behavior. However, such individual-level behavior changes are most likely to endure when analogous normative changes exist in the environmental context. This supposition is part of the foundation of social theories such as, "Diffusion of Innovations," which states that at least 15% of the members in a social context must be exposed to a behavioral change message in order for the message to diffuse through the environment and create a new norm that supports the new protective behaviors (14). Both individual behaviors and influencing normative beliefs, needless to say, can be difficult to impact, hence the importance and need for community-level interventions, as well as for multi-level interventions, which, when simultaneously implemented, can facilitate the desired change (see Chapter 2 of this book).

Examples of Interventions

Dyadic Interventions

Dyadic interventions focus on the salience of couple relationships or the sexual dyad as the contexts where social-behavioral and other factors shape sexual relations and the risk for STDs including HIV (15). These interventions differ from individual-level interventions in that they include both members of the sexual dyad in the behavior-change effort, occur in the context of relationship dynamics, and often focus on communication patterns between partners within the dyad (16–19). Because couple-based interventions encourage collaboration between members of the sexual dyad in addressing mutual needs, they may be more effective in fostering communication patterns that initiate and sustain HIV/STD prevention methods such as condom use (16–17). El-Bassel et al. (16) suggest that HIV/STD couple-based interventions delivered to the couple together may be more effective than those delivered to one partner alone because they provide a safer, less threatening environment for individuals to introduce safer sexual practices without fear of negative reactions, they eliminate the expectation for individuals to convey new knowledge and skills to their sexual partners, and may provide a supportive environment for partners to disclose personal information like extradyadic relationships and STD history.

There are unique challenges to successful implementation of dyadic interventions because they focus on both members of the sexual dyad. Successful implementation of these types of interventions is directly related to the stability and longevity of the relationship between the partners (18) and the ability to recruit both partners and particularly male sex partners of females into the intervention (18,20) Additionally, the study protocol must address issues that are unique to STD/HIV prevention efforts focused on couples, including gender-based issues of power and control in sexual relationships and methods for addressing concerns about infidelity and lack of trust and the threat of intimate partner violence that might occur because of the sensitive nature surrounding disclosure of STD/HIV risk behaviors (21,20). Finally, recruitment of couples into interventions can present major challenges to successful implementation especially for those interventions that target minority (i.e., African-American and Latino) couples. There are few published studies of effective recruitment strategies for couple-based interventions; most of the available literature has focused on marital and family therapy interventions that target Caucasian couples (20). Successful strategies for recruiting couples into interventions have elicited input and feedback from the target community, included cultural relevance in the recruitment strategies, utilized study protocols that were sensitive to participants' safety and confidentiality, and included recruitment schedules that were flexible for and accommodating of the target community (21).

There are few published studies of HIV/STD behavioral interventions that target couples; most have been conducted outside the United States (18). Four examples of published dyadic interventions are provided here. Two are couple-based STD/HIV behavioral interventions—Project Connect and the PARTNERS Project—and two are interventions that target HIV serodiscordant couples—the Voluntary Counseling and Testing Efficacy Study and the Zambia-UAB HIV Research Project. A more detailed description of each is provided in Table 1.

Project Connect (16) was a randomized clinical trial designed to test the efficacy of a six-session HIV/STD relationship-based intervention and examine whether the intervention was more effective when provided to couples or to the woman alone. The goal of the intervention was to increase condom use, decrease STD transmission and reduce the number of sexual partners among heterosexual couples. The intervention was based on the AIDS Risk-Reduction Model—a conceptual framework for organizing behavioral change information and HIV risk-reduction skills—and the ecological perspective—a perspective that emphasizes factors from the individual to macro level that influence behavior (16). Study findings from the three-month follow-up suggested that the intervention was efficacious in reducing the number of unprotected sexual acts and increasing the number of protected sexual acts. There was no significant difference, however, in the study outcomes between women who received the intervention alone and those who received it with their partners (16). Data from the 12-month follow-up provided evidence of sustained efficacy for the intervention over time as there was also a reduction in the number of unprotected sex acts at 12-months post-intervention (22). However, there was still no significant difference in this outcome between women who received the intervention alone and those who received it with their partners.

The PARTNERS Project (17) was a couple-based intervention designed to reduce the risk of STDs including HIV and unintended pregnancy among young Hispanic women and their male partners. Couples enrolled in the study received either a risk-reduction intervention or the community educational standard of care. The intervention was based on Fishbein's Integrated Behavior Change Model (23) and the Information-Motivation-Behavioral Skills Model of HIV/AIDS Risk Reduction (24), and it focused on skills training in risk reduction (condom use, mutual monogamy, use of effective contraceptives) and interactive skills-based activities including behavioral modeling and role-playing. The major behavioral outcomes were number of unprotected vaginal sex acts in the past 90 days and the consistency of condom and contraceptive use with the main partner. Study findings showed no significant intervention effect for condom or contraceptive use; both study groups reported increased condom and contraceptive use at follow-up.

The Voluntary HIV Counseling and Testing Efficacy Study (25,26) was a three-site randomized clinical trial designed to test the efficacy of voluntary HIV counseling and testing given to individuals and couples in reducing risk behavior associated with the sexual transmission of HIV-1 in developing countries. The trial was conducted between 1995 and 1998 in Kenya, Tanzania, and Trinidad, and the primary outcome was self-reported unprotected intercourse with a nonprimary partner. Couples in the study were randomly assigned to receive VCT or basic health information. VCT was based on the client-centered HIV-1 counseling model (25,26), which includes personalized risk assessment and development of a personalized risk assessment plan for each participant. Study findings showed that participants in the VCT group reduced the incidence of unprotected intercourse with their enrollment partners and

Table 1 Group interventions: table of evidence.

Study	Setting and study population	Study design	Intervention and control	Study outcome
Corey, Wald, Sacks, et al. (65)	1484 immunocompetent, heterosexual monogamous couples serodiscordant for HSV-2; 96 study sites in United States, Canada, Europe, Latin America, and Australia	Randomized, placebo-controlled trial; 2 groups	Intervention—500 mg of valacyclovir once daily; Comparison—placebo; both for 8 months	Risk of HSV-2 transmission significantly reduced in intervention group
The Voluntary HIV-1 Counseling and Testing Efficacy Study Group (26)	3120 individuals and 586 couples; three study sites—Kenya, Tanzania, and Trinidad	Randomized clinical trial; couples randomized together	Intervention—VCT (based on CDC client-centered HIV-1 counseling model); Control—health information video and discussion about HIV-1 transmission and condom use; biological samples for HIV-1 and STDs	Couples in VCT group reduced unprotected sex with enrolled partner; couples in which one or both partners were diagnosed with HIV-1 were more likely to reduce acts of unprotected intercourse.
Allen, Meinsen-Derr, Kautuzman, et al. (27)	963 cohabiting heterosexual HIV serodiscordant couples; VCT center, Lusaka, Zambia	Single-site clinical trial	Intervention-confidential VCT including free treatment for syphilis, condoms skills training and free condoms; Comparison group—concordant HIV-negative couples; biological markers	Sustained but imperfect condom use in HIV serodiscordant couples; biological markers showed underreporting of unprotected sex acts
El-Bassel, Witte, Gilbert, et al. (16)	217 heterosexual couples; hospital-based clinics in Bronx, New York.	Randomized clinical trial	6 session intervention with 3 conditions: 1) couple condition—women and partner receive intervention; 2) women-alone condition—only woman receives intervention; 3) education control condition—women alone in one HIV/STD information session	Reduced proportion of unprotected and increase proportion of protected sexual acts; no significant difference between couples who received the intervention together and women who received the intervention alone

(Continued)

Table 1 Group interventions: table of evidence.—Cont'd

Study	Study design	Setting and study population	Intervention and control	Study outcome
Harvey, Henderson, Thornburn, et al. (17)	Randomized behavioral trial	146 mostly Hispanic couples; Los Angeles and Oklahoma city	Intervention—3-session, couple-based, skills training, behavior modeling role-playing and games; Comparison—community educational standard of care for STD prevention and unintended pregnancy	No difference between the two groups in terms of consistent condom use, effective contraceptive use, and frequency of unprotected sex
Cohen, MacKinnon, Dent, Mason, Sullivan (66)	Single-session group discussion	426 adults, majority African American and men; waiting room of Los Angeles STD clinic	Intervention group –video group on condom use and a health educator-facilitated group discussion on STD prevention methods and condom use; Comparison group—usual STD services	Men in intervention group had lower STD reinfection rates; no evidence of change for women.
DiClemente, Wingood (30)	Randomized controlled behavioral trial	128, 18–29 year old sexually active African-American women; community center setting in Bayview-Hunter's Point, San Francisco	Intervention group—Five weekly 2-hour small group sessions on gender and ethnic pride, sexual decision making, sexual assertiveness and communication training, condom use and cognitive coping skills; intervention given to comparison group at later time	Women in intervention more likely to report consistent condom use with partners, negotiating condom use, and not having sex when condoms not available.
El-Bassel, Schilling (67)	Randomized behavioral trial	84 female methadone patients, African American and Hispanic; methadone maintenance clinics in New York City	Intervention—Five 2-hour sessions with information on AIDS transmission and prevention; condom use; and assertiveness training, problem solving and communication skills; Comparison–group HIV/AIDS information only	Significant increase in condom use with partners among women in intervention group

Kelly, Murphy, Washington, Wilson et al. (68)	Randomized behavioral trial	197 women, mostly African American; inner-city health clinics in Milwaukee	Intervention—4-weekly 90 minute sessions based on cognitive-behavioral and risk reduction skills training principles and peer support; Comparison group—family and child nutrition intervention	Increase in condom use with partners and decrease in frequency of engaging in unprotected sex for women in intervention group
O'Donnell, O'Donnell, San Doval, et al. (69)	Behavioral trial—Video Opportunities for Innovative Condom Education and Safer Sex (VOICES/VOCES)	2004 adult males, mostly African American and Hispanic; STD clinic in South Bronx	Intervention—20-minute video-based intervention in a 60-minute session included risk information, and culturally-specific strategies for encouraging condom use; Comparison—usual STD clinic services	Men in intervention group had significantly lower rates of new STD infections.
St. Lawrence, Brasfield, Jefferson, Alleyne, O'Bannon, Shirley (70)	Behavioral trial	246 inner-city African-American youths; public health clinic in Mississippi	Intervention—8 weekly 90–120 minute sessions based on social learning theory, sessions on AIDS education, sexual decision and values, technical competency skills, social competency skills, cognitive competency skills, and social support and empowerment; Comparison—AIDS education only	Significantly greater condom use and lower frequency of unprotected intercourse among youth in intervention group; delayed sexual onset for abstinent youth in the intervention group

that couples in which one or both members were infected with HIV-1 were more likely to reduce the incidence of unprotected intercourse than couples who were not infected; there were, however, no differences in unprotected intercourse with unenrolled partners (25,26).

The Zambia-UAB HIV Research Project (ZUHRP) was a single-site VCT intervention for cohabiting serodiscordant couples conducted in Lusaka, Zambia (27). The major assessments were condom use before and after VCT, patterns and correlates of condom use after VCT, and biological markers for STDs, including HIV. The study population included a comparison group of concordant HIV-negative couples. Study findings showed that discordant couples reported an increase in condom use after joint VCT and that they maintained the behavior for at least one year. Additionally, results from the biological markers showed that discordant couples underreported their numbers of unprotected sex acts.

Small-Group Interventions

Small groups in STD prevention are defined as collections of individuals (usually <20 members) (9) with similar backgrounds and/or risk profiles who are gathered together in the same place and/or at the same time (e.g., STD clinic patients, persons in drug treatment, incarcerated populations) (7). Small groups can be used as forums for information-exchange, problem-solving, and communication, as well as for providing social support for members (9). Additionally, small groups offer the advantages of face-to-face interaction with peers and an arena for practicing social skills like safer-sex negotiation with others (9). Different group configurations can be utilized, but most fall into the categories of a convenient or convened group.

Convenient groups exist prior to the introduction of an intervention and look more like small communities of people with shared experiences. Susser et al. (28) found considerable risk behaviors among homeless mentally ill men and subsequently initiated a condom-use training intervention with homeless shelter residents. Seal et al. (29) conducted qualitative focus groups with men who played basketball together. The benefit of convenient groups is that the individuals identify as group members and the group's cohesion can facilitate acquisition of skills and knowledge. Convened groups are those that are formed for the sole purpose of the intervention. In this case, the group format is used as an intervention modality where learning occurs via group interactions and activities such as role plays. Ehrhardt et al. (10) used small groups in their Future Is Ours intervention with women who utilized a family planning clinic. DiClemente and Wingood (30) used convened groups in their sexual risk-reduction intervention with African-American women.

Use of convenient and convened groups depends on the sample size, goals of the intervention study, and the theoretical constructs on which the intervention is based. Education-only interventions can be implemented individually or in a group setting. The type of group may not affect members' information acquisition. The same is true for interventions that include skill-building exercises, where members can learn from watching other members. Interventions that attempt to change norms or normative behavior are affected by the type of group utilized in the intervention. Pre-existing groups have pre-existing norms that may act as a barrier (or a facilitator) to behavioral and normative change.

Most STD/HIV prevention interventions that target small groups are based on constructs from social-cognitive and reasoned-action theories. They attempt to increase knowledge about prevention, strengthen behavior-change motivation, and teach risk-reduction skills (18). Additionally, small-group interventions usually are presented in multiple sessions that involve substantial amounts of contact time with participants (18), and are delivered by several methods including role play, group counseling, and interactive discussion (7). They are usually facilitated by a health professional or they are peer led (9). The expected immediate outcomes of these interventions are an increase in skill proficiency and an intention by the participants to use the skills in reducing or changing their STD risk-behavior.

Strengths of small group interventions include the following: 1) transportability to different settings; 2) well-defined protocols that can be implemented and adapted by providers; 3) an approach that allows participants to receive assistance and skills in making changes in complex risk behaviors; 4) the intimacy of individual counseling with the added benefits of peer support; and 5) the opportunity for face-to-face interaction with peers (9,18). Among the limitations are the time commitments required for participants and providers and the limited number of individuals that are reached by these interventions (9,18). Additionally, a major factor in the success of small-group interventions is the strength of the group facilitator (9).

Small-Group Intervention Implementation

Although "the group" is the intervention vehicle, prior to implementation, the intervention must be tailored to the group members. Intervention tailoring can be accomplished through formative work, specifically by matching the intervention with the goals of the study and the needs of the population. Tailored interventions attempt to facilitate risk-reduction change by identifying and utilizing the characteristics that are distinct to the targeted topic, context, and/or population as part of the intervention strategies. Interventions can be tailored to address a specific issue, such as tailoring the Popular Opinion Leader (POL) model (31) for HIV prevention to address syphilis prevention through the creation of syphilis prevention messages. Interventions can also be tailored to address a specific population; using the POL example again, the model was originally tested with gay men, but it can be and has been tailored for women.

Challenges to implementation can be logistical (e.g., timing of the group session) or circumstantial (e.g., group member life events or need), as well as structural (e.g., the location of the sessions) and personal (e.g., the inability of the facilitator to engage the participants). Such challenges, and how they can be addressed, support the importance of publishing lessons learned from both successful and unsuccessful intervention studies. Small-group interventions are ideally implemented in settings where the target group is likely to frequent. Although the health department might appear ideal, negative perceptions associated with attending a public health clinic may prohibit comfortable use by the target population. Thus, alternative settings may be more acceptable. In one study, which intended to enhance the self-protective sexual behaviors of African-American women, a neighborhood family planning clinic was used (10). In another intervention study that targeted gay, lesbian, and bisexual adolescents, gay and lesbian community centers were utilized (32).

Small-Group Intervention Examples

STD clinics are ideal for individual and small-group interventions. A visit to the STD clinic is a "teachable moment" where both infected and uninfected patients can benefit from an intervention effort. At a minimum, STD clinics should provide STD testing and treatment, counseling and testing for HIV services, and patient education materials (33). Although these are standard STD clinic services, if a patient does not test positive for an STD or request a HIV test, he/she may receive little counseling prior to or after STD testing.

Project Respect (34) was one of the few clinic-based intervention studies that demonstrated an effect on risk behavior. The purpose of this multi-method intervention was to compare the effects of two interactive HIV/STD counseling prevention interventions. Prior to this multi-center intervention, the efficacy of counseling to prevent STDs and HIV had not been clearly demonstrated. Participants who visited an STD clinic were randomized to one of three individualized interventions between 1993 and 1996. The intervention conditions consisted of 1) four enhanced counseling sessions, 2) two brief counseling sessions, or 3) two brief encounters analogous to current care. Assessment consisted of a baseline and follow-up questionnaires at 3, 6, 9, and 12 months post-intervention end and STD tests at 6 and 12 months. Using an intent-to-treat analysis, results indicated that self report 100% condom use at 3 and 6 months was higher ($p < .05$) in both the 1) enhanced counseling and 2) brief counseling conditions, compared with participants in condition 3) the brief encounters. Also, 30% fewer participants had new STDs in both the enhanced counseling (7.2%; $p = .002$) and brief counseling (7.3%; $p = .005$) arms compared with those in the didactic messages arm (10.4%) at the six-month STD diagnostic testing period. At the 12-month STD diagnostic, 20% fewer participants in conditions 1 and 2 had new STDs compared with those in condition 3 ($p = .008$). The findings were consistent across the five study sites, similar for men and women and greater for adolescents and persons with an STD diagnosed at enrollment.

Gender- and Age-Specific Group Interventions

Gender- and age-specific group interventions, at a minimum, can fulfill two goals. First, such interventions give participants the opportunity to engage, share, and learn with demographic peers. Second, if the participants have communities and/or networks in common, what is learned during the intervention could disseminate and have a broader effect. For women, one such intervention was "The Future Is Ours Project" (10). The Future Is Ours Project was a gender-specific group intervention for women, which intended to affect the unsafe sexual encounters and strategies of sexually active women. The participants were family planning clients from a high HIV sero-prevalence area in New York City. Women were randomized into one of three conditions: 1) an eight-session, 2) a four-session, or 3) a control condition. Participants were given a baseline assessment and follow-up assessments at 1, six, and 12 months post-intervention. Using an intention-to-treat analysis, women who were assigned to the eight-session group reported three-and-a-half ($p = 0.09$) and five ($p < 0.01$) fewer unprotected sex occasions, during the previous month, at both the 1- and 12-month follow-up. Women in the eight-session group also reported less unprotected vaginal and anal intercourse compared to controls at one month (odds ratio [OR] = 1.93, 95% confidence interval [CI] = 1.07, 3.48, $p = 0.03$) and at 12-month follow-up (OR = 1.65, 95% CI = 0.94, 2.90, $p = 0.08$). Women in the eight-session group also reduced the number of sex occasions at both follow-ups and had greater odds of first-time use of an alternative protective strategy (refusal, outercourse, mutual testing) at one-month follow-up. The authors conclude that gender-specific interventions of sufficient intensity can promote short- and long-term sexual risk reduction of women in a family planning setting.

An example of an intervention that targeted adolescents was conducted by Jemmott and colleagues (35). The intent of this intervention was to determine the efficacy of a skill-based HIV/STD risk-reduction intervention in reducing self-reported, unprotected sexual intercourse of African-American and Latino adolescent girls. Ethnic minority, sexually active adolescent girls were recruited from the adolescent medicine clinic and randomized to receive one of three interventions: 1) HIV/STD prevention information, 2) HIV/STD prevention information and skills, or 3) a control group that addressed health issues unrelated to sexual behavior. Adolescents were given assessments at baseline, 3, 6, and 12 months. Over 680 adolescents were recruited into the study; the retention rate was 88%. Results indicated that there were no differences between the information intervention and the health control condition. Participants in the skills-based intervention reported less unprotected sex than either information only or the control groups ($p = .03$ and $p = .002$, respectively). At the 12-month follow-up, participants in the skills-based group also reported fewer sexual partners ($p = .04$) and were less likely to test positive for STD ($p = .05$). Although no differences in the frequency of unprotected sexual intercourse, the number of partners, or the rate of STD were observed at the 3- or 6-month follow-up between participants in the three conditions, results suggest that skill-based HIV/STD interventions may have a long-term effect on sexual risk behaviors and STD rates of African-American and Latino adolescent girls in clinic settings.

Community-Level Interventions

Community as a concept is based on the notion that society cannot exist and progress without a set of mutual relationships expressing the obligations of individuals to each other and to groups of which they are a part (36). Definitions for "community" are based on geographical or territorial conceptualizations (i.e., people living in the same neighborhood, within the same city, state, or country) or from the perspective of social networks or relationships where people may have shared interests, norms, and values (37). In STD/HIV interventions, community can be the setting, the resource, the agent, or the target of the intervention. When community is the setting for the intervention, the intervention is described as community based (13). In this case, community is primarily defined from a territorial perspective and represents the location in which the intervention was implemented. An intervention is also community-based when the community is the resource for the intervention. Here the intent of the intervention is to mobilize community resources, and promote community participation and ownership in addressing health priorities. When the community is the agent of the intervention, the intent involves mobilization and use of community resources and focuses on working with community insiders. Members of the community take active part in identifying the needs of people in the community and in strategic planning and implementation of interventions and programs that promote the health of the entire community.

When the community serves as a target of the intervention, the intervention can be referred to as community-level intervention. In this case, intervention strategies are directed at entire communities with the aim of creating widespread and durable behavior change throughout the target population (11–13). Community-level interventions in STD/HIV prevention attempt to change norms, attitudes, collective self-efficacy, and risk behaviors in populations vulnerable to disease. They emphasize the use of education to empower people through mediating structures, networks, and community institutions. Community-wide change is achieved through an orchestrated effort aimed at the right target groups, with culturally appropriate messages, for a sustained period of time (2,38). The discussion in this chapter will focus on community-level interventions.

In community-level interventions, the community is recognized as a unit of identity. The health status characteristics of the community rather than individual behaviors and characteristics are targeted. The focus of the interventions is on changing the social milieu, including changing the norms of collectives around relevant risk behaviors. Community-level interventions aim to influence behaviors both by changing social norms regarding risk behaviors and by increasing the social acceptability and support for safer behaviors (39). The effort to promote safer behavior may entail creating a healthy community environment through broad systemic changes in public policy and community-wide institutions and services (13). Thus, community-level interventions may also target the laws, policies, and other structural factors that influence risk behaviors in the community.

Community-level interventions often involve the use of multi-component strategies. They may combine individual and environmental change strategies across multiple settings. For example, a community-level intervention targeting drug using populations for HIV prevention might combine HIV testing and counseling of individuals at a clinic or drug treatment site, social network strategies for promoting use of condoms and clean needles, and media advocacy for a change in policy regarding needle exchange.

Building community capacity is a necessary condition for the development, implementation, and maintenance of effective community-level interventions. Community-level interventions must aim at building or increasing the community's capacity to be self determining in specific community problems (40). A community's capacity may be defined in terms of accessing and effectively using needed financial and material resources (i.e., money, goods, and services); technical resources including individual skills and organizational capacities; and social resources (e.g., leaders, strong community-based institutions, coalition of community organizations, and high-level participation by community members) (40).

Benefits of community-level interventions include the ability to address contexts of risk behaviors and reach large numbers of individuals who are at risk. Additionally, these interventions may have longer lasting effects and the potential to be cost effective (2,12,13). Community-level interventions also face a number of challenges because they are known to be more difficult to implement, monitor, control, and evaluate. These challenges often raise questions about the validity and reliability of research methods used to evaluate the effects of community-level interventions. Some of the difficulties of methods for evaluating community-level interventions include the difficulty involved in randomizing entire communities appropriately, the difficulty in finding suitable (uncontaminated) comparison communities and problems in making connections between immediate outcomes of specific programs, given the limited number of communities typically examined by community-level interventions. Also, evaluation of community-level interventions often involves collecting multiple types of data (e.g., surveys, in-depth surveys, focus group interviews) from multiple sources (e.g., random sample of community members, community leaders, representative of community agencies). This increases the likelihood of obtaining different results, given that community groups may have divergent views of problems and concerns in the community. This poses a challenge to interpretation and decisions about how to integrate and prioritize the results (41). Kirkwood et al. (42) contend, however, that the best approach to designing a study to evaluate the effect of a community-level intervention is likely to come from a jigsaw from different and often imperfect design elements. These design elements help to paint a coherent picture of the intervention, so that what is achieved by the whole is greater than the individual parts (42).

There are a variety of approaches to delivering community-level interventions. These include outreach strategies (e.g., community outreach, peer and social networks strategies) and media campaigns including social marketing, entertainment education, and media advocacy. The Internet and other interactive media have also become important media for delivering community-level interventions to different population groups. A discussion including examples of the approaches for delivering community-level interventions follows.

Community outreach strategies have long been the mainstay of STD and HIV prevention efforts. Outreach interventions are generally conducted by peer or paraprofessional educators face-to-face with high-risk populations. They are conducted in a range of local settings with the intent of reaching people where they congregate, including street corners, gay bars, bath houses, parks, and selected areas throughout the community, and to provide immediate individual counseling or small group presentations, as well as peer education and specially designed workshops. They rely on outreach workers who typically are indigenous to the local community, familiar with the norms and practices of the community, and trusted as a source of information. Outreach workers are uniquely able to serve as role models, educators, and advocates who can provide people at risk with changing and accurate risk-reduction information in settings that are familiar to them and at times of greatest risk. While frequently used by community-based and grass root services organizations, community outreach has been tested and found to be an effective strategy for providing at-risk populations with the means for behavior change (e.g., HIV/AIDS educational materials, bleach kits for disinfecting injection equipment, condoms for safer sex) to reduce or eliminate their STD and HIV/AIDS transmission risk.

Examples of community outreach interventions include Community PROMISE and The Mpowerment Project. The Community PROMISE intervention used peer outreach and modeling strategies for HIV/AIDS risk-reduction for various at-risk populations, including injection drug users, their female sex partners, sex workers, non-gay identified MSM, high-risk youth, and residents in areas with high STD rates (43). The Mpowerment Project, a community-level HIV prevention intervention for young gay men, used a set of four integrated activities including formal and informal outreach to provide people with information and resources to prevent and help treat infectious diseases, especially HIV/AIDS, other STDs, and hepatitis (44).

The social network approach focuses intervention on high-risk social networks—a set of people (or organizations or other social entities) connected by a set of social relationships, such as friendship, sexual relationships, co-working, or information sharing (45). The social network strategy is based on the notion that individuals are linked together to form large social networks, and that diseases such as STDs/HIV and associated risk behaviors are often clustered in social networks. This approach provides an opportunity to target entire networks rather than just to change the behavior of individuals. It uses naturally existing leaders of the networks who are credible and who also have influence on the network members. Kelly's Popular Opinion Leader (46) intervention is a frequently cited example of a social network focused community-level intervention. Kelly and colleagues reported significant reduction in HIV risk behaviors of gay men who received HIV/AIDS prevention messages from reliably identified popular opinion leaders. These leaders served as behavior change endorsers to their peers (46). Additionally, Rothenberg et al. (47) used social network strategies during an outbreak of syphilis in a suburban Atlanta community. Disease investigators conducted interviews, used network diagrams to prioritize their work, and relied on network connections for finding hard-to-reach individuals (47). Finally, CDC recently (2003–2005) funded nine community-based organizations (CBOs) in seven U.S. cities to demonstrate the feasibility of using social network strategies to identify individuals with undiagnosed HIV infection (48). In this two-year project, HIV-seropositive and high-risk HIV-seronegative persons were enlisted to recruit members of their social, sexual, and drug-use networks for HIV counseling, testing, and referral services. Data from the first year of the project showed HIV rates for persons who were newly identified that were five times the average rates reported by publicly funded HIV counseling and testing sites (48). These data suggest that social network strategies may be effective in reaching and identifying persons with undiagnosed HIV infection.

The Internet and other interactive media channels have attracted considerable attention as potential vehicles for disseminating health interventions to targeted communities (see Chapter 9 in this book). Internet web sites and chat rooms, bulletin boards, kiosks, newsgroups, and listservs are electronic information sources that allow tailored messages and feedback to be delivered to and from intended audiences. They may also serve as vehicles for targeted messages to social networks or relationships developed over the Internet. It has been reported that one third of adults who visit the Internet are directed to sexually oriented web sites, chat rooms, and news groups (49) where they can observe sexual images or participate in sexual discussions with individuals or groups. While participation in virtual sexual discussions does not carry risk for STD and HIV in itself, it has been shown that individuals who use the Internet to find sex partners for actual sexual contact may be at risk for STDs, including HIV (50–52). This reality makes the Internet and other interactive media important channels for targeted HIV/STD prevention messages.

The San Francisco Department of Public Health used an Internet-based intervention, free online syphilis testing, to address a syphilis epidemic in men-who-have-sex-with-men (MSM) in San Francisco (53). The Health Department collaborated with a community-based organization, Internet Sexuality Information Services, Inc., to design an innovative, confidential, online testing service for syphilis. The intervention offered a free and convenient alternative for testing and an additional means for detecting syphilis cases.

The Entertainment-Education strategy is an additional approach for media campaigns/mass education targeting communities. Entertainment-Education (E-E) strategy links entertainment and education and is a process in which educational or motivational information is purposely embedded into entertainment media, in order to increase audience members' knowledge about an issue, create favorable attitudes, shift social norms, and change the overt behavior of individuals and communities (54). Programs are characterized by ongoing story lines with several concurrent plots linked together by the characters' personal relationships. Each episode ends with a hook or "cliffhanger" that creates interest in the next episode, and a brief epilogue that poses rhetorical questions or provides information, such as the number of telephone hotline (55). The E-E strategy utilizes the appeal of entertainment formats such as melodramas or soap operas to consciously address educational issues. They often engage audience members emotionally and may stimulate conversations and discussions by individuals on various topics including STDs/HIV. Such conversations and other social interactions generated by the E-E programs can create new impetus and opportunities for behavior change (54).

The Hollywood, Health & Society (HH&S) program at the Norman Lear Center, the University of Southern California, used the E-E approach. Funded by the Centers for Disease Control and Prevention (CDC) and the National Institute of Health's (NIH) National Cancer Institute (NCI), the project recognizes the profound effect that entertainment media have on behavior and provides expert consultation and resources for writers and producers who develop scripts with health story lines, including information on STDs and HIV/AIDS (56).

Media advocacy has also been used as a strategy for community-level interventions. Media advocacy is "the purposeful and planned use of mass media to bring problems and policy solutions to the attention of the community and local decision-makers" (57). It seeks to broaden the "frame" of the news presentations in the public debate. A successful media advocacy campaign targets three distinct groups that influence one another: opinion leaders, the public, and the media. Many opinion leaders will be more likely to support health initiatives when they believe the public agrees with their position. It is important for STD/HIV advocates to develop media advocacy skills in order to shape the stories and policy solutions conveyed by the media about STD/HIV issues. Additionally, the media can provide STD/HIV advocates and their organizations with visibility and credibility, and can contribute significantly to the successful promotion of progressive STD and HIV/AIDS advocacy agenda (58,59).

An example of a community-level intervention that used media advocacy is "Know HIV/AIDS." This Emmy and Peabody Award–winning initiative is a public education partnership of the Kaiser Family Foundation and Viacom and it uses targeted public service announcements (PSAs), HIV-themed programming, and free print and online information resources. To date, the campaign has incorporated HIV/AIDS story lines into more than 40 Viacom-produced TV shows that have been seen by millions worldwide. As part of the 2003 World AIDS Day activities, Viacom's cable networks aired nearly 20

HIV/AIDS-related specials and news updates, and gave *Know HIV/AIDS* PSAs prime placement and frequency across the company's television, radio, and outdoor properties. Viacom's properties include the broadcast networks CBS and UPN; cable networks MTV, BET, VH1, CMT: Country Music Television, TV Land, Nickelodeon, Nick at Nite, The N, Showtime, Spike TV, and Comedy Central; 185 Infinity Broadcasting radio stations in the top 50 markets; and billboards, buses, and bus shelter advertising faces in the nation's largest markets (60).

A final strategy for community-level interventions is social marketing. Social marketing, a mass communication strategy, applies marketing principles and tools to influence human behavior on a large scale for the benefit of society (61; also, see Chapter 6 in this book for additional information). It is a strategy that employs private sector approaches to produce, distribute, and promote products and services that are considered to be good for the public (61). The steps of social marketing are as follows: 1) conduct a needs assessment of the target audience; 2) design social marketing strategies and/or products based on results from the needs assessment; 3) pre-test the strategies and products using audience segmentation and incorporate audience feedback into the strategies and/or products; 4) implement the strategies; and 5) continuously monitor and evaluate the effect of the campaign.

Social marketing has played a significant role in promoting condom and contraceptive behavior change in developing countries (61,62), and has been wildly recognized as an important strategy for increasing STD/HIV prevention awareness and assisting in fostering community norms that support risk reduction and utilization of prevention resources. While not as widely adopted in the United States, a few published studies have reported the application of social marketing across the country.

Cohen et al. (2) report on the implementation of a 1993–1996 condom social marketing campaign in the state of Louisiana. This statewide campaign made condoms freely available in 93 clinics, 39 community mental health centers, 29 substance abuse treatment sites, and more than 1000 businesses in neighborhoods with high rates of STDs and HIV. The widespread availability of free condoms was associated with increased condom use, particularly by persons at high risk for STDs and HIV (2). Additionally, Kennedy and colleagues designed and evaluated the Prevention Marketing Initiative (PMI), a multimodal social market intervention aimed at reducing HIV transmission among adolescents in five U.S. cities—Nashville, Newark, northern Virginia, Phoenix, and Sacramento. They employed a coalition-based social marketing approach and found that social marketing combined with other methods reduced the STD/HIV risk behaviors of adolescents (63). Finally, Vega and colleagues (64) reviewed social marketing campaigns that were initiated in seven U.S. cities—Atlanta, Chicago, Ft. Lauderdale, Los Angeles, Miami, New York, and San Francisco—to address the high incidence rates of syphilis in MSM.

Conclusion

Given the challenges and limitations of each of the intervention approaches discussed in this chapter, an important consideration in STD/HIV prevention is deciding when best to apply strategies that target the individual, group, or the community (4). Several factors should guide this decision, including epidemiology; and broader social, political, economic, institutional, and cultural issues. Perhaps effective STD/HIV prevention requires a mix of individual, group, and community interventions. The challenge is how to combine them and how to ensure that economic, policy, or political support help to change the social environment in which STD/HIV risk takes place (4).

References

1. Sweat MD, Denison JA. Reducing HIV incidence in developing countries with structural and environmental interventions. *AIDS*. 1995;9(suppl A):S251–S257.
2. Kelly JA. Community-level interventions are needed to prevent new HIV INFECTIONS. *American Journal of Public Health*. 1999;89:299–301.
3. Cohen DA, Farley TA, Bedimo-Etame JR, Scribner R, Ward W, et al. Implementation of condom social marketing in Louisiana, 1993 to 1996. *American Journal of Public Health*. 1999;89:204–208.
4. Mayaud P, Mabey D. Approaches to the control of sexually transmitted infections in developing countries: old problems and modern challenges. *Sexually Transmitted Infections*. 2004;80:174–182.
5. Homan GC. *The Human Group*. New York, NY: Harcourt Brace Jovanovich; 1982.
6. Bormann EG. *Small Group Communication Theory and Practice*. New York, NY: Harper and Row; 1990.
7. Centers for Disease Control and Prevention. *Report: What We Have Learned 1990–1995, Behavioral Interventions and Research Branch, Division of STD/HIV Prevention*. Atlanta, GA: Centers for Disease Control; 1996.
8. Remien RH, Stirratt MJ, Dolezal C, et al. Couple-focused support to improve HIV medication adherence: a randomized controlled trial. *AIDS*. 2005;19:807–814.
9. Freudenberg N. AIDS prevention strategies in the United States: a selective review of the literature. In: Freudenberg N and Zimmerman MA, eds. *AIDS Prevention in the Community: Lessons from the first Decade*. Washington, DC: American Public Health Association; 1995:13–29.
10. Ehrhardt AA, Exner TM, Hoffman S, Silberman I, Leu CS, Mille, S, Levin B. A gender-specific HIV/STD risk reduction intervention for women in a health care setting: short- and long-term results of a randomized clinical trial. *AIDS Care*. 2002;14:147–161.
11. Miller RL, Kelly JG. Community-level approaches to preventing HIV: guest editors' introduction. *The Journal of Primary Prevention*. 2002;23:151–156.
12. Pinkerton SD, Kahn JG, Holtgrave DR. Cost effectiveness of community-level approaches to HIV prevention. *The Journal of Primary Prevention*. 2002;23:151–156.
13. McLeroy, KR, Norton BL, Kegler MC, Burdine JN, Sumaya C. Community-based interventions. *American Journal of Public Health*. 2003; 93:529–533.
14. Roger EM. *Diffusion of Innovations*. New York: The Free Press; 1983.
15. Painter T. Voluntary counseling and testing for couples: a high-leverage intervention for HIV/AIDS prevention in sub-Saharan Africa. *Social Science and Medicine*. 2001;53:1397–1411.
16. El-Bassel N, Witte SS, Gilbert L, et al. The efficacy of a relationship-based HIV/STD prevention program for heterosexual couples. *American Journal of Public Health*. 2003; 93:963–969.
17. Harvey S, Henderson JT, Thorburn S, et al. A randomized study of a pregnancy and disease prevention intervention for hispanic couples. *Perspectives on Sexual and Reproductive Health*. 2004; 36:192–196.

18. Kelly JA, Kalichman SC. Behavioral research in HIV/AIDS primary and secondary prevention: recent advances and future directions. *Journal of Consulting and Clinical Psychology*. 2002;70:626–639.

19. Misovich SJ, Fisher JD, Fisher WA. Close relationships and elevated HIV risk behavior: evidence and possible underlying psychological processes. *Review of General Psychology*. 1997;1:72–107.

20. Witte SS, El-Bassel NE, Gilbert L, Wu E, Chang M, Steinglass P. Recruitment of minority women and their main sexual partners in an HIV/STI prevention trial. *Journal of Women's Health*. 2004;13:1137–1147.

21. El-Bassel N, Gilbert L, Rajah V, Foleno A, Frye V. Fear and violence: raising the HIV stakes. *AIDS Education and Prevention*. 2000;12:154–170.

22. El-Bassel N, Witte SS, Gilbert L et al. Long-term effects of an HIV/STI sexual risk reduction intervention for heterosexual couples. *AIDS and Behavior*. 2005;9:1–13.

23. Fishbein M. The role of theory in HIV prevention. *AIDS Care*. 2000;12:273–278.

24. Fisher JD, Fisher WA. Changing AIDS-risk behavior. *Psychology Bulletin*. 1992;111:455–474.

25. The Voluntary HIV-1 Counseling and Testing Efficacy Study Group. The Voluntary HIV-1 Counseling and Testing Efficacy Study: design and method. *AIDS and Behavior*. 2000;4:5–14.

26. The Voluntary HIV-1 Counseling and Testing Efficacy Study Group. Efficacy of voluntary HIV-1 Counseling and Testing in Individuals and Couples in Kenya, Tanzania, and Trinidad: a randomized trial. *Lancet*. 2000;356:103–112.

27. Allen S, Meinzen-Derr J, Kautzman M, et al. Sexual behavior of HIV discordant couples after HIV counseling and testing. *AIDS*. 2003;17:33–740.

28. Susser E, Valencia E, Miller M, Tsai WY, Meyer-Bahlburg H, Conover S. Sexual behavior of homeless mentally ill men at risk for HIV. *American Journal of Psychiatry*. 1995;152:583–587.

29. Seal DW, Kelly JA, Bloom FR, Stevenson LY, Coley BI, Broyles LA. HIV prevention with young men who have sex with men: what young men themselves say is needed. Medical College of Wisconsin CITY Project Research Team. *AIDS Care*. 2000;12:6–26.

30. DiClemente RJ, Wingood GM. A randomized controlled trial of an HIV sexual risk-reduction intervention for young African-American Women. *Journal of the American Medical Association*. 1995;274:1271–1276.

31. Kelly JA, St. Lawrence JS, Diaz YE. Community AIDS/HIV risk reduction: the effects of endorsement by popular people in three cities. *American Journal of Public Health*. 1992;82:168–171.

32. Pratt D. Working it Out. Scenes from the Lives of Gay and Lesbian Youth. *Body Positive*. 2002;15(6) Accessible at: http://www.thebody.com/bp/nov02/working_it_out.html

33. Centers for Disease Control and Prevention. Program Operations Guidelines. 2004. Available at: http://www.cdc.gov/std/program/medlab/Ref-PGmedlab.htm.

34. Kamb ML, Fishbein M, Douglas JM, et al. Efficacy of risk-reduction counseling to prevention human immunodeficiency virus and sexually transmitted diseases: a randomized controlled trial. *Journal of the American Medical Association*. 1998;280:1161–1167.

35. Jemmott JB, Jemmott LS, Braverman PK, Fong GT. HIV/STD risk reduction interventions for African American and Latino adolescent girls at an adolescent medicine clinic: a randomized controlled trial. *Arch Pediatr Adolesc Med*. 2005;159:440–449.

36. Citrin T. Topics for our times: public health—community or commodity? Reflections on healthy communities. *American Journal of Public Health*. 1998;88:351–352.

37. Atienze AA, King AA. Community-based health intervention trials: an overview of methodological issues. *Epidemiologic Reviews*. 2002;24:72–79.

38. Revenson TA, Schiaffino KM. Community-based health interventions. In Rappaport J, Seidman E, eds. *Handbook of Community Psychology*. New York, NY: Kluwer Academic/Plenum; 2000.

39. Valdiserri RO, Ogden LL, McCray E. Accomplishments in HIV prevention science: implications for stemming the epidemic. *Nature Medicine*. 2003;9:881–886.

40. Beeker C, Guenther-Grey C, Raj A. Community empowerment paradigm drift and the primary prevention of HIV/AIDS. *Social Science and Medicine*. 1998;46:831–842.

41. Israel BA, Schulz AJ, Parker EA, Becker AB. Review of community-based research: assessing partnership approaches to improve public health. *Annual Review of Public Heath*. 1998;19:173–202.

42. Kirkwood BR, Cousens SN, Victora CG, de Zoysa I. Issues in design of studies to evaluate the impact of community-based intervention. *Tropical Medicine and International Health*. 1997;2:1022–1029.

43. CDC AIDS Community Demonstration Projects Research Group. Community-level HIV intervention in 5 cities: final outcome data from the CDC AIDS Community Demonstration Projects. *American Journal of Public Health*. 1999;89:336–345.

44. Kegeles SM, Hays RB, Coates TJ. The Mpowerment Project: a community-level HIV prevention intervention for young gay men. *Am J Public Health*. 1996;86(8 Pt 1):1129–1136.

45. Klovdahl AS, Graviss EA, Yaganehdoost A, et al. Networks and tuberculosis: an undetected community outbreak involving public places. *Social Science and Medicine*. 2001;52:681–694.

46. Kelly JA, St. Lawrence JS, Diaz YE, et al. HIV risk behavior reduction following intervention with key opinion leaders of a population: an experimental analysis. *American Journal of Public Health*. 1991;81:168–171.

47. Rothenberg R, Kimbrough L, Lewis-Hardy R, et al. Social network methods for endemic foci of syphilis: a pilot project. *Sexually Transmitted Diseases*. 2000;27:12–18.

48. Centers for Disease Control and Prevention. Use of social networks to identify persons with undiagnosed HIV infection—seven U.S. cities, October 2003–September 2004. *Morbidity and Mortality Weekly Report*. 2005;54:601–605.

49. Toomey KE, Rothenberg RB. Sex and cyberspace—virtual networks leading to high-risk sex. *Journal of the American Medical Association*. 2000;284:485–487.

50. Ashton M, Sopwith W, Clark P, McKelvey D, Lighton L, Mandal D. An outbreak no longer: factors contributing to the return of syphilis in Great Manchester. *Sexually Transmitted Infections*. 2003;79:291–293.

51. Bull SS, Lloyd L, McFarlane M, Rietmeijer CA. HIV and sexually transmitted infection risk behaviors among men seeking sex with men on-line. *American Journal of Public Health*. 2001;91:988–989.

52. McFarlane M, Bull SS, Rietmeijer CA. The internet as a newly emerging risk environment for sexually transmitted diseases. *Journal of the American Medical Association*. 2000;284:443–446.

53. Levine DK, Scott KC, Klausner JD. Online syphilis testing—confidential and convenient. *Sexually Transmitted Diseases*. 2005;32:139–141.

54. Kennedy MG, O'Leary A, Beck V, Pollard K, Simpson P. Increases in calls to the CDC National STD and AIDS Hotline following AIDS-related episodes in a soap opera. *Journal of Communication*. 2004;54:287–301.

55. Vaughan PW, Regis A, Catherine ES. Effect of entertainment-education radio soap opera on family planning and HIV prevention in St. Lucia. *International Family Planning Perspectives*. 2000;26:148–157.

56. The National Lear Center web site. Available at: http://learcenter.org/html/projects/?cm=hhs. Accessed April 25, 2005.

57. Holder HD, Treno AJ. Media advocacy in community prevention: news as a means to advance policy change. *Addiction.* 1997;92(suppl 2):189–199.
58. Freimuth VS, Quinn SC. The contributions of health communication to eliminating health disparities. *American Journal of Public Health.* 2004;94:2053–2055.
59. Dorfman L, Woodruff K, Chavez V, Wallack L. Youth and violence on local television news in California. *American Journal of Public Health.* 1997;87: 1311–1316.
60. Viacom web site. Available at: http://www.viacom.com/press.tin?ixPressRelease= 80254133. Accessed April 25, 2005.
61. Jacobs B, Kambugu FSK, Whitworth JAG, et al. Social marketing of prepackaged treatment for men with urethral discharge (Clear Seven) in Uganda. *International Journal of STD & AIDS.* 2003;14:216–221.
62. Meekers D. The role of social marketing in sexually transmitted diseases/HIV protection in 4600 sexual contacts in urban Zimbabwe. *AIDS.* 2001;15:285–287.
63. Kennedy MG, Mizuno Y, Seals BF, Myllyluoma J, Weeks-Norton K. Increasing condom use among adolescents with coalition-based social marketing. *AIDS.* 2000;14:1809–1818.
64. Vega MY, Roland EL. Social marketing techniques for public health communication: a review of syphilis awareness campaigns in 8 US cities. *Sexually Transmitted Diseases.* 2005;32:S30–S36.
65. Corey L, Wald A, Patel R, et al. Once-daily valacyclovir to reduce the risk of transmission of genital herpes. *New England Journal of Medicine.* 2004;350:11–20.
66. Cohen D, McKinnon DP, Dent C, Mason H, Sullivan E. Group counseling at STD clinics to promote use of condoms. *Public Health Reports.* 1992;107:727–731.
67. El-Bassel N, Schilling RF. 15-Month follow-up of women methadone patients taught skills to reduce heterosexual HIV transmission. *Public Health Reports.* 1992;107:500–504.
68. Kelley JA, Murphy DA, Washington CD, et al. The effects of HIV/AIDS intervention groups for high-risk women in urban clinics. *American Journal of Public Health.* 1994;86:1442–1445.
69. O'Donnell CR, O'Donnell L, San Doval A, Duran R, Labes K. Reductions in STD infections subsequent to an STD clinic visit: using video-based patient education to supplement provider interactions. *Sexually Transmitted Diseases.* 1998;25:161–168.
70. St. Lawrence JS, Brasfield TL, Jefferson KW, Alleyne E, O'Bannon RE, Shirley A. Cognitive-behavioral intervention to reduce African American adolescents' risk for HIV infection. *Journal of Consulting and Clinical Psychology.* 1995;63:221–237.

5

Structural Interventions

Frederick R. Bloom, R.N., Ph.D., and Deborah A. Cohen, M.D., M.P.H.

Overview and Summary of Review Methods

The term "structural intervention" is a relative newcomer to a longstanding mode of implementing changes beyond the individual in order to change health behaviors and health outcomes. As such, there remain variations in the precise definition of the term. In 1995 there was increasing use of the term applied to HIV/AIDS interventions. Sweat and Denison (1) differentiate structural levels of causation from other macro-levels in that structural interventions influence laws, policies, and standard operational procedures implemented through activism, lobbying, and changes in policy. Interventions that they review pair structural-level intervention with those that are environmental (influencing living conditions, resources and opportunities, and recognition of other levels of causation). O'Reilly and Piot (2) portray structural intervention as synonymous with "enabling approaches" (3). These are defined as interventions that change the social or physical environment to enable changes in determinates of risk. Interestingly, this is categorized as environmental intervention by Sweat and Denison (1). O'Reilly and Piot (2) differentiate structural interventions from other interventions including the community level, described as those pertaining to a fixed geographical area. More recent writers have included community-level interventions as a type of structural intervention (4). Thus, there is clearly disagreement in the limits of what may be considered a structural intervention.

Some of the difficulties in finding a clear definition of structural intervention are reflections of the multi-disciplinary aspects of public health, where different theoretical frameworks and terms refer to similar concepts (5). In addition, structural interventions may be linked to other levels of intervention either directly or indirectly. For example, implementation of a national immunization program might be considered a structural intervention because of the policy and organizational changes. However, this same intervention is dependent on 1) a biomedical intervention preventing infection by increasing host resistance to infection by altering biological factors; 2) community-level intervention using messages to increase vaccination acceptability; and 3) individual level intervention involving patient care by health care providers, and so on. These latter three interventions may have been developed independently

Behavioral Interventions for Prevention and Control of Sexually Transmitted Diseases. Aral SO, Douglas JM Jr, eds. Lipshutz JA, assoc ed. New York: Springer Science+ Business Media, LLC; 2007.

through research, indirectly instilling a multi-level approach to the program, or implemented as part of the structural intervention directly, as part of a multi-level intervention program.

In 1998, in an attempt to provide a clearer definition of structural intervention in the context of HIV prevention, an internal workgroup at the Centers for Disease Control and Prevention (CDC) endeavored to clarify the structural barriers and facilitators of HIV prevention (6). This resulted in a broad framework of nine systems (governments, service organizations, businesses, workforce organizations, faith communities, justice systems, media organizations, education systems, and health care systems) and four levels of barriers or facilitators for HIV prevention (economic resources, policy supports, societal attitudes, and organizational structures).

Working Definition of Structural Intervention

Blankenship et al. (6) also take a broad view of structural intervention, stating that structural interventions in public health alter "the context within which health is produced or reproduced." (We interpret the term *reproduced* to indicate restoration of optimal health when health is impaired.) The definition of structural intervention that we shall use in the following discussion will consider the "context" as the environmental factors that influence STD prevention. These systems will be divided into four broad categories of structural factors (7,8). The following is not a comprehensive list, but is presented to afford the reader a better understanding of this framework:

- product availability, e.g., interventions involving:
  - condoms, which may reduce risk
  - drug availability and use, which may increase risk
- social structures/policies, e.g., interventions focused on:
  - community social change/social norm change
  - political system change
  - legislative system change
- physical aspects of product or broader environment, e.g., interventions that address changing the physical environment, such as:
  - crack cocaine "shooting galleries"
  - sex clubs, bathhouses
- media and cultural messages, e.g., interventions that seek to change the cultural environment through:
  - media campaigns
  - local media (pamphlets, fliers)

Thus, structural interventions for STDs will be reviewed in terms of the primary target of an intervention as an (i.e., environmental factor based on the above four categories). However, structural interventions embedded within multi-level interventions have been equally important, both in their contribution to STD and HIV prevention, and as antecedents to today's structural intervention endeavors. Since structural intervention may be a compelling aspect of multilevel interventions in terms of broadening the effect on public health at a population level, we shall also provide a limited review of important historical examples of multilevel interventions with key structural intervention components.

In order to facilitate our review of structural intervention, we conducted database and library searches based on personal knowledge of structural intervention and related literature. In addition, database searches were conducted using MEDLINE, PSYCHLIT, SOCIOFILE, CINAHL, AIDSLINE, and PUBMED. Relevant articles were reviewed and antecedent articles were identified from citations. The following discussion will begin with a historical perspective on structural intervention and will reveal how structural interventions have been critical to the development of public health in general and STD prevention more specifically.

Historical Perspective

Early Antecedents to Structural Intervention

Though the term *structural intervention* is relatively new, structural interventions in terms of policy change and manipulation of societal and cultural level factors are not. Efforts to improve health and control disease through manipulation of the environment or changes in policy are longstanding (though not uniformly effective) in human history. For example, the first efforts for sanitation and irrigation date back to the ancient Greeks and Romans who developed aqueducts to benefit the entire population (influence product availability). Efforts to control plague in 1600s through the extermination of rodent populations in Frankfurt (9) are another early example (changing the physical or broader environment). The development of what we now call structural intervention, as a key element of public health practice, has more recent antecedents in social hygiene, social medicine, and human ecology as early as the mid-1800s.

In the latter half of the 19th century, European scientists began to include the environment as a key factor in epidemiology and began to recommend or employ structural interventions to improve health on a population level (10). In an effort to improve social welfare and health, Virchow, working with typhus in 1848, recommended improvements in education and policy, alleviation of poverty, and intervention in social structure and policy (11). John Snow's efforts to control cholera in London through improvements in sanitation and provision of clean water from 1854 to 1856 are well known (12,13), primarily intervening in physical structure. Some of the most impressive and successful public health efforts through implementation of structural interventions were those implemented by Florence Nightingale between 1854 and 1898. Shortly after her arrival at the hospital at Scutari during the Crimean War, Nightingale implemented changes to the physical structure that housed the sick and procedural changes for their care and cleanliness. Following her return to England, she worked to improve health care for British soldiers through structural and policy changes in health care services and prevention through improved sanitation, nutrition, and care (14).

Public Health in the 20th Century: Structural Components and Multilevel Interventions

Structural interventions continued to be important internationally, through the turn of the century, with the Yellow Fever eradication efforts led by Walter Reed and others in Cuba and Panama, and Malarial Control efforts in the United States and abroad (relying strongly on changing physical aspects of the environment—mosquito control). Structural intervention has been used effectively as a means of sustaining biomedical interventions through policy change or institutionalization of systems of biomedical or community-level interventions. The development of the Polela (also Pholela) Community Health Centers by Sidney and Emily Kark and John Cassel in South Africa during the 1930s and 1940s was one such intervention.

The Polela Center program was a national health care program that has served as a model for subsequent community health centers development. It was arguably one of the first attempts to integrate system-wide, structural changes on social and cultural levels with biomedical intervention(11,15). The Polela Health Center interventions were enacted as a coordinated pilot project designed to deliver health care to rural South African communities (16,17). This program was a multilevel intervention of structural, biomedical, community, and behavioral components. However, the most innovative features of this program were the structural interventions employed to overcome societal barriers to the provision of existing interventions for rural South Africans.

These innovative interventions involved changes to the physical environment, national policy and infrastructure, and social structure, as follows. Structural intervention on the physical environment was changed by building of a network of clinics in rural areas previously without clinics coupled with the development of community gardens. The former improved health care access, while the latter enhanced nutrition through increasing the availability of garden produce otherwise unavailable. Structural intervention through changes in national policy and infrastructure development were essential to the facilitation and delivery of biomedical intervention (clinical care and treatment, nutritional improvement), community-level intervention (coordinated clinic facilities located to serve geographical communities), and behavioral intervention (changing health-seeking practices toward clinic attendance, for instance, and facilitating use of community gardens for better nutrition). Structural intervention to influence the social structure was critical to interventions addressing STD prevention, as follows:

Sidney Kark suggested a structural intervention component for STDs including recommendations for social norm and behavioral changes to reduce syphilis incidence in Africans whose lives were transformed by diamond and gold mining, with the resultant social destabilization of existing communities (18). Unfortunately, this early attempt at structural intervention for STD (and the Polela Health Community Health Center project as a whole) was never adopted by the South African government because of political barriers including apartheid and the election of a new, less sympathetic government (19). Importantly, the scientists who worked on the Polela project continued to exert a great influence on public health; Cassel coming to the United States (UNC at Chapel Hill) to continue to integrate the idea of social determinants of health into epidemiology (20,21), and the Karks emigrating to Israel, continuing their work on community-oriented primary care (22). Their work in Polela and afterward served as a model for community health centers.

Similarly, between 1936 and 1947, Thomas Parran's work on syphilis included policy and program changes paralleling some aspects of the Polela Centers with the 1937 syphilis control program in the United States and the

Rapid Treatment Centers (RTCs) of the mid-1940s. Like the Polela projects, the RTCs were an innovative structural component of a multilevel intervention with biomedical and individual-level interventions. RTCs offered a newly designated physical space and policy that, to an otherwise unknown extent, provided STD treatment and counseling as a public health program. A national plan for the Syphilis Control Program and the institutionalization of the RTCs through structural intervention at the legislative level (National Venereal Disease Control Act of 1938) provided infrastructure and sustainability through policy change. Knowledge and awareness were targeted through a media campaign. Changes in the physical structure of STD treatment (development of Rapid Treatment Centers designated for STD treatment) provided the setting and a program (a set of policies and procedures) for biomedical and behavioral intervention based on traditional social work. Structural (or system-level) components of multi-level interventions continued to be widely implemented in international health from the 1950s through the 1980s covering a broad range of health concerns (23).

The use of structural interventions continued to expand following the WHO/UNICEF Alma Ata declaration of 1978 that linked health to structural conditions including political, social, and economic reform (24). This sparked a number of broad multilevel intervention programs targeting diarrheal diseases (insuring access to clean water), and respiratory diseases (reducing the prevalence of tobacco use, clean air standards) (23,25,26).

The HIV Pandemic: Structural Level as Primary Intervention

Though there is a rich literature on structural factors contributing to HIV/AIDS during the first decade of the epidemic, there is limited publication of structural interventions (5). Notable exceptions to this include documentation of grassroots social norm changes of reduced sexual risk in gay communities (community-level social-structure change), policy change at governmental levels, and physical structure changes such as the closing of bathhouses in the San Francisco (27). In addition, the 100% condom use program for commercial sex workers and their clients in Thailand was a structural intervention based on policy change, product availability (condoms), and change in the physical environment through monitoring of brothels (1). By 1995, structural intervention for HIV prevention in developing countries was well entrenched (1,3). During this same time period, Holmes called for intervention on the environment of health (from a human ecology perspective) to prevent bacterial STD transmission in developing countries and in the United States (28). This ecological perspective brought the health environment, and thus structural intervention, to the forefront as a means to alter the environment in which STD transmission occurs.

In the 1990s and through the present, structural interventions (though not always defined as such) became more evident in HIV and STD prevention internationally and domestically. For instance, policy changes that increased access to clean syringes were implemented in Australia, several European nations, and a few U.S. cities to reduce HIV transmission risk for intravenous drug users (IDUs) (29). A variety of public policy interventions for bathhouses were implemented as structural interventions to reduce sexual risk, though one analysis of these sometimes conflicting policies found them to be ineffective at reducing sexual risk (30).

Description of the Types of Structural Intervention Currently for STD/HIV

Structural interventions should be used whenever the desired process or mechanism involves a change in the environment or ecology within which health and illness are embedded. This implies that one or more given factors that influence health and illness have been identified, that a target population can be influenced by such change, and that a mechanism for structural intervention can be identified or developed. For example, structural interventions to reduce syphilis in gay men have been employed in Los Angeles, California, with some immediate success (31). Interventions included a media campaign and increased condom availability in community settings serving high-risk individuals, such as bars and nightclubs.

In addition to the previously mentioned Thai intervention for brothels, legislation and policy have been shown to be key elements in prevention for injection drug users, whether in relation to laws governing pharmacies or operational procedures employed by pharmacies (32,33). Use of the Internet to facilitate the availability of laboratory testing for STDs in an area with increasing syphilis for gay men is an innovative structural intervention using internet technology to increase product availability (lab testing initiation, lab results, and STD prevention information) (34). The following sections will provide detail relating to structural information across the four categories discussed: product availability, policy and social structures, media and cultural messages, and physical structures.

Product Availability

Condom Availability

Condom availability simply provides access to condoms and does not necessarily require overt motivational or educational messages. The rationale for these programs is that by simply increasing the number of condoms available and accessibility to them, condom use will increase. Usually, however, condom availability is coupled with some motivational or marketing message, to increase awareness and to make condoms appear to be socially acceptable and desirable. Globally, condom social marketing, condom subsidies, and condom availability have been the cornerstones of HIV prevention campaigns. In the United States, condom availability has been an explicit component of 1) condom social marketing programs, 2) school-based condom availability programs and 3) clinic- and community-based condom availability programs. In contrast, condom availability is often an unacknowledged component in 1) group, peer, and street outreach interventions, and 2) individual and group counseling, with or without HIV testing (37–43).

Expected proximate outcomes: Increase in proportion of sexual encounters in which a condom is used.

Needle Exchange Programs

Needle/syringe exchange programs provide sterile needles to individuals who return used needles in exchange, thereby reducing the likelihood of reuse of an infected needle. These programs have the added advantage that they may reduce the number of discarded needles and syringes on streets. Needle exchange programs (NEPs) are in operation in many states and cities in the

United States. They operate through fixed or mobile sites and can include van stops, scheduled street exchange sites, or even provide delivery services. Almost all U.S. needle exchange programs (NEP) provide only one syringe for each syringe brought in to the NEP, but many provide small numbers of syringes to IDUs making their first visit to the NEP (44–47).

Expected proximate outcomes: Reduction in proportion of drug injections in which a previously used syringe is used.

Needle Deregulation
In many states there are laws and regulations that inhibit availability of sterile needles and syringes to IDU. These include laws requiring prescriptions for needles/syringes and laws banning the possession of needles/syringes as "drug paraphernalia." These laws are not present or are not enforced in many states, and some states have passed laws that make explicit exemptions in them to increase the availability of sterile needles/syringes to IDU. By allowing IDU to purchase their own sterile needles/syringes, needle deregulation efforts should reduce the likelihood that IDU will reuse infected needles/syringes from others (33,48–51).

Expected proximate outcomes: Reduction in the proportion of drug injections in which a previously used syringe is used.

Alcohol Taxes
Alcohol use has been associated with high-risk behaviors in many studies, including high-risk sexual behavior. While reducing alcohol availability is not usually considered as an HIV prevention strategy for individuals, it may be a useful tool to reducing HIV transmission in populations. Alcohol availability is determined by a variety of factors, including the strictness and strength of enforcement of alcohol beverage control laws, the price of alcohol (often associated with alcohol taxes), the number and type of outlets where alcohol can be purchased, and the places where alcohol consumption is permitted (e.g., in public settings, cars, or clubs). Increases in alcohol taxes have specifically been followed by reductions in STDs (50,51).

Expected proximate outcomes: Reduction in number of sex partners, increase in proportion of sexual encounters in which a condom is used.

Policy and Social Structures

Community Mobilization and Street Outreach Programs
Outreach to persons at risk can be conducted in a variety of ways and for various purposes, including its use as a mechanism to bring people in to receive other interventions. In this context, however, we use the term *Street Outreach* to describe a community-based strategy in which the risk-reduction intervention is delivered in community settings, usually outdoors in high-incidence neighborhoods. The goal of the intervention is to reduce the spread of HIV and STDs by increasing condom use, reducing the sharing of needles, and increasing HIV testing (and STD testing in some cases). Street outreach is usually conducted by peers from the community in which it is undertaken and involves a face-to-face personal interaction with high-risk persons. Community mobilization campaigns, on the other hand, also involve street contacts by peer educators, but the aim is to change the norms of risky behavior for an entire community. However, the two programs in practice may be similar, because people with whom outreach workers have contact may continue to spread

risk-reduction messages; thus, individuals in the target communities who have not been personally reached by outreach workers still get messages about safer sex and drug use through others (52,53).

Expected proximate outcomes: Reduction in the number of sex partners, increase in proportion of sexual encounters in which a condom is used, reduction in the proportion of drug injections in which a previously used needle is used; increase in number of individuals tested for HIV, STD, or both.

Opinion Leader Programs

These programs identify, train, and enlist the help of key opinion leaders to change risky sexual norms and behaviors; they have been well evaluated only as they have been applied to men who have sex with men (MSM). The program is based on diffusion of innovation/social influence principles, which states that trends and innovations are often initiated by a relatively small segment of opinion leaders in the population. Once innovations are visibly modeled and accepted, they then diffuse throughout a population, influencing others. Their ultimate goal is reduction of sexual risk behavior in MSM (55–57).

Expected proximate outcomes: Reduction in the number of sex partners, increase in proportion of sexual encounters in which a condom is used.

Supervised Activities for Youth

If youth are supervised, in theory they have less time to engage in high-risk behaviors. There are many types of programs that involve youth in supervised activities. Very few studies have evaluated the impact of supervised activities on HIV risk behaviors. However, one program that placed youth in community service activities showed a reduction in unprotected sex (57).

Expected proximate outcomes: Reduction in the number of sex partners, reduction in the frequency of sexual intercourse.

STD National Policy-Level Interventions

Policy changes at the federal level of public health in terms of STD Program Operations Guidelines are intended to drive modifications in standard of care as practiced by state and locally funded clinics, while treatment and lab testing guidelines focus on establishing a policy for best practices for individual care-providers thus influencing practice in the private sector as well, though these national guidelines have not been evaluated. Although increasing condom availability is a critical component of HIV/STD interventions, there are currently no federal guidelines that specify that all STD and HIV clinics should provide condoms to their clients. Such a policy could influence the two million patients seen in public STD clinics annually, and the estimated 500,000 HIV patients receiving medical care.

Expected proximate outcomes: Increase in awareness of changes to STD best practices for health care providers; increase in proportion of sexual encounters in which a condom is used.

Legal and Legislative-Level Interventions

California, Tennessee, Colorado, and Wisconsin have legal and regulatory environments that specifically allow partner-delivered medication (PDM) to treat specified STDs. Other states do not specifically allow this practice, while some clearly restrict partner-delivered medication. Golden et al. demonstrated the efficacy of having patients infected with gonorrhea and chlamydia deliver medication to their partners to provide presumptive treatment and prevent reinfection in the initially diagnosed patients (58). State laws facilitate (or hinder) implementation of this biomedical intervention through manipulation of the legislative environment, and are potent sustained structural interventions. However, their effect on STD transmission depends on their primary intent, and other factors in the environment. For instance, laws that restrict partner-delivered medications have, as their primary intent, the protection of patients from adverse effects related to partner use of medication without medical supervision. This restriction, while being very effective at preventing adverse reactions to pharmaceutical agents, limits efforts to reduce STD reinfection.

Expected proximate outcomes: Reduction in the rates of gonorrhea and Chlamydia reinfection.

Media and Cultural Messages

Media Campaigns

Media interventions are efforts to use both small and large media to promote products or behaviors related to HIV prevention and are discussed in greater depth in Chapter 6 in this volume. Nevertheless, they are structural interventions designed to alter the social environment as a means of health improvement or disease prevention. Media campaigns promoting condom use have been very successful in Europe and in developing countries. Large-scale media campaigns have not been used for condom promotion in the United States to date. Because HIV and the behaviors associated with its transmission are often stigmatized in the United States, large-scale campaigns have been very general, information-based, or fear-based and have not been found effective. Campaigns using small media have been much more commonly employed, and these include the distribution of novellas, posters, flyers, and other promotional items. These smaller campaigns can be less visible to the general public and more targeted at a variety of subgroups. However, intervention effectiveness has not been well documented. Media campaigns as intervention are discussed in greater detail in Chapter 6 (59,60).

Expected proximate outcomes: Reduction in the number of sex partners, increase in proportion of sexual encounters in which a condom is used.

Physical Structures

Bathhouse Regulations/Closure

Bathhouses are establishments for men to have sex (often anonymously) with other men. Many establishments have rules that require condoms be used during sex, but these policies may not be enforced. The enhanced opportunities for sex with many individuals increase the risk of disease transmission. Recently, syphilis outbreaks have been traced to bathhouses. Bathhouses can be further regulated to enforce condom use or be closed if condom use is not routine. This intervention was used in some cities in the 1980s, but it has not been evaluated (30,61,62).

Expected proximate outcomes: Reduction in the number of sex partners, increase in proportion of sexual encounters in which a condom is used.

Crackhouse or Shooting Gallery Regulation or Closure

Crackhouses and shooting galleries serve as places for people to engage in sex, non-injection drug use, injection drug use, or all of these. These establishments exist outside of the law, but in theory may be identifiable and subject to regulation or closure. This intervention has not been evaluated (64,65).

Expected proximate outcomes: Reduction in the number of sex partners, increase in proportion of sexual encounters in which a condom is used, reduction in the proportion of drug injections in which a previously used syringe is used.

Closure of Alcohol Outlets

Given that the properties around alcohol outlets are often venues for loitering and antisocial behaviors, such as public drinking or even drug use and drug sales, particularly in low-income, minority neighborhoods, closure of these outlets may eliminate opportunities for people to meet each other and engage in - high-risk behaviors. A study of the effects of closing alcohol outlets in the wake of the 1992 Los Angeles Civil Unrest indicated a greater decline in gonorrhea cases in neighborhoods where alcohol outlets were closed compared to neighborhoods where they remained open (66).

Feasibility and Barriers

Policy Changes, Politics, and Social Norms

A key element in the feasibility of conducting a structural intervention is the support or lack thereof at the level of intervention, whether governmental, societal, or institutional level. If the political climate is in opposition to any facet of the policy change or the intended outcome, feasibility of implementation is decreased. This complexity cannot be overestimated. Stakeholders, leaders, social norms, and the changing nature of policy over time all play a part in feasibility of successful implementation of structural intervention. Considering the Polela example previously mentioned, the governmental policy toward indigenous peoples in 1945 supported structural intervention to improve their health and health care, only to reverse this decision in 1948 with the election of the Nation Party government.

In the case of NEPs, the feasibility of implementation is lessened related to whether states have laws prohibiting possession of hypodermic needles. Interestingly, as mentioned, some states with laws that prohibit possession of needles do not enforce those laws, and those states have existing NEPs despite what appears to be a barrier to feasibility. School systems and parents of children enrolled in schools are formidable facilitators or opponents of structural interventions based on their disapproval or encouragement of school-based intervention (see Chapter 12 in this volume). Both respond to and support social norms for child-rearing, education, and responsibility for a child's health.

Unintended Consequences

In addition to the feasibility of structural intervention implementation, consideration of unintended consequences has several important ramifications. Bloom et al. call for ongoing evaluation of structural interventions to help respond to and interrupt unintended consequences (67). They discuss how efforts to reduce HIV transmission may have contributed to the more recent rise in syphilis infections in HIV-infected gay men. Policy and media interventions were employed at various societal levels to implement the need for all sexually active persons to "know your HIV status," "know your partner," and adopt safer sex strategies (e.g., abstinence is safest, condom use provides some safety, oral sex is less risky than anal sex). This set of messages was well suited to HIV prevention, and there is evidence that gay men engage in HIV sero-sorting to reduce HIV transmission risk. However, Bloom, et al. found that some men contracted syphilis because they considered only their risk for HIV transmission based on HIV sero-sorting and other HIV prevention strategies (e.g., the perception that unprotected oral sex is at low risk for transmission of HIV) while ignoring other prevention strategies (abstinence, consistent condom use) (67). This unintended consequence could be ameliorated through ongoing evaluation and follow-up intervention to respond to gay men's selection of HIV prevention strategies that places them at risk for other STDs (67).

Cost Effectiveness

An analysis of the cost effectiveness of structural level HIV/STD interventions indicates that structural interventions are generally more cost effective than individual level interventions (Table 1) (68). The reason has to do with the large number of people that can be reached with a structural intervention and the relatively low cost per person reached. Structural interventions are generally more cost effective when they are targeted in geographical areas with a high prevalence of HIV or STD. For this reason, interventions targeting high school youth in the United States are generally not cost effective in the short term because the HIV prevalence is so low. Similarly, even high-risk women in the United States tend to have a relatively low prevalence of HIV, so in order for any intervention to be cost effective for the purposes of preventing HIV transmission, the interventions have to be very inexpensive.

Table 1 Cost effectiveness of HIV prevention structural interventions.

Intervention	Cost per infection prevented
Videos in STD clinics, single session[*]	$4,700
Community mobilization (Mpowerment) (53)	$12,000
Needle exchange-high prevalence areas (42)	$13,000
Mass media campaigns (59)	$18,000
Opinion leader programs (54)	$23,000
Needle exchange-medium prevalence areas (42)	$47,000
Condom availability/accessibility (36)	$47,000
Street outreach[†]	$110,000
Youth supervision programs (57)	$3,100,000
Street outreach targeting women in low-income housing[‡]	$3,400,000

[*]O'Donnell CR, O'Donnell, L, et al. Reductions in STD infections subsequent to an STD clinic visit: using video-based patient education to supplement provider interactions. *Sexually Transmitted Diseases*. 1998;25:161–168.
[†]Wendell DA, Cohen, DA, et al. Street outreach for HIV prevention: effectiveness of a state-wide program. *International Journal of STD & AIDS*. 2003;14:334–340.
[‡]Sikkema KJ, Kelly, JA, et al. Outcomes of a randomized community-level HIV prevention intervention for women living in 18 low-income housing developments. *American Journal of Public Health*. 2000;90:57–63.

Benefits and Challenges

As has been shown, structural interventions are quite varied in scale, population or system targeted, and in the methods used to enact change. Methods by necessity must be different when lobbying for and enacting legislation or other government policy, implementing media campaigns at a variety of population levels, changing aspects of the provision of goods and services, changing the social and physical environment, or for other efforts. Formal evaluation is not always practical for large-scale structural intervention. That is, structural interventions are often enacted in an environment with many confounding variables present or emerging.

For instance, consider the following scenario for a given locale: A peer opinion leader intervention may be initiated by a community agency, while a media campaign is undertaken by a health department, and legislative changes are enacted. Regardless of whether STD rates fall, rise, or remain constant following these interventions, determining how these or other structural interventions contribute to STD prevention cannot always be accomplished through standard research protocols.

When evaluation is not feasible, reassessment of the local population to gain an understanding of social norms and risk behavior, knowledge and awareness of STDs, access to services, and other factors is needed. Since structural interventions apply to continually evolving systems, the need for recurrent and responsive interventions should always be considered. One of the strongest benefits of structural intervention is the capacity of such interventions to reach large numbers of people without an inordinately high cost. In addition, some structural interventions can be sustained over an extended period of time (e.g., legislation and documented policy changes in particular). However, there is always potential for structural intervention to become outmoded if not responsive to the changing environment. The difficulty in evaluating such large-scale intervention in a natural and changing environment is an important limitation but can be moderated through continued involvement and assessment of affected populations and structural aspects of systems in their environment.

As has been seen in the previous discussion of complex changes in risk behavior through social norm change (know your partner, know your HIV-status, use condoms, choose safer sex options), once these concepts are adopted by a group, there is potential for drift and reshuffling of key directives, that in this case, provided a less risky environment for HIV transmission, yet increased risk for syphilis or other STDs (67).

Structural intervention has several compelling aspects. making it an important tool for public health and STD prevention:

• Potential for low-cost intervention reaching relatively high numbers of persons
• Potential sustainability of changes in health systems

At the same time, there are serious challenges and limitations:

• Formal evaluation may be costly and time consuming
• Evaluation may be difficult or impossible relating to confounding variables

- System-level changes, though sustained, may drift over time, requiring some plan for reassessment and subsequent intervention to refocus or shift changes to minimize unintended consequences
- Unintended consequences may be large in proportion to the reach of intervention

Recommendations for Practice

When designing structural interventions, the benefits and challenges described in the previous section should all be considered. A broad assessment of the geographic community should be conducted, including populations at risk and the local health systems (public, private, community-based, or traditional/lay health). By gaining a better understanding of these aspects, potentially undesirable consequences can be identified and possibly averted. For instance, a health clinic may wish to improve access to care for a particular population. An assessment can provide information as to the barriers to access for that population, and, if broadly conducted, provide information on potential barriers to care for other populations that may be currently using the clinical facilities. If we understand the varying and sometimes conflicting needs of the said populations, we can make certain that one group's access to care will not be improved at the expense of another. The structural intervention can be tailored to provide the best access for all populations served.

In addition, a clear understanding of what is within a given entity's locus of control will assist in planning a successful intervention. One possibility to address this, a logic model of local STD prevention, may serve as a guide to help identify what system-level interventions are possible, and whether those changes have the potential to influence the desired outcome. Alternatively, a taxonomy of factors influencing a particular problem area, developed during assessment activities, may elucidate similar information. For instance, if an entity planning a structural intervention cannot influence laws nor legislation that restrict needle-exchange, it is irrelevant whether the capacity is there, whether training for outreach workers is developed, whether there is adequate availability of these potential services, or whether facilities exist or can be modified to provide the service. Identification of product availability, social structure and policy, and physical structures mentioned previously may also help to better define the desired outcomes of the intervention and potential influences on success.

Whenever feasible, a formal evaluation plan can be developed along with planning for structural intervention, and implemented as part of the process. A number of structural interventions have successfully been evaluated as previously discussed. However, regardless of whether formal evaluation is or is not possible, follow-up assessments conducted at set intervals will help to identify areas of further concern. Doing so will not prevent unanticipated consequences of intervention but will help to identify such consequences so that additional intervention may be implemented as indicated. In addition, valuable feedback may be provided without the additional delay of waiting for surveillance data to show a recurring or secondary problem.

In summary, structural interventions, whether implemented as part of a multi-level intervention or developed as a sole intervention, are integral to

STD and HIV prevention specifically and public health in general. These potentially low-cost, high-effect interventions can be of great value to programs with limited (or more expansive) resources, provided there is a willingness to attend to the recommendations made in this chapter (e.g., preliminary and follow-up assessments and evaluation whenever possible). In many cases, structural interventions have been shown to be successful and cost effective and should be considered as a proven public health tool. Each situation requiring structural intervention may have unique features in terms of population diversity, health system characteristics, and social and material resources or challenges. Because of this variability, there remains a need to evaluate proven models of structural interventions applied in a variety of circumstances (after tailoring to local conditions). In addition to this, other promising or widely used interventions would also benefit from further research as to the possibilities and limits for wider dissemination.

References

1. Sweat MD, Denison JA. Reducing HIV incidence in developing countries with structural and environmental interventions. *AIDS*. 1995;(suppl A):S251–S257.
2. O'Reilly KR, Piot P. International perspectives on individual and community approaches to the prevention of sexually transmitted disease and human immunodeficiency virus infection. *J Infect Dis*. 1996;174(suppl. 2):S214–S222.
3. Tawil O, Verster A, O'Reilly, KR. Enabling approaches for HIV/AIDS prevention: can we modify the environment and minimize the risk. *AIDS*. 1995;9:1299–1306.
4. Manhart LE, Holmes KK. Randomized controlled trials of individual-level, population level, and multilevel interventions for preventing sexually transmitted infections: what has worked? *J Infect Dis*. 2005; 191(suppl 1):S1–S178.
5. Parker RG, Easton D, Klein CH. Structural barriers and facilitators in HIV prevention: a review of international research. *AIDS*. 2000;14(suppl 1):S22–S32.
6. Blankenship KM, Bray SJ, Merson MH. Structural interventions in public health. AIDS 2000;14(suppl. 1):S11–S21.
7. Cohen DA, Scribner R. An STD/HIV prevention intervention framework. *AIDS Patient Care and STDS*. 2000;14:37–45.
8. Cohen DA, Scribner RA, Farley TA. A structural model of health behavior: a pragmatic approach to explain and influence health behaviors at the population level. *Preventive Med*. 2000;30:146–154.
9. Forsyth A. The plague within: why the lessons of ecology not modern medicine hold the solution to the current AIDS epidemic. *Equinox*. 1987;Nov/Dec:136–152.
10. Susser M. *Causal Thinking in the Health Sciences*. Oxford University Press: London, 1973.
11. Trostle J. Early work in anthropology and epidemiology: from social medicine to the germ theory, 1840-1920. In: Janes CR, Stall R, Gifford SM, eds. *Anthropology and Epidemiology*. The Netherlands: D Reidel; 1986; p. 35–57.
12. Centers for Disease Control and Prevention. 150th anniversary of John Snow and the pump handle. *MMWR Morb Mortal Wkly Rep*. 2004;53:783.
13. Lilienfeld DE. John Snow: the first hired gun? *American Journal of Epidemiology*. 2000;152:4–9.
14. Gill G. Nightingales: the extraordinary upbringing and curious life of Miss Florence Nightingale. New York: Ballantine Books; 2004.
15. Geiger HJ. Community-oriented primary care: a path to community development. *Am J Public Health*. 2002;92:1713–1716.
16. Anderson MR, Smith L, Sidel VW. What is social medicine? *Monthly Review*. 2005;56:27–34.

17. Trostle J. Anthropology and epidemiology in the twentieth century: a selective history of collaborative projects and theoretical affinities. 1920 to 1970. In: Janes CR, Stall R, Gifford SM, eds. *Anthropology and Epidemiology*. The Netherlands: D. Reidel; 1986. p. 59–94.

18. Kark S. The social pathology of syphilis in Africans (Reprinted from *South African Medical Journal* 23:77–84). *International Journal of Epidemiology*. 2003 [1949]; 32:181–186.

19. Reddy PS, Mbewu AD, Nogoduka CM. Commentary: Sexually transmitted infection in South Africa: 50 years after Sidney Kark. *International Journal of Epidemiology*. 2003;2:189–192.

20. Cassel JC. The contribution of the social environment to host resistance. *American Journal of Epidemiology*. 1976;104:107–123.

21. Cassel JC, Patrick RC Jr, Jenkins CD. Epidemiology analysis of the health implications of culture change: a conceptual model. *Annals of the New York Academy of Sciences*. 1960;84:938–949.

22. Mullan F. Community-oriented primary care: an agenda for the '80s. *New England Journal of Medicine*. 1982;307:1076–1078.

23. Mull JD. The primary health care dialectic: history, rhetoric, and reality. In Coreil J, Mull JD, eds. *Anthropology and Primary Health Care*. Boulder, CO: Westview Press; 1990.

24. Kendall C. The implementation of a diarrheal disease control program in Honduras: is it 'selective primary health care' or 'integrated primary health care.' *Social Science and Medicine*. 1988;27:17–23.

25. Coreil J. The evolution of anthropology in international health. In: Coreil J, Mull JD, eds. *Anthropology and Primary Health Care*. San Francisco: Westview Press, 1990.

26. Foster G. Applied anthropology and international health: retrospect and prospect. *Human Organization*. 1982;41:189–197.

27. Shilts R. *And the Band Played On*. New York: St. Martin's Press; 1987.

28. Holmes KK. Human ecology and behavior and sexually transmitted bacterial infections. *Proceedings of the National Academy of Science*. 1994;91: 2448–2455.

29. Taussig JA, Weinstein B, Burris S, Jones TS. Syringe laws and pharmacy regulations are structural constraints on HIV prevention in the US. *AIDS*. 2000;14(suppl. 1): S47–S51.

30. Woods WJ, Binson D, Pollack LM, Wohlfeiler D, Stall RD, Catania JA. Public policy regulating private and public space in gay bathhouses. *Journal of AIDS*. 2003;32:417–423.

31. Chen JL, Kodagoda D, Lawrence AM, Kerndt PR. Rapid public health interventions in response to an outbreak of syphilis in Los Angeles. *Sexually Transmitted Diseases*. 2002;29:277–284.

32. Groseclose SL, Weinstein B, Jones TS, Valleroy LA, Fehrs LJ, Kassler WJ. Impact of increased legal access to needles and syringes on practices of injecting-drug users and police officers—Connecticut. *Journal of AIDS and Human Retrovirology*. 1995;10:82–89.

33. Taussig J, Junge B, Burris S, Jones TS, Sterk CE. Individual and structural influences shaping pharmacists' decisions to sell syringes to injection drug users in Atlanta, Georgia. *Journal of American Pharmacological Association*. 2002;42(6 suppl 2):S40–S45.

34. Haines E. San Francisco to use web site in effort to promote syphilis testing, treatment. *Los Angeles Times*. June 21, 2003.

35. Arnold CB, Cogswell BE. A condom distribution program for adolescents: the findings of a feasibility study! *American Journal of Public Health*. 1971;61:739–750

36. Bedimo AL, Pinkerton SD, Cohen DA, Gray B, Farley TA. Condom distribution: a cost-utility analysis. *International Journal of STD & AIDS*. 2002;13:384–392.

37. Calsyn DA, Meinecke C, Saxon AJ, Stanton V. Risk reduction in sexual behavior: a condom giveaway program in a drug abuse treatment clinic. *American Journal of Pubic Health*. 1992;82:1536–1538.

38. Cohen DA, Nsuami M, Martin DH, Farley TA. Repeated school-based screening for sexually transmitted diseases: a feasibility strategy for reaching adolescents. *The American Academy of Pediatrics*. 1999;104:1281–1285.

39. Hanenberg R, Rojanapithayakorn W, Kunasol P, Sokal D. The impact of Thailand's HIV control programme, as indicated by the decline of sexually transmitted diseases. *Lancet*. 1994;344:243–245.

40. Robinson NJ, Silarug N, Suraiengsunk S, Auvert B, Hanenberg R. Two million HIV infections prevented in Thailand: estimate of the impact of increased condom use. Program and abstracts of the XI International conference on AIDS; 1996; Vancouver, British Columbia, Canada.

41. Rojanapithayakorn W, Hanenberg R. The 100% Condom Program in Thailand. *AIDS*. 1996;10:1–7.

42. Heimer R, Khoshnood K, Bigg D, Guydish J, Junge B. Syringe use and reuse: effects of syringe exchange programs in four cities. *Journal of AIDS and Human Retrovirology*. 1998;18(suppl 1):S37–S44.

43. Jacobs P, Calder P, Taylor M, Houston S, Saunders LD, Albert T. Cost effectiveness of Streetworks' needle exchange program of Edmonton. *Canadian Journal of Public Health*. 1999;90:168–171.

44. Kaplan EH. Economic analysis of needle exchange. *AIDS*. 1995;9:1113–1119.

45. Kaplan EH, Heimer R. A model-based estimate of HIV infectivity via needle sharing. *Journal of Acquired Immune Deficiency Syndromes*. 1992;5:1116–1118.

46. Centers for Disease Control and Prevention (CDC). Assessment of street outreach for HIV prevention—selected sites, 1991-1993. *Journal of the American Medical Association*. 1993;270:2675.

47. Calsyn DA, Saxon AJ, Freeman G, Whittaker S. Needle-use practices among intravenous drug users in an area where needle purchase is legal. *AIDS*. 1991;5:187–193.

48. Cotten-Oldenburg NU, Carr P, DeBoer JM, Collison EK, Novotny G. Impact of pharmacy-based syringe access on injection practices among injecting drug users in Minnesota, 1998 to 1999. *Journal of Acquired Immune Deficiency Syndromes and Human Retrovirology*. 2001;27:183–192.

49. Holtgrave DR, Pinkerton SD, Jones TS, Lurie P, Vlahov D. Cost and cost-effectiveness of increasing access to sterile syringes and needles as an HIV prevention intervention in the United States. *Journal of Acquired Immune Deficiency Syndromes & Human Retrovirology*. 1998;18(suppl 1):S133–S138.

50. Chesson H, Harrison P, Kassler WJ. Sex under the influence: the effect of alcohol policy on sexually transmitted disease rates in the United States. *Journal of Law and Economics*. 2000;XLIII:215–238.

51. Scribner R, Cohen D, Farley T. Geographic relation between alcohol availability and gonorrhea rates. *Sexually Transmitted Disease*. 1998;25:544–548.

52. Kahn JG, Kegeles SM, Hays R, Beltzer N. Cost-effectiveness of the Mpowerment Project, a community-level intervention for young gay men. *Journal of Acquired Immune Deficiency Syndromes & Human Retrovirology*. 2001;27:482–491.

53. Kegeles SM, Hays RB, Coates TJ. The Mpowerment Project: a community-level HIV prevention intervention for young gay men. *American Journal of Public Health*. 1996;86(8 Pt 1):1129–1136.

54. Kelly JA, St. Lawrence JS, Stevenson LY, Hauth AC, Kalichman SC, Diaz YE, Brasfield TL, Koob JJ, Morgan MG. Community AIDS/HIV risk reduction: the effects of endorsements by popular people in three cities. *American Journal of Public Health*. 1992;82:1483–1489.

55. Kelly JA, St. Lawrence JS, Diaz YE, Stevenson LY, Hauth AC, Brasfield TL, Kalichman SC, Smith JE, Andrew ME. HIV risk behavior reduction following intervention with key opinion leaders of population: an experimental analysis. *American Journal of Public Health.* 1991;81:168–171.

56. Pinkerton SD, Holtgrave DR, DiFranceisco WJ, Stevenson LY, Kelly JA. Cost-effectiveness of a community-level HIV risk reduction intervention. *American Journal of Public Health.* 1998;88:1239–1242.

57. O'Donnell L, Stueve A, San Doval A, Duran R, Haber D, Atnafou R, Johnson N, Grant U, Murray H, Juhn G, Tang J, Piessens P. The effectiveness of the Reach for Health Community Youth Service Learning Program in reducing early and unprotected sex among urban middle school students. *American Journal of Public Health.* 1999;89:176–181.

58. Golden MR, Whittington WLH, Handsfield HH, Hughes JP, Stamm WE, Hogben M, Clark A, Malinski C, Helmers JRL, Thomas KK, and Holmes KK. Effect of expedited treatment of sex partners on recurrent or persistent gonorrhea or chlamydial infection. *New England Journal of Medicine.* 2005;352:676–685.

59. Dubois-Arber F, Jeannin A, Konings E, Paccaud F. Increased condom use without other major changes in sexual behavior among the general population in Switzerland. *American Journal of Public Health.* 1997;87:558–566.

60. Lehmann P, Hausser D, Somaini B, Gutzwiller F. Campaign against AIDS in Switzerland: evaluation of a nationwide educational programme. *British Medical Journal.* 1987;295:1118–1120.

61. Farley TA. Cruise control: bathhouses are reigniting the AIDS crisis. It's time to shut them down. *Washington Monthly.* 2002;Nov.

62. Mutchler MG, Bingham T, Chion M, Jenkins RA, Klosinski LE, Secura G. Comparing sexual behavioral patterns between two bathhouses: implications for HIV prevention intervention policy. *Journal of Homosexuality.* 2003;44:221–242.

63. Green TC, Hankins CA, Palmer D, Boivin JF, Platt, R. My place, your place, or a safer place: the intention among Montreal injecting drug users to use supervised injecting facilities. *Canadian Journal of Public Health.* 2004;95:110–114.

64. Kerr T, Wood E, Small D, Palepu A, Tyndall MW. Potential use of safer injecting facilities among injection drug users in Vancouver's Downtown Eastside. *Canadian Medical Association Journal.* 2003;169:759–763.

65. Wood E, Kerr T, Spittal PM, Li K, Small W, Tyndall MW, Hogg RS, O'Shaughnessy MV, Schechter MT. The potential public health and community impacts of safer injecting facilities: evidence from a cohort of injection drug users. *Journal of Acquired Immune Deficiency Syndrome.* 2003;32:2–8.

66. Cohen DA, Ghosh-Dastidar B, Bluthenthal R, Scribner R, Farley TA, Robinson P, Scott M, Miu A, Kerndt PR. Gonorrhea and the 1992 Civil Unrest in Los Angeles. Program and abstracts of the XV International Conference on AIDS; July, 2004; Bangkok, Thailand.

67. Bloom FR, Whittier DK, Leichliter JS, McGrath JW. Gay men, syphilis, and HIV: the biological impact of social stress. In Feldman D, ed. *AIDS, Culture, and Gay Men.* Gainesville, FL: University Press of Florida (*in press*).

68. Cohen DA, Wu SY, Farley TA. Comparing the cost-effectiveness of HIV prevention interventions. *Journal of AIDS.* 2004;37:1404–1414.

6

STD Prevention Communication: Using Social Marketing Techniques with an Eye on Behavioral Change

Miriam Y. Vega, Ph.D., and Khalil G. Ghanem, M.D.

Behavior change is an effective strategy in curbing the spread of sexually transmitted infections (STIs). As a first step, we must communicate healthful behaviors to the public. Unfortunately, research has repeatedly shown that knowledge alone is not always enough (1–3): Being aware of a healthful behavior does not necessarily translate into engaging in it. Sexual behavior, in particular, has strong social components that involve a web of social relations, expectations, issues regarding confidence in one's abilities, beliefs about risk, and the perceived severity of STIs and their sequelae. Therefore, a successful prevention campaign must not only be educational, but also persuasive.

The goal of changing sexual behaviors is to ultimately decrease the rate of disease transmission. Transmissibility can be decreased by correct and consistent condom use, delaying the initiation of sexual activity, mutual monogamy, decreasing numbers of sex partners, no concurrency, and promoting use of available vaccines against STIs (e.g., hepatitis B) (4). Duration of infectiousness can be reduced by promoting rapid health evaluations for symptoms of STI and by screening high-risk asymptomatic populations. Therefore, to decrease the rate of spread, we have to target social behaviors explicitly by using persuasive communication to instill behavior change. This approach is at the core of disease prevention—halting the spread of communicable diseases (whether curable, incurable, or chronic) by changing behaviors as a primary prevention strategy, or changing behaviors after infection to prevent further spread. In both instances, social marketing, concretely based on researched theories of behavior change, is a necessary step in order to maximize effectiveness of prevention campaigns.

This chapter is not meant to be a systematic or exhaustive review of the literature on mass media campaigns, as those already exist (5). The primary purpose of this chapter is to identify factors, other than knowledge, that influence the adoption of healthful behaviors and to develop social marketing frameworks to help public health officials optimize public health campaigns aimed at preventing STIs, including HIV. We will use social marketing examples and

Behavioral Interventions for Prevention and Control of Sexually Transmitted Diseases. Aral SO, Douglas JM Jr, eds. Lipshutz JA, assoc ed. New York: Springer Science+Business Media, LLC; 2007.

highlight the different characteristics of STIs, which may have an effect on message development.

General Definition of Social Marketing

The goal of health communication is to bring about improvements in health-related practices and, in turn, health status (6). Social marketing and behavior change are integral components of health communication. Social marketing, generally, is a planned process for influencing social change. Social marketing borrows more conventional techniques from its ostensible parent, consumer marketing, including marketing and consumer research, advertising and promotion (segmentation, message design and testing, media strategy, and evaluation), and couples them with social scientific theories of behavior change. This creates a hybrid form of communication designed not to sell a product or service, but to affect awareness, attitudes, beliefs, and, consequently, behaviors. Meta-analyses have shown that health communication campaigns do have a small but tangible effect on behavior change (5). In summary, social marketing is defined as "the application of commercial marketing technologies to the analysis, planning, execution, and evaluation of programs designed to influence the voluntary behavior of target audiences in order to improve their personal welfare and that of their society" (7).

Health promotion campaigns use various mass media channels, including newspapers, magazines, radio, television, and, more recently, the Internet, to convey messages to the public. The motivation for campaign researchers to work with commercial mass media originates from consistent research, showing that mass media is often the primary source of consumer health information (8). In terms of language, social marketing refers to people as consumers, audience members, or target audiences. Behaviors may be referred to as the products being promoted. The use of mass media has become increasingly sophisticated, especially in the past few decades, and we have seen the increasing implementation of social scientific theories in the service of prevention campaign design. The increased sophistication of social marketing has led to the derivation of a corpus of best practices tenets that prevents us from having to reinvent the wheel as future prevention campaigns are conceived. In conducting a social marketing campaign, a set of logical components must be considered; we have highlighted these in the following sections. We will begin by reviewing behavioral change theories, which have a direct effect on prevention messages.

Theories of Behavior Change

Conventional wisdom holds that knowledge directly correlates with the adoption of health behaviors. Thus, health advocates spend a great deal of time and effort optimizing message design, presentation, and distribution. However, research indicates that knowledge does not necessarily result in the adoption of positive behaviors; in order to reduce morbidity and mortality, health communication must go beyond education (6). This forces us to ask the question, how do we change health behaviors when education alone does not seem to be adequate to the task? Well-known theories of behavior change can provide guidance.

The five most commonly cited theories of behavior change are the Health Belief Model (9), the Theory of Planned Behavior (10), Stages of Change (11), Social Cognitive Theory (12), and Diffusion of Innovation (13). We will broadly address these theories as they relate to social marketing; for a more in-depth review of the theories please refer to Chapter 2. Each social-psychological theory provides a framework applicable to the conception, design, and implementation of public health campaigns, and offers valuable insights into what purely informative campaigns may be lacking. These theories address broad realms of perceived susceptibility of the individual to an illness or disease, individuals' attitudes toward a behavior, perceived norms, influence by the group and the community environment, and self-efficacy (an individual's confidence in performing the behavior). Obviously, no theory is all encompassing. Interdisciplinary borrowing of techniques suggests that new insights are found in a multitude of voices, and one must consider the applicability of a given theoretical model to a particular circumstance.

First, let us consider the broader context in which we intend to examine these models, i.e. the purpose of health promotion campaigns. Health campaigns strive for a sustained public health effect. This is achieved through lasting behavior changes. Lasting change is a result of voluntary behavior change at the individual level. To facilitate this, a campaign must appeal to the values and cost-benefit evaluation of each targeted group, emphasizing short-term salient benefits rather than the long-term abstract collective benefits. Likewise, messages must be customized in such a way that they are interesting, relevant, and captivating to the audience(s). Messages should be clear, easy-to-understand, and easy to act on. Unless people remember how, when, and what to do, it's unlikely that a health communication campaign will be successful. Social marketing techniques applied to health communication campaigns have been shown to be effective in crafting health messages that "speak" to target audiences. No matter how well crafted a campaign is from a theoretical perspective, if it cannot "reach" the audience, it will not have an effect. Cultural competence and an understanding—both qualitative and quantitative—of target audiences are essential precursors to applying theories of behavior change to prevention campaigns effectively.

The Health Belief Model

The most influential theory of why people practice or fail to practice health behaviors is the Health Belief Model (HBM) (9). This model attempts to predict the practice of health behaviors on the basis of beliefs about a particular health threat and about the likelihood that a particular health behavior will lead to a reduction of that threat. In terms of social marketing, the HBM suggests that "consumers" are more likely to adopt a new behavior as recommended in a campaign if a) individuals feel threatened by the disease, and b) if they perceive that the benefits outweigh the barriers that are present. In terms of perceived costs and benefits, this factor refers to how an individual assesses the advantages and disadvantages of a particular, recommended course of action. In social marketing terminology, this is the "price." If one expects the benefits to exceed costs, then one is more likely to adopt recommended behaviors. This is especially important to consider with behaviors that involve less tangible social situations.

Messages should be designed to arouse appropriate levels of concern while considering the targets' beliefs about the price of the recommended action.

The use of comparisons, statistical data, and testimonies are techniques that may be applied to either stimulate feelings of concern where too few exist, or to allay risk perceptions when they are excessive. Risk perceptions or feelings of concern are needed to motivate change, but excessive depictions of risk in health messages can lead to avoidance, denial, and other maladaptive responses. For example, if an individual feels a consequence is inevitable, there is little incentive to adopt a preventive strategy. This model is tied to the notion of response efficacy, meaning that one believes the recommended response will mitigate negative outcomes. If one doubts the efficacy of the recommended behavior, the benefits hardly seem worth the effort. Therefore, successful health communication messages should heighten perceived benefits of recommendations while diminishing the perceived costs of their adoption.

Social Cognitive Theory

Social cognitive theory (SCT), also called social learning theory states, quite simply, that we learn how to behave in social situations by watching others; through witnessing behaviors performed by others, there is an increased sense that we can perform the behaviors efficaciously. Perhaps most prominent with respect to influencing health behavior is the concept of self-efficacy. Self-efficacy is the conviction that one can successfully execute the behavior required to produce outcomes (12).

Higher perception of self-efficacy to perform an action correlates with the likelihood of action, because when self-efficacy is low, people rarely attempt behavior change (14,15). Therefore, campaign messages should bolster people's belief that they can successfully adopt the recommended behavior. Techniques for bolstering self-efficacy might include emphasizing capability or demonstrating that recommended behaviors are easily accomplished.

Theory of Planned Behavior

The Theory of Planned Behavior (TPB) integrates attitudinal and behavioral factors, positing that the immediate antecedent of any behavior is the intention to perform it (10). The theory suggests that expected outcomes of the behavior, beliefs about what significant others think about the behavior in question, and perceived control over the behavior shape intentions. Consumers' attitudes are influenced both by perceived broad societal norms and more immediate influences such as family members. For example, a social marketing message promoting condom use may be rejected if one's social network downplays the importance of condom use.

In trying to promote chlamydia screening, campaign planners utilized TPB. They suggested that the social norm was to get screened for chlamydia (16). The campaign was reportedly successful in encouraging those exposed to it over the radio and television to call a hotline. This model suggests that making a behavior seem socially desirable, rather than aberrant, will more likely lead to its adoption.

Diffusion of Innovation Model

The Diffusion of Innovation Model (DIM) looks at how new ideas are communicated to, and accepted by, members of a group or population (13). A major component of the theory is the recognition of the utility of highly visible and respected opinion leaders who can assist in dispensing a message.

In terms of prevention campaigns, campaign planners could enlist members of status (celebrity, social involvement) within a particular community, to disseminate and personally endorse messages. Mobilizing the support of opinion leaders significantly improves chances of successful innovation because they use their ability to influence the community and facilitate changes in social norms and behaviors by sharing factual information, expressing their concern for prevention, and endorsing and modeling effective behavior change strategies within their social and sexual networks.

Stages of Change

The Stages of Change (SOC) model addresses a person's readiness to respond to a lifestyle change, moving through a series of five stages as they adopt or alter a behavior pattern (11). The SOC maintains that movement through the stages varies from person to person. While these stages may not accurately describe the behavior change process in all situations or different cultures, understanding these stages can provide yet another framework for developing communication programs.

Again, this model reinforces the notion that information dissemination alone does not constitute an effective prevention communication. Enhanced awareness and knowledge of risks are important conditions for change; however, knowledge is not always the chief motivator for change. A program that starts with skills (e.g., how to use a condom), before individuals accept that they are at risk, may fail. Individuals in pre-contemplation and contemplation stages should receive messages that increase awareness, in addition to susceptibility, benefits, and emotional setbacks that others have experienced. Those that are in preparation and action should receive messages reinforcing new behaviors and modeling skills needed for the behavior, which in turn enhances self-efficacy.

Integrating Insights of Behavioral Change Theories to Prevention Campaigns

STIs are socially transmitted diseases in as far as sexual behavior is social behavior. Behavior changes that not only minimize physical risks, but also account for social components of transmission, represent the greatest promise of controlling the spread of STIs. These theoretical models have been advanced in health-risk research as useful in understanding and predicting preventive health behaviors within social contexts. They differ, while building upon each other, and commonly emphasize decision-making processes leading to healthful behaviors. These models suggest perceived costs are weighed against perceived benefits and that the decision-maker is acutely aware of vulnerability, as well as being capable or willing to make choices that minimize risk or optimize protection. Importantly, decisions to adopt preventive behaviors are not made in a vacuum; rather, they are generated within a social context.

In order to change, individuals must perceive the following: 1) They are at personal risk; 2) changing their behavior will result in benefits that are relevant to them; 3) social norms will support their actions at each stage of behavioral change; 4) they have the skills and resources needed to make the changes; and 5) they are ready for change. This suggests that a complex approach is needed when designing a campaign to encourage preventive health behaviors. To be effective, the campaign should attend to elements not only of information, but also perceived vulnerability, self-efficacy, response efficacy (benefits outweigh costs, both personal and social), readiness to change, intention and motivation to change, potential skills deficits (e.g., negotiation skills in a relationship), peer group norms and support, self-knowledge, and critical awareness of social and cultural forces. In Table 1, we highlight some campaign examples. The main purpose of using behavior change theories is to optimize the conditions needed for people to make healthy choices.

As we elaborate on social marketing techniques, several questions are vital. How, in creating a social marketing campaign around STI prevention, can we a) speak directly to the target population, raising personal awareness; and b) encourage community-wide dialogue about STIs, thus changing the cultural norms?

Table 1 Theories of behavior change and some applications.

	Definition	Example of social marketing component
Health Belief Model (HBM)	People engage in a new behavior depending on their perception of risk for a certain condition (disease X): how serious disease X is, its consequences, and belief in the efficacy of the behavior to reduce risk or severity of effect.	• To increase sense of vulnerability in the target population, use someone who "looks" and has a similar background to the target audience. Arouse fear but provide a clear solution.
Theory of Reasoned Action (TRA)	Subjective norms dictate whether a person will engage in a new behavior—namely, their beliefs about how people around them will view the behavior in question.	• Suggesting that others are engaged in the behavior being promoted. • The University of North Carolina, Chapel Hill, (2003, 2004) conducted a social norms marketing campaign for first-year students with the theme: "Whether it's Thursday, Friday, or Saturday night, 2 out of 3 UNC students return home with a .00 blood alcohol concentration." They used actual blood alcohol level data.
Social Cognitive Theory (SCT)	People acquire new patterns of behavior by observing or learning from others and building a sense of self-efficacy—a belief that one can do the behavior.	• Having someone model the new behavior. • Instead of just saying that people should negotiate condom use, can actually show a couple discussing condom use.
Stages of Change (SOC)	People do not change their behavior overnight. Instead, they go through a series of stages: from not thinking about making a change, to considering the change, to finally changing a specific behavior.	• Targeting people at different stages and providing cues that may help them move along those stages. • Individuals just contemplating starting a new behavior may need only to read a brochure or watch a brief video. • To help someone move from contemplation to action, can highlight how the new behavior will have a direct effect on those around them.

(Continued)

Table 1 Theories of behavior change and some applications. — Cont'd

	Definition	Example of social marketing component
Diffusion of Innovation (DOI)	A new idea or behavior is circulated by a respected community leader and accepted by the community members over time.	• Having a community leader advocate the behavior being promoted. • In Seattle a "manifesto" was put together by key members of the MSM community and was circulated throughout the neighborhoods and in local media. • Can have key community members wearing promotional items such as T-shirts and caps carrying messages about contraceptive use.

Social Marketing Techniques

A behavior change communication program, besides utilizing behavioral theories of change, needs to draw upon well-tested and practiced contemporary marketing principles. These principles entail 1) segmenting the target audience by variables including age, sex, socioeconomic levels, psychographics (i.e., attitudes, values, outlook); 2) audience research to assess actual attitudes, perceptions, knowledge, and behavior as well as nuanced aspects of culture for a particular target population; 3) concept development and pre-testing to ensure strategies and materials are effective and relevant; messages should target various segments of the audience, because one message rarely moves everyone; 4) addressing benefits meaningful to the audience; and 5) evaluation. See Table 2 for an outline of these steps. Campaign planners can use results of epidemiological studies to define relevant health problems, conduct interviews and focus groups to learn how people conceive of STIs and health problems, and make use of various mass media channels to cause change.

As with all endeavors, clear goals and objectives help focus the direction of thought, research, and resources in the design and implementation of prevention campaigns. A widely known means for setting out realistic prevention campaign goals (known by the acronym SMART) is used frequently in the prevention field and is useful to consider. SMART campaigns are 1) Specific (identify what will be done to whom, when, and where); 2) Measurable (identify when and how many); 3) Attainable (achievable: Are you attempting too much?); 4) Realistic (can it be done with available resources—including staff and technologies?); 5) Time-phased (identify a specified time; when you will achieve the objective). A basic formula for objectives could be, "By (date), XX% of the (demographic or psychological segments) in (community) will (be aware of, believe that, do ...)," or more concretely, "By the year 2007, 75% of Spanish-speaking women in the South Bronx will understand what a Pap smear is used for." Along with SMART objectives, it is important to outline a campaign's performance indicators. Performance indicators are measures of inputs, processes, outputs, outcomes, and effects for development of programs. When supported with sound data and reporting, indicators enable managers to track progress, demonstrate results, and take corrective action to improve delivery. Participation of key stakeholders in defining indicators is important, as they are then more likely to understand and use indicators for making management decisions. To establish performance indicators, one can develop

Table 2 Social marketing techniques.

	Methods	Accomplishes	Questions that should be answered
Establishing SMART goals	Review of epidemiological & demographic profiles Creating an evaluation and communication plan Developing a logic model	An assessment of the problem, available resources, funding, and target audience. Sets performance indicators to help assess progress of campaign	What is the problem? What are your objectives? Do your objectives target a specific audience? Are the objectives measurable, attainable, timely, and realistic? Which resources will be needed for the campaign? What are future steps?
Conducting formative evaluation	Focus groups Community mapping Community observation Key informant interviews Surveys	Identification of the target audience, their attitudes, beliefs & knowledge along with their actions, & locations of relevance.	What does your target audience know? What does your target audience believe? At what locations can your target audience be found? What behaviors does your target audience engage in?
Developing messages	Analyze formative evaluation results Review theoretical models Develop tag lines Consult with key informants	Identification of the messages that are needed and how to word those messages in a theoretically sound and culturally appropriate manner	Which theoretical models will help address the target's beliefs, attitudes and knowledge in a culturally responsive manner?
Designing campaign materials	Determine channels and formats to reach audience.	Development of draft materials. Assessment of how to deliver messages (poster, radio spot, palm cards, fotonovelas, manifesto).	What information should be presented? What appeal should be used? How will you reach the audience?
Test marketing	Focus groups Key informant interviews	Assessment of reaction to the messages and concepts. Assessment of theory	How will your audience react to the materials? Will they understand the Message?
Dissemination of materials to target population	Utilizing community leaders and stakeholders Creating media buzz	Distribution of materials within relevant locations Receiving free media exposure.	How to reach audience? Where will audience be exposed to message?
Evaluation of campaign	Process evaluation Outcome evaluation Impact evaluation	Assessment of the challenges of implementing the campaign and analyses including obstacles and facilitators. Assessment of how the campaign is affecting beliefs, knowledge, attitudes, and/or behaviors of the target audience. Assessment of campaign awareness and recall.	Was the campaign implemented as originally planned? Does your target audience recall the campaign? Have those who have seen/heard the campaign engaged in the proposed behavior (i.e. testing)? Are there measurable outcomes such as changes in incidence?
Refining campaign	Interpret and draw conclusions from what has been evaluated.	Assessment of what has been learned through the various evaluation methods. Campaign evolvement.	Can and should the campaign be changed?

a logic model. The logic model clarifies objectives of any project, program, or policy. It aids in the identification of expected causal links—the "program logic"—in the following results chain: inputs, processes, outputs (including coverage or "reach" across beneficiary groups), outcomes, and impact. It leads to the identification of performance indicators at each stage in this chain, as well as impediments in the attainment of the objectives. The logic model is also a vehicle for engaging partners in clarifying objectives and designing activities. During implementation of the campaign, the logic model serves as a useful tool to review progress and take corrective action. This can also guide evaluation—a step that many perceive as being at the end of a sequential process, but a step that we posit needs to be conceived of at the beginning of the social marketing process, as it affects every step of the social marketing campaign.

Evaluation

Evaluation is a continual process of judging value on what a project or program has achieved, particularly in relation to activities planned and overall objectives. Evaluation is important because it helps identify the constraints or bottlenecks. Solutions to constraints can then be identified and implemented. Evaluation starts at the beginning. Recall that we mentioned that SMART objectives must be measurable so that they may be continually evaluated. Evaluation starts with objectives and should take place throughout. This enables project planners and implementers to progressively review strategies according to changing circumstances to attain the desired objectives.

Types and stages of evaluation vary across fields. For social marketing purposes, three types of evaluation are especially relevant: formative (evaluating who the target audience is); process monitoring (did the campaign reach the intended audience?); and outcome monitoring (did the intended audience's behavior change as a result?).

Formative evaluation focuses on the pre-implementation phase and lays the foundation for a campaign. This is groundwork for the development of campaign messages, placement, and design. During this stage, we ask what the extent of the problem is; we review the demographics of the problem; we research knowledge, attitudes and practices; and contributing influences. Formative evaluation informs you about the target audience (where they spend time, what they do with their time, what they read, what television shows they watch). What you learn about the problem during the formative stage will help you decide which audience your program will focus on. The channels of communication you disseminate messages through will depend on where the individuals within your target audience get information.

Process evaluation is a structured way to provide program staff members with additional feedback about their work. This feedback is primarily designed to fine-tune implementation of the program, and often includes information that is purely for internal use by program managers. Process evaluation centers around two issues: 1) did the program involve the targeted audience; and 2) were the planned activities actually carried out? During process evaluation, we ask who the targeted audience was and whether they participated. In other words, what was delivered to whom and when. Again, this takes you back to the SMART objectives and performance indicators.

Outcome monitoring is more complex than process monitoring. Outcome monitoring seeks to define the extent to which the campaign has met anticipated outcomes. Outcome evaluation addresses the results of a program and measures the effects on the target population.

Imagine you are putting together a campaign targeting college-aged women regarding chlamydia:

1. What was their baseline knowledge of chlamydia (i.e. formative evaluation)?
2. What was their knowledge after the communication program (i.e. process evaluation)?
3. Did the women go and get tested (i.e. outcome evaluation)?

You will also need to assess exposure to the campaign messages. Though exposure to the campaign messages by itself does not guarantee changes in behavior, the probability of success is enhanced. Recall and recognition are measures that specifically determine whether audiences are seeing campaign messages or logos or brand names. Respondents are asked to recall whether they have seen, heard, or read anything on the campaign topic and, if so, the medium in which they have seen or heard or read the message. Attention is measured by asking the respondents specific questions about the campaign. For recall, you do not want just to ask "do you remember this campaign"; you should ask "can you name the characters?" or "can you name three specific items from the campaign?" If, for example, a campaign included a hotline number, one can measure how many calls come into the hotline before, during, and after the campaign. Evaluation is a constant that helps form and improve a campaign, and it is important to continually ask the question of how goals and objectives can be measured.

Target Segmentation

A core principle in social marketing is targeting campaigns to carefully selected segments of a larger audience. Targeting refers to the practice of segmenting the population into unique and distinguishable groups to which specific products, services, or messages are directed (17). Audience segmentation is based on selected variables such as demographics (e.g., age and sex), health status (STD- or HIV-positive), geographic dispersion, and values. Targeting allows planners to select appropriate messages, message sources, and channels for each audience segment. Few practice this as effectively as the television and movie industry, and this is, of course, how the coveted 18–35-year-old demographic came into common awareness. A portion of the population was identified demographically as most likely to possess the expendable income, buying power, and consumer habits that would result in the most profitable return for an advertiser's money; much of television is geared towards capturing the attention of this particular group and affecting their consumer behavior. There is an important lesson for social marketers to learn from this: When considering the design of a prevention campaign, we are looking for the most return on our investment. Our gains are measured in the reduction of the spread of disease, and, following this model, we profit by isolating a high-risk demographic and targeting them in a manner that will be most effective.

Target segmentation involves grouping people on the basis of common characteristics. The purpose of grouping people together from a communication context is to identify audiences whose similar characteristics are considered important to the communication of prevention messages. What works with one group may not work with another, and only a clear understanding based on research into the target population can uncover the specifics. For example, the cities of San Francisco and Los Angeles are both in California and both used the same advertising agency in recent syphilis prevention campaigns targeting men having sex with men (MSMs). The campaigns, very similarly conceived initially, were designed to incorporate "mascots" Phil the Sore (as part of the *Stop the Sores* Campaign) and The Healthy Penis (featured in promotional materials and costumed outreach workers). Formative research on the target population in Los Angeles indicated that the "Healthy Penis" image conveyed a negative message, which labeled MSM as "dicks" and sex-crazed. Thus, Los Angeles chose "Phil the Sore." In San Francisco, the sore character has not been as popular as the "Healthy Penis," reflecting a preference for a sex-positive image, which was noted in pre-testing (18).

Target segmentation entails developing an audience-centered orientation, rather than focusing solely on the conveyed message. This orientation is achieved by formative research into the audience profile (needs, wants, perceptions, lifestyles, living environment, and media habits). This is why extensive research on the target audience should be conducted before messages are developed to determine the existing attitudes and social norms concerning targeted behaviors. This research should a) identify the beliefs that differentiate members of the target audience who do and do not perform the desired behavior and b) determine whether the target population has the capacity to perform the desired behavior.

What do you want your target audiences to know, think, and do (adopt behaviors or policies; make donations or decisions; subscriptions, etc.)? Be specific about what you want them to "do," since it is the most important component when analyzing target audiences. You may want to divide information between different segments in each audience: Those who have already adopted the behaviors or actions and those who have not. Some of these persons may be against the idea. However, most of them are probably receptive, but face real or perceived barriers. Understanding this population/audience segment (those who have not adopted the behavior or action) is essential to the rest of your plan. Social marketers should not assume that what worked with some people will work with everyone. In some sense, generalizations are necessary, but inattention to the level of generalizations being made about target populations can be the difference between success and failure.

There are numerous examples of nationally directed social marketing campaigns, but just as all politics are local, so too should be social marketing campaigns. Identification of the activity that needs to be promoted (testing, healthful choices), local epidemiology, local barriers to engaging in promoted behaviors, and identifying ways around those barriers by using structural and psychological methods are necessary steps for any well-conceived campaign. For example, an evaluation was conducted of HIV testing rates during the three months immediately before and after London's 1994 World AIDS Day (a very general campaign to raise AIDS awareness). Participants were stratified according to sex, sexual orientation, and the reasons for testing. Findings were compared with data from the initial HIV awareness campaign in 1986–1987 to see whether there were any differences in the two separate one-day social marketing campaigns in terms of increasing rates of testing and identifying positive test takers. There were no significant differences across time periods in rates of testing. Furthermore, there were no differences in numbers of individuals testing positive within specific segments of the population (heterosexual, bisexual, gay) before and after World AIDS Day. This example demonstrates the limitations of a general campaign that targets multiple heterogeneous at-risk groups and it highlights the importance of targeting the campaign in order to ensure a successful outcome in the population of interest.

In 1988, the *America Responds to AIDS* campaign was developed, consisting of public service announcements (PSAs), a telephone hotline, and brochures (19). PSAs showed an individual who knew someone with AIDS discussing the disease, trying to instill fear to motivate behavior change, and emphasizing preventive measures. The brochure was sent to all U.S. households to increase knowledge. While fear was raised, and the campaign was found to have increased calls to an information hotline, the campaign ultimately fizzled. There was no target segmentation, diffusion of information through community leaders was not achieved, and the information was not propagated through informal community channels (19).

It is especially useful to consider the Diffusion of Innovation theory with regards to target segmentation. Preventive innovations are typically difficult to diffuse within most social systems (13). However, it appears that positive, dense networks (e.g., strong supervisory and peer relations), along with broad interpersonal communication channels (e.g., multiple, diverse number of friends, acquaintances, and colleagues), result in an increased possibility for the acceptance of preventive innovations. Thus, local segmentation can aid in identifying the most effective targets to initiate the diffusion of prevention messages.

While target segmentation is necessary, it does not mean that a prevention campaign should pick one high-risk population exclusively as its target. Even if only one population is being targeted, it does not mean that direct marketing to that population alone is the most effective way of designing a campaign. Effective social marketing campaigns often have multiple target audiences, which usually include the affected population and other individuals and groups that influence the environment of the affected population. While prudent to target a very specific population, there are often multiple avenues to communicate messages to that population.

Pretesting Materials

Understanding a target audience entails knowing their epidemiology, needs, and predispositions towards the campaign planner's issues of interest; it also entails knowing what they think about the actual materials and messages proposed for distribution. Social marketing revolves around the audience. Pretesting is a type of research that involves systematically gathering target reactions to messages and materials before they are produced in final form. Testing involves selecting a group of individuals that share the key characteristics of the target group. For example, if the social marketing campaign is targeting young gay males, focus groups should consist of young gay males. The object is to determine whether the reaction of the test group meets the predetermined objectives and goals for the intervention. In other words, are we saying what we think we are saying? Some questions to consider: 1) How does the test group feel about, respond to, or change as a result of participating in different intervention activities? 2) Does the activity effectively convey the message? 3) Assess comprehension: Does it make sense to the target audience? Before the target audience can accept your message, they have to be able to understand it. 4) Determine personal relevance: Will the target audience perceive the message as relevant? For the message to be effective, the audience must feel that it is talking to someone like them.

In terms of campaign design, testing can help determine whether the materials are appealing to the targeted populations and will generate interest in each group. Pre-testing can detect overlooked aspects as well, such as the adequacy of the reading level of materials. Pre-testing could also suggest more mundane and straightforward marketing issues; for example, whether the addition of more graphics is needed to garner greater attention. Essentially, the core of pre-testing is to determine whether the material or strategy is both appropriate and acceptable to the intended audience in a "real-life" test. Because health behaviors are imbedded in social beliefs, values, and traditions, it is important to use materials and strategies that are consistent with the cultural norms of the particular community or group. Pre-testing often reveals whether a message, material, or channel is culturally acceptable, or it may help define how it can be made more so.

Channel Mixing

In selecting channels—the methods of message delivery (choices about how to reach a target audience) will be made. Information from the process of target segmentation and pre-testing is of use in identifying effective means for reaching a target population. Determining not only what types of media are popular, but specifically which brands, titles, and establishments are frequented are details of great importance. It does no good to advertise in the *Washington Times*, when a target population reads the *Washington Post*. What newspapers are read, what TV shows are watched, which churches are attended, which agencies are used, what recreational activities are engaged in, and what businesses are patronized—this information helps define a "culture." From a social scientific standpoint, this information will provide more data about the target population, and from a practical standpoint this information is absolutely necessary to determine how to efficiently get information to its target.

Campaigns that use multiple channels at different times to deliver messages are more effective at changing behaviors than those that rely on a single modality (20–22). Furthermore, the most successful health communication campaigns involve a "systems approach" that combines multiple mass media approaches (TV, radio, print, etc.), booklets, direct mail, community partnerships, training efforts, and activities by grass roots organizations that have credibility with the target audience(s). These efforts, combined together in an effective and coordinated manner, can attract more attention, and can reach more people.

The key is using multiple communication formats and changing messages to match changing needs and interests of different target audiences. The methods selected should be based on an analysis of the target groups' profiles. For example, print materials serve best as tools for raising awareness, reinforcing a certain behavior, or as a reminder. Radio and television can serve to disseminate information very quickly to many people simultaneously. Developing and distributing target-audience-specific print materials on STIs (informational brochures, disease-specific fact sheets, treatment guidelines, talk boards, billboards, posters, etc.) should be part of a continuing effort. Visual materials help individuals remember important information better than just reading or hearing alone. Audiovisual materials such as videotapes are useful in disseminating messages and ideas to audiences and can be especially useful for demonstrating or modeling a specific behavior.

Regardless of the media outlet used, campaigns should be clear, consistent, and credible. Clarity is a function not just of language, but also of visual elements. All messages should be consistent with one another and with program objectives, regardless of format. Sources that your audience believe and trust have a great effect. Family or extended family members, peers, slightly older peers, and successful role models are all possibilities for spokespersons. Again, careful audience research should be the guide. For some audiences, trust is a major issue. Credibility is an issue that was highlighted in the diffusion of innovations theory, noting that government agencies, for some target groups, may not be viewed as credible.

New Frontiers

The goal of the social marketing campaigns around STI prevention is to create and apply a range of communication strategies, research designs, and theories of behavior that can lead to behavior changes in large numbers of people. One should not limit oneself to PSAs when considering mass media outlets. There may be opportunities to get messages into news and entertainment programming as well.

Media advocacy is the strategic use of news-making through TV, radio, and newspapers to promote public debate, and generate community support for changes in community norms and policies (23). Throughout the *Stop the Sores* syphilis campaign, planners engaged in media advocacy by looking for opportunities to create news to support their awareness campaigns. Campaign representatives presented formative research findings, campaign design, and outcome evaluations at national conferences where press picked up on the findings for a news story. Additionally, the campaign was evocative, and thus engendered media coverage on its own. The *Stop the Sores* campaign was featured on "The Tonight Show" on NBC and on "The Daily Show" on Comedy Central. Furthermore, the *Stop the Sores* campaign planners intentionally sent out press releases during "sweeps" month when more viewers tend to tune in. This media coverage allowed the awareness campaigns to get increased publicity at no additional cost.

Entertainment education, also known as enter-educate, pro-social entertainment, or edu-tainment is used throughout the world to put educational content into entertainment formats to increase knowledge, create favorable attitudes, and change overt behavior concern over a health issue (24). Edu-tainment, is popular entertainment imbedded with health or social messages. Edu-tainment can model desired behavior (SCT), provide lessons on the rewards of a new behavior and the disadvantages of an old one (HBM) and create new norms (TPB).

Entertainment-education story lines have been imbedded in television shows for several decades. When sitcom "All in the Family"'s Edith Bunker discovered a lump in her breast and went to get a mammogram, there was a reported increase in the number of women seeking breast exams (25). A more recent example occurred on the sitcom "Friends." The episode focused on pregnancy resulting from condom failure. One of the characters, Rachel, experiences an unplanned pregnancy after a one-night stand with Ross, another main character. In the episode, Rachel tells Ross about the pregnancy. Ross responds with disbelief and exclaims, "But we used a condom!" Two subsequent messages that "condoms are only 97% effective" reinforced the condom use and condom failure elements. Thus, the possibility of condom failure and the resulting consequence of pregnancy were communicated to a very large adolescent audience in a vivid manner (on its first airing, the episode drew 1.7 million U.S. viewers between 12 and 17 years old) (26). In a nationwide telephone survey conducted after the episode aired, 27% of the 506 teens polled had seen it, and 65% of them recalled the sex education message about condom failure (26). The youths who talked to an adult about the episode were more likely to report learning about condoms than teens that didn't. These teens were also less likely to reduce their perception of condom efficacy after the episode.

These examples demonstrate possibilities for delivery of important health messages to a large audience through edu-tainment. They also indicate a potential for influencing awareness, knowledge, and beliefs. Working closely with scriptwriters and producers, STI-related information can be written into the story lines of popular sitcoms and soap operas. This not only helps raise awareness, but may also change social norms over a period of time. One can create story lines out of real life cases from agencies and communities. Such story lines may be referred to as "log lines" and can be pitched to studio executives or series' scriptwriters more effectively during the summer (27).

Research Methods

Various research methods described above provide social marketers with data and feedback on the campaign and the content of the messages. There is a particular emphasis on the use of focus groups, community observation, community mapping, and street intercepts. Focus groups are used to explore issues, describe context and findings, and discover new ideas, issues, concerns, and connections. Focus groups are not polls, but in-depth, qualitative interviews with a small number of carefully selected people brought together to discuss a host of topics ranging from pizza to safe sex. The composition of a focus group is usually based on similarity of the group members. Bringing people with common interests or experiences together makes it easier for them to carry on a productive discussion. The focus groups can be used throughout all phases of the campaign, from formative evaluation, to pre-testing materials and subsequent modifications. In a smoking prevention campaign targeting adolescents, campaign researchers observed a message recognition rate of 61% among Arizona adolescents after 18 months, which was attributed to the use of focus groups (28). Specifically, focus groups evaluated the effectiveness of message content and style before implementing a smoking prevention activity.

Mapping is the visual representation of data by geography or location—the linking of information to place. Community mapping does this in order to illustrate social and economic change on a community level. Mapping is a powerful tool in two ways: 1) it makes patterns and trends based on place easier to identify and analyze; and 2) it provides a visual way of communicating those patterns to a broad audience, quickly, and dramatically. Increasingly, community practitioners are using Geographic Information Systems (GIS) to carry out community mapping projects. Limited funds may preclude the use of advanced technologies. However, for a social marketing project carried out with limited funds, you can have outreach staff members go out into the neighborhood to discover the community's assets.

Unobtrusive observational studies are conducted by observing the target audience's behavior while it is happening. In a syphilis elimination social marketing campaign in Houston during 2003, campaign planners used community-mapping techniques to locate sites where MSM met for anonymous sex. Over 70 anonymous-sex venues were located (e.g., adult book/video stores, bathhouses, public restrooms, fitness centers). Observations at these sites revealed the type of clients, behaviors, and availability of health information. Subsequently, street intercepts administered at some venues provided information about clients' knowledge of STIs, community norms and attitudes, and sex and drug-using behaviors. The resulting campaign reported the number of MSM tested for syphilis increased by 22% from the previous year.

Street intercepts involve approaching likely target members at a certain time and place, asking a few qualification or screening questions, then asking for permission to deliver a questionnaire in return for a small incentive. Intercept surveys have great advantages in terms of low expense, speed of data collection, and collecting a range of views. They are typically used to assess awareness and recall of a campaign. You can use street intercepts after community observation to better understand observed behaviors after campaign implementation or to assess outcomes.

The *Stop the Sores* campaign in Los Angeles was implemented in 2002 and 2003. It was developed to address a resurgence of syphilis in MSM in 2001, which increased 80%, from 126 cases in 2000 to 227 in 2001. The campaign used the following channels: magazines targeting MSM, campaign-linked outreach events, "Phil the Sore"–costumed outreach workers, posters, and media advocacy. Immediately after roll-out, MSM were sampled, primarily at coffee shops, sidewalks, strip malls, parks, and laundromats over a two-month period. Of those sampled, 62% were exposed to the campaign, and, of those, 57% got tested. On average, respondents reported seeing the campaign 15 times. After controlling for ethnicity/race, age, HIV status, number of anonymous partners, and number of commercial sex venue visits in the foregoing month, men who were aware of the campaign were three times more likely to have been tested for syphilis in the foregoing six months. The top four perceived messages of the campaign included practice safe sex, get tested, learn about syphilis, and use condoms.

Message Content and Characteristics

Beyond developing messages that provide information, campaign developers need to take into account the behavior theories reviewed earlier by addressing perceptions of risks, perceptions of self, one's physical and social environments, and the costs and benefits of recommendations. The identification of the factors likely to influence preventive health outcomes allows for the development of five general frameworks of message design:

1. Messages should communicate levels of risk.
2. Messages should bolster a sense of self-efficacy.
3. Messages should promote efficacy of recommendations.
4. Messages should encourage consumers to visualize a new norm.
5. Messages should promote benefits and minimize costs.

How messages in campaigns are framed in terms of appeal is also important. Emotional appeals may make a message attention-getting and memorable; strong emotional appeals may backfire if not done carefully. One of the most controversial emotional appeals is fear (29). Fear appeals attempt to elicit a response from the target audience using fear as a motivator (e.g., fear of injury, illness, loss of life). The key to ensuring successful fear tactic campaigns is to give individuals specific information about the effectiveness of a recommended action as well as clear information on how to actually do what is recommended (30). If no such information is given about a desired health behavior change, scare tactic campaigns may cause people to deny they're at risk for health hazards. People who are threatened will take one of two courses of action: danger control or fear control (30). Danger control seeks to reduce the risk. Fear control seeks to reduce the perception of risk. Danger control is outer-focused towards a solution. Fear control is inner-focused away from a solution. For danger control to be selected, a person needs to perceive that an effective response is available (response efficacy) and that they are capable of utilizing this to reduce the risk (self-efficacy). If danger control is not available or selected, then action defaults to fear control.

A meta-analysis suggests that strong fear appeals produce high levels of perceived severity and susceptibility to a particular disease, and that they are more persuasive than low or weak fear appeals (30). The results also indicate that fear appeals motivate both adaptive danger control actions such as message acceptance and maladaptive fear control actions such as defensive avoidance. It appears that strong fear appeals and high-efficacy messages produce the greatest behavior change, while strong fear appeals with low-efficacy messages produce the greatest levels of defensive responses.

Along with cautious use of fear, appeals can frame messages to emphasize what a person can lose if they do not engage in preventive behaviors that are sometimes considered risky (e.g., talking to a partner about using condoms). It has been argued that it may be better to focus on those that did not engage in healthful behaviors (did not use a condom) and contracted an STI (31). The degree to which messages should attend to specific factors depends on those targeted and on the results of the formative research.

STI Characteristics

The relation between perceived vulnerability, perceived severity of the STI, and preventive behaviors is a central component of health communication and thus of message development. We have discussed the behavioral theories and social marketing techniques, alluding to STIs in general. Let us look now at how specific STI characteristics need to be taken into account when developing messages targeted at particular infections. We should note that, in general, people tend to underestimate their vulnerability to adverse (negative) health events (32).

HIV poses a serious threat to health; it also has a prolonged incubation period. Transmission of HIV, is a function of a combination of factors, including the infectivity of the donor, characteristics of the recipient, and the nature of the frequency of the risk behaviors (33). As a result, some people who engage in high-risk behaviors do not contract the virus, whereas others appear to contract it from a single exposure. Therefore, perceived vulnerability will vary greatly. Also, HIV is highly stigmatized, which may cause denial of vulnerability. In all, social marketing campaigns need to take into account the fear surrounding HIV and perhaps the denial of personal susceptibility as a result of that fear.

In 1987, Australia released the "Grim Reaper" advertisement, in which the Reaper knocked down men, women, and children in a bowling alley. While the advertisement garnered media attention, it may have led some to see those with HIV as the reaper instead of the dead (the original intent) (34). The advertisement did increase awareness; however, a cohort of gay men exposed to the campaign were later found to have reduced safe sex behaviors (35). One hypothesis is that the campaign may have motivated maladaptive fear control responses such as denial. Furthermore, the advertisement raised the anxiety level and the rates of testing among an unintended population: low risk heterosexuals-especially women (36). What was ineffectual about the ad was not that it induced fear; rather, it did not provide an appropriate context in which to raise a sense of personal threat and efficacy in its target audience. Similarly, the 1988 *America Responds to AIDS* campaign presented a heterosexual family and a slogan stating: "AIDS—Protect yourself and your family—get the facts." Awareness was increased; however, the message did not provide a concrete plan to prevent HIV, and consequently the campaign did not lead to specific behavior changes (37).

Taking into account the behavioral theories discussed thus far, a social marketing campaign around testing could try to promote the positive outcomes of counseling and testing (that is, peace of mind and opportunity for early medical intervention). It could also change the perception of the social norm by suggesting that many members of the target audience are being counseled and tested. Because HIV is highly stigmatized, there would be a need to emphasize and diffuse a new testing norm. Creating a sense of personal vulnerability can be done by increasing the personal relevance of messages, taking into account cultural sensitivity, or presenting a source similar to the target audience. Personal vulnerability must be accompanied by recommendations about how to avoid the threat.

The issues associated with human papillomavirus (HPV) are varied and complex. Although HPV is the most prevalent STI in the United States, fewer than one third of men in the general population have heard of it; similarly, lack of knowledge has been reported among women in general, and high school and college-aged women in particular (38,39). Of those who have heard of HPV, few are aware that it is associated with cervical carcinoma; that it can be present without symptoms; or that it can be transmitted by genital contact. Furthermore, even amongst those who regularly get Papanicolaou (Pap) smears, there is a lack of knowledge as to its purpose (40). Many women who reject the Pap test do so because of the necessary pelvic examination (41)—this is particularly true of Hispanic women (42,43). In a study assessing perceived risks and beliefs, the majority of women attributed negative emotions (guilt, anxiety, regretful, dirty) to hypothetically testing positive for HPV (44). Research on women who have received abnormal cervical smear results indicates that they often experience psychological consequences, including anxiety, fears about cancer, sexual difficulties, changes in body image, and concerns about the loss of reproductive functions (45). Thus, there are emotional costs associated with HPV testing. Furthermore, there are conflicting messages about HPV: it is extremely common, and it could lead to cervical cancer, yet most women spontaneously clear the infection (46). Women struggle to balance the understanding that HPV usually regresses without treatment with the knowledge that HPV can, in some cases, progress to cervical cancer (47). Therefore, we must develop campaigns that are cognizant of these issues and that attempt to minimize women's confusion, guilt, anxiety, and psychological distress (48). Because HPV is common, and because those at highest risk of developing cervical cancer are women who have not had consistent Pap screenings, it would make sense to focus a campaign on those who do not get frequent Pap smears.

Some women diagnosed with chlamydia experience concern about future reproductive morbidity and anxiety about negative reactions from friends, family, and sex partners (49). Current knowledge of the natural course of chlamydia is insufficient to provide complete reassurance about an individual's future reproductive health. It is imperative that care be taken to ensure that women do not develop unrealistic expectations of chlamydia screening. For example, campaigns should not inadvertently imply that diagnosis and treatment of chlamydia will prevent infertility. Indeed, given the current state of knowledge about chlamydia, some uncertainty about future reproductive health may be an inevitable cost of screening those who test positive; this should be made clear to women before their participation (49). Whereas women feel anxious about their future reproductive health, fear stigmatization, and blame themselves for contracting chlamydia, men generally report less concern, are unwilling to disclose their condition to sex partners, and some project attributions of blame onto their partners (50). Delays in seeking care appeared to be related to perceptions that chlamydia is a relatively minor infection, particularly in men. Thus, health promotion campaigns need to reflect sex and age differences, emphasizing the negative consequences of delayed clinic attendance and exposure to repeat infections.

Although approximately 20% of the population is infected with HSV-2, 80% of these infections are unrecognized or asymptomatic (51). However, even asymptomatic infections have been associated with shedding of the virus from the genital tract, thereby increasing the risk of transmission. There has been concern that HSV-2 testing of persons without symptoms will cause substantial psychosocial harm. However, recent research has shown that there is no apparent lasting adverse psychosocial effect of detecting HSV-2 infection of people without a history of genital herpes who also are seeking herpes testing at an STD clinic (52). Furthermore, HSV-2-specific related concerns include fear of telling future partners, concern about transmitting to a sex partner, feeling sexually undesirable, feeling socially stigmatized, feeling like "damaged goods," sex avoidance owing to social responsibility, fear of transmitting to a newborn, and relationship concerns relating to the diagnosis (53). Unlike chlamydia, which is curable with antibiotics, HSV-2 is not curable; it can, and often does recur, thus "disclosing" itself to a sex partner. People with HSV-2 may see themselves as a "walking disease." Therefore, communications regarding HSV-2 should highlight the asymptomatic nature of infection, and the potential for transmission despite a lack of symptoms. Researchers have found that tying the importance of getting tested to the goal of protecting the health of sex partners is associated with increased intentions of getting tested (54).

Prior to the introduction of effective antimicrobial therapy, syphilis was correctly perceived as a very serious infection. With the advent of penicillin therapy, and the resulting paucity in incidence of long-term sequelae, many now view syphilis as a less serious problem. Unfortunately, there has been a recent upsurge in the number of syphilis cases associated with HIV infection (55). Syphilis is highly infectious during its early stages. However, initial skin lesions may not be apparent or may be too mild to cause discomfort, and these lesions often regress without therapy. This may cause significant time to elapse between infection and diagnosis. During this lag time, a person has the opportunity to infect others. Misperception that people cannot get syphilis through oral sex seems be fueling some of the recent rise in syphilis. Because the risk for HIV transmission through oral sex is much lower than the risk through anal or vaginal sex, people might incorrectly consider unprotected oral sex to be a safer practice for all STIs (56). Therefore, syphilis campaigns need to inform the target audience about the routes of transmission; symptoms associated with each stage (or lack thereof); information about diagnosis, treatment, and cure; and information about the untreated sequelae. It would also be appropriate for campaign planners to alert the target audience that syphilis may facilitate HIV transmission (57).

Case Studies of Special Populations: Latinos/Hispanics and MSM

Because of cultural differences, preventive interventions may need to be tailored to specific ethnic groups and often to specific subgroups within an ethnic group (e.g., recent immigrants from Mexico versus highly acculturated Mexican Americans). A combination of economic, institutional, religious, cultural, and political barriers make it difficult for Hispanics to get health care and seek screening. Studies have shown that a lower percentage of Hispanic women compared with Caucasian women have had a Pap screening within the past three years (58). Hispanic adolescent females are found to have significantly less knowledge of what Pap screenings are than Caucasians or African Americans (59). Furthermore, level of assimilation, education, and embarrassment has been found to be associated with Pap smear screening (60). Targeting a primarily Hispanic audience raises a number of issues. Data from the U.S. census show that the majority of Hispanics speak Spanish rather than English. There are data suggesting that the younger audience preferentially speaks English, though Spanish may be spoken at home (60). Therefore, a bilingual communication campaign with a particular emphasis on graphics may be most effective. Edutainment and the use of fotonovelas are two potentially favorable channels that may be used to target a Hispanic audience.

Fotonovelas are a popular genre of comic strips in Latin America that apply pictures of real people to illustrate narrative plots similar to those in soap operas. The story in each is told by means of illustrated panels with bubble dialog, sometimes supplemented by a line of text to set the scene. Most fotonovelas are about 100 pages long. In Spanish-speaking communities, they can be bought at neighborhood grocery and general stores, beauty parlors, drugstores, gas stations, etc. They have a broad readership, and for many recent immigrants to the United States they are a welcome link to home. Fotonovelas are generally most effective in communities that are familiar with the medium. When designing a fotonovela, four basic elements must be considered: plot, dialogue, characters, and visual content. The plot, or story line, should be developed with the message woven in as part of the story. Scene changes should be clearly marked to help the reader follow the story. The dialogue between characters in the story consists of short sentences in words that are familiar to the reader located in "balloons" within each frame. The characters in the fotonovela should be based on thorough research. They play a critical role in conveying the message to the reader. The visuals, whether photographs or drawings, should appeal to the intended audience. They should motivate readers to pick up the fotonovela. The visual on the cover is important in motivating the reader to pick up and read the story. Fotonovelas are used throughout the United States in various prevention campaigns targeting Hispanics. For example, one campaign trying to raise awareness of HIV/STD risk among Hispanic day laborers used a fotonovela called "It looks like rain . . . Put on your hat, my friend" (61). Through focus groups, the fotonovela was found to help diffuse the message of condom use in the tight network of day laborers and to increase perceived susceptibility.

Men Who Have Sex with Men

Men who have sex with men (MSM) have been the target of STI (predominantly HIV) prevention campaigns for over two decades. After the epidemic years of 1986 through 1990, rates of syphilis steadily declined in the United States to an all-time low of 2.5 cases per 100,000 in 1999 (MMWR 1999). However, recent outbreaks in the MSM community have led to renewed concerns. Because it is not often clear whether these new infections are occurring among self-described gay, bisexual, or heterosexual MSM (e.g., men on the down-low), it is important to fashion messages to try to reach all of these men without alienating a subset. For example, a campaign that focuses on "gay men" may not engage self-described heterosexual MSM. This increases the likelihood that such a campaign would not meet its goals. To ensure successful interventions, it is vital to develop new ways to engage the targeted community. This often requires the establishment of a relationship based on trust and an open, nonjudgmental dialogue between community members and the public health community.

In gay men, self-acceptance is associated with reports of engaging in fewer high-risk sexual behaviors and a greater commitment to a social network of gay people (62,63). Self-acceptance in gay men is associated with a greater likelihood of seeking information regarding HIV and other STDs and with a greater sense of self-efficacy at being able to enact those prevention behaviors. When targeting MSM in social marketing efforts, messages should raise awareness of the increase of HIV and syphilis infections in MSM; encourage the adoption or re-adoption of risk reduction or safer sex practices; provide support for those who would like to practice safer sex; and make safer sex practices a priority health consideration. Communication campaigns targeting MSM should take into account the cohesiveness of the gay community (64). For MSM living in a more cohesive community, campaign planners may wish to highlight norms around safer sex and make use of influential opinion leaders within that community to disseminate safe sex messages, utilizing the diffusion of innovation theory. In cities where there is not a cohesive MSM community, diffusion of innovation may not be appropriate and therefore campaign planners may wish to highlight benefits of condom use. Thus, campaign planners may wish to focus on messages that, for example, eroticize safe sex (65).

To better highlight these strategies; let us focus on the gay community in Seattle. In 2003, a group of gay men in Seattle issued a "community manifesto" (referring to STIs and HIV) that challenged MSM to "act against the behaviors and attitudes responsible for the spread of these diseases." The manifesto asserted that every MSM was "responsible for the health and well-being of the community." This campaign's focus was to change the norms of the community (TPB) by placing the burden of health of the community as a whole on the shoulders of each individual member of the community. The manifesto also stated that all MSM must "care about their health—their own, the community's and each person's—as an act of self and an affirmation of self worth," thus framing the use of condoms by members of the MSM community as a way to show self-respect. The manifesto was distributed through full-page ads in local targeted media and press conferences. Gatekeepers were also solicited as "endorsers," exemplifying diffusion of innovation. At the national STD prevention conference in 2004, researchers presented data suggesting that safe sex was the norm in Seattle—they conducted a telephone survey of 400 men and found that only 1 in 5 gay men said they had had unprotected sex (66). Whether this is a direct result of the manifesto needs further study. However, this example demonstrates how a city with a fairly cohesive MSM community can diffuse and model safer sex norms.

New Technologies, Remaining Questions

In recent years, there has been a proliferation of new tests and medications that enable early detection and chronic management of diseases. While public health officials are trying to "market" healthful behaviors to the general public, a new phenomenon of direct-to-consumer advertising (DTCA) of new products by the industry has emerged. Until the end of the last decade, consumers received information about prescription drugs from physicians or other health care professionals. Today, pharmaceutical companies spend several billion dollars a year to advertise directly to these consumers. Advertisements for pain medications, antihistamines, and medications targeting erectile dysfunction are ubiquitous. New Zealand and the United States are the only industrialized nations that permit direct-to-consumer advertising (67). From 1997 to 2001, spending on research and development in the United States increased 59% while spending on DCTA increased by 145% (68). In 2000, 91% of individuals in the United States reported having seen DCTAs (69). The U.S.

General Accounting Office estimates that 8.5 million consumers annually request and receive from their physician a prescription for a particular drug in response to seeing a direct-to-consumer advertisement (68). In a cross-sectional survey conducted in 2001 (70), researchers found that lower socioeconomic status was associated with requesting preventive measures (such as a screening) as a result of information gleaned from a DTCA. Hispanics, people who had not completed high school and those with chronic diseases were more likely to seek preventive care as a result of DTCA.

While it may be argued that DTCA provides consumers with a greater sense of control when visiting their provider, the effect that it has on issues of prevention is unclear. For example, the introduction of highly active antiretroviral therapy (HAART) has led to dramatic reductions in HIV morbidity and mortality. However, concerns have surfaced regarding an increase in unsafe sexual practices because of the widespread availability and effectiveness of HAART. In a survey of 997 male patients in an STD clinic in San Francisco, some respondents were less likely to practice safe sex because DTCA for several antiretroviral drugs (which used images of fit individuals engaged in strenuous physical activities) suggested that HIV could be easily controlled and was therefore a condition that no longer warranted heightened vigilance (71).

In early 2005, *OUT* magazine featured an advertisement for the drug Reyataz. An electronic chip was embedded in the magazine; when the cover was opened, the sound of a ringing phone was followed by a male voice saying that he was having too much fun to worry about his chronic illness (72). The same company's web site (www.reyataz.com) relayed the following message: "Ask your doctor how REYATZ, in combination therapy, can help you FIGHT HIV YOUR WAY." These two examples highlight how DTCA may not only fail to educate, but may also encourage risky behaviors by decreasing perceived severity of threat. It is worth noting that the advent of HAART, independent of DTCA, may be associated with increased unsafe sexual practices of MSM. The perception of decreased threat from HIV with the advent of HAART and younger age have been associated with a higher incidence of STIs (73). In a meta-analysis, persons who believed that receiving HAART or having an undetectable viral load protected against transmitting HIV were more likely to engage in unsafe sexual practices (74). While research continues to investigate these associations, it appears that the resulting optimism and improved health status produced by HAART may have contributed to unanticipated consequences in MSM: lack of fear of acquiring and transmitting HIV, an increase in high-risk sexual behaviors, and a resurgence of gonorrhea and syphilis. Other factors, such as the increasing use of the internet as a venue to find sex partners may also be playing a role.

DTCAs are not limited just to drugs. There are also DCTAs related to HPV testing. Digene released a DTCA (both in PSA and magazine format) about their new HPV DNA test. Digene advertisements suggest that the Pap smear alone is not enough to detect cervical cancers, and that high-risk HPV testing in combination with the Pap smear is indicated for all women. The PSAs use the following tag lines: "Ask your doctor and tell your friends. Everyone we know should know." The web site's written materials (www.hpvtest.com) state: "You're not failing your Pap test but it might be failing you . . . if you're a gambling woman, then getting just a Pap test is fine." Although most women who are sexually active will get HPV at some point, very few women with HPV will develop cervical cancer. No single public health entity currently recommends the blanket use of HPV testing for all women. Aside from the financial, emotional, and clinical consequences for women, how this advertising strategy will affect attitudes towards HPV, and consequently behavior, is still unclear.

Some Practical Considerations

Effective relationships and partnerships with community leaders, policy makers, and other key individuals can strengthen health communication campaigns. Those who have influence in the community can be critical in establishing grassroots receptivity to STI prevention campaigns. They can also help secure additional untapped resources. Partners are essential vehicles to funnel information and to give a new voice to an old message. In many cases, partnering with community leaders, stakeholders, and coalitions has helped generate community support for the effort and has served to make the issue "local" or immediate. Partnering with organizations promotes "buy-in" and expands the campaign's reach. For example, in Georgia's syphilis campaign (2003–2005), organizers were able to spend the bulk of their funds on disseminating educational materials instead of material development. Public health officials partnered with local community-based organizations serving the local target populations of interest (e.g.. African-American MSM organizations, etc.) that were able to provide in-kind services for message development.

The process of developing a new social marketing campaign can be time-consuming and resource-intensive. If funding resources are few, adapting existing materials and making them appropriate for your specific program objectives may be the most prudent course. However, the adaptation process also entails a formative evaluation process and pre-testing. Adaptation generally requires less time and fewer resources than does starting from scratch. Often, a piece of the material contains some useful information but is not written at an appropriate reading level or contains too many concepts. It may contain suitable visuals or graphics, or a unique approach to presentation, without the appropriate message. Adaptation to meet the needs of a new audience should be a thoughtfully planned process.

As a final note, attention must be paid to the degree of explicitness that government or media standards allow. Conversely, many community activists often call for more direct and explicit messages. A mass media campaign dealing with a controversial topic must continually deal with the delicate balance between content that is approved by government/media and an effective message. Over time, levels of acceptability do change. San Francisco Department of Health officials collaborated on their syphilis awareness campaign called "Healthy Penis," with local printing business owners helping to produce some of the more graphic materials.

Conclusion

Successful health communication campaigns are based on systematic planning efforts and on communication objectives that are attainable, measurable, clear, and time-limited. Successful campaigns develop and deliver health messages that are tailored to specific target audiences. Widely disseminated generic health messages aimed at increasing knowledge about certain issues have been shown to be less effective than more targeted efforts. Health communication efforts with a "consumer-perspective" are much more effective at motivating target audiences. This requires designing and delivering messages that are adapted to the needs, perceptions, preferences, and situations of the intended audiences, rather than the needs and goals of the message designers or institutions.

References

1. Braun J, Burkhalter B, Jimerson A, Keith N, Porter B. BASICS Strategy Paper: BASICS Communication Strategy. Arlington, VA: Basics; 1994.
2. Diaz RM. *Latino Gay Men and HIV: Culture, Sexuality, and Risk Behavior*. New York: Routledge, 1998.
3. Sheeran P, Abraham C, Orbell S. Psychosocial correlates of heterosexual condom use: a meta-analysis. *Psychological Bulletin*. 1999;125:90–132.
4. Anderson RM, Blythe SP, Gupta S, Konings E. The transmission dynamics of the human immunodeficiency virus type 1 in the male homosexual community in the United Kingdom: the influence of changes in sexual behaviour. *Philos Trans R Soc Lond B Biol Sci*. 1989;325:45–98.
5. Snyder LB, Hamilton MA, Mitchell EW, Kiwanuka-Tondo J, Fleming-Milici F, Proctor D. A meta-analysis of the effect of mediated health communication campaigns on behavior change in the United States. *J Health Commun*. 2004;9(suppl 1):71–96.
6. Graeff JA, Elder JP, Booth EM. *Communication for Health and Behavior Changes: A Developing Country Perspective*. San Francisco: Jossey Bass; 1993.
7. Andreasen A. *Marketing Social Change: Changing Behavior to Promote Health, Social Development and the Environment*. San Francisco: Jossey Bass; 1995.
8. Salmon C. *Information Campaigns: Balancing Social Values and Social Change*. Newbury Park: Sage, 1992.
9. Rosenstock IM. The health belief model and nutrition education. *J Can Diet Assoc*. 1982;43:184–192.
10. Ajzen I, Fishbein M. *Understanding Attitudes and Predicting Social Behavior*. Englewood Cliffs, NJ: Prentice-Hall, 1980.
11. Prochaska JO, DiClemente CC, Norcross JC. In search of how people change: applications to addictive behaviors. *American Psychologist*. 1992;47:1102–1114.
12. Bandura A. Self-efficacy: toward a unifying theory of behavioral change. *Psychological Review*. 1977;84:191–215.
13. Rogers EM. *Diffusion of Innovations*, 4th ed. New York: The Free Press, 1995.
14. Cecil H, Pinkerton SD. Reliability and validity of a self-efficacy instrument for protective sexual behaviors. *J Am Coll Health*. 1998;47:113–121.
15. Smith PB, Weinman ML, Parrilli J. The role of condom motivation education in the reduction of new and reinfection rates of sexually transmitted diseases among inner-city female adolescents. *Patient Educ Couns*. 1997;31:77–81.
16. Oh MK, Grimley DM, Merchant JS, Brown PR, Cecil H, Hook EW, 3rd. Mass media as a population-level intervention tool for *Chlamydia trachomatis* screening: report of a pilot study. *J Adolesc Health*. 2002;31:40–47.
17. Dahl DW, Gorn GJ, Weinberg CB. Marketing, safer sex, and condom acquisition. In: Goldberg ME, Fishbein M, Middlestadt SE, eds. *Social Marketing: Theoretical and Practical Perspectives*. Mahwah, NJ: Lawrence Erlbaum Associates, 1997:169–185.
18. Montoya JA, Rotblatt H, Mall KL, Klausner J, Kerndt PR. Evaluating "Stop the Sores," A community-led social marketing campaign to prevent syphilis among men who have sex with men, Los Angeles County 2002-03. International Society for Sexually Transmitted Disease Research Congress. Ottawa, Canada, 2003.

19. Winett RA, Altman DG, King AC. Conceptual and strategic foundations for effective media campaigns for preventing the spread of HIV infection. *Evaluation and Program Planning* 1990;13:91–104.

20. Dignan M, Michielutte R, Wells HB, Bahnson J. The Forsyth County cervical cancer prevention project: I. Cervical cancer screening for Black women. *Health Education Research*. 1994;9:411–420.

21. Blohm M, Herlitz J, Hartford M, Karlson BW, Risenfors M, Luepker RV, et al. Consequences of a media campaign focusing on delay in acute myocardial infarction. *American Journal of Cardiology*. 1992;69:411–413.

22. Flay BR. Evaluation of the development, dissemination, and effectiveness of mass media health programming. *Health Educ Behav*. 1987;2:123–129.

23. Wallack L, Dorfman L. Media advocacy: a strategy for advancing policy and promoting health. *Health Educ Q*. 1996;23:293–317.

24. Singhal A, Rogers EM. *Entertainment-Education: A Communication Strategy for Social Change*. Mahwah, NJ: Lawrence Erlbaum Associates, 1999.

25. Bryant J. Message features and entertainment effects. In: Bradac JP, ed. M*essage Effects in Communication Science*. Newbury Park, CA: Sage, 1989:231–262.

26. Collins RL, Elliott MN, Berry SH, Kanouse DE, Hunter SB. Entertainment television as a healthy sex educator: the impact of condom-efficacy information in an episode of Friends. *Pediatrics*. 2003;112:1115–1121.

27. Glik D, Berkanovic E, Stone K, Ibarra L, Jones MC, Rosen B, Schreibman M, Gordon L, Minassian L, Richardes D. Health education goes Hollywood: working with prime-time and daytime entertainment television for immunization promotion. *J Health Commun*. 1998;3:263–282.

28. Riester T, Linton M. Designing an effective counteradvertising campaign—Arizona. *Cancer* 1998;83:2746–2751.

29. Latour M, Rotfield H. There are threats and (maybe) fear-caused arousal: theory and confusions of appeals to fear and fear arousal itself. *Journal of Advertising Research*. 1997;26:45–67.

30. Witte K, Allen M. A meta-analysis of fear appeals: implications for effective public health campaigns. *Health Educ Behav*. 2000;27:591–615.

31. Thompson SC, Kent DR, Thomas C, Vrungos S. Real and illusory control over exposure to HIV in college students and gay men. *Journal of Applied Social Psychology*. 1999;26:189–210.

32. Perloff LS, Fetzer BK. Self-other judgments and perceived vulnerability to victimization. *Journal of Personality and Social Psychology*. 1986;50:502–510.

33. Lawrence D, Jason J, Holman R, Murphy J. HIV transmission from hemophilic men to their heterosexual wives. In: Alexander N, Gabelnick H, Hodgen G, Spieler J, eds. *The Heterosexual Transmission of AIDS: Proceedings of the CONRAD 2nd International Workshop*. New York: Alan R. Liss, 1991:35–57.

34. Lupton DA. From complacency to panic: AIDS and heterosexuals in the Australian press, July 1986 to June 1988. *Health Educ Res*. 1992;7:9–20.

35. Rosser BS. The effects of using fear in public AIDS education on the behaviours of homosexually active men. *Journal of Psychology and Human Sexuality*. 1991; 4:123–134.

36. Morlet A, Guinan JJ, Diefenthaler I, Gold J. The impact of the "grim reaper" national AIDS educational campaign on the Albion Street (AIDS) Centre and the AIDS Hotline. *Med J Aust*. 1988;148:282–286.

37. Kenny J. Fear and humor in prevention campaigns. In: Paalman M, ed. *Promoting Safer Sex: Prevention of Sexual Transmission of AIDS and Other STD*. Amsterdam: Swets & Zeitlinger, 1990:75–80.

38. Kaiser Family Foundation. National Survey of Public Knowledge of HPV, the Human Papillomavirus. Kaiser Family Foundation: Menlo Park, CA; February 17, 2000. Accessible at: www.kff.org. Accessed January 16, 2007.

39. Mays RM, Zimet GD, Winston Y, Kee R, Dickes J, Su L. Human Papillomavirus, genital warts, pap smears, and cervical cancer: knowledge and beliefs of adolescent and adult women. *Health Care Women Int*. 2000;21:361–374.

40. Burak LJ, Meyer M. Using the health belief model to examine and predict college women's cervical cancer screening beliefs and behavior. *Health Care Women Int*. 1997;18:251–262.

41. Dzuba IG, Diaz EY, Allen B, Leonard YF, Lazcano Ponce EC, Shah KV, Bishai D, Lorincz A, Ferris D, Turnbull B, Hernandez Avila M, Salmeron J. The acceptability of self-collected samples for HPV testing vs. the Pap test as alternatives in cervical cancer screening. *J Womens Health Gend Based Med*. 2002;11:265–275.

42. Fernandez MA, Tortolero-Luna G, Gold RS. Mammography and Pap test screening among low-income foreign-born Hispanic women in USA. *Cad Saude Publica*. 1998;14(suppl 3):133–147.

43. Martin LM, Calle EE, Wingo PA, Heath CW, Jr. Comparison of mammography and Pap test use from the 1987 and 1992 National Health Interview Surveys: are we closing the gaps? *Am J Prev Med*. 1996;12:82–90.

44. Ramirez JE, Ramos DM, Clayton L, Kanowitz S, Moscicki AB. Genital human papillomavirus infections: knowledge, perception of risk, and actual risk in a non-clinic population of young women. *J Womens Health*. 1997;6:113–121.

45. Anhang R, Goodman A, Goldie SJ. HPV communication: review of existing research and recommendations for patient education. *CA Cancer J Clin*. 2004;54:248–259.

46. Cockburn J, White DM, Hirst S, Hill D. Response of older rural women to a cervical screening campaign. *Health Promot Journal of Australia*. 1991;1:29–34.

47. Anhang R, Wright TCJ, Smock L, Goldie SJ. Women's desired information about human papillomavirus. *Cancer*. 2004;100:315–320.

48. Harper DM. Why am i scared of HPV? *CA Cancer J Clin*. 2004;54:245–247.

49. Duncan B, Hart G, Scoular A, Bigrigg A. Qualitative analysis of psychosocial impact of diagnosis of Chlamydia trachomatis: implications for screening. *BMJ*. 2001;322:195–199.

50. Darroch J, Myers L, Cassell J. Sex differences in the experience of testing positive for genital chlamydia infection: a qualitative study with implications for public health and for a national screening programme. *Sex Transm Infect*. 2003;79:372–373.

51. Fleming DT, McQuillan GM, Johnson RE, Nahmias AJ, Aral SO, Lee FK, St Louis ME. Herpes simplex virus type 2 in the United States, 1976 to 1994. *N Engl J Med*. 1997;337:1105–1111.

52. Miyai T, Turner KR, Kent CK, Klausner J. The psychosocial impact of testing individuals with no history of genital herpes for herpes simplex virus type 2. *Sex Transm Dis*. 2004;31:517–521.

53. Melville J, Sniffen S, Crosby R, Salazar L, Whittington W, Dithmer-Schreck D, DiClemente R, Wald A. Psychosocial impact of serological diagnosis of herpes simplex virus type 2: a qualitative assessment. *Sex Transm Infect*. 2003;79:280–285.

54. Hullett CR. Using functional theory to promote sexually transmitted diseases (STD) testing: the impact of value-expressive messages and guilt. *Communication Research*. 2004;31:363–396.

55. High-Risk Sexual Behavior by HIV-Positive Men Who Have Sex with Men—16 Sites, United States, 2000–2002 CDC. *MMWR Morb Mortal Wkly Rep* 2004;53:891–894.

56. Varghese B, Maher JE, Peterman TA, Branson BM, Steketee RW. Reducing the risk of sexual HIV transmission: quantifying the per-act risk for HIV on the basis of choice of partner, sex act, and condom use. *Sex Transm Dis*. 2002;10:386.

57. Nusbaum MR, Wallace RR, Slatt LM, Kondrad EC. Sexually transmitted infections and increased risk of co-infection with human immunodeficiency virus. *J Am Osteopath Assoc*. 2004;104:527–535.

58. Behbakht K, Lynch A, Teal S, Degeest K, Massad S. Social and cultural barriers to Papanicolaou test screening in an urban population. *Obstet Gynecol.* 2004;104: 1355–1361.
59. Smith P, Weinman M, Mumford D. Knowledge, beliefs, and behavioral risk factors for human immunodeficiency virus infection in inner city adolescent females. *Sex Transm Dis.* 1992;19:19–24.
60. Coronado GD, Thompson B, Koepsell TD, Schwartz SM, McLerran D. Use of Pap test among Hispanics and non-Hispanic whites in a rural setting. *Prev Med.* 2004;38:713–722.
61. Estremera DY, Arevalo M, Armbruster J, Kerndt P. Parece que va a llover, compadre, ponte el sombrero (It looks like rain, put on your hat, my friend): An HIV/STD risk awareness fotonovela for Latino day laborers. The 130th Annual Meeting of APHA, 2002.
62. Fisher JD, Fisher WA, Misovich SJ, Kimble DL, Malloy TE. Changing AIDS risk behavior: effects of an intervention emphasizing AIDS risk reduction information, motivation, and behavioral skills in a college student population. *Health Psychol.* 1996;15:114–123.
63. Fisher JD, Misovich SJ. Evolution of college students' AIDS-related behavioral responses, attitudes, knowledge, and fear. *AIDS Educ Prev.* 1990;2:322–337.
64. Fishbein M, Chan DK-S, O'Reilley K, Schnell D, Wood R, Beeker C, Cohn D. Attitudinal and normative factors as determinants of gay men's intentions to perform AIDs-related sexual behaviors: a multisite analysis. *Journal of Applied Social Psychology.* 1992;22:999–1011.
65. Perloff RM. *Persuading People to Have Safer Sex: Applications of Social Science to the AIDS Crisis.* Mahwah, NJ: Lawrence Erlbaum Associates, 2001.
66. Brewer DD, Golden MR, Handsfield HH. Factors associated with potential exposure to and transmission of HIV in a probability sample of men who have sex with men. Abstract presented at National STD Prevention Conference, March 8-11, 2004, Philadelphia, PA.
67. Marks JH. The price of seduction: direct-to-consumer advertising of prescription drugs in the US. *NC Med J.* 2003;64:292–295.
68. *Prescription Drugs: FDA Oversight of Direct-to-Consumer Advertising Has Its Limitations.* Washington, DC: United States General Accounting Office, 2002.
69. Mello MM, Rosenthal M, Neumann PJ. Direct to consumer advertising and shared liability for pharmaceutical manufacturers. *JAMA.* 2003;289:477–481.
70. Murray E, Lo B, Pollack L, Donelan K, Lee K. Direct-to-consumer advertising: public perceptions of its effects on health behaviors, health care, and the doctor-patient relationship. *J Am Board Fam Pract.* 2004;17:6–18.
71. Klausner JD, Kim A, Kent C. Are HIV drug advertisements contributing to increases in risk behavior among men in San Francisco. *AIDS.* 2001;16:2349–2950.
72. Jacobs A. AIDS fighters face a resistant form of apathy. *New York Times.* April 13, 2005;A25.
73. van der Snoek EM, de Wit JB, Mulder PG, van der Meijden WI. Incidence of sexually transmitted diseases and HIV infection related to perceived HIV/AIDS threat since highly active antiretroviral therapy availability in men who have sex with men. *Sex Transm Dis.* 2005;32:170–175.
74. Crepaz N, Hart TA, Marks G. Highly active antiretroviral therapy and sexual risk behavior: a meta-analytic review. *JAMA.* 2004;292:224–236.

7

Partner Notification and Management Interventions

Matthew Hogben, Ph.D., Devon D. Brewer, Ph.D.,
and Matthew R. Golden, M.D., M.P.H.

Partner notification (PN) for STDs is widely acknowledged as a cornerstone of STD control, although suitable evaluation data are generally sparser than one would like for programs of national scope. The basic rationale for PN is that the sex partners of patients infected with STD ought to be notified of their exposure to STD, followed by evaluation and treatment (1). Public health professionals (provider referral) or infected patients (patient referral) are the two principal groups of people through which partners can be notified. Ideally, notification is accompanied by various forms of education and counseling pertaining to disease and means of exposure (1–3). Education and counseling, however, are by no means assured.

We begin this chapter with a description of PN history and current practice in the United States and review studies of its effectiveness to provide context for the interventions we describe in subsequent sections. After background comments, the chapter is organized around interventions requiring public health professional involvement followed by interventions that do not. Although the main focus of the chapter is on PN in the United States, we have not ignored studies conducted elsewhere.

A Short History of and Rationale for Partner Notification

American PN efforts, also known as contact tracing, derive from Thomas Parran's tenure as Surgeon General in the 1920s and 1930s, when syphilis was endemic at substantially higher rates than today and was incurable, albeit not untreatable. Arsenic-based therapies were not ideal treatments (when they were applied), and the only plausible alternative for controlling the spread of syphilis was to break the chain of infection through notification of sex partners of infected persons, hoping that behavioral change would follow. The advent of effective treatment (i.e., penicillin) simply added a new goal of curing infected persons. One unintended consequence of effective treatment was occasionally perceived as decreased need for behavioral change.

Behavioral Interventions for Prevention and Control of Sexually Transmitted Diseases.
Aral SO, Douglas JM Jr, eds. Lipshutz JA, assoc ed. New York: Springer Science+ Business Media, LLC; 2007.

The logic from the preceding paragraph is applicable to other curable STD, such as gonorrheal and chlamydial infections—the two most common reportable diseases in the United States (4). One of the primary goals of partner notification is to treat exposed partners (4,5). In principle, such treatment reduces disease incidence and prevalence, apart from the effects of STD introduced from other populations and geographic areas (6,7). Further useful purposes addressed by PN include fulfillment of the health care provider's "duty to warn," and the collection of epidemiologic data (8–10). For HIV infection, the only viral STD for which there is any organized attempt to provide PN, the primary goal of treating infected partners is modified to bringing infected partners to continuing care. The duty to warn is, of course, vital, although HIV partner notification remains controversial in some circles (11,10).

Current Status and Effectiveness of Partner Notification

Status

PN has traditionally involved two options for notification—either by a public health professional (provider referral) or by the patient (patient referral, also known as self-referral). The public health professional is frequently a person who has been trained to elicit numbers of partners, use varying amounts and qualities of locating information to find partners and notify them of their exposure, and to convince notified partners to seek evaluation and treatment. Such professionals have several titles across the country, the most common of which is Disease Intervention Specialist (DIS). The infected patient whom the DIS is interviewing for partners and locating information is most commonly known as the index case, although the term "original patient" is also widespread.

Provider referral begins when a DIS interviews an index case to elicit partners and associated identifying, locating, and exposure information. The DIS then uses this information to find partners, notify them of their exposure confidentially, and facilitate their examination and treatment. In subsequent sections, we describe the interview and notification process in more detail. Patient referral places responsibility for notifying partners on the index case (responsibility for convincing partners to seek evaluation and treatment is unclear). Standard implementation of patient referral is for the health care provider or DIS simply to tell index cases to notify their partners—this exhortation from providers is frequently perfunctory, especially if the STD has relatively little historical association with partner notification (e.g., chlamydial infection).

Effectiveness

Data on the effectiveness of PN are limited, and no data on PN process outcomes have been compiled or reported at the national level for several decades. Brewer (12) and Golden et al. (13,14) recently reviewed process measures of partner notification for syphilis, gonorrhea, chlamydial infection, and HIV. Of reports in the literature and from surveyed health departments (14–38, depending on the disease), the median numbers of new cases of STD diagnosed per index case interviewed were 0.22 for syphilis, 0.25 for gonorrhea, 0.22 for chlamydial infection, and 0.07–0.13 for HIV. The ranges around these medians were quite broad. Of partners whom the DIS or patient attempted to notify, the median percentages who were undiagnosed positives were 8% for syphilis and HIV and 18% for chlamydia and gonorrhea. In two surveys of health departments nationwide, selected for high morbidity, Golden et al. (13,14) found that 89% of people with syphilis were interviewed for partners, compared with 32–52% of HIV cases (dependent on the survey) and 12–17% of chlamydial and gonorrheal cases, respectively.

Systematic reviews of the relatively few trials and evaluations (12,15–17) indicate that provider referral is more effective than patient referral in notifying partners and identifying new cases for most STD. Provider referral is, however, substantially more expensive than patient referral, which not only suggests cost-effectiveness can be an issue in choosing notification strategies, but also that widespread provider referral is sometimes not economically feasible.

HIV presents somewhat different contingencies to bacterial STD. In terms of partner notification, one difference is that case-finding (i.e., new HIV cases) yields compared with STD case-finding can reasonably be expected to be lower because a person can only have a new case of HIV once. Few trials of partner notification effectiveness for HIV exist (18). Landis et al. (19) conducted a small trial of 74 HIV-infected patients randomized to either patient (35) or provider (39) referral, which became the principal reference for the HIV Partner Counseling and Referral Services (PCRS) manual (2). More partners in the provider referral condition than in the patient referral condition were counseled and tested (23% versus 16%), with similar proportions of each number tested having new HIV-positive cases (25% versus 20%). These proportions, however, represented low case-finding numbers: new cases formed only 3–6% of the 310 partners named.

Few attempts have been made to evaluate the effect of PN on disease transmission. Potterat and colleagues have assessed the effects of augmenting and redirecting PN on gonorrhea and chlamydia transmission in Colorado Springs in three separate reports covering different time periods between 1971 and 1998. During the periods of intensified PN, disease incidence or complications from disease declined relative to the period preceding the intensified PN (20,21). Other observational evidence of the effect of PN comes from New York State (Du et al., unpublished data). Multivariate analyses of county-level data on gonorrhea from 1992 to 2002 showed that the extent of PN coverage and success of PN (percentages of partners identified, located, and presumptively treated) at one point in time were independently associated with future incidence rates. Similarly, Han et al. (22) found that targeting partner notification services for gonorrhea on "core" geographic areas in a county—those accounting for 50% of the county caseload—was associated with a greater decline in incidence between 1983 and 1997 than that in a morbidity-, geography-, and sex case ratio–matched comparison county. However, rigorously designed community-level trials of PN (12) are needed to determine the effect of PN on incidence with appropriate confidence.

Interventions Requiring DIS Involvement

We first focus on interventions that entail some degree of DIS involvement in the partner notification process, and then discuss interventions that can be implemented independently of DIS or of dedicated public health staff.

We note, however, that among the latter group of interventions, DIS may be the most suitable candidates to operate the intervention programs.

Provider Referral

The basic interview process for provider referral and its variants was originally designed for interviewing people with syphilis and is outlined in two documents prepared by the Centers for Disease Control (CDC) to guide U.S. STD program operations: the Program Operation Guidelines (1) and the STD Employee Development Guide (23). Data collected during the partner notification process are shown in Table 1. During an interview, the first task of the DIS is to establish how many sex partners the index case claims during the appropriate interview window (typically 60–90 days for STD other than syphilis and HIV; the window varies up to a year according to stage of syphilis) (1). The number of partners claimed is most often known as the number of period partners. The DIS then attempts to collect identifying and locating information on each partner with a view to contacting and notifying each of those named. When an index case provides sufficient locating information about a contact to give a DIS a reasonable chance of finding that contact, the case is "initiated." Process statistics are generally calculated with reference to the index case, so the "contact index" for a given location or timeframe is the number of period partners whom the DIS will try to locate divided by the number of index cases: generally equivalent to cases initiated divided by index cases. As shown in Table 1, one can also measure initiated case dispositions after notification: contacts tested, treated and new cases found are the most relevant to the fundamental principles of treating infected persons and providing prophylaxis.

Other useful statistics calculable from the data collected in Table 1 are indexes with reference to the number of partners initiated. Any PN program should be interested in the proportions of traceable contacts who are notified, tested, and treated. A program should also maintain some knowledge of the proportion of period partners who are initiated as contacts. This is most salient when small proportions of period partners are initiated as cases. For example, during syphilis outbreaks in men having sex with men (MSM) in several U.S. cities beginning circa 2000 (25), numbers notified per index case were quite high by recent standards (>1.2) in some cities, although the median brought-to-treatment index was only 0.09. But index cases claimed numerous partners, with mean partners claimed per index case ranging between 3.0 and 10.0. The median proportion of partners contacted was 14% (range = 8–48%), and the median proportion of period partners claimed who were new cases was only 1%.

Macke, Hennessy, and McFarlane (26) followed 40 DIS in one of the few recent formal evaluations of process. They concluded that DIS-based partner notification was labor-intensive and that factors not overtly related to PN accounted for the majority of DIS time. HIV cases and post-primary and post-secondary syphilis cases took up the most time by disease, as did clients classifiable as both index cases and contacts. Time spent on HIV and syphilis cases compared with others may be due to DIS handling patient care issues not addressed by medical providers. That is, some DIS time is spent attending to patients' individual health and not public health.

Table 1 Main partner elicitation and provider referral data.

Data collected (per index case)	Terminology and statistics
Interview	
Number of sex partners claimed	Period partners
Number of partners with identifying and locating information	Cases initiated /index cases = *Contact index* /period partners
Notification	
Number of partners contacted	N contacted /index patients = *Notification index* /cases initiated /period partners
Post-notification	
Number of partners tested	N tested /index patients /cases initiated /period partners
Number of partners treated	N treated /index patients = *Treatment index* (*Epidemiologic index*) /cases initiated /period partners
Number of partners found to be infected	N positive /index cases = *Case-finding index* (*Brought-to-treatment index*)[*] /period partners
Common Dispositions	

Contacted, treated, tested, found to be infected = *Treating infections* (fundamental principle of partner notification).

Contacted, treated, infection status negative or undetermined = *Prophylactic treatment* (fundamental principle).

Could not be contacted.

Contacted, refused evaluation and/or treatment.

[*]The inverse of this figure gives the number of index cases needed to interview (NNTI) to find a new case of the STD in question. The NNTI is another commonly reported statistic. The treatment and case-finding indices together are sometimes known as the *Intervention index*.

Improving the Process of Provider Referral

Contract Referral

In contract, or conditional, referral, a public health professional elicits partners' names and locating information from the index case, but arranges a time frame with the index case during which that person will notify the named partners. If the index case does so, and the partners present for evaluation, program staff time and costs can be spared to some extent. If the index case fails to notify partners, or if those partners do not present for evaluation, the program staff will attempt to notify the partners.

The mere fact that the index case knows that a DIS can notify partners may stimulate greater index case notification rates, which would enhance the effectiveness of the method. The test of this hypothesis would be a comparison of unaided notification rates for contract referral with partner referral, but these data have not been collected. Two conditions assessed in Cleveland's unpublished trial (16,17) came close. Contract referral with a three-day window for gonorrhea-infected index cases to notify named partners yielded 0.62 partners per index case who presented for evaluation, versus 0.37 for patient referral (with or without educational pamphlets). The difference of 0.25 was statistically different from 0 (95% confidence interval = 0.17 to 0.33). The outcome variable was a treatment index rather than a notification index and the proportion of partners in the contract condition who had to be notified by DIS is unknown.

Peterman et al. (27) tested contract referral against provider referral (with or without blood draws in the field) for syphilis. After randomizing 1,966 people to one of the three conditions, they found broadly similar proportions of partners who were located (1.1–1.2 per index case), tested (0.86–0.92), and treated (0.61–0.67). Brought-to-treatment indices were also close, ranging from 0.18 for both provider referral conditions to 0.20 for contract referral. Almost identical proportions of period partners were found via contract (19%) versus provider referral (20% average across the two conditions). Costs were lower for contract referral: $317 per partner treated, versus $343 to $362 for the provider referral conditions.

Increasing Case-Finding and Epidemiologic Yield

The case-finding and epidemiologic yield from partner notification via provider and contract referral can, in principle, be improved by a) eliciting partners more fully; b) obtaining more comprehensive and accurate locating, identifying, and exposure information on elicited partners; c) using such information more effectively in finding partners; and d) increasing the efficiency and speed with which notified partners are examined and treated. We examine interventions that focus on each of these steps in the partner notification process in turn.

Eliciting Partners

There are many possible reasons why people may not report all of their partners when asked to recall them in an interview with a DIS, including real or perceived consequences of diagnosis and the partner notification process, as well as issues related to self-presentation to DIS, privacy, motivation, and memory (28,29). Research shows that people do indeed underreport their partners when asked to recall them, and forgetting appears to be a primary factor (28,30). Individuals who report many partners are the most likely to forget partners. In addition, recalled and forgotten partners are generally similar on key epidemiologic variables, such as frequency and recency of exposure (28).

Brewer and colleagues developed several techniques for eliciting sex and drug-injection partners based on how people naturally recall them (31) and then evaluated these procedures in research and partner notification settings. In one randomized trial, asking individuals to report their sex partners in reverse chronological order, commonly thought to be best practice, elicited essentially the same number of sex partners as recalling partners in a free, unconstrained order (30). Although standard practice of DIS typically has been restricted to this basic form of elicitation, research shows that elicitation can be enhanced substantially with supplementary questioning procedures.

After an interviewee has been asked about how many partners he or she has and has indicated that he or she did not have or cannot recall any more, one simple strategy to boost reporting is to prompt nonspecifically (e.g., ask "Who else have you had sex with in the last 12 months?"). After such prompting and any additional responses elicited, an interviewer can read the list of partners already elicited back to the interviewee slowly to ensure that all partners were correctly recorded and prompt nonspecifically again. Nonspecific prompting and reading back the list of elicited partners each elicited 5–10% additional partners beyond those already mentioned in the interview, on average (28,30).

Particular types of recall cues, administered after such prompting, provide the largest increases in the number of partners elicited. Sets of cues referring to locations where people have sexual contact with their partners or first meet their partners and first names each elicit approximately 10–20% additional sex partners (30,32). Parallel location cues and network cues focused on eliciting partners socially connected to partners already elicited are even more effective in boosting recall of injection partners (30). In these studies, other types of cues (e.g., based on individual characteristics, role relationships, significant personal events) were not as effective in eliciting additional sex or injection partners. Interviewees who recalled many partners on their own tended to forget the most partners (28). Few individuals who recalled only one partner on their own listed any additional partners in response to the cues. Also, cue-elicited and freely recalled partners did not differ meaningfully on epidemiologically significant variables. In a randomized trial of various recall cues administered in routine STD PN, the supplementary techniques (nonspecific prompting, reading back the list of elicited partners, and recall cues [including the comparatively ineffective ones]) increased the number of new STD cases found (i.e., brought to treatment) by 12% (32).

Other approaches to partner elicitation have also been examined systematically. In one observational study, contact interviews conducted by telephone elicited similar numbers of partners on average as interviews conducted in person (29). HIV contact interviews conducted in confidential HIV testing sites result in more partners elicited and more new cases found per case interviewed than contact interviews performed with clients at anonymous testing sites (33). Reinterviewing also yields additional elicited partners (29,34,35) as does extending interview (or recall) periods beyond the ordinarily recommended lengths (35–37). Furthermore, trained contact interviewers elicit more partners than untrained interviewers (35,38), and there appear to be no meaningful differences between trained interviewers in the number of partners they elicit (39).

Reporting of Partners' Identifying, Locating, and Exposure Information

To our knowledge, there have been no evaluations of interventions designed to increase the comprehensiveness or accuracy of identifying, locating, and exposure information about elicited partners. The available evidence indicates that people report information about partner demographics (6,40) and partnership dates of first and last exposure (41) reliably. However, in one study (40), index cases reported information about their partners' risks for transmission (number of partners, involvement in commercial sex, bisexual behavior, and injection drug use) with only low to moderate reliability.

Finding Partners

Tomnay, Pitts, and Fairley (42) suggested the use of new communication technology for PN. They identified mobile phones, text messaging, and other electronic communication as methods for reducing the costs of provider referral, although reductions on notification and case-finding effectiveness would also have to be measured. Tomnay et al. also noted privacy concerns, citing the need for secure web sites and a general assurance that electronic notification will go to and be read by only the exposed partner. The latter is especially difficult to assure, but is required as maintenance of confidentiality, which is guaranteed by law in most areas and strongly endorsed by CDC for both STD and HIV partner notification (1,2).

Two evaluations of electronic referral mechanisms have been conducted, both in California (43,44). Klausner et al. describe a 1999 San Francisco outbreak of syphilis in men using an Internet chat room, noting that identifying and locating information was limited to "screen names." While DIS can often quite easily obtain this particular piece of identifying information, having a screen name often precludes the need for sex partners to learn much else about each other's identity. Nevertheless, health department personnel sent e-mail messages to partners with chat room screen names, comparing replies against a list of screen names provided by the two index cases originating the outbreak investigation. If a respondent's screen name matched a screen name on the list provided by the index cases, the contact was considered notified. From this process and subsequent presentations for evaluation, five cases (four new, one from earlier in 1999) were identified. Klausner et al. reported a contact index of 12.4, with 42% of "named" partners notified, as described above. Cases with many partners had a higher proportion of untested partners than cases reporting few partners. On a smaller scale in Los Angeles, two unrelated cases of syphilis were attributed to internet contacts (43). Together these two cases reported 150 partners, and at least 36 were notified via e-mail. The main deficiency of Internet-based PN compared with in-person provider referral is the reduced ability to persuade a partner to seek evaluation. However, Internet-based PN clearly has promise, given that the alternative to Internet partner notification by DIS here was simply patient referral.

Testing and Treating Partners

Aside from patient-delivered therapy, or expedited partner therapy (discussed in a subsequent section), we are not aware of any systematic research on interventions focused on increasing the efficiency and speed with which notified partners are examined and treated.

Alternatives and Adjuncts to Provider and Contract Referral

Cluster/Social Network Investigation

Cluster investigation is a cousin of PN and has almost as long a history in STD control. Usually, cluster investigations for STD (typically syphilis) occur parallel to PN and entail interviewing cases and their partners to elicit persons who have symptoms of STD, are partners of STD cases, or who may otherwise benefit from screening. Such persons named by cases are called "suspects" and those named by uninfected partners are called "associates." The case-finding yield for cluster investigation in the last 20 years is substantially less than that for PN (with the brought-to-treatment index ranging from 0.002 to 0.11 and the percentage of suspects/associates who are new diagnoses ranging from 0.3 to 9 across four reports) and lower than that for cluster investigation in earlier years of syphilis control, when syphilis prevalence was many times higher than in recent decades (12).

Recently, some investigators have modified and extended the traditional approach to cluster investigation for bacterial STD. This newer approach involves tracing the sexual or social contacts of cases, and sometimes of uninfected persons also. Such tracing can continue for several generations (or steps) beyond the initial persons interviewed, and may also entail ethnographic fieldwork to identify other promising persons to interview and social settings to investigate for disease control. Rothenberg and colleagues (45) applied all aspects of this approach in 1998 to curb syphilis transmission in a zip code in Atlanta with hyperendemic early syphilis. Had this approach not been implemented, as few as 38% of the new cases ultimately detected would have been found. Similar applications of related techniques helped describe and likely contain rapidly expanding epidemics of syphilis and penicillin-resistant gonorrhea elsewhere (46–49). However, the success of cluster investigation and related approaches appears to be closely tied to high disease incidence, and they tend to be unproductive in settings with low to moderate incidence (12).

Infected persons are potential candidates for conducting cluster referral, having some knowledge of who of their social as well as their sex partners is likely to be infected. In Los Angeles (50), peer "recruiters" from an HIV clinic who referred others produced 0.61 infected persons per recruiter (essentially the brought-to-treatment index, Table 1). Another recently concluded program included MSM as recruiters drawn from various clinical and community sources in Seattle (Golden et al., unpublished data) with a lower yield of new HIV infections per recruiter (0.08), but not all of the recruiters were HIV positive. Plausibly, new recruiters who occupy positions in the social network of persons at risk different from other recruiters must be enrolled on a continual basis, thereby preventing significant "saturation" of recruiters' peers.

Interventions Not Requiring DIS Involvement

The conduct of provider referral is predicated on having the resources to interview patients presenting with STD for their partners. Without interviews, one cannot tell how many partners have been exposed, much less locate and inform them. As a general rule, however, U.S. health departments and other organizations lack the resources to interview patients infected with STD other than syphilis, regardless of putative cost-effectiveness at a societal level (13,51). With HIV, the resources may exist and many see the value (11), but attitudes toward partner notification are often mixed (52), and the current CDC guidance on HIV Partner Counseling and Referral Services (PCRS) (2) emphasizes voluntary patient referral over partner elicitation.

Golden et al. (13) found that, among 60 health departments in areas of high morbidity (i.e., top 50 in at least one of syphilis, HIV, chlamydial infections, gonorrhea), 89% of syphilis cases were interviewed, against 52% of HIV cases and only 17% of gonorrhea cases and 12% of chlamydial cases. With further data in a subsequent survey, the estimated proportion of HIV cases interviewed for partners dropped to 32% (14). Golden et al. also found that resources were negatively correlated with proportions interviewed, so higher proportions of gonorrhea and chlamydial cases may have been interviewed in lower prevalence settings. Nevertheless, the point remains that program cannot rely on provider-based referral mechanisms for many STD cases—and the reader should bear in mind that the ratios of reported gonorrhea and chlamydial cases alone to reported primary and secondary syphilis are approximately 41:1 and 116:1 (53). In similar fashion, Rogstad and Henton (54) asked 155 U.K. general practitioners about partner notification practices. Only 10% of the 88 respondents replied they would undertake partner notification, citing training and funding barriers, as well as time and perceived lack of demand.

Finally, many index cases prefer alternatives to provider referral, although these preferences vary. A Swedish study showed high acceptability for provider-based referral (55), but a survey in Australia showed only 33% of respondents preferred provider referral (56). Golden, Hopkins, Morris, Holmes, and Handsfield (57) surveyed HIV-infected persons at an HIV/AIDS care clinic, finding that 84% of the sample thought provider referral should be offered, while only 20% actually requested help notifying partners.

Patient Referral

In both public and private settings the most common alternative to provider referral is patient referral, practiced by 79–84% of physicians responding to a national probability sample (the range is a function of the STD) in both public and private settings (58,59). Physicians rated patient referral as favorably as provider referral on several dimensions, including its effectiveness for infection control (60). Some studies of patients suggest the majority of patients prefer at least the option of patient referral over provider referral (61,62). Partner violence is one aspect of patient referral that might give program managers and providers pause for thought, with Maher et al. (63) reporting 24% of women fearing some violence related to telling partners if they had HIV (hypothetically). However, of the 32 who had actually practiced patient referral previously for an STD, only 1 reported a violent response. More research into the actual levels of violence attributable to patient referral is needed.

Effectiveness

Patient referral effectiveness can theoretically be measured by the same statistics presented in Table 1. However, some of those statistics rely on having a professional present to collect them, which is typically not the case for patient referral. Index case patient report is one substitute (and it is a useful substitute), while proxy data can be gathered from people who seek treatment and acknowledge being contacts.

Few U.S. data speak to the determinants of effective patient referral. Internationally, two studies from Uganda report such determinants in detail (64,65). Qualitative results from interviews and focus groups, total $N = 148$, indicated high acceptance of patient referral in terms of importance and responsibility, but also citation of negative consequences (e.g., mistrust, relationship ending, quarrelling). In quantitative findings, 426 participants claimed 518 partners, for a partner index of 1.22. The authors found that past successful referral (odd ratio [OR] = 17.1 for women and 14.9 for men, both $p < .001$), but also intentions (OR = 2.7 for women, $p < .001$ and 1.2 for men, $p < .01$, per point on 7-point scales) and self-efficacy (OR = 1.8 for women, $p < .05$ but 1.2, NS for men) were predictors of patient referral. One general point is that those who are willing to refer partners before being asked can be counted on to some extent to refer partners when they are asked. But two other general points are that odds ratios reflect that previous behavior was a far stronger predictor than dispositions and that overall patient referral effectiveness measured by the proportion of partners referred, 32.8%, or by the contact index, 0.40, was low. Turning to characteristics of the partner rather than the index case, Warszawski and Meyer (66) reported from a French population-based survey that patients were less likely to notify casual partners than main partners (27% of adults and 14% of adolescents notified casual partners against 92% and 68%, respectively, for main partners).

Interventions

Interventions in patient referral pertain to enhancements to basic referral instructions that could improve either notification or reduce index case infection. Kissinger et al. (67) recently completed a trial including a test of patient referral and counseling against patient referral and counseling and a booklet of referral cards. The trial also included a condition in which patients were given medications for partners; see below under "Expedited Partner Therapy" for discussion of those outcomes. The trial was conducted in New Orleans, enrolling 977 men with clinically diagnosed with urethritis (subsequent lab testing showed the urethritis was predominantly driven by gonorrhea: > 60%). Overall follow-up was 79%, but only 38% of these (30% of the full sample) agreed to provide urine for biologic testing. There was no clear-cut reason for this low rate, but the investigators surmised general reluctance, possibly fears of drug testing, alleviated only by participants' suspicions they were (re)infected. Notification rates per partner of those given booklets were similar to those receiving patient referral, 53% versus 48% (identical proportions, 54%, saw their partners at all). Nonsignificantly higher proportions in the booklet arm "gave the intervention" to their partners, 58% versus 48%, with the difference between intervention adherence and notification by men in the booklet arm (58% versus 53%) probably due to leaving a referral card without talking to the partner. In contrast to the relatively similar notification behaviors, infections at follow-up in those in the booklet arm were substantially lower than in the control arm, OR = 0.22 (95% CI = 0.11–0.44). Infection rates were high in both arms: 14.3% for the booklet arm, and 42.7% for the control arm. This led the investigators to suspect that the men agreed to be tested only if they thought they might have an STD. On an intention to treat basis, the rates were 4.6% versus 12.3%, still significantly different at $p < .01$. In summary, provision of the booklet was no more than equivalent to patient referral in producing notification, but was associated with reduced reinfection of index cases.

In two randomized trials in Denmark, chlamydial cases either gave urine sample collection kits to their partners (who were to mail samples to the laboratory in prepaid envelopes) or referred their partners to examination with a package containing a urethral swab and prepaid envelope for mailing to the laboratory (68,69). The case-finding yield from cases given urine collection kits was approximately twice as large as that for cases asked to refer partners to examination. A higher proportion of partners was tested with the urine collection kits and such partners were tested earlier on average than were partners referred to examination. An unknown number of partners referred to examination may have been examined but not recorded as such if they did not bring the swab to their examinations.

Other patient referral interventions draw on African populations, where lack of resources means provider referral is not an option for HIV or any STD (65). Basic clinic training with simple written instructions can improve case management: Harrison et al. (70) reported a large increase in correct case management after brief health worker training sessions. Specifically, correct management, including providing patient referral cards and instructions, rose from 5% to 12% of patients' visits in control clinics, but from 14% to 83% in intervention clinics, $p < .01$. Unfortunately, referral management was not separated from other case management activities. Mathews et al. (71) evaluated a video designed to improve notification rates. The video was developed by a national mass media company that already produced a popular soap opera. The video was set in a community analogous to the study site (an urban township with a busy community health center), featuring a dramatic love affair, followed by diagnosis, treatment, and partner notification. The principal outcome measure was referral cards given to index cases to give to their partners (this outcome measure relies on the partner seeking evaluation after notification, so the outcome measure is biased downwards throughout the study). Compared with a pre-intervention baseline rate of 0.20 cards returned per index case— that is, the estimated treatment index and the minimum possible contact index—the return rate rose to 0.27 during the intervention phase. Although the difference of 0.07 was not statistically different from 0 (95% CI = −0.05 to 0.17), the authors felt the result was promising. In particular, women seeing the video were most likely to believe they could find their partners (97% versus 83%, $p < .01$).

Expedited Partner Therapy

Expedited partner therapy (EPT) is a broad term covering methods whereby partners of index cases receive treatment before a personal evaluation. We note the process is *not* supposed to be in lieu of personal evaluation. Therefore, although this process technically does not require DIS involvement, we note that management of EPT by a public health program (and including managing cooperation with private providers) is amenable to DIS skills and experience.

The rationale for treatment without knowing that the partner has an STD is the principle of prophylactic treatment. Both the local surveys of practitioners (61,72,73) and the results from a national survey of physicians (74) suggest that approximately half of those surveyed have ever given STD patients medications for their partners and that 10–15% do so regularly (i.e., endorsing terms such as "usually" or "always"). Hogben et al. found that usage was both widespread and sporadic, appearing to correlate weakly with using partner management strategies more intensive than patient referral instructions, which were also widespread.

Most experimental interventions (67,75,76) and evaluations (77) have studied using index cases as the sole means of bringing therapy to partners, although one trial (75) incorporated DIS assistance when requested. What is delivered to the partner may be medication directly, or a prescription for medication. Kissinger et al.'s (77) observational study was based on a cohort of

256 women with chlamydial infection at a family planning clinic, for whom there were follow-up data for 70% within a year. Women were allowed to take medications for their partners if they chose, along with patient-referral cards, with others receiving referral cards alone. Of the comparison group receiving patient referral instructions alone, 25.5% were reinfected within a year. Only 11.5% of those accepting medications were reinfected, OR = 0.37 (95% CI = 0.15–0.97). Although women who chose EPT in this non-randomized study were plausibly more effective at compliance than those who did not, this result could well represent a typical effect in a setting where EPT is voluntary—which would be the programmatic norm. An earlier retrospective cohort analysis from Sweden (78) had also found reduced rates of reinfection in women who chose to take medications to partners (2% reinfection versus 8% for patient referral).

Three randomized controlled trials have been conducted since the Kissinger et al. (77) evaluation, one assessing women with chlamydial infection (76); one assessing men and women with either or both of chlamydial infection and gonorrhea (75); and one assessing men diagnosed with urethritis (67). Schillinger et al. enrolled 1,787 women from five U.S. cities, with 81% follow-up for reinfection at up to three months. Women in the control condition received written and verbal instruction to refer partners (patient referral); those in the experimental condition received medications in addition to the same referral instructions as controls. Cumulative infections by three months were 15% in the control group and 12% in the group receiving medication, OR = 0.80 (95% CI = 0.62–1.05).

Seattle-King County's effort (75) to test EPT for chlamydial infection and gonorrhea drew participants from private as well as public clinic (e.g., STD, family planning) settings, with 2,105 women and 646 men enrolled (68% follow-up at 18 weeks). At follow-up, EPT recipients were significantly less likely to be infected with STD, $RR = 0.76$ (95 CI = 0.59–0.98). As the primary biologic outcome for which the study was powered, the 24% reduction is the most germane figure, but subanalyses indicated a substantially larger reduction for gonorrhea, $RR = 0.32$ (95% CI = 0.13–0.77), than for chlamydial infection, $RR = 0.82$ (95% CI = 0.62–1.07). Moreover, the relative risk for chlamydial infection is almost identical to that reported by Schillinger et al. (expressed as an odds ratio, the Seattle-King County statistic was exactly the same: 0.80).

We have described the final trial involving EPT previously under patient referral interventions (67), because the trial included booklet-enhanced patient referral as well as an EPT condition. Follow-up prevalence of men assigned to patient-delivered medication was 24%, compared with 43% for patient referral, OR = 0.38 (95% CI = 0.19–0.74). The prevalence of the former did not differ statistically from booklet referral, for which prevalence at follow-up was 14%. Had larger numbers been tested however, the difference may have become meaningful (a difference of 14% versus 23% becomes detectable at $p < .05$ with power = .80 when total $N = 582$).

Reinfection rates, however, are only one of the appropriate outcome tests for a PN intervention. As with many of the other interventions reviewed in this chapter, the behavioral outcomes are also essential as indicators of the prevention of transmission to persons other than the index case. In behavioral terms, EPT as it has been most commonly tested, comprises patient referral plus provision of medication. That is, the index case is enjoined to notify his or her partners and, in fact, refer them for evaluation, just as one would for patient referral. Based on the partner follow-up model described earlier in this chapter, the principal behaviors of interest are notification and treatment, with some studies also reporting sexual behaviors of index cases and partners during the notification and treatment phases.

Having medications to deliver results consistently in equivalent or higher notification rates. Schillinger et al. (76) reported that women randomized to EPT were more likely to "comply with the intervention"; that is, notify and refer partners, 85% versus 75%, $p < .01$. Golden et al. (75), however, reported almost identical notification rates for patient referral and EPT across gender: 78% versus 77%. Kissinger et al. (67), studying men, reported a substantial increment in notification rates: 71% versus 48%, $p < .001$, for talking to the partner about the infection. Notably, the 71% rate was also significantly higher than that for men in the booklet-enhanced referral arm (53%), $p < .001$. The 75–78% notification rates in the patient referral arms were higher than many estimates of the proportions of partners who present for evaluation and who may represent an estimate of the deficit between notification and seeking evaluation and treatment by patient-referred partners.

Next is the question of treatment rates, and, here, EPT appears to increase partner treatment rates consistently compared to patient referral. Both Golden et al. and Kissinger et al. reported substantial increments in the proportions of partners receiving treatment via EPT compared with via patient referral. In Golden et al., 61% of participants in the EPT arm reported all partners were "very likely" treated, versus 49% in the patient referral arm, $p < .01$. On a similar question, whether the partner was "very likely" to have been treated or tested negative for STD, 64% of those in the EPT arm agreed, versus 52% of those in the patient referral arm, $p < .01$. Kissinger et al. (67) found that 56% of men randomized to give medications to their partners reported that their partners told them they took the medication, while 48% also reported seeing the partner take the medications. Corresponding percentages in the patient referral arm were 45% and 32%, both $p < .001$.

The increments in patient-reported partner treatment are between 20% and 50%, depending on the study and question. Golden et al. also found only 6% of those in the EPT arm reported sex with a partner not believed "very likely" to either have been treated or tested negative, versus 12% of the patient referral arm, $p < .01$, while, comparing EPT to patient referral participants, Kissinger et al. found less unprotected sex prior to partner treatment, 28% versus 37%, $p < .05$, and slightly less overall unprotected sex between treatment and follow-up (with any partner), 29% versus 34%, $p = .05$. Although all of these data are patients' reports rather than direct observation (e.g., by DIS), the important comparisons are between groups, and patients' reporting biases and social desirability should be spread across those groups.

As a highly promising but relatively newly studied series of interventions, albeit not a novel practice (74), unintended consequences of EPT need to be explored. Those cited include the possibility of partners avoiding evaluation because they have been treated—a point that is particularly salient with respect to missed co-morbidity (especially HIV co-morbidity) and to women with early pelvic inflammatory disease (PID). Stekler et al. (79) reported from a multi-city survey that HIV co-morbidity in MSM may be high enough (at least in some locations) for MSM with STD to be a high priority for DIS-based partner management. A smaller survey of STD clinic patients (80) reported 10% or higher co-morbidity for trichomoniasis in patients infected with gonorrhea or chlamydia. Chlamydial and gonococcal co-morbidity were combined with gonorrheal infection alone in the study, so the actual level of co-morbidity between these two infections could not be determined. However, co-treatment for chlamydial infection of those also infected with gonorrhea is common and likely warranted, so untreated infections are unlikely for this combination. There is no evidence to suggest that providing medication either facilitates or retards evaluation-seeking by partners, so additional research on this topic is an important priority.

For that matter, direct estimates of the effect of patient referral upon evaluation-seeking are needed. Therefore, any inhibiting effect of EPT upon partner presentation for evaluation has to outweigh the higher notification rates achieved with EPT. There are competing logic models supporting both circumstances, and various factors may interact with EPT to produce a facilitating effect for some and an inhibiting effect for others. Both logic models can be described within the popular Health Belief Model (HBM) (81,82). In the HBM, positive health behaviors depend upon two important factors, the perceived susceptibility to a negative health outcome and the perceived severity of that outcome. The just-notified partner will be more likely to seek evaluation (the positive health behavior) if the medication prompts a sense of increased susceptibility via an increased strength of belief that he or she could have an STD and even via increased perceived severity if the medication prompts thoughts about disease outcomes. But the just-notified partner might also perceive diminished severity by taking the medication and might then be less likely to seek evaluation.

Both missed morbidity and progress to PID increase the need for personal evaluations. Therefore, medication should be accompanied by instructions to seek evaluation and to avoid sex during the course of medication, among other health education instructions. Of course, the same ought to be true of instructions accompanying patient referral, because these issues apply equally to both strategies. Finally, the presence of the intervention as an option and the typically favorable responses of patients to the prospect (83) does not mean that every patient will actually choose to take medications to partners or that all providers will choose to dispense them for all patients. In San Francisco, Klausner and Chaw (84) reported patient-delivered partner therapy was the partner management of choice for 23% of chlamydial infection cases—the authors still concluded the option was useful.

Conclusions

In spite of the lack of high-quality national data, there is substantial intervention research on STD partner management, including notification. In the spirit of providing more tools for improving management rather than fewer, and providing avenues rather than directives, we suggest that the following interventions have merit, but ought to be assessed for appropriateness to individual programs. Assuming that syphilis (and, one hopes, HIV) remain priorities for DIS services, gonorrheal and chlamydial infections may be managed via patient referral, enhanced ether with referral cards, EPT, or both (the constraints already discussed notwithstanding). In view of the fact that some referral card-based interventions were accompanied by counseling, a trained person who can offer such counseling is warranted where resources permit. Auxiliary efforts such as peer-driven cluster referral are inexpensive to operate and produce cases that by definition are unlikely to be found through DIS-based provider referral. Evaluation of any of these approaches on a continuing basis is recommended.

We close this chapter with some broader points about where partner management can take place. Most STD is diagnosed and treated outside public settings (59,85). Golden et al. (83) demonstrated the scope and value of a "treatment community-level" partnership for STD partner management in Seattle. On these lines, Evans et al. (86) in the United Kingdom evaluated family planning clinic-based treatment and management of STD, as an alternative to care in overburdened specialist genitourinary medicine clinics. They found that, with training and some marketing (to providers), clinics documented patient referral instructions for index cases, including referral cards, for 84% of their chlamydia-infected patients (and their contacts). The study is a small-scale evaluation, but is, with the other material cited above, yet another example of how open-minded and innovative approaches can make some form of partner management available wherever STDs are found.

References

1. Centers for Disease Control and Prevention. Partner services. In: *Program Operation Guidelines for STD Prevention*. Atlanta, GA: CDC; 2001.
2. Centers for Disease Control and Prevention. HIV partner counseling and referral services: Guidance. December 1998. Available at: http://www.cdc.gov/hiv/pubs/pcrs.htm.
3. Potterat JJ, Mehus A, Gallwey J. Partner notification: operational considerations. *International Journal of STD & AIDS*. 1991;2:411–415.
4. Centers for Disease Control and Prevention. *Sexually Transmitted Disease Surveillance, 2003*. Atlanta, GA; CDC; 2004.
5. Rothenberg R, Potterat JJ. Partner notification for sexually transmitted diseases and HIV infection. In Holmes KK, Sparling PF, Mardh PA, eds. *Sexually Transmitted Diseases*, 3rd ed. New York, NY: McGraw-Hill; 1999:745–752.
6. Aral SO, Hughes JP, Stoner B, Whittington W, et al. Sexual mixing patterns in the spread of gonococcal and chlamydial infections. *American Journal of Public Health*. 1999;89:825–833.
7. Kerani RP, Golden MR, Whittington WLM, Handsfield HH, Hogben M, Holmes KK. Spatial bridges for the importation of gonorrhea and chlamydial infection. *Sexually Transmitted Diseases*. 2003;30:742–749.
8. Clark EG. Studies in the epidemiology of syphilis: epidemiologic investigations in a series of 996 cases of acquired syphilis. *Venereal Disease Information*. 1940;21:349–369.
9. Potterat JJ. Contact tracing's price is not its value. *Sexually Transmitted Diseases*. 1997;24:519–521.
10. Potterat JJ, Muth SQ, Muth JB. Partner notification early in the AIDS era: Misconstruing contact tracers as bedroom police. In: Margolis E, ed. *AIDS Research/AIDS Policy: Competing Paradigms of Science and Public Policy*. Greenwich, CT: JAI Press; 1998:1–15.
11. Golden MR. HIV partner notification: a neglected intervention. *Sexually Transmitted Diseases*. 2002;29:472–475.
12. Brewer DD. Case-finding effectiveness of partner notification and cluster investigation for sexually transmitted diseases/HIV. *Sexually Transmitted Diseases*. 2005;32:78–83.

13. Golden MR, Hogben M, Handsfield HH, St. Lawrence JS, Potterat JJ, Holmes KK. Partner notification for HIV and STD in the United States: Low coverage for gonorrhea, chlamydial infection, and HIV. *Sexually Transmitted Diseases.* 2003;30:490–496.

14. Golden MR, Hogben M, Potterat JJ, Handsfield HH. HIV partner notification in the United States: a national survey of program coverage and outcomes. *Sexually Transmitted Diseases.* 2004;31:709–712.

15. Macke BA, Maher, JE. Partner notification in the United States: an evidence-based review. *American Journal of Preventive Medicine.* 1999;17:230–242.

16. Mathews C, Coetzee N, Zwarenstein M, et al. A systematic review of strategies for partner notification for sexually transmitted diseases, including HIV/AIDS. *International Journal of STD & AIDS.* 2002;13:285–300.

17. Oxman A, Scott EAF, Sellors JW, et al. Partner notification for sexually transmitted diseases: an overview of the evidence. *Canadian Journal of Public Health.* 1994;85:127–132.

18. Fenton KA, Peterman TA. HIV partner notification: taking a new look. *AIDS.* 1997;11:1–12.

19. Landis SE, Schoenbach VJ, Weber DJ, et al. Results of a randomized trial of partner notification in cases of HIV infections in North Carolina. *New England Journal of Medicine.* 1992;326:101–106.

20. Potterat JJ, Muth SQ, Rothenberg RB, et al. Sexual network structure as an indicator of epidemic phase. *Sexually Transmitted Infections.* 2002;78(S1):i152–i158.

21. Woodhouse DE, Potterat JJ, Muth JB, Pratts CI, Rothenberg RB, Fogle JS. A civilian-military partnership to reduce the incidence of gonorrhea. *Public Health Reports.* 1985;100:61–68.

22. Han Y, Coles B, Muse A, Hipp S. Assessment of a geographically targeted field intervention on gonorrhea incidence in two New York state counties. *Sexually Transmitted Diseases.* 1999;26:296–302.

23. Centers for Disease Control and Prevention. *STD Employee Development Guide.* Atlanta, GA: CDC; 1992.

25. Hogben M, Paffel J, Broussard D, et al. Syphilis partner notification with men who have sex with men: a review and commentary. *Sexually Transmitted Diseases.* 2005;32(Suppl):S43–S47.

26. Macke BA, Hennessy MH, McFarlane M. Predictors of time spent on partner notification on four US sites. *Sexually Transmitted Infections.* 2000;76:371–374.

27. Peterman TA, Toomey KT, Dicker LW, Zaidi AA, Wroten JE, Carolina J. Partner notification for syphilis: a randomized, controlled trial of three approaches. *Sexually Transmitted Diseases.* 1997;24:511–521.

28. Brewer DD, Garrett SB, Kulasingam S. Forgetting as a cause of incomplete reporting of sexual and drug injection partners. *Sexually Transmitted Diseases.* 1999;26:166–176.

29. Brewer DD. Interviewing practices in partner notification for STD and HIV. Abridged report to the Division of STD Prevention, Centers for Disease Control and Prevention. 2006. Available at: http://www.interscientific.net/reprints/CDCreport.pdf.

30. Brewer DD, Garrett SB. Evaluation of interviewing techniques to enhance recall of sexual and drug injection partners. *Sexually Transmitted Diseases.* 2001;28:666–677.

31. Brewer DD, Garrett SB, Rinaldi G. Free-listed items are effective cues for eliciting additional items in semantic domains. *Applied Cognitive Psychology.* 2002;16:343–358.

32. Brewer DD, Potterat JJ, Muth SQ, et al. Randomized trial of supplementary interviewing techniques to enhance recall of sexual partners in contact interviews. *Sexually Transmitted Diseases.* 2005;32:189–193.

33. Hoffman RE, Spencer NE, Miller LA. Comparison of partner notification at anonymous and confidential HIV test sites in Colorado. *Journal of Acquired Immune Deficiency Syndrome & Human Retrovirology.* 1995;8:406–410.

34. Doering VE, Elste G, Lehmann-Franken, et al. Improvement of infection control research with gonorrhea patients through reinterviews. *Dermatologische Monatsshrift.* 1979;165:41–45.

35. Stuart J. Venereal disease contact investigation. *Journal of Venereal Disease Information.* 1951;32:242–247.

36. Starcher ET, Kramer MA, Carlota-Orduna B, Lundberg DF. Establishing efficient interview periods for gonorrhea patients. *American Journal of Public Health.* 1983;73:1381–1384.

37. Zimmerman-Rogers H, Potterat JJ, Muth SQ, et al. Establishing efficient partner notification periods for patients with chlamydia. *Sexually Transmitted Diseases.* 1999;26:49–54.

38. Alary M, Joly JR, Poulin C. Gonorrhea and chlamydial infection: comparison of contact tracing performed by physicians or by a specialized service. *Canadian Journal of Public Health.* 1991;82:132–134.

39. Brewer DD, Potterat JJ, Muth SQ. Interviewer effects in the elicitation of sexual and drug injection partners. Paper presented at the 24th International Sunbelt Social Network Conference, Portoroz, Slovenia, May 2004.

40. Stoner BP, Whittington WLM, Aral SO, Hughes JP, Handsfield HH, Holmes KK. Avoiding risky sex partners: perception of partners' risks v partners' self reported risks. *Sexually Transmitted Infections.* 2003;79:197–201.

41. Brewer DD, Rothenberg RB, Muth SQ, Roberts JM, Jr, Potterat JJ. Agreement in reported sexual partnership dates and implications for measuring concurrency. *Sexually Transmitted Diseases.* 2006;33:277–283.

42. Tomnay JE, Pitts MK, Fairley CK. New technology and partner notification—why aren't we using them? *International Journal of STD & AIDS.* 2005;16:19–22.

43. Centers for Disease Control and Prevention. Using the internet for partner notification of sexually transmitted diseases‡Los Angeles County, California, 2003. *Morbidity and Mortality Weekly Report.* 2004;53:129–131.

44. Klausner JD, Wolf W, Fischer-Ponce L, Zolt I, Katz MH. Tracing a syphilis outbreak through cyberspace. *Journal of the American Medical Association.* 2000;284:447–449.

45. Rothenberg R, Kimbrough L, Lewis-Hardy R, et al. Social network methods for endemic foci of syphilis: a pilot project. *Sexually Transmitted Diseases.* 2000;27:12–18.

46. Centers for Disease Control and Prevention. Gang-related outbreak of penicillinase-producing *Neisseria gonorrhoeae* and other sexually transmitted diseases: Colorado Springs, Colorado, 1989–1991. *Morbidity and Mortality Weekly Report.* 1993;42:25–28.

47. Gerber AR, King LC, Dunleavy GJ, Novick L. An outbreak of syphilis on an Indian reservation: descriptive epidemiology and disease-control measures. *American Journal of Public Health.* 1989;79:83–85.

48. Potterat JJ, Muth SQ, Bethea RP. Chronicle of a gang STD outbreak foretold. *Free Inquiry and Creative Sociology.* 1996;24:11–16.

49. Rothenberg RB, Sterk C, Toomey KE, et al. Using social network and ethnographic tools to evaluate syphilis transmission. *Sexually Transmitted Diseases.* 1998;25:154–160.

50. Jordan WC, Tolbert L, Smith R. Partner notification and focused intervention as a means of identifying HIV-positive patients. *Journal of the National Medical Association.* 1998;90:542–546.

51. Pourat N, Brown ER, Razack N, Kassler W. Medicaid managed care and STDs: Missed opportunities to control the epidemic. *Health Affairs.* 2002;21:228–239.

52. Potterat JJ. Partner notification for HIV: Running out of excuses. *Sexually Transmitted Diseases.* 2003;30:89–90.

53. Centers for Disease Control and Prevention. *Sexually Transmitted Disease Surveillance, 2004.* Atlanta, GA: CDC; 2005.

54. Rogstad KE, Henton L. General practitioners and the National Strategy on Sexual Health and HIV. *International Journal of STD & AIDS.* 2004;15:169–172.

55. Tyden T, Ramstedt K. A survey of patients with *Chlamydia trachomatis* infection: Sexual behaviour and perceptions about contact tracing. *International Journal of STD and AIDS.* 2000;11:92–95.

56. Tomnay JE, Pitts K, Fairley CK. Partner notification: Preferences of Melbourne clients and the estimated proportion of sexual partners they can contact. *International Journal of STD & AIDS.* 2004;15:415–418.

57. Golden MR, Hopkins SG, Morris M, Holmes KK, Handsfield HH. Support among persons infected with HIV for routine health department contact for partner notification. *Journal of Acquired Immune Deficiency Syndromes.* 2003;32:196–202.

58. McCree DH, Liddon NC, Hogben M, St. Lawrence, JS. National survey of doctors' actions following the diagnosis of a bacterial STD. *Sexually Transmitted Infections.* 2003;79:254–256.

59. St. Lawrence JS, Montano DE, Kasprzyk D, Phillips WR, Armstrong K, Leichliter JS. STD screening, testing, case reporting, and clinical and partner notification practices: a national survey of US physicians. *American Journal of Public Health.* 2002;92:1784–1788.

60. Hogben M, St. Lawrence JS, Montano DE, Kasprzyk D, Leichliter JS, Phillips WR. Physicians' opinions about partner notification methods: case reporting, patient referral, and provider referral. *Sexually Transmitted Infections.* 2004;80:30–34.

61. Golden MR, Whittington WLM, Gorbach PM, Coronado N, Boyd MA, Holmes KK. Partner notification among private providers for chlamydial infections in Seattle-King County: a clinician and patient survey. *Sexually Transmitted Diseases.* 1999;26:543–547.

62. Potterat JJ, Rothenberg R. The case-finding effectiveness of a self-referral system for gonorrhea: a preliminary report. *American Journal of Public Health.* 1977;67:174–176.

63. Maher JE, Peterson J, Hastings K, et al. Partner violence, partner notification, and women's decisions to have an HIV test. *Journal of Acquired Immune Deficiency Syndromes.* 2000;25:276–282.

64. Nuwaha F, Faxelid E, Neema S, Eriksson C, Hoje B. Psychosocial determinants for sexual partner referral in Uganda: qualitative results. *International Journal of STD & AIDS.* 2000;11:156–161.

65. Nuwaha F, Faxelid E, Wabwire-Mangen F, Eriksson C, Hoje B. Psycho-social determinants for sexual partner referral in Uganda: quantitative results. *Social Science & Medicine.* 2001;53:1287–1301.

66. Warszawski J, Meyer L. Sex differences in partner notification: results from three population based surveys in France. *Sexually Transmitted Infections.* 2002;78: 45–49.

67. Kissinger PK, Mohammed H, Richardson-Alston G, et al. Patient-delivered partner treatment for male urethritis: a randomized controlled trial. *Clinical Infectious Diseases.* 2005;41:623–629.

68. Anderson B, Ostergaard L, Moller F, Olesen JK. Home sampling versus conventional contact tracing for detecting *Chlamydia trachomatis* infection in male partners of infected women: randomised study. *British Medical Journal.* 1998;316: 350–351.

69. Ostergaard L, Andersen B, Moller JK, Olesen F, Worm AM. Managing partners of people diagnosed with *Chlamydia trachomatis*: a comparison of two partner testing methods. *Sexually Transmitted Infections.* 2003;79:358–361.

70. Harrison A, Karin SA, Floyd K, et al. Syndrome packets and health worker training improve sexually transmitted disease case management in rural South Africa: Randomized controlled trial. *AIDS*. 2000;14:2769–2779.

71. Mathews C, Guttmacher SJ, Coetzee N, et al. Evaluation of a video based health education strategy to improve sexually transmitted disease partner notification in South Africa. *Sexually Transmitted Infections*. 2002;78:53–57.

72. Niccolai LM, Winston DM. Physicians' opinions on partner management for non-viral sexually transmitted infections. *American Journal of Preventive Medicine*. 2005;28:229–233.

73. Packel LJ, Guerry S, Bauer HM, et al. Patient-delivered partner therapy for chlamydial infections: attitudes and practices of California physicians and nurse practitioners. *Sexually Transmitted Diseases*. 2006;33:458–463.

74. Hogben M, McCree DH, Golden MR. Patient-delivered partner therapy for sexually transmitted diseases as practiced by U.S. physicians. *Sexually Transmitted Diseases*. 2005;32:101–105.

75. Golden MR, Whittington WLM, Handsfield HH, et al. Effect of expedited treatment of sex partners on recurrent or persistent gonorrhea or chlamydial infection. *New England Journal of Medicine*. 2005;352:676–685.

76. Schillinger JA, Kissinger PK, Calvet H, et al. Patient-delivered partner treatment with azithromycin to prevent repeated *Chlamydia trachomatis* infection among women. *Sexually Transmitted Diseases*. 2003;30:49–56.

77. Kissinger PK, Brown R, Reed K, et al. Effectiveness of patient delivered partner medication for preventing recurrent *Chlamydia trachomatis*. *Sexually Transmitted Infections*. 1998;74:331–333.

78. Ramstedt K, Forssman L, Johannisson G. Contact tracing in the control of genital *chlamydia trachomatis* infection. *International Journal of STD & AIDS*. 1991;2: 116–118.

79. Stekler J, Bachmann L, Brotman RM, et al. Concurrent sexually transmitted infections (STIs) in sex partners of patients with selected STIs: implications for patient-delivered partner therapy. *Clinical Infectious Diseases*. 2005;40:787–793.

80. Khan A, Fortenberry JD, Juliar BE, Tu W, Orr DP, Batteiger BE. The prevalence of chlamydia, gonorrhea, and trichomonas in sexual partnerships: implications for partner notification and treatment. *Sexually Transmitted Diseases*. 2005;32: 260–264.

81. Becker MH. The health belief model and personal health behavior. *Health Education Monographs*. 1974;2:324–508.

82. Becker MH. AIDS and behavior change. *Public Health Reviews*. 1988;16:1–11.

83. Golden MR, Whittington WLM, Handsfield HH, et al. Partner management for gonococcal and chlamydial infection: expansion of public health services to the private sector and expedited sex partner treatment through a partnership with commercial pharmacies. *Sexually Transmitted Diseases*. 2001;28:658–665.

84. Klausner JD, Chaw JK. Patient-delivered therapy for chlamydia: putting research into practice. *Sexually Transmitted Diseases*. 2003;30:509–511.

85. Brackbill RM, Sternberg MR, Fishbein M. Where do people go for treatment of sexually transmitted diseases? *Family Planning Perspectives*. 1999;31:10–15.

86. Evans J, Baraitser P, Cross J, Bacon L, Piper J. Managing genital infection in community family planning clinics: an alternative approach to holistic sexual health service provision. *Sexually Transmitted Infections*. 2004;80:142–144.

8

Interventions in Sexual Health Care–Seeking and Provision at Multiple Levels of the U.S. Health Care System

Matthew Hogben, Ph.D., and Lydia A. Shrier, M.D., M.P.H.

Much of the time, the popular construction of health care is reactive—a woman is hit by a car, the ambulance arrives within a certain time, the medics have suitable training, and the hospital has the staff with the necessary skills and the best equipment for them to use. But, as the old proverb reminds us, an ounce of prevention is worth a pound of cure. Routine health care–seeking and provision is part of that ounce, and sexual health care, here, mainly for disease or infection control, is part of high-quality comprehensive health care (1,2).

For this chapter, we will focus on sexual health care–seeking and provision both in the sense of a recommended routine event (e.g., a yearly check-up) and as a reaction to suspicion of a sexually transmitted infection or disease, including human immunodeficiency virus (HIV) infection. HIV transmission presents perhaps the most critical rationale for improved health care–seeking and provision because unrecognized HIV infection persists in part due to lack of routine testing (3) and, in turn, increases the risk of complications and further transmission. We also include studies from the perspectives of the provider and system, as well as the patient, so some interventions covered herein optimized health care–seeking through improving access and availability.

We have left questions about the quality of health care for STD aside, except as perceptions about getting appropriate care pertain to actual health care–*seeking*. Care may entail screening and treatment—screening is the topic of another chapter in this volume; treatment falls outside the scope of this chapter. This chapter examines the factors that lead to provision of sexual health care, with interventions using patients and providers as intervention targets, and both groups and system-level changes as the agents of change.

Defining a Framework for Sexual Health Care–Seeking and Provision

The principal organizing framework for this chapter is drawn from Aral and Wasserheit's (4) Person-Time of Infectiousness (PTI) model. The full model explains delays in health care–seeking and service delivery between STD

Behavioral Interventions for Prevention and Control of Sexually Transmitted Diseases.
Aral SO, Douglas JM Jr, eds. Lipshutz JA, assoc ed. New York: Springer Science+Business Media, LLC; 2007.

onset and secondary prevention and how delays affect the proportion of people affected and the duration of infectiousness. Health care–seeking delays comprise the second component of this model—the first is loss to detection, the subsequent three (diagnostic, treatment, and prevention delays) pertain to delays that follow actual entry into the health care system and therefore fall outside the scope of this chapter. Each of the components contains references to various potential targets of intervention and agents of change: pathogen, individual (both characteristics and behaviors), provider, and health system/societal parameters. The topic material of the interventions we discuss can be classified into these parameters; this constitutes the organization of our sections on interventions, but also on correlates of health care–seeking and provision. To the extent the data permit, we also discuss the interactions among these parameters, although there is little true multilevel research on sexual health care–seeking or provision.

A separate chapter in this volume examines screening interventions as a stand-alone topic. However, screening for STD is typically an integral part of systemic and provider-level interventions promoting health care provision; for example, a provider who eschews STD screening as part of sexual health care can hardly be said to be contributing to a patient's health care–seeking. Consequently, we have included studies with screening as an outcome variable, but only when this outcome is presented in the context of overall improved sexual health care.

Extent and Common Correlates of Health Care–Seeking and Provision

To guide intervention efforts, one would like to know what proportion of a given target population actually receives routine health care and which variables are related to health care–seeking and provision. Numerous surveys and cohort studies have yielded many more calls for interventions to improve sexual health care–seeking and provision than there are actual interventions. However, such studies are helpful to intervention research in that they reveal important variables to consider as subject matter for intervention. They comprise, in effect, the broadest type of formative research (but we are not suggesting they replace formative research for any given intervention!). Table 1 provides a summary of factors found in this section of the chapter.

Extent of Sexual Health Care–Seeking

Estimating the extent of sexual health care–seeking relies on two sources of information: estimates of how many people seek care and which providers include appropriate sexual health care as part of health care provision (which can occur without health care–seeking). In 2002, 84.1% of the general population (75.2% of 18–24 year olds; 78.2% of 25–44 year olds) made at least one health care visit to a doctor's office or emergency department, or received a home visit from a doctor, but causes and content of such visits were not broken down (5). Uninsured persons were substantially less likely to seek care and Hispanic or Latino persons were the least likely of any race or ethnicity to have a regular source of health care (5). Compared with their insured peers, adolescents who lack health insurance are more likely to have health

Table 1 Health care-seeking parameters from the person-time infectiousness model and relevant topic areas: correlates.

Content factors	Parameters			
	Pathogen	Individual	Provider	Health system
Symptom seriousness and duration	Conflicting findings, may depend on perceptions of STD outcomes		Providers who do not take sexual histories miss asymptomatic disease	
Sociodemographic variation		Minorities receive fewer services, adolescents and young adults less likely to have sought routine care		Availability diminished for uninsured persons; sexual health care rarer than other health care; minorities overrepresented in public care settings
Self-treatment		Self-treaters took longer to access care; HIV-infected users of complementary medicine used health care more frequently than others		
Health literacy	Names and characteristics of STD often unfamiliar to patients	Low literacy inhibits health care-seeking		
Perceived stigma		Those perceiving stigma may turn to self-treatment and alternative therapies		Perceived discrimination inhibits care-seeking; so does lack of confidentiality (minors)
Sustaining health care		Returning for HIV test results negatively correlated with male gender, married status, requesting STD testing; positively correlated with being an STD contact	Provider-patient rapport sometimes helps, but provider-patient continuity negatively correlated with screening	Ease of return appointments, cost, hours, testing strategies improve return rates

(Continued)

Table 1 Health care-seeking parameters from the person-time infectiousness model and relevant topic areas: correlates. —Cont'd

	Parameters			
Content factors	Pathogen	Individual	Provider	Health system
Provider actions			Recommending tests influences patient acceptance	Formal guidance for sexual histories varies by country, generally not shown in provider surveys; (female) screening guidelines more common and more commonly adhered to
Accessibility and waiting time		Lack of knowledge about services diminishes care-seeking		Long wait times sometimes reduce care-seeking and return rates; short distances from regular locations, urine tests, extended hours help
Perceived staff competence		Quality of care correlates with health care-seeking	Trained providers more likely to take sexual histories and screen on the basis of one	Clinic protocols promote better sexual health care provision

problems (6,7), including chlamydial infection (8), and less likely to receive preventive health care (9), have physician contact at least annually, and have a usual source of health care (7).

Substantially smaller fractions of the population receive sexual health care than receive health care services overall. In Colorado, 72% of youth had accessed health care services in the past year, but only 39% had ever had an STD evaluation (10). A report from managed care organizations estimated that at least half of female patients in King County, Washington, had been asked about sexual activity, a reasonable precursor to a full sexual history (11). A more specific estimate is not possible because data were often inconsistently recorded. Finally, a STD clinic survey revealed that 81% of respondents had accessed non-STD medical care in the past three years, and 46% identified a routine health care visit (12). In sum, a majority of Americans had some sort of health care visit in the preceding year, and many women are at least asked about sexual activity.

On provider behavior, widespread sociopolitical norms may dictate which provider behaviors in health care visits are approved (especially where adolescents are concerned), although guidance is less formal than for screening and treatment (13). U.K. guidance clarifies good practice in sexual health care for adolescents—promoting honesty, no-judgmental questioning, and confidentiality (14). Endorsing such practice, however, is easier than the actual practice itself, which is borne out in U.S. studies. For example, in primary care provider visits by adolescents, missed opportunities to talk about sexual health behaviors appear frequent (15). Surveys from Colorado (16) and Quebec (17) found similar deficits; all but Maheux focused on the existence of adolescent sexual health care. Screening provides an indirect estimate of comprehensive sexual health care. Screening rates, too, suggest missed opportunities; adherence to screening guidelines for females is inconsistent (18–21). Little guidance exists for male screening for any STD in the United States, and the practice is rare. College students have some access to sexual health care; Koumans et al. (22) estimated that 73% of college students attended a school with available personal STD education (but only 60% of schools had health centers). Finally, testing for HIV in those infected with STD and vice versa is also inconsistent (23).

Correlates of Sexual Health Care–Seeking

Pathogens
Data pertaining to the effects of pathogens on health care–seeking yield no coherent portrait. Some literature suggests that STD that are perceived as more serious (24) are more likely to produce health care–seeking than other STD. Short or nonexistent symptom durations may also reduce the likelihood of seeking health care (25). These ostensibly logical relationships, however, are not immutable; a qualitative study of females suggested severity could actually inhibit health care–seeking if the putative patient becomes too worried about consequences to explore them (26). Moreover, Fortenberry (27) reported that females (mean age = 17.6 years) who were symptomatic required more time to seek care than those who were asymptomatic; Hightow et al. (28) reported that symptomatic persons were less likely to return for HIV test results than were those without symptoms. Awareness of STD infection may drive two opposing reactions: one urging treatment-seeking to reduce the negative effects of infection, the other urging avoidance of negative perceptions of a health visit experience (e.g., stigma). This area clearly deserves further research into the complexity of reasons for health care-seeking (29).

Individuals
Across studies, black (8 of 12 studies) and Hispanic (6 of 11 studies) youth typically received fewer general health care services than others (30). Importantly, these effects are independent of socioeconomic status. Comparing rates of health care–seeking for adults by racial and ethnic category is often confounded by differential racial and ethnic prevalences of STD, but an Institute of Medicine report (31) noted widespread racial disparities in overall health care.

While minorities are underrepresented in general health–care seeking and provision, they are overrepresented in the public sector sexual health care environment. Clinic attendees (N = 2,490) from five geographically disparate urban STD clinics were disproportionately of minority status (48% non-Hispanic African American versus 36% non-Hispanic white), typically young (< 25 years) and poor (67% with annual household incomes < $20,000) (12). Interestingly, 77% had a high school education (32%) or better (45%), suggesting education was not the only impediment to income (the unemployment rate was 43%, with only 35% in full-time employment). This finding speaks to unmeasured structural variables such as insurance availability and quality (itself partially dependent on employment), rather than simply to racial/ethnic status. The most significant bias in the study with respect to inferring characteristics of all STD clinic patients is the urban setting of each clinic.

Celum et al. (12) found 58% of the patients they surveyed had no insurance at all (only 14% had Medicaid). Costs have also formed a barrier to sexual health care–seeking in women enrolled in Women, Infants and Children (WIC) programs (25). Nearly two-thirds of those women (64%) preferred their own doctors, followed by community health centers and family planning clinics (15–17%): only 5% preferred an STD clinic.

Those who avoided self-treatment were more likely to seek care in a timely fashion (24). Self-treatment may be a technique that temporarily satisfies the two reactions we discussed above: relief from disease while avoiding an anticipated aversive experience. Complementary and alternative medicine (CAM) use, on the other hand, has been associated with more frequent health care–seeking (means of 8.4 visits versus 6.2 visits to specialists, $p < .05$), although this finding is confined to HIV-infected persons (33). Use of CAM may have been a function of poorer overall health; Burg et al. also found CAM users had more mean disability days in the previous four weeks (2.5 versus 1.3, $p < .05$).

Low health literacy (33) can inhibit health care-seeking and add to a negative experience while seeking health care, although Fortenberry et al. (34) also found that the effect of low literacy was attenuated by individual-level variables, such as self-rated health, and structural variables, such as health care costs. High levels of perceived stigma (35,36) can lower rates of health care–seeking, with such behaviors sometimes replaced by self-treatment and alternative therapies (37).

Finally, a person may initiate health care–seeking, but not sustain it. For example, some individuals get tested for STD, but do not find out their test results. Correlates of failure to return for results of HIV testing include male gender, married status, and diagnosis with something other than an STD (28). Interestingly, those who simply requested STD testing were less likely to return for results than those who were tested for STD-related reasons, including being a sexual contact of someone else diagnosed with an STD.

Providers and Systems

We have collapsed these categories for this section alone because so many studies of correlates rely on data from the point of view of the prospective patient, who experiences the provider as part of the system. There are numerous barriers to health care–seeking. In focus group surveys of adolescents and young adults, lack of knowledge about services and STDs, costs, shame, waiting times, and discrimination were all cited as barriers to health care-seeking (38). Waiting time is also a barrier in U.K. primary care practice, while extended hours, urine-based testing, and clinic locations short distances from "familiar places" are examples of facilitating factors (39). Patients do attend to clinician recommendations. For example, clinician recommendations for hepatitis B vaccine at a New York STD clinic were correlated with acceptance, controlling for knowing a vaccinated person and the perceived risks of the disease and the vaccine (40).

The barriers cited in Tilson et al. (38) notwithstanding, perceived quality of care remains an important factor in care-seeking, at least for U.S. clinic patients and members of high endemicity communities. Qualitative and quantitative data suggest the perceived process and quality of care at an STD clinic are more closely related to health care–seeking, in this case for gonorrhea, than either barriers in getting to care or fear that family or others would find out the respondent had an STD (41). Analysis of qualitative answers from separate respondents bore out these findings. Related to perceived quality of care, a sense of personal readiness among HIV-infected persons, itself influenced by trust in physicians, was a predictor of care-seeking according to one review (42). A relationship with a given physician, however, may not be necessary; Reid et al. (43) reported that young women in a health maintenance organization were *more* likely to be screened if they saw different providers over the course of two years, odds ratio (OR) = 1.41 (95% confidence interval [CI] = 1.14–1.76).

Purely structural conditions also affect health care. In a survey of HIV clinics in Los Angeles County, clinics with a written protocol for STD treatment (including an accurate and current sexual history) were more likely to ask patients about unsafe sexual behavior at each visit (prevalence ratio [PR] = 2.2, $p < .001$) and to screen on the basis of a sexual history (PR = 1.7, $p < .01$) (44). But structural conditions can also inhibit health care–seeking. Eighty percent of adolescents enrolled in HMOs in one study went "out of plan" to obtain contraceptives and, of those tested for an STD, 40% were tested out of plan (45). Many adolescents, who cited convenient access and confidentiality as barriers to using their HMO, may simply have failed to seek care at all. We examine the importance of confidentiality as a cross-cutting element of interventions later in this chapter.

Interventions at Each Level of the Person-Time Infectiousness Model

Having shown which characteristics of diseases, persons, and systems are consistently related to health care–seeking and provision, we now turn to interventions at the various levels of the PTI (4). We note here that the potential for interactions among levels as described by Aral and Wasserheit mean that many interventions have effects across levels of the PTI, regardless of the level at which the intervention was implemented. Some of these effects are purely collateral in nature (and intervention with providers may have effects on patient behavior). Others are putatively intended by those conducting the intervention (a system-level change in screening policy could be measured in individual physician behaviors). Table 2 provides a summary of intervention content found in this section of the chapter.

Pathogens

A direct intervention upon the characteristics of the pathogen is inherently not behavioral and therefore beyond the scope of this chapter. Interventions designed specifically to increase symptom recognition are rare, although women with ostensibly asymptomatic or unrecognized HSV-2 infection have been taught to recognize symptoms to some extent (46). In this study, about 50% of these women actually had recognizable symptoms and were successfully taught to recognize them. At the time, the authors speculated widespread education might reduce HSV-2 transmission, although later research focused upon genuinely asymptomatic viral shedding and suppressive therapy (47). Other interventions

Table 2 Health care-seeking parameters from the person-time infectiousness model and relevant topic areas: interventions.

Interventions content	Parameters			
	Pathogen	**Individual**	**Provider**	**Health system**
Symptom/ status awareness	HIV status awareness and GC/CT awareness campaigns raise profiles of respective diseases, symptom recognition may aid HSV-related care-seeking			Screening programs and protocols uncover STD
Health care-seeking promotion and skills training		Adolescents in small-group intervention change attitudes toward health care-seeking, females seek care; single sessions improve patient willingness to discuss sexual health	Providers can be trained to screen and take confidential sexual histories with more comfort; nurse training as useful as physician training	System-level sustained intervention (including provider-driven) increases screening; lack of confidentiality reduces care-seeking and disclosure (adolescents)
Home testing and screening	Urine tests for GC/CT make home testing more feasible	Acceptability high (70%+); uptake can be low (<10%), and varies by intensity of original contact, gender, and ease of return		Availability of home-based testing improves rescreening rates; improved access to urine tests increases screening
Case management and sustained care	Case management studies dominated by HIV	HIV+ people with active case managers improved care-seeking over those in passive referral; STD-infected persons in post-treatment counseling groups improved routine care-seeking; Patients receiving phone reminder or motivational interviews had improved retesting rates	Lack of interventions to improve case management of HIV other than for MSM; trained pharmacists can deliver health care on the basis of sexual histories and testing	Engaging non-governmental organizations can improve care-seeking through reach to infected and susceptible persons

(Continued)

Table 2 Health care-seeking parameters from the person-time infectiousness model and relevant topic areas: interventions.—Cont'd

Interventions content	Parameters			
	Pathogen	Individual	Provider	Health system
Tailored testing and screening			Health educators to link testing and care in high morbidity settings improves health care	Geographically and institution-ally-based (e.g., EDs, correctional facilities) testing and screening finds cases
Costs				Increasing co-payments reduces numbers of persons seeking care; ED screening in high morbidity settings is cost-effective; as are phone reminders and motivational interviews for rescreening
Community level variables		Favorable community norms can improve individual care-seeking and maintenance	Community partici-pation, including public-private collaboration, can lessen distrust of providers and services; related to improved cultural competence	School and community service-based learning are avenues to care-seeking and pro-vision; so can integrated services (including across gender)

may incorporate symptom recognition, as can basic health education, but measurement of increased symptom recognition as an outcome is rare. Moreover, the overlaps among symptoms of STD and other conditions may make relying on patient recognition without some prior reason to suspect disease insufficiently sensitive (e.g., the patients in Langenberg et al. had been evaluated for HSV-2).

While interventions in symptom recognition are rare, there are several interventions to promote awareness of the existence of pathogens, both in prospective patients and health care providers. HIV prevention programs have been interested in ensuring people know their HIV status because knowledge does appear to be correlated with reduced risk behaviors (48). A community awareness campaign (49) in Los Angeles that aimed to stimulate knowledge about STDs and increase knowledge of facilities &&& suitable for adolescents. Youth and young adults aged 17 to 21 years were hired as peer health advocates, were trained on STDs and other health related topics, and provided outreach to their peers on a daily basis. Recognition of campaign materials (e.g., palm cards with role model stories about sexual health care–seeking and provision that were written by local adolescents) increased across the span of the intervention period, from 8% at baseline to 77% at the 18-month post-test; corresponding levels at a comparison site stayed below 5% recognition. These findings illustrate the use of a low-cost, community-participatory awareness campaign, but awareness campaigns rarely produce significant behavioral change by themselves. Instead, they facilitate other interventions by reinforcing positive norms, in this case, for health care-seeking.

Individuals

Adolescents, Young Adults, and Routine Care-Seeking

Interventions to improve routine health care-seeking are promoted as proper preventive care, and can also serve in lieu of relying on patients to diagnose acute problems (i.e., recognize symptoms with adequate sensitivity). Many such interventions have been targeted toward adolescents and young adults, who comprise a high prevalence age group. Adolescents in one intervention (mean age = 15.8 years) enrolled in small, gender-specific groups operated by community-based organizations (CBOs) cooperating with academic researchers and local health departments (50). The three-session intervention used didactics, question and answer sessions, and role plays to (a) outline the benefits of and barriers to receiving a comprehensive health check-up (including a full and accurate sexual history), (b) practice talking to professionals and to friends and family about the need for comprehensive and confidential health care, (c) show practical options for care, for example, where to go and how to navigate through the relevant organization; and, finally, (d) form a specific plan to seek care. Each session was followed by "homework," for example, talking to a parent about health care. Outcomes were what proportion of those enrolled in each condition (a) talked to friends and/or family about health care, (b) made appointments for care, and (c) kept those appointments (in a three-month window). Females in the intervention condition were more likely than those in the control condition to do all three, with odds ratios, respectively, of 4.50, 3.04, and 2.87, all $p < .001$. Males, however, were not, with corresponding odds ratios of 1.13, 0.84, and 0.74, all ns, although they did show changes on the psychosocial variables targeted by the intervention (51). Either the intervention was not strong enough to affect male behavior or an unmeasured environmental variable interfered with the relationship between psychosocial and behavioral change.

Self-testing and self-collected specimen kits are typically favorably received by patients and provide a means to get health care to the individual, as an alternative to getting the individual to health care. In one study of adolescent detainees, 85% of those approached for self-testing with vaginal swabs agreed to do so, while only 22% of sexually active females examined by a physician received a pelvic exam (a further 16% declined an exam) (52). Twenty-eight (21%) of 133 females using the self-test were diagnosed with an STD, compared to 5 (4%) of 113 assigned to physician care. The five adolescents diagnosed represented 20% of those who were examined (which suggests physician criteria for examination had no discriminatory value at all). However, four females receiving pelvic exams were found to have abnormal Pap tests, and three were diagnosed with pelvic inflammatory disease. None of these conditions would have been recognized with a self-test without at least an accompanying sexual history. The high acceptability of self-testing is analogous to that found by Bradshaw et al. (53) in their examination of self-testing (and street outreach) in Australian injection drug users. Bradshaw et al. reported 76% acceptance of self-testing for *Chlamydia trachomatis, Neisseria gonorrhoeae*, and *Trichomonas vaginalis* versus 9% acceptance for practitioner-directed sampling, $p < .001$. One might reasonably suggest that the detained females in Holland-Hall et al. provided a biased sample, but Tebb et al. (54) found the same results when asking female adolescents in Northern California teen clinics to rank self-collected specimens (urines or swabs) against clinical pelvic exams. Adolescents in that study actually preferred urine samples to swabs, $p < .01$, but also preferred home swabs to clinical exams, $p < .01$.

In Seattle, patients infected with either gonorrhea or chlamydial infection were randomized to receive clinic rescreening or to choose between rescreening in the clinic versus with a home-based kit (55). The trial was underpowered (N = 122), but the rescreening rates by condition warrant further study. Of those randomized to the choice condition, 45% were rescreened in less than 28 days from enrollment against 32% of those randomized to the clinic condition. Within the choice condition, 61% of those who chose home testing were rescreened within 28 days against 38% of those choosing the clinic as a venue, $p = .10$. However, participation rates in a British sample of young men and women (39% for women, 46% for men) who were asked in writing if they would take a home-based chlamydia screening test suggest that uptake is not necessarily assured without some initial face to face contact (56). The authors found lack of response was far more common than refusal to participate. Recent data gathered from US men in a managed care setting support Stephenson et al.'s findings in that less than 8% of men returned urine-based specimen kits for assessing chlamydial infection that were mailed to them (57).

Ongoing Care-Seeking and Provision: Case Management

HIV counseling and testing and case management models are another source of individual-level interventions. Wolitski, MacGowan, Higgin, and Jorgensen (58) reviewed 35 studies of counseling and testing across four populations with and without HIV (MSM, drug users, women and heterosexual couples, and mixed populations). With respect to "help-seeking" from medical professionals, they found some differences in MSM, but not in other populations. Indeed, they found no studies even addressed help-seeking in women and heterosexual couples and noted help-seeking in MSM may have been related to stage of disease, not counseling and testing.

Nevertheless, case management can improve sexual health care-seeking, including when sexual care provision is integrated with other health care provision. HIV-positive patients who made up to five visits to a case manager over 90 days (reasonably brief by management standards for many chronic conditions) were more likely to visit a clinician for care at least once within 6 months (78% versus 60%, $p < .001$) and at least twice within 12 months (64% versus 49%, $p < .001$), compared to those randomized to a passive referral system (59). The effect of both methods attenuated slightly over time as shown by the lower percentages over 12 versus 6 months, with the case management condition attenuating slightly more slowly. Gore-Felton et al. (60) enrolled 943 HIV-positive people from a broad spectrum (both genders, heterosexuals and sexual minorities, and geographically, racially and ethnically diverse) into an ongoing trial designed to maximize quality of life for people living with HIV. The intervention targeted multiple outcomes, in them adherence to medication and to ongoing health care advice from providers (which entails routine and sustained health care-seeking and provision). The protocol was intensive, involving 15 90-minute sessions divided equally into coping and adjustment, risk behaviors, and health behaviors. An effective intervention of even this length is possible for an HIV care facility that expects extended contact with its patients. (One might even suggest that retention in a 15-session intervention constitutes improved health care-seeking and provision.)

One more intervention deserves attention in this section, although it is not strictly a health care intervention. Shain and colleagues (61,62) have evaluated a risk reduction intervention based in part around peer support groups added to interactive STD counseling. One of the counseling goals was "vigilant" health care-seeking. Support groups conferred some additional initial protection as measured by gonococcal or chlamydial incidence, although the effect was confined to the first year of follow-up (attendance at more sessions was also helpful). Health care-seeking need not be entirely confined to interventions delivered via a formal health care program.

Providers

For provider-focused interventions, the patient is no longer the target or the agent of change, so the outcomes for these interventions are relevant in that they increase the odds that providers will initiate sexual health care provision (e.g., asking for a sexual history), facilitate a better sexual health care experience (e.g., provider skills training), or both. Shafer et al. (63) implemented a team-based screening program in a health maintenance organization, in which a team of physicians provided intervention leadership (thus engaging the attentions of the physicians in general), information-sharing reviewed on an ongoing basis, and a model for incorporating adolescent STD screening into health care provision. Comparisons of subsequent screening in five clinics assigned to the experimental condition against five control clinics showed that screening rates were consistently higher in experimental clinics, $p < .001$, by 18 months after the intervention.

Simply providing a route for providers to use up-to-date technology (urine-based screening) and single-session interventions on such aspects of STD as the need for screening can produce greater levels of screening. Introduction of urine-based screening methods for adolescents in a high STD prevalence adolescent clinic resulted in a near doubling of the number of cases of chlamydial infection detected (47% of all cases were due to screening asymptomatic patients) (Van Devanter et al., unpublished data).

Tailored information for adolescents and young adults is generally recommended (64) with data suggesting adolescents are most comfortable discussing sexual information in the context of routine health care (65). Skills-building and feedback to increase motivation and behavior centered around asking about HIV risk and discussion of behavior change (if warranted) can increase such discussion. Patients exposed to a single-session skills building intervention with feedback reported an increase in asking about risk and discussing risk reduction, albeit with the greatest effects for low risk patients (66). Similar to Shafer et al. (63), continued intervention reinforcement maintained the post-intervention effect (which appeared to drift downward after the reinforcement ended). Dodge et al. included a broader training for nurses, which brings up the important point that health care provision interventions with nurses and other non-physician providers are equally relevant (67).

Systems

System-level, or structural interventions, may be especially useful for increasing health care-seeking and care provision and may provide the best overall effects on population-level heath in the long term. To make an analogy with writing about the determinants of phase-specific approaches to STD control (68) and intervention strategies, health care-seeking and provision are like endemic prevalence and incidence – they are spread throughout the population at a relatively stable level. Structural interventions matched to such endemicity are aimed more at community-level efforts and even at shifting population behaviors than at high risk individuals. True, many of the system-level interventions were aimed at, or at least tested on, high prevalence groups. But the principle remains population-level behavioral change – increased overall health care-seeking, and better overall health care provision.

Structural Interventions in Formal Settings

In 2002, the Massachusetts Department of Health identified the 15 cities in the state with the highest HIV prevalences. People attending one of the four health care settings with the highest combination of patient volume and morbidity in each city were offered a visit with a "health educator," who offered HIV testing and linkage to care for those who were already HIV-positive (69). Prevalence in the 3,068 persons who accepted testing (of 10,352 offered testing) was 2%, of whom 82% received their results and were linked to care. The larger underlying principle is to match service provision to high morbidity locations. Correctional facilities (70) and emergency departments (EDs) in high prevalence areas (71) provide other examples of the introduction of structural interventions. Mehta et al. (72) were even able to demonstrate that ED screening was cost-effective.

Sansom, Rudy, Strine, and Douglas (73) provide one example of the effect of a structural intervention on an "endemic" behavior – accepting a vaccine. They randomized clients of a sexual health program to either a generic appointment reminder card or to telephone contact (both a reminder and a follow-up if the appointment was missed) in order to improve rates of receiving a second dose of hepatitis B vaccine. By an intent-to-treat analysis, 87% of clients in the experimental condition received a second dose, versus 80% of the control group, $p < .05$. Of clients in the experimental condition who received the full intervention, 90% received a second dose. In short, the intervention cut missed appointments almost in half. Analogous findings were visible in an intervention aimed at increasing follow-up visits for retesting in clients of two STD clinic clients (suburban Maryland and Los Angeles) diagnosed with gonorrhea or chlamydial infections (74). Malotte and colleagues tested (a) a standard reminder card against (b) the card plus a $20 incentive and against (c) a card, telephone contact, and a motivational interview. The interview/phone conditions produced higher return rates than a reminder card alone, $OR = 2.6$, 95% CI = 1.3–5.0, although the incentive condition did not differ from a card alone, $OR = 1.2$, 95% CI = 0.6–2.5. A follow-up study comparing the telephone reminder alone against the motivational interview alone suggested the telephone reminder was sufficient (74). Gift et al. (75) showed the telephone reminder alone was more cost-effective than any other method; Malotte et al. recommended the more expensive motivational interview when telephone contact was not likely to be assured. Notably, these studies have relied on urine-based screening, frequently via nucleic acid amplification testing. This structural change alone has facilitated testing outside of clinic settings; future research should help determine its most effective use (76). We also note that rescreening interventions can also be combined with home-based specimen collection as discussed earlier in this chapter (55,54).

In resource-poor areas, pharmacists may even serve as adjunct health care providers, although most need training on proper diagnosis and/or treatment (77,78). Kwema et al. observed that 60% to 80% of pharmacy staff correctly diagnosed symptoms from simulated patients. The need for further training on correct treatments was, however, equally apparent; hardly any prescribed first line treatments and many pharmacists were willing to sell partial doses (thus undertreating). Garcia et al.'s educational intervention substantially improved counseling, but the authors noted diagnosis and treatment in the trial location, Peru, was still inconsistent.

Structural Interventions Beyond Formal Settings

So far under system-level interventions, we have confined ourselves to the formal health care system – clinics and pharmacies. Next, we examine interventions that rely on community members for structural change – these usually incorporate health care-seeking and provision rather than focus upon it. Women's non-governmental organizations (NGOs) across Africa have roles in finding health care information (often via the Internet) and translating and disseminating messages to improve health care for women (79). The NGOs were assisted by some US institutions in a community-academic partnership that yielded increased capacity in the NGOs, including health care-seeking, by the end of the project. Other community partnerships have included anti-stigma campaigns, including prejudice directed at HIV/AIDS care providers (80) and models for national-level capacity-building for service delivery (81).

Structural Changes that Increase Barriers to Health Care-Seeking and Provision

We also examine the effects of a "negative" intervention, specifically, the introduction of a putative barrier to health care-seeking and provision. Rietmeijer et al. (82) reported that budget shortfalls in Denver brought about the 2003 introduction of a $15 co-payment for services at the STI clinic of the Denver Metro Health area. Non-residents were charged up to $65 for the same services. Overall visits declined 28.5% between 2002 and 2003, with STD diagnoses dropping in commensurate fashion (28% to 38% declines in chlamydial infections and gonorrhea, respectively). The effect was particularly pronounced for those below the Federal poverty lines – such persons dropped from 60% to 29% of cases. As context, case reports in Colorado declined by

11% for chlamydial infections and by 24% for gonorrhea between 2002–2003 (83,84); these figures include the Denver numbers.

Interactions Among Health Care-Seeking Interventions

Interactions Defined by PTI Levels

Encouragingly, interventions exist at all levels of the health care system as described in Aral and Wasserheit (4). However, none has been a true multi-level intervention in which intervention at one level is crossed factorially with intervention at another level. Intervention at multiple levels has been endorsed by public health experts, most notably by the Institute of Medicine (85). Multilevel interventions are visible in such areas as stroke recovery (86) and cancer control (87), but not in sexual health care-seeking and service provision.

We can reasonably say that several interventions produced changes at more than one level of the PTI model, even if the intervention was delivered to only one level. For example, physicians have been encouraged to screen (63) and were therefore the target of intervention, but the intervention effects were also seen in the structure of health care provision in the HMO they studied. The GCAP interventions were not formally linked as a multilevel intervention (this would have entailed randomizing adolescents to levels of their intervention, but also within communities with or without an awareness campaign and so forth), but they did use similar attitudinal and behavioral measures across a range of interventions and sites, so one could observe the effects of intervention at different levels on the same variables. And, finally, some interventions such as the Massachusetts study offering a visit with a health educator to people in selected clinics (69) used a structural intervention to affect individual behavior as an outcome variable for evaluating the intervention. In fact, several interventions we reviewed might reasonably have been categorized in different levels from those we selected.

As a final word in interactions, we look at the contribution of the increasingly popular internet (88) as a source of health information. Tietz, Davies, and Moran (89) reviewed web-based STD resources, finding that "reliable information" and "authoritative recommendations" were available for patients and providers, but immersed in outdated and inaccurate information. Government-sponsored sites were the most accurate (including www.cdc.gov/std). Beyond information provision, the potential interactions between web-based portals of information and subsequent health care-seeking and provision at individual, provider, and system levels remain to be explored on any widespread basis, although recommendations for constructing and tailoring websites exist (90). Interventions in web-based sexual health care-seeking and provision may be an especially salient area for further study.

Interactions as Cross-Cutting Elements of Interventions

Community Involvement

We have already cited Shain et al. (61) as an example of involving community members to improve health care-seeking. Interventions based around lay health advisors (91) provide examples of improving health care provision and access to care. A review of behavioral interventions for adolescents (92) cited community-relevant variables such as community service learning and school councils as intervention content delivery mechanisms. A review of clinic patients (93) also emphasized the importance of learning from clients (i.e., community members). Community involvement can also contribute to culturally sensitive health care provision and consequent lessening of distrust of health care providers, two factors posited to increase health care-seeking (94,95). These factors are often associated with black/African-American and Hispanic/Latino-identified persons, but should not be exclusively associated with any particular sociodemographically defined group. Although the importance of quality care to patients and community members (41) should not be discounted, culturally competent health care remains a facet of sexual health care for which there is much room for improvement (96). In particular, varying cultural contingencies can produce different effects by cultural group if those contingencies are not taken into account when tailoring the intervention (96).

VanDevanter et al. (97) presented a logic model for "community-academic-health department" collaborative partnerships in health care-seeking and provision interventions based on Florin et al.'s (98) staged model of developing community partnerships. Four stages included building on established partnerships (initial mobilization); setting up permanent organizational structure with goal-directed subcommittees reporting to a main advisory board; capacity building; and planning. Questions, answers, and incorporation of answers into policies are expected from all three parties. The desired outcome is, of course, an intervention in which all parties have vested interests. The inclusion of community and health department members also aids sustainability, especially when data from interventions and program evaluations are used to guide future decisions, as suggested for HIV Prevention Community Planning (99).

Integrated Sexual Health Care

Virtually any person engaged in community involvement will find some interest in integrated health care provision. Stein (100) and Duerr et al. (101) have both recommended the integration of family planning with STD/HIV services (the latter for HIV-infected women). Peck et al. (102) reported a 15-year effort in Haiti to integrate primary care with HIV counseling and testing, suggesting the integrated approach reduced the amount of infection one would otherwise expect. Family planning services often offer STD/HIV services, but most often serve a predominantly female population (e.g., Planned Parenthood).

Integrated sexual health care should also consider providing STI services for both men and women. Men's health care needs are often unmet, especially in adolescents (103,104), and, as noted above, health care-seeking interventions sometimes seem to have better effects for females than for males. In largely heterosexually transmitted STD (e.g., chlamydial infections), attention to disease in men may be important. Raine, Marcell, Rocca, and Harper (105) reported that, in a San Francisco family planning clinic that began taking male clients, 110 males made an initial visit (88% for STD treatment and mostly learning about the source of health care via word of mouth) without damaging female client satisfaction dramatically ("very" or "mostly" satisfied overall rates dropped from 98% to 92%; complete satisfaction with quality of care dropped from 100% to 99%).

Public Versus Private Considerations

Brackbill, Sternberg, and Fishbein (106) have shown that a substantial proportion of STDs are seen in the private sector, suggesting that health care provision interventions might be directed toward providers in private settings as profitably as in public settings. Brugha and Zwi (107) have noted the patients often find private sector services more attractive across a range of communicable diseases and international settings, but also that quality of services may actually be inconsistent. Collaborative structures such as that described by Golden et al. (108; see above under system-level interventions) may well improve service provision while fulfilling the needs of patients and both the public and private sectors of the health care system.

Privacy and Confidentiality

Confidential services are a cornerstone of most STD and HIV health care provision; the Health Information Portability and Accountability Act (HIPAA) is the latest manifestation of the attention paid to the confidentiality of medical records. (The consequences, intended and unintended, are beyond the scope of this chapter.) There is one notable exception to the presumption of confidentiality: health care for minors. Virtually every jurisdiction permits minors from the mid-teens (most often 15 or 16 years) to seek care independent of an adult, but not all places guarantee the provision of care will remain confidential from any adult guardian. For example, Texas requires that providers report to police the identity of all persons under 17 whom providers find are sexually active (109). Aside from the effect of this law on physician-patient relationships, Franzini et al. modeled projected economic costs based on levels of diminished health care-seeking. They estimated that loss of confidentiality in a cohort of 72,000 adolescent females < 17 years would amount to over $43 million in increased health care costs. Ford, Millstein, Halpern-Fescher, and Irwin (110) conducted a trial of the effect of hearing different forms of a confidentiality guarantee (none, conditional, unconditional) during a health care visit upon adolescents' willingness to disclose information about sensitive issues, including sexuality. They found that assuring confidentiality increased willingness to disclose from 39% to 46.5%, $p < .05$, and increased the number willing to seek future health care from 53% to 67%, $p < .001$. When comparing the unconditional confidentiality to a conditional version, willingness to return increased from 62% to 72%, $p < .01$. Several interventions described in this chapter rely on confidential health care, and some even teach the importance of confidentiality as part of the intervention (50).

Conclusions

We conclude by presenting some principles and elements of interventions and their interactions that we suggest are relevant to clinical managers. The crosscutting elements just described also serve as reasonable principles for clinical management. That is, a health care facility that prizes community collaboration, that values privacy and confidentiality, that addresses sexual health care in public and private settings and that provides sexual health care in the context of other health care (i.e., integration) is likely to provide a successful program. Any clinic can be part of a community-health department-academic partnership.

What are feasible directions in which these principles can be put into practice? We suggest clinic participation in large scale activities such as community awareness campaigns and other norm-generating activities is frequently inexpensive and sustainable, if the awareness campaigns are carefully targeted and tailored. It may be rarer for clinics to actively run health care-seeking and provision interventions, but they can foster linkage between their facilities and organizations that do intervene to promote health care-seeking. Hotlines and websites with advice and information can be administered by health care facilities, or at least such facilities can participate in their content and construction.

Training for providers so they take sensitive, but accurate and comprehensive sexual histories is also helpful. Feasibility data (unpublished) from GCAP showed that a supportive management structure in a managed care setting produced swift and useful training with role plays as well as didactic information – this information can be kept up to date if health care facilities and epidemiologic data-collecting organizations (state health departments, CDC) communicate with one another. In settings with small groups of providers, GCAP staff went to practices to train providers. As with Shafer et al. (63), facility staff who can "champion" the importance of training is helpful.

Structural changes include flexible opening hours and mobile care units. The principle of the Bloodmobile is applicable in concept, even if the scale would be smaller! Local disease epidemiology and sociodemographic circumstances can inform precise practices – this includes where to locate sexual health services in care facilities other than HIV/STD clinics and reproductive health settings.

We close with an example of a broad scale collaborative structural intervention from a different topic area (STD partner management). Golden et al. (108) reported the mechanics of an intervention aimed at testing the effects of expedited partner therapy (see Chapter 7 in this volume) on chlamydial and gonococcal infections. The public health service in Seattle asked all private providers to report cases and to give permission to contact partners (preferring a cooperative model to a directive one). At the time analyses were reported, over 700 private providers in the catchment area as well as eight emergency room and nine private sector clinics had given blanket permission to contact infected patients for sex partner referral. These permissions, with case-by-case permission, translated into over 90% of all potentially eligible patients. Of those contacted, 65% reported at least one untreated partner (although many preferred to notify partners themselves). Twelve commercial pharmacies in Seattle agreed to stock the treatment regimens prescribed by the STD clinic and to distribute them for a $4.00 fee. What this project demonstrates is that, with patience and application, a health care facility can collaborate with providers in public and private settings and with commercial entities and other professionals (pharmacies and pharmacists) on a county-wide scale representing over 1.7 million people (Bureau of the Census, 2000). There is no conceptual reason the model cannot be generalized to other forms of sexual health care.

References

1. Chaulk CP, Zenilman J. Sexually transmitted disease control in the era of managed care: "magic bullet" or "shadow on the land"? *Journal of Public Health Management and Practice*. 1997;3:61–70.
2. Institute of Medicine. *The Hidden Epidemic: Confronting Sexually Transmitted Diseases*. Washington, DC: National Academy Press; 1997.
3. MacKellar DA, Valleroy LA, Secura GM, et al. Unrecognized HIV infection, risk behaviors, and perceptions of risk among young men who have sex with men. *Journal of Acquired Immune Deficiency Syndrome*. 2005;38:603–614.
4. Aral SO, Wasserheit JN. STD-related health care seeking and health service delivery. In: KK Holmes, Sparling PF, Mardh P, et al., eds., *Sexually Transmitted Diseases,* 3rd ed. New York: McGraw-Hill; 1999:1295–1305.
5. National Center for Health Statistics. *Health, United States, 2004: With Chartbook on Trends in the Health of Americans*. Hyattsville, MD: Department of Health and Human Services.
6. Ford CA, Bearman PS, Moody J. Foregone health care among adolescents. *Journal of the American Medical Association*. 1999;282:2227–2234.
7. Newacheck PW, Brindis CD, Cart CU, et al. Adolescent health insurance coverage: recent changes and access to care. *Pediatrics*. 1999;104:195–202.
8. Geisler WM, Ma LC, Kusonoki Y, Upchurch DM, Hook III EW. Health insurance coverage, health care-seeking behaviors, and genital chlamydial infection prevalence in sexually active young adults. *Sexually Transmitted Diseases*. 2006;33:389–396.
9. Yu SM, Bellamy HA, Schwalberg RH, Drum MA. Factors associated with use of preventive dental and health services among U.S. adolescents. *Journal of Adolescent Health*. 2001;29:395–405.
10. Rietmeijer CA, Bull SS, Ortiz CG, Leroux T, Douglas JM Jr. Patterns of general health care and STD services use among high-risk youth in Denver participating in community-based urine chlamydia screening. *Sexually Transmitted Diseases*. 1998;25:457–463.
11. Downey L, Lafferty WE, Tao G, Irwin KL. Evaluating the quality of sexual health care provided to adolescents in Medicaid Managed Care: a comparison of two data sources. *American Journal of Medical Quality*. 2004;19:2–11.
12. Celum CL, Bolan G, Krone M, et al. Patients attending STD clinics in an evolving health care environment. *Sexually Transmitted Diseases*. 1997;24:599–605.
13. Centers for Disease Control and Prevention. STD Treatment Guidelines 2002. *MMWR*. 2002;51 (No. RR-6).
14. Free C. Advice about sexual health for young people. *British Medical Journal*. 2005;330:107–108.
15. Burstein GR, Lowry R, Klein JD, et al. Missed opportunities for sexually transmitted diseases, human immunodeficiency virus, and pregnancy prevention services during adolescent health supervision visits. *Pediatrics*. 2004;111:996–1001.
16. Torkko KC, Gershman K, Crane LA, et al. Testing for chlamydia and sexual history taking in adolescent females: results from a statewide survey of Colorado primary care providers. *Pediatrics*. 2000;106:E32.
17. Maheux B, Haley N, Rivard M, et al. Do physicians assess lifestyle health risks during general medical examinations? A survey of general practitioners and obstetrician-gynecologists in Quebec. *Canadian Medical Association Journal*. 1999;160:1830–1834.
18. Centers for Disease Control and Prevention. Chlamydia screening among sexually active young female enrollees of health plans—United States, 1999–2001. *Morbidity and Mortality Weekly Report*. 2004;53:983–985.

19. Fiscus LC, Ford CA, Miller WC. Infrequency of sexually transmitted disease screening among sexually experienced US female adolescents. *Perspectives on Sexual and Reproductive Health*. 2004;36:233–238.

20. Hogben M, St. Lawrence JS, Kasprzyk D, et al. Sexually transmitted disease screening in the United States by obstetricians and gynecologists. *Obstetrics and Gynecology*. 2002;100:801–807.

21. Levine WC, Dicker LW, Devine O, et al. Indirect estimation of chlamydia screening coverage using public health surveillance data. *American Journal of Epidemiology*. 2004;160:91–96.

22. Koumans EH, Sternberg MR, Mohamed C, Kohl K, Schillinger JA, Markowitz LE. Sexually transmitted disease services at US colleges and universities. *Journal of American College Health*. 2005;53:211–217.

23. Sena AC, Mertz KJ, Thomas D, Wells D, Costa S, Levine WC. A survey of sexually transmitted diseases/HIV coinfection testing and reporting practices among health care providers in New Jersey. *Sexually Transmitted Diseases*. 2005;32: 406–412.

24. Meyer-Weitz A, Reddy P, Van Den Borne HW, Kok G, Pietersen J. The determinants of health care seeking behaviour of adolescents attending STD clinics in South Africa. *Journal of Adolescence*. 2000;23:741–752.

25. Crosby RA, Yarber WL, Meyerson B. Perceived monogamy and type of clinic as barriers to seeking care for suspected STD or HIV infection: Results from a brief survey of low-income women attending Women, Infants, and Children (WIC) clinics in Missouri. *Sexually Transmitted Diseases*. 1999;26:399–403.

26. Cunningham SD, Kerrigan D, Pillay KB, Ellen JM. Understanding the role of perceived severity in STD-related care-seeking delays. *Journal of Adolescent Health*. 2005;37:69–74.

27. Fortenberry JD. Health care seeking behaviors related to sexually transmitted diseases among adolescents. *American Journal of Public Health*. 1997;87:417–420.

28. Hightow LB, Miller WC, Leone PA, Wohl D, Smurzynski M, Kaplan AH. Failure to return for HIV posttest counseling in an STD clinic population. *AIDS Education and Prevention*. 2003;15:282–290.

29. Ward H, Mertens TE, & Thomas C. Health seeking behaviour and the control of sexually transmitted disease. *Health Policy & Planning*. 1997;12:19–28.

30. Elster A, Jarosik J, VanGeest J, Fleming M. Racial and ethnic disparities in health care for adolescents. *Archives of Pediatric and Adolescent Medicine*. 2003;157:867–874.

31. Institute of Medicine. *Unequal Treatment: Confronting Racial and Ethnic Disparities in Health Care*. Washington, DC: National Academy Press; 2002.

32. Burg MA, Uphold CR, Finley K, Reid K. Complementary and alternative medicine use among HIV-infected patients attending three outpatient clinics in the Southeastern United States. *International Journal of STD & AIDS*. 2005;16: 112–116.

33. Brandt HM, McCree DH, Lindley LL, Shapre PA, Hutto BE. An evaluation of HPV educational materials. *Cancer Control*. 2005;12(Suppl 2):103–106.

34. Fortenberry JD, McFarlane MM, Hennessy M, et al. Relation of health literacy to gonorrhoea related care. *Sexually Transmitted Infections*. 2001;77:206–211.

35. Fortenberry JD, McFarlane M, Bleakley A, et al. Relationships of stigma and sham to gonorrhea and human immunodeficiency virus screening. *American Journal of Public Health*. 2002;92:378–381.

36. Lichtenstein B. Stigma as a barrier to treatment of sexually transmitted infection in the American Deep South: issues of race, gender and poverty. *Social Science and Medicine*. 2003;57:2435–2445.

37. Fortenberry JD. The effects of stigma on genital herpes care-seeking behaviors. *Herpes*. 2004;11:8–11.

38. Tilson EC, Sanchez V, Ford CL, et al. Barriers to asymptomatic screening and other STD services for adolescents and young adults: focus group discussions. *BMC Public Health.* 2004;4:21.

39. Griffiths V, Ahmed-Jushuf I, Cassell JA, Association for Genitourinary Medicine. Understanding access to genitourinary medicine services. *International Journal of STD & AIDS.* 2004;15:587–589.

40. Samoff E, Dunn A, VanDevanter N, Blank S, Weisfuse IB. Predictors of acceptance of hepatitis B vaccination in an urban sexually transmitted diseases clinic. *Sexually Transmitted Diseases.* 2004;31:415–420.

41. Hogben M, Bloom F, McFarlane M, et al. Factors associated with sexually transmitted disease clinic attendance. *International Journal of Nursing Studies.* 2004;41:911–920.

42. Nordqvist O, Sodergard B, Tully MP, Sonnerborg A, Lindblad AK. Assessing and achieving readiness to initiate HIV medication. *Patient Education & Counseling.* 2006;62:21–30.

43. Reid RJ, Scholes D, Grothaus L, Truelove Y, Fishman P, McClure J, Grafton J, Thompson RS. Is provider continuity associated with chlamydia screening for adolescent and young adult women? *Preventive Medicine.* 2005; 41:865–872.

44. Taylor MM, McClain T, Javanbakht M, et al. Sexually transmitted disease testing protocols, sexually transmitted disease testing, and discussion of sexual behaviors in HIV clinics in Los Angeles County. *Sexually Transmitted Diseases.* 2005;32:341–345.

45. Civic D, Scholes D, Grothaus L, McBride C. Adolescent HMO enrollees' utilization of out-of-plan services. *Journal of Adolescent Health.* 2001;28:491–496.

46. Langenberg A, Benedetti J, Jenkins J, Ashley R, Winter C, Corey L. Development of clinically recognizable genital lesions among women previously identified as having "asymptomatic" herpes simplex virus type 2 infection. *Annals of Internal Medicine.* 1989;110:882–887.

47. Corey L, Wald A, Patel R, et al. Once-daily valacyclovir to reduce the risk of transmission of genital herpes. *New England Journal of Medicine.* 2004;350:11–20.

48. Marks G, Crepaz N, Senterfitt W, Janssen RS. Meta-analysis of high-risk sexual behavior in persons aware and unaware they are infected with HIV in the United States. *Journal of Acquired Immune Deficiency Syndromes.* 2005;39:446–453.

49. Larro M, Malotte CK, Penniman T, et al. Outcomes from the Gonorrhea Community Action Project (GCAP) small media community awareness intervention in Los Angeles County, California. 2006:*Manuscript under review.*

50. VanDevanter NL, Messeri P, Middlestadt SE, et al. A community-based intervention designed to increase preventive health care seeking among adolescents: the Gonorrhea Community Action Project. *American Journal of Public Health.* 2005;95:331–337.

51. Hogben M, Ledsky R, Middlestadt S, et al. Psychological mediating factors in an intervention to promote adolescent health care-seeking. *Psychology, Health, & Medicine.* 2005;10:64–77.

52. Holland-Hall CM, Wiesenfeld HC, Murray PJ. Self-collected vaginal swabs for the detection of multiple sexually transmitted infections in adolescent girls. *Journal of Pediatric and Adolescent Gynecology.* 2002;15:307–313.

53. Bradshaw CS, Pierce LI, Tabrizi SN, Fairely CK, Garland SM. Screening injecting drug users for sexually transmitted infections and blood borne viruses using street outreach and self collected sampling. *Sexually Transmitted Infections.* 2005;81:53–58.

54. Tebb KP, Paukku MH, Pai-Dhungat MR, Gyami A-A, Shafer MB. Home STI testing: the adolescent female's opinion. *Journal of Adolescent Health.* 2004;35: 462–467.

55. Sparks R, Helmers JR, Handsfield HH, et al. Rescreening for gonorrhea and chlamydial infection through the mail: a randomized trial. *Sexually Transmitted Diseases.* 2004;31:113–116.

56. Stephenson J, Carder C, Copas A, Robinson A, Ridgway G, Haines A. Home screening for chlamydial genital infection: is it acceptable to young men and women? *Sexually Transmitted Infections.* 2000;76:25–27.

57. Scholes D, Marrazzo JM, Heidrich F, Lindenbaum J, Yarbro P, Farrell-Ross M Outreach Strategies for Chlamydia Screening: Results from a Population-Based Screening Feasibility Trial in Male Managed Care Enrollees. 15th Biennial Congress of the International Society for Sexually Transmitted Diseases Research. 2003 July 27–30; Ottawa, Canada.

58. Wolitski RJ, MacGowan RJ, Higgins DL, Jorgensen CM. The effects of HIV counseling and testing on risk-related practices and help-seeking behavior. *AIDS Education and Prevention.* 1997;9(Suppl. B):52–67.

59. Gardner LI, Metsch LR, Anderson-Mahoney P, et al. Efficacy of a brief case management intervention to link recently diagnosed HIV-infected persons to care. *AIDS.* 2004;19:423–431.

60. Gore-Felton C, Rotherham-Borus MJ, Weinhardt LS, et al. The Health Living project: an individually-tailored, multidimensional intervention for HIV-infected persons. *AIDS Education and Prevention.* 2005;17(Suppl. A):21–39.

61. Shain RN, Piper JM, Holden AEC, et al. Prevention of gonorrhea and chlamydia through behavioral intervention. *Sexually Transmitted Diseases.* 2004;31:401–408.

62. Shain RN, Holden AEC, Piper JM, et al. Efficacy of Two Project Safe Behavioral Interventions During 3 Follow-Up Years: Results of a Randomized Trial. Paper presented at the Biennial Meeting of the International Society for STD Research. 2005 July; Amsterdam, Netherlands.

63. Shafer MA, Tebb KP, Pantell RH, et al. Effect of a clinical practice improvement intervention on chlamydial screening among adolescent girls. *Journal of the American Medical Association.* 2002;288:2846–2852.

64. Boekeloo BO, Schamus LA, Simmens SJ, Cheng TL. Tailoring STD/HIV prevention messages for young adolescents. *Academic Medicine.* 1996;(10 Suppl): S97–S99.

65. Boekeloo BO, Schamus LA, Cheng TL, Simmens SJ. Young adolescents' comfort with discussion about sexual problems with their physician. *Archives of Pediatric and Adolescent Medicine.* 1996;150:1146–1152.

66. Dodge WT, Bluespruce J, Grothaus L, et al. Enhancing primary care HIV prevention. *American Journal of Preventive Medicine.* 2001;20:177–183.

67. Miles K, Knight V, Cairo I, King I. Nurse-led sexual health care: international perspectives. *International Journal of STD and AIDS.* 2003;14:243–247.

68. Aral SO. Determinants of STD epidemics: implications for phase appropriate intervention strategies. *Sexually Transmitted Infections.* 2002;78(Suppl. 1):i3–i13.

69. Centers for Disease Control and Prevention. Voluntary HIV testing as part of routine medical care—Massachusetts, 2002. *Morbidity and Mortality Weekly Report.* 2004;53:523–526.

70. Arriola KR, Braithwaite RL, Kennedy S, et al. A collaborative effort to enhance HIV/STI screening in five county jails. *Public Health Reports.* 2001;116:520–529.

71. Mehta SD, Rothman RE, Kellen GD, et al. Unsuspected gonorrhea and chlamydia in patients of an urban adults emergency department: a critical population for STD control intervention. *Sexually Transmitted Diseases.* 2001;28:33–39.

72. Mehta SD, Bishai T, Howell MR, et al. Cost-effectiveness of five strategies for gonorrhea and chlamydia control among female and male emergency department patients. *Sexually Transmitted Diseases.,* 2002;29:83–90.

73. Sansom S, Rudy E, Strine T, Douglas W. Hepatitis A and B vaccination in a sexually transmitted disease clinic for men who have sex with men. *Sexually Transmitted Diseases.* 2003;30:685–688.

74. Malotte CK, Ledsky R, Hogben M, et al. Comparison of methods to increase repeat testing in persons treated for gonorrhea and/or chlamydia at public sexually transmitted disease clinics. *Sexually Transmitted Diseases.* 2004; 31:637–642.

75. Gift TL, Malotte CK, Ledsky R, et al. A cost-effectiveness analysis of interventions to increase repeat testing in patients treated for gonorrhea or chlamydia at public sexually transmitted disease clinics. *Sexually Transmitted Diseases.* 2005;32:542–549.

76. Ford CA, Viadro CI, Miller WC. Testing for chlamydial and gonorrheal infections outside of clinic settings: A summary of the literature. *Sexually Transmitted Diseases.* 2004;31:38–51.

77. Garcia PJ, Gotuzzo E, Hughes JP, Holmes KK. Syndromic management of STDs in pharmacies: evaluation and randomised intervention trial. *Sexually Transmitted Infections.* 1998;74(suppl. 1):S153–S158.

78. Kwema A, Sharma A, Muga C, Wamae N, Bukusi E. The Competence of Pharmacy Staff in Managing STDs of Self-Medicating Patients in Nairobi. Paper presented at the Annual Meeting of the International Society for STD Research. 2005 July; Amsterdam, Netherlands.

79. Pillsbury B, Mayer D. Women connect! Strengthening communications to meet sexual and reproductive health challenges. *Journal of Health Communication.* 2005;10:361–371.

80. Rutledge SE, Abell N. Awareness, acceptance, and action: An emerging framework for understanding AIDS stigmatizing attitudes among community leaders in Barbados. *AIDS Patient Care and STDs.* 2005;19:186–199.

81. Johnson K, Kennedy SB, Harris AO, Lincoln A, Neace W, Collins D. Strengthening the HIV/AIDS service delivery system in Liberia: an international research capacity-building strategy. *Journal of Evaluation in Clinical Practice.* 2005;11:257–273.

82. Rietmeijer CA, Alfonis GA, Douglas JM, Lloyd LV, Richardson DB, Judson FN. Trends in clinic visits and diagnosed *Chlamydia trachomatis* and *Neisseria gonorrhoeae* after the introduction of a copayment in a sexually transmitted disease clinic. *Sexually Transmitted Diseases.* 2005;32:243–246.

83. Centers for Disease Control and Prevention. *Sexually Transmitted Disease Surveillance, 2002.* Atlanta, GA: Department of Health and Human Services; 2003.

84. Centers for Disease Control and Prevention. *Sexually Transmitted Disease Surveillance, 2003.* Atlanta, GA: Department of Health and Human Services; 2004.

85. Institute of Medicine. *The Future of the Public's Health in the 21st Century.* Washington, DC: National Academy Press; 2002.

86. Morgenstern LB, Staub L, Chan W, et al. Improving delivery of acute stroke therapy: the TLL Temple Foundation Stroke Project. *Stroke.* 2002;33:160–166.

87. Lowe JI, Barg FK, Norman S, McCorkle R. An urban intergenerational program for cancer control education. *Journal of Cancer Education.* 1997;12:233–239.

88. Bleakley A, Merzel C, VanDevanter NL, Messeri P. Computer access and internet use among urban youths. *American Journal of Public Health.* 2004;94:744–746.

89. Tietz A, Davies SC, Moran JS. Guide to sexually transmitted disease services on the internet. *Clinical Infectious Diseases.* 2004;38:1304–1310.

90. Gilbert LK, Temby JR, Rogers SE. Evaluating a teen STD prevention website. *Journal of Adolescent Health.* 2005;37:236–242.

91. Thomas JC, Eng E, Earp JA, Ellis H. Trust and collaboration in the prevention of sexually transmitted diseases. *Public Health Reports.* 2001;116:540–547.

92. Robin L, Dittus P, Whitaker D, et al. Behavioral interventions to reduce incidence of HIV, STD, and pregnancy among adolescents: a decade in review. *Journal of Adolescent Health.* 2004;34:3–26.

93. Greenberg JB, Bloom FR, Coles FB, et al. Learning from clients: an opportunity for sexually transmitted disease programs. *Journal of Public Health Management & Practice.* 2002;83:59–68.

94. Butcher RO, Hood RG, Jordan WC. Optimizing treatment for African Americans and Latinos with HIV/AIDS. *Journal of the National Medical Association.* 2005;97:1093–1100.

95. Morrison-Beedy D, Carey MP, Aronowitz T, Mkandawire L, Dyne J. Adolescents' input on the development of an HIV risk reduction intervention. *J Assoc Nurses AIDS Care*. 2002;131:21–27.

96. Landrine H, Klonoff EA. Culture change and ethnic-minority health behavior: an operant theory of acculturation. *Journal of Behavioral Medicine*. 2004;27: 527–555.

97. VanDevanter N, Hennessy M, Howard JM, et al. Developing a collaborative, academic, health department partnership for STD prevention: the Gonorrhea Community Action Project in Harlem. *Journal of Public Health Management & Practice*. 2002;86:62–68.

98. Florin P, Mitchell R, Stevenson J. Identifying training and technical assistance needs in community coalitions: a developmental approach. *Health Education Research*. 1993;8:417–432.

99. Jenkins RA, Averbach AR, Robbins A, et al. Improving the use of data for HIV prevention decision-making: lessons learned. *AIDS & Behavior*. 2005;9(Suppl.): S87–S99.

100. Stein Z. Family planning, sexually transmitted diseases, and the prevention of AIDS—divided we fail? *American Journal of Public Health*. 1996;86:783–784.

101. Duerr A, Hurst S, Kourtis AP, Rutenberg N, Jamieson DJ. Integrating family planning and prevention of mother-to-child HIV transmission in resource-limited settings. *Lancet*. 2005;366:261–263.

101. Peck R, Fitzgerald DW, Liautaud B, et al. The feasibility, demand, and effect of integrating primary care services with HIV voluntary counseling and testing: evaluation of a 15-year experience in Haiti, 1985-2000. *Journal of Acquired Immune Deficiency Syndromes*. 2003; 33:470–475.

103. Juszczak L, Cooper K. Improving the health and well-being of adolescent boys. *Nursing Clinics of North America*. 2002;37:433–442.

104. Porter LE, Ku L. Use of reproductive health services among young men, 1995. *Journal of Adolescent Health*. 2000;273:186–194.

105. Raine T, Marcell AV, Rocca CH, Harper CC. The other half of the equation: serving young men in a young women's reproductive health clinic. *Perspectives on Sexual and Reproductive Health*. 2003;355:208–214.

106. Brackbill R, Sternberg M, Fishbein M. Where do people go for treatment of sexually transmitted diseases? *Family Planning Perspectives*. 1999;311:10–15.

107. Brugha R, Zwi A. Improving the quality of private sector delivery of public health services: challenges and strategies. *Health Policy and Planning*. 1998;13: 107–120.

108. Golden MR, Whittington WLH, Handsfield HH, et al. Partner management for gonococcal and chlamydial infection: Expansion of public health services to the private sector and expedited sex partner treatment through a partnership with commercial pharmacies. *Sexually Transmitted Diseases*. 2001;28, 658–665.

109. Franzini L, Marks E, Cromwell PF, et al. Projected economic costs due to health consequences of teenagers' loss of confidentiality in obtaining reproductive health care services in Texas. *Archives of Pediatric and Adolescent Medicine*. 2004;158:1140–1146.

110. Ford CA, Millstein SG, Halpern-Felsher BL, Irwin CE. Influence of physician confidentiality assurances on adolescents' willingness to disclose information and seek future health care: a randomized controlled trial. *Journal of the American Medical Association*. 1997;278:1029–1034.

9

Use of the Internet in STD/HIV Prevention

Mary McFarlane, Ph.D., and Sheana S. Bull, Ph.D., M.P.H.

The Internet has been identified as a risk environment for STDs, including HIV, for several years. Like the HIV epidemic itself, this online risk environment rapidly increased in importance, and revealed critical areas of the public health infrastructure that require new expertise and support. In the first section of this chapter, we will discuss the risk environment of the Internet, with most of the focus on men who have sex with men (MSM). The second half of the chapter will focus on the potential of the Internet for facilitating STD/HIV prevention, health education, outbreak awareness, and other public health interventions. In times of rapid change, public health officials often learn by trial and error in the interest of expediency, rather than taking the time to establish careful, scientific evaluations of new interventions. Such is the case with the Internet; thus, while we describe many Internet-based interventions here, we have very little data to support the feasibility, acceptability, efficacy, cost-effectiveness, and generalizability of these efforts.

The Risk Environment: History and Motivations

We will soon show that the Internet is a new risk environment for STDS, including HIV. First, it is important to understand how the Internet itself arose, and why people use it for facilitating sexual risk behavior. Historically, any new communications medium is soon used for sexual purposes, such as pornography, dating, prostitution, or facilitating sexual encounters between anonymous or casual partners (1). Gackenbach and Ellerman (2) point out that, as early as 1986, groups of electronic communicators were gathering online for sexual discussions under the newly created Usenet venues of alt.sex, alt.drugs, and other, similar channels. The World Wide Web as we know it was born in March 1989, and freely available software for viewing web pages quickly ignited the Internet craze. As computers and software increased in speed and decreased in cost over the subsequent decade, electronic communication became faster, included photos, and even incorporated video and audio streaming. All of these capabilities combined to provide users with a social network that could be visited without leaving the comfort of one's own home.

Behavioral Interventions for Prevention and Control of Sexually Transmitted Diseases. Aral SO, Douglas JM Jr, eds. Lipshutz JA, assoc ed. New York: Springer Science+ Business Media, LLC; 2007.

Soon, electronic communications technology improved to the point that Internet sites could be accessed from cell phones; additionally, Bluetooth devices can be used to communicate with like-minded persons within very close proximity, such as on a commuter train.

Cooper and his colleagues (3) suggested years ago that the accessibility, affordability, and perceived anonymity of the Internet are the "triple-A engine" that drives sexual disinhibition online. In the years since he suggested this terminology, the accessibility and affordability have increased exponentially. A number of others have emphasized other characteristics of the Internet, such as the ability to rapidly find a group of people with similar (sexual) interests, and to engage those people in "conversation"—and sexual negotiation—with a potentially low level of social anxiety.

Risks Presented by the Internet

The vast majority of research regarding sexual behavior and the Internet has focused on MSM. In early research (4), investigators showed that among HIV-testing patients in Denver, Colorado, Internet sex-seekers were more likely to be male and to have partners of either the same or both sexes. For purposes of this exposition, we will call this group RSM±W (respondents who have sex with men or with men *and* women). A much higher percentage of RSM±W were Internet sex-seekers when compared with exclusively heterosexual respondents. Internet sex-seekers were more likely to have had a past STD, and were more likely to have had sex with someone they knew to be HIV-positive. (Note that these were patients in an HIV-testing clinic, nearly 98% of whom were HIV-negative; thus, exposure to HIV-positive partners does not represent serosorting in this population.) Internet sex-seekers had more lifetime and past-year partners than respondents who found their sex partners offline. While this study presented data showing a relationship between online sex-seeking and STD/HIV risk behaviors, it has been criticized for involving a specialized, localized sample. In addition, due to the relatively homogenous demographics of the sample, the study did not examine differences by race or ethnicity.

A study of Atlanta Gay Pride attendees (5) found that 34% of respondents had had sex with someone whom they had initially met online. As is often the case with convenience samples, the majority of participants in online sexual partnerships were white (84%) and younger than respondents who met their sex partners elsewhere. Importantly, this study examined the relationship between meeting sex partners online and having unprotected anal intercourse with two or more partners in the past six months. The relationship was adjusted for age, education, ethnic status, AIDS knowledge, condom attitudes, and use of cocaine, marijuana, methamphetamines, and nitrites. Meeting sex partners over the Internet was shown to be related to the risky behavior even after adjusting for all these factors. The analysis was replicated for four subsets of men: HIV seropositive men, HIV seronegative men, men who reported ever accessing a gay-oriented web site, and men who reported sexual activity in the past six months. Meeting sex partners over the Internet continued to be independently related to the outcome variable except in the HIV seropositive men.

We have presented only two studies of STD/HIV risk behavior related to the Internet. There are many more such studies, some with data collected online, and others with data collected in person (5–12). A few studies attempt to compare data from in-person surveys to data from online surveys. For example, Rhodes et al. (10) performed a survey of MSM in two venues: the Internet and bars. In this case, the Internet sample was older, more educated, and more likely to report being bisexual (versus exclusively gay). Controlling for age and education, the Internet sample was far more likely to report a history of STD and to be HIV-infected. Interestingly, bar respondents were more likely to report engaging in anal sex in the past year, though this difference is between two very high proportions (88% vs. 97%).

Does the Internet somehow enhance a given person's willingness to be risky, or does the Internet merely attract persons who already engage in risk behaviors? Data to support either assertion are difficult to obtain. Most studies of risky behavior of Internet sex-seekers ask about Internet sex and about overall risk in the past several months. For example, Hirshfield et al. (13) found that men who met their partners both online and offline were more likely than "offline only" men to have engaged in unprotected anal intercourse in the study time period. The data do not show, however, that men engage in riskier behavior with their online vs. offline partners. Very few studies have asked questions about sexual behaviors with both Internet partners and non-Internet partners. In part, this is because a survey asking about both sets of partners is very cumbersome and repetitive, a poor measurement strategy when assessing samples of people who may have limited interest in responding to long, drawn-out questionnaires.

Despite these difficulties, Bolding et al. (14) studied this very question with MSM in a London HIV treatment clinic, HIV testing clinic, gyms, and on UK Internet sites devoted to gay men. They found that, in their sample, men met "casual UAI partners" (casual partners with whom they engaged in unprotected anal intercourse) of the same HIV status through the Internet. They were no more likely to meet serodiscordant casual UAI partners, or casual UAI partners of unknown status online than offline. The notion that the Internet contributes to HIV serosorting is intriguing. While HIV serosorting may present reduced risk for HIV transmission, its effects on STD transmission potentially could be harmful.

Is the Internet adding to the overall risk of the MSM population, or does it simply replace bars, bathhouses, and clubs for some MSM? Again, this is difficult to answer, but we have some data to suggest an additive effect of the Internet on population sexual behavior. In interviews with patients with early syphilis in San Francisco over the years 2001–2003 (15), public health officials found that the proportion reporting meeting partners at bars, bathhouses, etc., remained fairly constant. The Internet, however, increased in importance as a partner-seeking venue over that time period. This implies that, while the Internet is growing, other risk venues do not appear to have suffered a drop-off in their attendance. It is important to note that these data are from San Francisco, which is not representative of the rest of the United States. However, the Internet may be a venue of similar or greater importance in very rural areas, such as Wyoming (11), where bricks-and-mortar gay social venues are few or nonexistent. Other data (16) show that a significant percentage of Internet sex-seekers have traveled 100 miles or more to meet an online sex partner. The potential for rapid disease transmission represented by this type of Internet-facilitated partnership would have been unthinkable in the pre-Internet age.

Much remains to be done in assessing the true nature of the Internet as a risk venue. Some unanswered questions present real challenges to researchers who are accustomed to traditional epidemiology and assessment. For instance, how can we determine whether the online population is growing when it is difficult to assess how big it is at any time? How can we know how many people are using the Internet sex sites at any given time, when one person can be logged onto several such sites simultaneously? How can we be sure that people are providing us with valid data during online interviews? An interim answer to many of these questions is to use multiple methods and multiple disciplines to address the problem. Marketing specialists are aware of the size and demographics of many Internet groups. Internet service providers (ISP) and web-site owners are aware of how many unique subscribers log on to their services. Computer scientists have developed methods of searching the Internet for discussions of potential risk behaviors and outbreaks. Epidemiologists and behavioral scientists can collaborate to collect data from clinic patients, from outreach samples, and from Internet users. When these data converge (or diverge), we advance our knowledge of the credibility of the conclusions drawn. This multidisciplinary, multimethod approach to the Internet is essential not only in the assessment of risk, but in the efforts to perform online disease control and health promotion.

Why Use the Internet for Disease Control and Health Promotion?

The Internet has ample potential to facilitate interventions that can promote STD/HIV control and prevention. The medium can be used to promote disease prevention as a stand-alone intervention (i.e., all intervention components would be delivered online to a "virtual" audience, and no contact with public health clinical staff would occur). The medium can also be used to complement existing interventions by way of a "hybrid" intervention that combines the convenience of the Internet with existing clinic services. The advantages of using the Internet either as a stand-alone or hybrid intervention for STD prevention are numerous. The medium offers unprecedented reach to populations with potential risk for STD. The unique opportunity for interactivity online means the Internet can deliver sophisticated messages tailored to specific individual risk behaviors in a way no broadcast message can, and the Internet can serve as an avenue for social support to online communities and individuals at possible risk for STD.

Reach of the Internet

According to the PEW Internet and American Life Project, 66% of male and 61% of female adult Americans (defined as aged 18 and older) are now Internet users, and 78% of 18–29 year olds use the Internet. Although digital divide issues with regard to user race/ethnicity, education, and income persist, these divides have been continuously shrinking. Current data show that 43% of Black Americans use the Internet, 59% of Latinos/Hispanics, and 50% of rural residents, with anticipation that more and more of the American public will be wired in the near future (17). We can reach people online in much higher numbers than through any face-to-face campaign. In addition, the advance of such technologies as geo-targeting can allow us to target our efforts online to particular geographic areas where we know incidence and prevalence of disease is higher, or where there is a higher concentration of people with a particular STD risk profile. Such geo-targeting allows the use of banner ads or other information sharing online to be targeted to a given geographic area, allowing more judicious use of online advertising resources.

Why is reach important? Given the literature on sexual networks (18), it is clear that we are unlikely to identify all the "core" transmitters for various STD by relying on them to show up in a publicly funded STD clinic. Also, given the rise in sex partner seeking online, particularly among men who have sex with men (MSM) (16), it becomes imperative to consider multiple ways to share messages about STD risk and prevention to large numbers of people who would otherwise might not see them. For example, studies of MSM who use the Internet have shown them to be affluent, well educated, and largely covered by health insurance (11,16). If infected with STD or exposed to STD infection, they may not be aware of it, and may not be exposed to community or clinic level educational interventions that target lower income areas or publicly funded health clinics. Also, we can simply get messages to a much larger number of people online than in any clinic or community setting.

Examples of Programmatic Efforts: Overview

Current Internet-based programmatic efforts can be divided into several categories. In general, local efforts begin in the context of an Internet-implicated outbreak. Disease intervention specialists (DIS), tasked with finding partners of persons diagnosed with syphilis, are often provided with only an e-mail address or a chat-room nickname or "handle" for one or more partners. DIS must then find, or convince the patient to find, those partners in the Internet milieu. In one city, automated, anonymous "greeting cards" notifying partners of exposure can be sent. In some instances, chat rooms are used to raise outbreak awareness and augment partner notification strategies. To further facilitate testing, one city has implemented online "test slips," i.e., a signed, online order for a laboratory to perform a syphilis test that can be redeemed in the local jurisdiction. In conjunction with these techniques, some health departments or community-based organizations (CBOs) have negotiated for banner advertisements in various chat rooms and Internet venues. Banner advertisements generally direct the user to a web site that contains standard, didactic health communications, speaking to the need for interactive, targeted interventions. Because these have been the steps followed by several health departments with varying degrees of success, we will address each step in turn: online partner notification, chat-room outreach, online test slips, banner advertisements, and interactive, targeted interventions.

Internet-Based Partner Notification

Many STD programs have been forced to adapt traditional, face-to-face, partner-notification strategies to the Internet. In some cities, health department staff is restricted from performing online partner notification by lack of computer access in clinics, lack of access to the Internet in most offices, firewalls protecting any Internet-enabled computers from gaining access to "sexual" web sites, and local policy restricting use of the Internet by city employees for activities that can be construed as sexual. Fortunately, local CBO partners may not be so restricted, and may work with the health department to assist with online efforts. Staff at health departments and CBOs use e-mail and chat rooms to perform partner notification when warranted.

The use of e-mail is often preferable to the use of live chat, because the two strategies require vastly different investments of staff time for finding partners. E-mail can be accomplished passively (i.e., an e-mail message can be sent and the DIS can move on to other tasks while awaiting a response); however, locating someone in a chat room requires "lurking" for long periods in the chat rooms, hoping that the "target" person will enter the room. The chat room window may be placed in the "background" of the computer, but still, the DIS need to be at the computer until the task is complete. The task is complicated if the only locating information is a chat-room handle. In such cases, it may be difficult to identify people at all, as many online sex seekers use multiple handles. Once online contact is made with a partner, staff typically do not reveal to contacts that they have been exposed to syphilis, nor that they have been exposed to a disease at all. Rather, online contacts are told that staff have "important health information for you" and are encouraged to call or visit a local facility. Syphilis is mentioned only on the phone or face-to-face, after the identity of the contact has been verified.

Though some evaluation data have been gathered from programs conducting online partner notification, the data collection has been sporadic and no formal evaluation system exists. Of an initial 10 "online contacts" named during syphilis case interviews in Chicago, 8 were found by CBO partners in chat rooms, and 7 of those presented to the DIS for diagnosis and treatment. Two tested positive for syphilis. Most DIS will recognize these as particularly good contact rates for syphilis partners; however, without systematic evaluation, it is difficult to tell if these results are typical.

In order for evaluations to be successful, it is helpful for program staff to routinely request e-contact information during partner elicitation interviews. In one syphilis case-management interview, a patient provided over 200 names of online contacts. Because of the hours that may be required to reach patients' partners, high-volume cases such as this one may require alternative or additional efforts, such as general awareness campaigns to promote STD testing within a geographic region. Again, no formal evaluation of the partner-interview or partner-notification systems exists, but anecdotes indicate that the success of online partner notification is greatly enhanced when the original patient sends personal e-mail to the contacts.

Some local governments, department heads, health commissioners, and patients may have concerns about, or negative reactions to, online partner-notification efforts. Some concern has been expressed by local governments that violations of privacy regulations potentially could result from these efforts. Local areas have reported a wide range of number and proportion of partners found via online partner-notification efforts; of course, mixed results are often encountered in face-to-face partner notification as well. In the course of their pioneering, Internet-based efforts, the San Francisco Department of Health has learned several important lessons regarding online partner notification (19).

These include asking the original patient to notify partners before contact by public health personnel; sending e-mail messages from within, rather than from outside, the target's Internet service provider (such as AOL or Mindspring); using credible e-mail accounts with Department of Health logos; noting in the subject line that the e-mail is about an urgent health matter; protecting privacy by sending only individual (not group) messages; and gathering alternate, non-Internet contact information from respondents.

inSPOT

One method of allowing patients with sexually transmitted infections to notify their partners in a web-based, anonymous manner has been developed in San Francisco by Internet Sexuality Information Services (ISIS), Inc. The system is accessible at inSPOT.org, and allows users to send electronic greeting cards to sex partners. The cards can be sent anonymously (i.e., with no indication of the sender's identity or e-mail address), and can include a personally created message in addition to the standard text of the card. The cards notify partners that they may be infected with an STD, and urge partners to seek testing and treatment. As of November 2005 (Deb Levine, personal communication, November 2005), inSPOT.org was visited by an average of 750 people per day. Approximately 200 people send cards each month, and people send cards to an average of 2.5 partners, for an average of 500 cards per month. The anonymity of the system is clearly appealing, as 80% of cards are sent without any identification of the sender. However, 80% of the cards do include a personal message of some kind, which may provide some identifying information. About half (51%) of recipients clicked on the included web-link to the health department to find out more information about testing and treatment. Other cities, such as Los Angeles, recently have launched inSPOT in their cities.

Online Prescriptions

In 2005, San Francisco launched a program associated with inSPOT that allows e-card recipients to print their own prescriptions for antibiotics for the treatment of gonorrhea and chlamydia. The program is in its early stages of implementation at this writing, and has not been evaluated. To date, researchers in San Francisco have relied on pharmacists to send faxes regarding inSPOT prescriptions to the prescribing doctor. However, this system has not worked well, and new evaluation methods are being developed (Jeffrey Klausner, personal communication, January 2006).

Chat-Room Outreach

Chat-room outreach currently occurs in many areas, often in the context of community-based organization (CBO) efforts. Because chat rooms may not be active or "crowded" during the day, chat-room outreach often must occur at night. This can be difficult logistically for health departments. Outreach in chat rooms may have many components, but generally involves individual staff members logging into chat rooms, often with a handle (or nickname) such as "letstalkaboutsex" or "askmeaboutSTD." Staff members create "profiles" (self-descriptions registered with the Internet service provider) that explain the purpose of their visit to the chat rooms, the types of questions they can answer, and referral information for testing and treatment. Sometimes, to establish credibility, the staff member may reveal his or her sexual orientation, race/

ethnicity, or other pertinent characteristics. For the majority of efforts, the outreach staff are fairly passive in the chat rooms, with the exception of sending welcome messages to new arrivals and occasionally posting a brief line such as, "IM [instant message] me for sexual health info." This passivity prevents the chatters from becoming annoyed with the outreach staff, as has occurred in more active efforts. In addition, this passivity is more in line with the requirements of the ISPs who own the chat rooms.

When conducting online outreach, it is important that the staff member fully understand the nature of the online venue. For example, an outreach working in Atlanta may have questions and concerns from chatters in nearby states such as Alabama, Tennessee, and North and South Carolina. Thus, the outreach staff member must be equipped to answer questions and provide referrals for individuals from these nearby areas. Answering questions can be a difficult adventure, because chatters can and do ask disturbing or explicit questions. Questions can also be very specific, such as, "Can you get an STD from urine?" Thus, the outreach worker has to be well-versed in STD/HIV transmission, in chat-room parlance and etiquette, and in referrals to STD/HIV services. Referrals may not necessarily be limited to STD/HIV, but may also include drug treatment or detoxification referral and mental health emergency hotlines.

Howard Brown Health Center in Chicago, Illinois, conducts outreach in venues such as manhunt.net, gay.com, and America OnLine (AOL) chat rooms. Outreach staff announce their presence and state that they are there to answer questions. The outreach staff target syphilis in particular, but are trained to answer questions regarding any STD. Though no evaluation has been conducted, an evaluation plan includes counting the number of contacts made during various times of day, descriptions of encounters, and number of referrals made. Because Chicago chat-rooms often include participants from other parts of Illinois, as well as Wisconsin and Indiana, it may not be possible to evaluate whether referrals result in clinic attendance at nearby clinics.

In Houston, Montrose Clinic staff conduct online outreach as part of Project CORE (Cyber OutReach Education). A handbook has been developed for staff performing online interventions (20). The handbook contains material contributed by other sites, and is a valuable resource for the project staff. The chat-room outreach in Houston is slightly more active than in Chicago, in the sense that staff will occasionally post a topic, question, or statistic in an effort to generate contact with chatters. Staff use instant messaging, private chat, and larger "group" chat to accomplish their outreach. Referrals are made to other online resources, such as gayhealth.com, and to the Project CORE web site with its full list of referrals. The web site address is listed in the staff member's signature and profile.

One method of evaluating the Project CORE outreach includes counting the number of hits on Project CORE's web site. A more intricate evaluation, involving qualitative analysis of all online conversations (saved electronically and without identifiers), is planned. As a major focus of the outreach is referral for STD testing, it is hoped that the referral system can be evaluated.

The most formal evaluation of chat-room outreach to date comes from San Francisco. In San Francisco during two months of 2002, health professionals and staff from Internet Sexuality Information Services, Inc. (ISIS) conducted chat-room outreach in three venues. These venues were AOL chat-rooms specific to San Francisco, Craigslist (San Francisco), and M4M4Sex. Topics in the outreach program included symptoms, transmission, and treatment of syphilis (as well as other STDs, including HIV), and referral to testing. Health professionals responded to questions and provided syphilis fact sheets and online coupons for syphilis testing at the public STD clinic.

During the two-month outreach period, San Francisco staff spent 57 hours conducting outreach in the three online venues. They logged 212 interactions (67 on M4M4Sex, 21 on Craigslist, 124 on AOL). The rate of coupon redemption for clinic-based testing was 16% (35 coupons redeemed).

Additional San Francisco efforts include an "ask the expert" function on the San Francisco City Clinic's web page. The physician's photograph is posted online in order to increase the user's awareness that the posted queries are delivered to a real person. Users can type in any question, which will be forwarded to the physician and answered promptly. Similar web sites abound on the Internet, many of them including a "Frequently Asked Questions" section.

Auditorium-Style Chat

In another form of online outreach, San Francisco Department of Public Health (SFDPH) collaborated with ISIS to establish seven auditorium-style chats with online visitors to gay.com. In auditorium-style chats, many audience members can pose questions to the "expert" but not to each other. These sessions were real-time, one-hour interactions facilitated by a physician from SFDPH. Online chatters entered questions that were then selected by a moderator for expert response. The moderator posted the question, and the expert then posted an answer as quickly as possible. The software for conducting auditorium chat recorded the number of participants at any given time, and transcripts were reviewed and edited for clarity and removal of personal identifiers. Edited transcripts were posted on gay.com. During the seven, one-hour auditorium chats, approximately 120 visitors per session attended, with 10 to 50 people in the room at any given time. Questions were answered at the rate of 15 per hour. It is not clear whether participants were from the San Francisco area, or from elsewhere. This can be considered a drawback of the Internet for some program operations: it is impossible to tell if Internet users are physically located in the relevant city, or even in the country.

In Florida, United Foundation for AIDS (UFA) actively conducts Internet-based outreach to MSM. One focus of this CBO outreach is to communicate with users of crystal methamphetamine ("crystal meth"). UFA, in collaboration with an advisory board of former meth users, developed the Crystal Alert program, focused on Internet users who use crystal meth, to get users to meet face-to-face to address risk issues. The daily meetings have grown from approximately 7–10 members to 25–30 attendees. Other UFA outreach focuses on bringing MSM to the health department for STD and HIV testing. The Miami outreach is possibly the most intensely personal type of outreach, occasionally going so far as to send staff members to drive people to the clinic for testing. When appropriate, outreach staff follow up with chatters who have been tested, and provide a type of support throughout the process. During the chats, staff have noted a desire on the part of chatters to understand what sexual behaviors are less risky than others (e.g., "Is a top less risky than a bottom? Is oral sex likely to get me infected?"). These and other questions about the risks associated with particular sexual behaviors speak to the need for well-trained, expert outreach workers. They also speak to a willingness on the part of users to consider safer sexual activity.

Online Testing

The San Francisco Department of Public Health (SFDPH) launched its online syphilis testing program in June 2003. Persons can log on to stdtest.org to obtain a physician-ordered (and signed) laboratory requisition ("lab slip") and a unique identification number. The lab slip, once printed by the user, can be taken to a number of local laboratories for specimen collection and analysis. When testing is complete, the results are provided to SFDPH, who takes responsibility for posting the results with the identification number on the web site. The site also provides syphilis-related educational information, including signs, symptoms, and recommendations for future screening. Through mid-January of 2004, thousands of visits were logged on stdtest.org, but only 140 completed syphilis testing. Of the participants who completed testing, six (4.3%) had new syphilis infections (four infectious, two latent). Five of these infected patients were gay men. Of the gay men, one was HIV-positive, two were HIV-negative, and two were of unknown HIV serostatus. All infected patients received medical evaluation and treatment (21).

Banner Advertisements

Considering that the Internet is a multimedia environment with vast reach to the U.S. and international population, it is natural to consider broad-based, public-health communications online. Banner advertisements represent one such broad-based communication option. Banner advertisements are analogous to billboards, in that they are generally rectangular advertisements, often approximately one to two inches high and three to five inches wide or larger, placed in high-traffic areas of the Internet. Clicking on a banner advertisement results in a transfer to the web page of the advertiser's specification. One advantage of banner ads over traditional billboards is the ability to more effectively target advertising. For example, running a banner ad aimed at southern MSM in gay-oriented web venues is potentially more efficient than placing a billboard along southern highways.

The sale of banner advertisements is a major source of revenue for online entities, similar to the sale of radio and television advertising time. Banner advertisements are sold by quantities of "impressions," or the number of times an advertisement appears on the web page, and costs can range from $1000 per month to $10,000 per month. Usually, an advertiser purchases thousands or millions of impressions. Popular locations for banner advertising include gay.com, AOL, manhunt.net, craigslist.com, and similar venues. Some site owners may allow for the placement of banner advertisements for free in "remnant" space, i.e., space that hasn't been sold and would otherwise be unused. This remnant space is likely to be at lower traffic times and days (e.g., after midnight on weekdays).

The evaluation of banner ads is slightly less difficult than the evaluation of other interventions. It is fairly easy to count the number of people who click on the banner; in fact, some advertisers pay for the number of click-throughs, rather than the number of impressions. Once a user has clicked on the banner, however, it can be difficult to determine what effect the information on the linked web page has on behavior. In some instances, the owner of the linked web page may be able to track the "click trails" of viewers, or may incorporate redeemable coupons on the web page.

In San Francisco, SFDPH conducted an online banner-advertising campaign on gay.com and on AOL. Nine separate advertisements were run, for a total of more than 33 million impressions. The advertisements yielded 32,270 clicks to SFDPH web sites with syphilis information, for a click-through rate of 0.1%. The cost per click-through ranged from $0.05 to $10, depending on the host site and ad placement. Data on the amount of time spent on SFDPH web sites are not yet available. Additionally, there is no information regarding the acceptability or perceived utility of the information found on the SFDPH site.

Some organizations can be persuaded to provide online advertising for reduced or no cost, as a service to the public-health community. This practice has not been widespread among online venue owners. However, in recent months, officials from manhunt.net, an online sex-seeking venue, have contacted local public health partners in Houston (i.e., Montrose Clinic) to offer some free services such as online accounts for outreach workers, banner advertising, etc. Manhunt.net staff continue to contact local health departments in areas to which they are expanding their market. The company reports mixed responses from health departments, with some not returning phone calls. The owners of manhunt.net are trying to establish a community norm among venue owners; that is, they hope that by turning their subscribers' attention to public health and continuing to amass profit, they will show other owners that working with public health is not a detriment to business. Other web-site owners have been willing to work with researchers or health officials in localized areas, but not necessarily on a national basis.

Tailoring Online

Health promotion online has so far failed to take advantage of one of the primary benefits of the Internet—interactivity. Tailoring is a key component of interactivity, i.e., the capability to tailor messages to an individual based on their responses to a survey or questionnaire online. Tailoring has been utilized for many years to improve printed health education material—one investigation of patient health risk assessments for multiple risk behaviors including smoking, diet, and physical activity showed that persons receiving tailored feedback on risk assessment were 18% more likely to change at least one risk behavior compared to persons who received standardized or no feedback (22).

Tailoring is an ideal interactive component of the Internet. We can make messages relevant to a given demographic or behavioral risk characteristic by asking people to tell us a little bit about themselves before being exposed to an STD prevention message. Preprogrammed algorithms can also be used to provide message content that is relevant to a specific risk behavior. For example, if a participant in an online education intervention completes a survey documenting that they have been in a new sexual relationship (i.e., three months long) and recently decided to stop using condoms with their partner, the message about risk could differ from that delivered to the participant indicating they have had three new partners in the past six months. Programs can also be used to deliver messages using role models that can be selected to match a participant race/ethnicity, gender, or age. Thus, tailoring assists us to deliver messages firmly grounded in social and behavioral science. For example, if a person receives a message that addresses their personal behavior from someone who looks like him or her, there is an increased likelihood that the message will have more personal relevance, and will be more likely to promote behavior change (23–28). Unfortunately, few sites related to health are taking regular advantage of the potential of the Internet to tailor information. A recent review of 87 publicly available web sites devoted to improving diabetes self-management, for example, found that less than 10% had tailoring functions offering feedback on any type of behavioral assessment (29).

Social Support Online

Another interactive component of the Internet that is promising but somewhat underutilized and not well evaluated for health promotion is social support. The Internet is filled with sites that include chat rooms, "ask the expert" message boards, and web logs or "blogs," where people diary about any topic imaginable. Currently, we know there has been a proliferation of chat room–based sex education interventions developed and implemented by outreach workers in AIDS service organizations (ASO). Rhodes (30) described such an online HIV education process through chat rooms, and suggested that both the anonymity offered to chatters and the relationship established by the educator contributed to regular participation by chatters. We also know there have been randomized trials of Internet-related systems that utilize group visits online or chat rooms and have shown the approach has efficacy for increasing knowledge about disease, adherence to medications, and reduction in social isolation (31,32). The Comprehensive Health Enhancement Support System (CHESS) developed for cancer and chronic disease patients is perhaps one of the best-researched such interventions, and shows that online social support—in the context of a comprehensive online system that also includes access to web-based information, a library, and an "ask an expert" e-mail feature—is an effective approach for increasing participation in care among African American and White women with breast cancer (33).

We need to consider what new innovation the Internet offers to STD prevention initiatives; reach and interactivity suggest there are many promising interventions that can be developed and evaluated to capitalize on tailoring and social support capabilities of the medium.

While we are eager to embrace the Internet for STD/HIV prevention, we still have relatively little data on efficacy of the medium. Researchers have advocated taking a multi-level, or "social ecological" approach to health behavior change (34,35), arguing that the emphasis on psychological individual level behavior change interventions has missed important opportunities to consider influencing change by contemporaneously intervening at social, organizational and environmental levels (36–38). If we take this broad approach and consider any intervention at any of these levels could be informative for future Internet-based efforts to prevent STD, several studies of interest emerge.

Evidence from a recent study intervening at the organizational level to change physician behaviors is promising. The study compared the use of a multi-component Internet-based continuing education intervention specific to chlamydia (CT) symptoms, complications, diagnosis and treatment to a more generalized Internet-based continuing education program on women's health for physicians to increase chlamydia screening. Physicians in the multi-component Internet-based intervention had significantly higher CT screening than those completing the more general women's health module (39).

Another study of organizational level factors looked at outcomes when Investigators placed computers in the homes of persons infected with HIV and provided them with Internet access and regular electronic communication with clinic staff. This increase in access to care showed both increased use of computers and self-disclosure of risk behaviors for patients with HIV for the intervention group (40).

Looking at a multi-level intervention for STD prevention, a randomized control trial focused on providing both increased access to systems (i.e., organizational level) and social support to persons with HIV showed participants had greater satisfaction with HIV-related care; greater confidence in medical-related decision making; and decreased perception of social isolation (32).

It is interesting to note that the predominant trend emphasizing individual level interventions to promote behavior change for health interventions historically is so far not being replicated for online interventions, because there have been few randomized controlled trials of STD/HIV individual level prevention behaviors online that have incontrovertible findings. We do have some evidence from recently completed studies or studies that are in progress that can offer a glimpse of what might be possible online. A study of a tailored risk reduction message following completion of a sexual risk behavior assessment for MSM had high attrition, making interpretation of study results problematic, but investigators did document a trend in increased HIV testing among MSM assigned to the intervention group in this study (41). A study of rural MSM of an online education program to increase knowledge about HIV risk with a wait list control showed efficacy for increasing knowledge over a one week follow-up period (42). As of early 2007, data from 3 randomized trials involving web sites (funded by National Institute of Mental Health) are being evaluated. These web sites target a) MSM seeking sex partners online with a highly interactive e-learning application designed to increase knowledge, awareness of HIV risk and skills in reducing risk (Simon Rosser, PI-University of Minnesota); b) a web site testing the efficacy of tailored HIV prevention messages for youth (men and women, hetero- and homosexual) aged 18–24 at risk for HIV (Sheana Bull, PI-University of Colorado); and c) a comparison of efficacy of an online adaptation of the Popular Opinion Leader (POL) as an HIV educator versus the use of a traditional health educator in chat rooms online (Eric Benotsch, PI-University of Colorado).

What We Can Learn from Other Online Interventions

The results from these randomized controlled trials will not be available for at least one year. In the meantime, it can be instructional to consider ways the Internet has been used specifically to promote behavior change to address other health concerns. Data from a randomized trial using the Internet to deliver a behavioral weight loss program show that people will enroll, return frequently to the intervention web site, and derive benefits (i.e., significantly greater weight loss) from participation in an interactive Internet program (43). This program focused on the use of e-mail between participants and counselors during the weight loss program. Another weight loss program using a hybrid approach, where Internet-based counseling supplemented face-to-face counseling, showed significant weight loss among adults in the Internet program and adults and adolescents both demonstrated significant decreases in fat intake when compared with those in a face-to-face counseling program only (44). Studies of diabetes self-management interventions have demonstrated that recipients of tailored self-management messages online will improve self-management (45). McMahon et al. (46) showed that when participants could regularly upload their blood glucose readings to a clinic web site they had significantly lower A1C levels compared with those not accessing the web-based clinic system. Data from a randomized control trial on the effects of a tailored nutrition-education intervention online showed that people who receive these tailored messages make more steps toward improved nutrition than those receiving non-tailored messages (47). A study of youth in New Zealand showed that university students who accessed a student health center and subsequently participated in a behavioral screening with tailored feedback had significantly higher levels of physical activity and fruit and vegetable consumption than students who did not complete web-based activities (48). Randomized controlled trials of Internet-based treatment for chronic headache have shown promising results in reduction in headache symptoms and disability, but these studies, like others, had very high attrition (56–65%) (49,50). Finally, studies published on the efficacy of group level mental health interventions delivered online showed significant reductions in related distress, depression and ratings of annoyance (these investigators, too, showed attrition levels higher than those seen in traditional randomized controlled trials, i.e., 50%), and improved body image (52).

In summary, while we do see substantial proliferation in literature related to the development of Internet-based approaches to health promotion, we still have a very limited number of completed studies using a randomized controlled trial to test efficacy of interventions. From what we have presented here regarding both STD/HIV-related and other health behavior interventions at multiple levels, we have learned the following:

1. Interventions to change physician behaviors can be implemented to promote STD prevention;
2. Interventions that enhance access to systems or organizations may be valuable to consider for STD prevention;
3. People can generate a sense of social support and increased satisfaction with health care through use of Internet-based interventions;
4. Programs that utilize e-mail as the primary mechanism for counseling can be effective in changing behaviors;
5. Programs that use tailoring to individualize and personalize messages can be effective in changing behaviors.

This review suggests many promising opportunities for program planners involved in STD prevention efforts. Clinicians should consider options to link Internet to existing clinic services—web pages online can offer specific detail about services offered, and links to other information about STDs. STD risk assessments online that offer tailored feedback to individual responses—available either through a kiosk in clinic waiting rooms and/or via the World Wide Web—can standardize information that patients receive and save valuable clinician time in covering "standard" STD messages. Follow-up with clinic staff via e-mail or chat room discussions can be used to reinforce messages delivered in the clinic setting.

Clinicians may also want to consider technologies in addition to the Internet that can enhance clinical care and promote STD prevention. The use of text messaging via cell phones has been pilot tested and shown promising in an effort to reduce smoking among college students (53), and cell phones may offer a promising new platform for interventions, especially since they are even more ubiquitous than the Internet, and issues of digital divide appear to be less prominent for cell phone than Internet users. Likewise, the use of interactive voice recognition (IVR) automated telephone systems has been shown to have efficacy for increasing chronic illness prevention behaviors and access to care in diverse groups (54,55).

Certainly while we have little evidence of intervention efficacy available, it is challenging to identify specific strategies that are likely to have the greatest effect in STD prevention. However, it may be worth considering a more comprehensive approach like the CHESS system, which combines multiple offerings simultaneously in a web site, such as information access, "ask an expert," online access to medical record and social support. The SFDPH has implemented a number of different strategies for STD prevention online—perhaps their endeavors could serve as a blueprint for how to make interventions more comprehensive.

Finally, the work forthcoming that adapts efficacious community-, individual-, and group-level STD prevention interventions for the online environment may be instructive in illustrating the extent to which we may be able to borrow from "what works" in the real world and apply it to strategies online.

It is clear that the Internet is now and will continue to be an integral part of clinics and individual lives. While much has been written about how the Internet can fuel risk for STD, we have substantial optimism that the technology is available to exploit for innovative, far-reaching intervention.

References

1. Noonan R. The psychology of sex: a mirror from the Internet. In: Gackenbach J, ed. *Psychology and the Internet: Intrapersonal, Interpersonal, and Transpersonal Implications*. San Diego, CA: Academic Press; 1998.
2. Gackenbach J, Ellerman E. Introduction to psychological aspects of internet use In: Gackenbach J, ed. *Psychology and the Internet: Intrapersonal, Interpersonal, and Transpersonal Implications*. San Diego, CA: Academic Press; 1998.
3. Cooper A, McLoughlin I, Campbell K. Sexuality in cyberspace: update for the 21st century. *CyberPsychology & Behavior*. 2000;3:521–536.
4. McFarlane M, Bull SS, Rietmeijer CA. The Internet as a newly emerging risk environment for sexually transmitted diseases. *JAMA*. 2000;284:443–446.
5. Benotsch EG, Kalichman SC, Cage M. Men who have met sex partners via the Internet: prevalence, predictors, and implications for HIV prevention. *Archives of Sexual Behavior*. 2002;31:177–183.
6. Elford J, Bolding G, Sherr L. Seeking sex on the Internet and sexual risk behaviour among gay men using London gyms. *AIDS*. 2001;15:1409–1415.
7. Hospers HJ, Harterink Pl, Van Der Hoek K, Veenstra J. Chatters on the Internet: a special target for HIV prevention. *AIDS Care*. 2002;14:539–544.
8. Klausner JD, Wolf W, Fischer-Ponce L, Zolt I, Katz MH. Tracing a syphilis outbreak through cyberspace. *JAMA*. 2000;284:447–449.
9. Rhodes SD, DiClemente RJ, Yee LJ, Hergenrather KC. Correlates of Hepatitis B vaccination in a high risk population. An Internet sample. *Am J Med*. 2001;110:628–632.
10. Rhodes SD, DiClemente RJ, Cecil H, Hergenrather KC, Yee LJ. Risk among men who have sex with men in the United States: a comparison of an Internet sample and a conventional outreach sample. *AIDS Educ Prev*. 2002;14:41–50.

11. Williams ML, Bowen AM, Horvath KJ. The social/sexual environment of gay men residing in a rural frontier state: implications for the development of HIV prevention programs. *J Rural Health*. 2005:21:48–55.

12. Ross MW, Rosser BR, Stanton J. Beliefs about cybersex and Internet-mediated sex of Latino men who have Internet sex with men: relationships with sexual practices in cybersex and in real life. *AIDS Care*. 2004;16:1002–1011.

13. Hirshfield S, Remien, RH, Humberstone M, Walavalkar I, Chiasson MA. Substance use and high-risk sex among men who have sex with men: a national online study in the USA. *AIDS Care*. 2004;16:1036–1048.

14. Bolding G, Davis M, Hart G, Sherr L, Elford J. Gay men who look for sex on the Internet: is there more HIV/STI risk with online partners? *AIDS*. 2005;19:961–968.

15. Lo TQ, Samuel MC. State of California syphilis elimination surveillance data (through December 31, 2003). Internal report for the California Department of Health Services. 2004; accessible at http://www.dhs.ca.gov/ or by request from the Department.

16. Bull SS, McFarlane M, Rietmeijer CA. HIV/STI risk behaviors among men seeking sex with men online. *Am J Public Health*. 2001;91:988–989.

17. Pew Internet & American Life Project. Available at: http://www.pewinternet.org/trends/DemographicsofInternetUsers.htm. Accessed January 17, 2006.

18. Brewer DD, Potterat JJ, Muth SQ, Malone PZ, Montoya P, Green DL, Rogers HL, Cox P. Randomized trial of supplementary interviewing techniques to enhance recall of sexual partners in partner notification contact interviews. *Sex Trans Dis*. 2005;32:189–193.

19. Centers for Disease Control and Prevention. Internet use and early syphilis infection among men who have sex with men—San Francisco, California, 1999–2003. *MMWR*. 2003;52:1229–1232.

20. Roland E. *Cyber Health Educator Handbook*. Houston, TX: Montrose Clinic; 2005.

21. McFarlane M, Kachur R, Klausner JD, Roland E, Cohen M. Internet-based health promotion and disease control in the 8 cities: successes, barriers, and future plans. *Sex Transm Dis*. 2005;32(10 Suppl):S60–S64.

22. Kreuter MW, Strecher VJ. Do tailored behavior change messages enhance the effectiveness of health risk appraisals? Results from a randomized trial. *Health Educ Res*. 1996;11:97–105.

23. Bental DS, Cawsey A, Jones R. Patient information systems that tailor to the individual. *Patient Educ Couns*. 1999;2:171–180.

24. Campbell MK, DeVellis BM, Strecher VJ, Ammerman AS, DeVellis RF, Sandler RS. Improving dietary behavior: the effectiveness of tailored messages in primary care settings. *Am J Public Health*. 1994;84:783–787.

25. De Vries H, Brug J. Computer-tailored interventions motivating people to adopt health promoting behaviors: introduction to a new approach. *Patient Educ Couns*. 1999;36:99–105.

26. Kreuter MW, Strecher VJ. Changing inaccurate perceptions of health risk: results from a randomized trial. *Health Psychol*. 1995;14:56–63.

27. Lipkus IM, Lyna PR, Rimer BK. Using tailored interventions to enhance smoking cessation among African-Americans at a community health center. *Nicotine Tob Res*. 1999;1:77–85.

28. Marcus BH, Emmons KM, Simkin-Silverman LR, et al. Evaluation of motivationally tailored vs. standard self-help physical activity interventions at the workplace. *Am J Health Promo*. 1998;12:246–253.

29. Bull SS, Gaglio B, Garth MH, Glasgow RE. Harnessing the potential of the Internet to promote chronic illness self-management: diabetes as an example of how well we are doing. *Chronic Illness*. 2005;1:143–155.

30. Rhodes SD. Hookups or health promotion? An exploratory study of a chat room-based HIV prevention intervention for men who have sex with men. *AIDS Educ Prev* 2004;16:315–327.

31. Gustafson DH, Hawkins R, Boberg E, et al. Impact of a patient-centered, computer-based health information/support system. *Am J Prev Med.* 1999;16:1–9.
32. Flately Brennan P. Computer network home care demonstration: a randomized trial in persons living with AIDS. *Computers in Biology* 1998;28:489–508.
33. Gustafson DH, McTavish FM, Stengle W, et al. Use and impact of e-health system by low-income women with breast cancer. *J Health Commun.* 2005;10(s1): 195–218.
34. Brofenbrenner U. *The Ecology of Human Development: Experiments by Nature and Design.* Cambridge, MA: Harvard University Press; 1979.
35. Grzywacz J, Fuqua J. The social ecology of health: leverage points and linkages. *Behav Med.* 2000;26:101–115.
36. Breslow L. Social ecological strategies for promoting healthy lifestyles. *Am J Health Promot.* 1996;10:253–257.
37. Green LW, Richard L, Potvin L. Ecological foundations of health promotion. *Am J Health Promot.* 1996;10:270–281.
38. Stokols D, Allen J, Bellingham RL. The social ecology of health promotion: implications for research and practice. *Am J Health Promot.* 1996;10:247–251.
39. Allison JJ, Kiefe CI, Wall T, et al. Multicomponent Internet continuing medical education to promote chlamydia screening. *Health Reports.* 2001;116(1 Supp): 216–222.
40. Gustafson DH, Robinson TN, Ansley D, Adler L, Brennan PF. Consumers and evaluation of interactive health communication applications. The Science Panel on Interactive Communication and Health. *Am J Prev Med.* 1999;16:23–29.
41. Bull SS, Lloyd L, Rietmeijer CA, McFarlane M. Recruitment and retention of an online sample for an HIV prevention intervention targeting men who have sex with men: the Smart Sex Quest project. *AIDS Care.* 2004;16:931–943.
42. Bowen AM, Horvath KJ, Williams ML. A randomized control trial of Internet-delivered HIV prevention targeting rural MSM. *Health Educ Res.* 2007;22: 128–138. [Epub ahead of print].
43. Tate DF, Wing RR, Winette RA. Using Internet technology to deliver a behavioral weight loss program. *JAMA.* 2001;285:1172–1177.
44. Williamson DA, Martin PD, White MA, et al. Efficacy of an internet-based behavioral weight loss program for overweight adolescent African-American girls. *Eat Weight Disorder.* 2005;(3):193–203.
45. Stevens VJ, Glasgow RE, Toobert DJ, Karanja N, Smith KS. One-year results from a brief, computer-assisted intervention to decrease consumption of fat and increase consumption of fruits and vegetables. *Prev Med.* 2003;36:594–600.
46. McMahon GT, Gomes HE, Hickson Hohne S, Hu TM, Levine BA, Conlin PR. Web-based care management in patients with poorly controlled diabetes. *Diabetes Care.* 2005;28:1624–1629.
47. Oenema A, Brug J, Lechner L. Web-based tailored nutrition education: results of a randomized controlled trial. *Health Educ Res.* 2001;16:647–660.
48. Kypri K, McAnally HM. Randomized controlled trial of a web-based primary care intervention for multiple health risk behaviors. *Prev Med.* 2005; 41:761–766.
49. Strom L, Pettersson R, Andersson G. A controlled trial of self-help treatment of recurrent headache conducted via the Internet. *J Consult Clin Psychol.* 2000;68:722–727.
50. Devineni T, Blanchard EB. A randomized controlled trial of an internet-based treatment for chronic headache. *Behav Res Ther.* 2005;43:277–292.
51. Andersson G, Lindvall N, Hursti T, Carlbring P. Hypersensitivity to sound (hyperacusis): a prevalence study conducted via the Internet and post. *Int J Audiol.* 2002;41:545–554.
52. Winzelberg AJ, Eppstein D, Eldredge KL, et al. Effectiveness of an Internet-based program for reducing risk factors for eating disorders. *J Consult Clin Psychol.* 2000;68:346–350.

53. Obermayer JL, Riley WT, Asif O, Jean-Mary J. College smoking-cessation using cell phone text messaging. *J Am Coll Health*. 2004;53:71–78.
54. Piette JD, Weinberger M, McPhee SJ, Mah CA, Kraemer FB, Crapo LM. Do automated calls with nurse follow-up improve self-care and glycemic control amount vulnerable patients with diabetes? *Am J Med*. 2000;108:20–27.
55. Piette JD. Satisfaction with automated telephone disease management calls and its relationship to their use. *Diabetes Educator*. 2000;26:1003–1010.

10

Male Condoms

Lee Warner, Ph.D., M.P.H., and Katherine M. Stone, M.D.

Approximately 19 million cases of sexually transmitted infections (STIs), occur in the United States each year (1). For sexually active persons, male latex condoms remain the most widely available and commonly used barrier method for prevention of STI (2). When used consistently and correctly, male condoms reduce the risk of pregnancy and most STIs, including HIV, according to results of laboratory and clinical studies. Levels of condom use have continued to increase in recent years, as shown in national surveys of adolescents and adults (3–6), largely in response to the HIV epidemic. Condom use at last intercourse, for example, has now risen to more than 60% among adolescents (4) and adults at risk (6). Moreover, according to the 2002 National Survey of Family Growth (NSFG) (3), more than 13 million reproductive age women currently use condoms for contraception or protection from STIs, an increase from 9 million in the 1995 survey (7). Condom use thus continues to be an important part of public health efforts to prevent acquisition of STIs.

While there is general consensus that condoms must play a central role in any STI/HIV prevention program (8), how strongly condoms should be recommended to sexually active persons and those contemplating sexual activity remains controversial. Despite recent increases in condom use, current levels of use are likely insufficient for effective prevention of STIs. Questions about the effectiveness of condoms for STI prevention have also raised concerns regarding public health recommendations for their use (9–11).

In this chapter, we provide an overview of the role of male latex condom use for prevention of STIs. We first describe the mechanism of action and biologic plausibility for condoms to reduce the risk of STIs, and review both laboratory and clinical evidence on their effectiveness for STI prevention. We discuss the effectiveness of interventions promoting condom use, efforts to target condom promotion to specific settings and populations, and the surrounding controversies. We conclude by discussing areas of future research related to the use, effectiveness, and promotion of condoms.

Behavioral Interventions for Prevention and Control of Sexually Transmitted Diseases.
Aral SO, Douglas JM Jr, eds. Lipshutz JA, assoc ed. New York: Springer Science+ Business Media, LLC; 2007.

Mechanism of Action and Condom Types

Mechanism of Action

The male condom acts as a physical barrier by covering the penile urethra, foreskin, glans, and shaft, which are the major portals of entry and exit for many STI pathogens. When condoms are placed on the penis before any genital contact, used throughout intercourse, and remain intact, they protect the wearer's penis from direct contact with a partner's infectious cervical, vaginal, vulvar, or anal lesions, subclinical viral shedding, discharges, or fluids. They also protect the wearer's partner from direct contact with semen and urethral discharges or fluids, as well as lesions and subclinical viral shedding on the foreskin, glans, and shaft. Because of their coital-dependent nature, condoms must be used properly with each act of intercourse to be effective.

Condom Types

Approximately 97% of condoms available in the United States are manufactured from natural rubber latex ("rubber" condoms) (12). A small proportion are made from the intestinal caecum of lambs ("natural membrane," "natural skin," or "lambskin" condoms). Unlike latex condoms, natural membrane condoms contain small pores in the surface that may permit the passage of viruses, including hepatitis B virus, herpes simplex virus, and HIV (13,14). Because of this porosity, natural membrane condoms may not provide the same level of protection against STIs as latex condoms (15). No clinical data are available on contraceptive or STI prevention effectiveness for natural membrane condoms, however. Some condoms are manufactured from polyurethane or other synthetic materials. Compared with latex condoms, synthetic condoms are more resistant to deterioration, have a longer shelf-life, are non-allergenic, and are generally compatible with both oil-based and water-based lubricants (16). Three synthetic condoms have been cleared by the Food and Drug Administration (FDA) and are commercially available (Avanti™, Trojan Supra™, and eZ·on™).[1] The effectiveness of synthetic condoms to prevent STI has not been studied, and FDA labeling restricts their recommended use to latex-sensitive or allergic persons; however, synthetic condoms are believed to provide STI and contraception protection similar to latex condoms (17).

Spermicidal Condoms

Condoms lubricated with a small amount of the spermicide, nonoxynol-9 (N-9), ranging in concentration from 1% to 12%, have been available in the United States since 1983. However, their use is not recommended because spermicidal condoms are no more effective than other lubricated condoms in protecting against transmission of HIV and other STIs (2,18). Concerns also have been raised about N-9 products in general, since high frequency use of vaginal spermicidal N-9 products may cause genital ulceration and irritation and facilitate transmission of STIs including HIV (18,19). Since the amounts of N-9 contained in a spermicidal condom are much lower than those found in separately applied spermicide (2), they are probably less likely to cause

---

[1] Use of trade names and commercial sources is for identification only and does not imply endorsement by the U.S. Department of Health and Human Services.

adverse effects; however, spermicidal condom use was associated with increased risk of urinary tract infections in young women in one study (20).

Effectiveness Against STI and HIV

Laboratory Effectiveness

Condoms are regulated as Class II medical devices by the U.S. FDA (21). Every condom manufactured in the United States is tested electronically for holes and weak spots before it is packaged and released for sale. Each lot of condoms is also tested according to voluntary performance standards established by the American Society for Testing and Materials (ASTM) and International Standards Organization (ISO). As new technologies and testing procedures develop, these standards undergo periodic review.

Samples of condoms from each lot that pass electronic testing also undergo a series of additional laboratory tests for leakage, strength, dimensional requirements, and package integrity (22). If the sample condoms fail any of these tests, the entire lot is rejected and destroyed to prevent access by the public. Imported condoms are required to comply with the same performance requirements as domestic condoms and should be equally safe. A recent Consumer Reports survey showed that all condoms tested met industry standards, and that test performance did not vary with price, thickness, or country of manufacture (15). In vitro laboratory studies indicate that latex condoms provide an effective physical barrier against passage of even the smallest sexually transmitted pathogen (hepatitis B) (13,23–29).

Clinical Effectiveness

Factors Influencing Effectiveness

In clinical studies, the protection observed for condoms likely varies by STI because STIs vary in their routes of transmission, infectivity, and prevalence (17,30–32). Condom use should reduce the risk of STIs that are transmitted primarily to or from the penile urethra, such as gonorrhea, chlamydia, trichomoniasis, hepatitis B virus, and HIV. Condoms should also reduce the risk of STI that are transmitted primarily through contact with skin or mucosal surfaces to the extent that these areas are covered by the condom, such as genital herpes, human papillomavirus (HPV), syphilis, and chancroid (2,17,30–32). Protection may be less when these STIs involve areas not covered by the condom; however, the penis is the most common site of infection in men for chancroid (33), syphilis (34), and genital herpes (35). For HPV, the penis is the most common site of genital warts and subclinical HPV-associated epithelial lesions (36–41) and HPV DNA is detected most commonly from penile sites; however, the scrotum may also harbor HPV (42–44).

Condom effectiveness also could vary among STIs because of differences in the risk of transmission per sexual contact and number of sexual contacts with an infected partner (31,45–47), although this information frequently is not known. The probability of acquiring infection from a single sexual act depends on the prevalence of infection in the population (46,48) and the infectivity of the STI, both of which vary for different infections. Estimates of the transmission risk per unprotected sex act with an infected partner are approximately

0.001 for HIV (49,50), 0.20–0.50 for gonorrhea (51,52), 0.45 for chlamydia (53), and 0.70 for chancroid (54) and may vary according to other factors, including stage or severity of infection, presence of other STIs, and age and sex (55). If condoms are less than 100% effective, the cumulative risk of infection for both condom users and nonusers, given exposure to an infected partner, will increase more rapidly for relatively infectious STIs than for those that are less infectious (31,45,47). Consequently, studies comparing users and nonusers will demonstrate less protection for condoms against highly infectious STI (such as gonorrhea) than for less infectious STIs (such as HIV), even when the number of exposures to an infected partner is the same. Similarly, differences in numbers of sex acts with infected partners could explain variations in condom effectiveness estimates observed across studies against a specific STI, particularly one with high infectivity. Specifically, studies with short observation periods may provide higher effectiveness estimates for condom use (i.e., more suggestive of protection) than studies of longer duration, simply because the number of sex acts occurring with infected partners is lower (31).

Observed effectiveness also may vary within studies according to how well key design and measurement factors were assessed by investigators. For example, differences in how rigorously investigators ascertain participant exposure to STI-infected partners, whether condom use was consistent and correct and accurately reported, how infection status was assessed, and the temporal relationship between condom use and onset of infection undoubtedly affect condom effectiveness estimates (12,31,56–72). Although some studies combine different STI outcomes to increase statistical power, the heterogeneity of most STIs with respect to infectivity, population prevalence, and route of transmission complicates interpretation of effectiveness estimates. Disease-specific estimates of condom effectiveness are preferable, where possible (12,31,60). The overall strength of clinical studies to assess risk reduction associated with condom use has varied widely for different STIs based on recent reviews (12,31,70,71,73–78), making interpretation of effectiveness estimates challenging.

In summary, any factor that alters the likelihood of transmission, measurement of infection, or measurement of condom use can alter the estimate of condom effectiveness observed in a clinical study. While estimates of condom effectiveness are thus subject to considerable imprecision, clinical studies provide useful information regarding the general direction and magnitude of risk reduction against STIs associated with condom use.

Results of Clinical Studies

The highest quality clinical studies of condom effectiveness pertain to HIV infection. Numerous clinical studies have shown latex condom use to be highly effective for preventing sexually acquired HIV infection. Studies of discordant couples (where one partner is infected and the other is not) consistently demonstrate that condom use provides effective protection against HIV. Two meta-analyses of clinical studies of discordant couples estimate that consistent condom use reduces the risk of HIV transmission by 80–94% (74,75). No studies of discordant couples have evaluated correctness of use, which was associated with reduced HIV incidence in one study (79). The most recent meta-analysis (74) of discordant couples illustrates that transmission of HIV infection among consistent condom users is infrequent. Across 13 cohort studies reviewed, there were only 11 seroconversions among 587 self-reported consistent users, with many individual studies finding no seroconversions. This degree of protection suggests that condoms should be promoted to sexually active persons at risk for STIs for this reason alone (9).

The overall quality of clinical studies to assess the effectiveness of condoms against STIs other than HIV is considerably weaker. Unlike studies of HIV infection, clinical studies have shown inconsistent protective effects for condoms for most STIs. Interpretation of this literature has been difficult, however, due to inadequately designed studies to assess condom effectiveness, combined with inadequate numbers of studies to evaluate effectiveness against some STIs. Systematic literature reviews (31,70,71,73,76–78) have been conducted for clinical studies for several individual STIs, including gonorrhea, chlamydia, genital herpes, and HPV. These reviews document that only a small proportion of clinical studies measured factors critical to assessing condom effectiveness, such as exposure to infected partners, consistent and correct condom use, and incident infection. Additional concerns surround the impact of inaccurate reporting of condom use (48,57,58,63,64,68–70, 80–83) and imperfect performance of STD diagnostic tests (58,63,84) on effectiveness estimates. Because these limitations tend to underestimate condom effectiveness (31,56–58,61–63,69,71,80,81) the protective effects for condoms observed in clinical studies are likely to be lower (i.e., weaker) than the true protective effect, as has been documented by recent analyses (56–62,65).

For gonorrhea and chlamydia, most studies have demonstrated that condom use reduces infection risk in men and women (31), although the magnitude of protection provided has varied widely. Few studies have been adequately designed to evaluate condom effectiveness. A recent review of 45 studies of condom use and gonorrhea and chlamydia found, however, that studies that utilized better designs and analytic approaches to assess effectiveness were more likely to report statistically significant protective effects for condoms (31). This review also concluded that condom effectiveness likely is underestimated because of limitations in design, specifically from the inability to assess whether condom users and nonusers were exposed to partners who were STI-infected. Recent studies (61,62,65) of gonorrhea and chlamydia restricted to STD clinic patients with known exposure to infected partners, for example, documented protective effects for condom use that were markedly stronger than those reported for patients with unknown exposure.

For HPV, two systematic reviews of more than 40 clinical studies (71,78) concluded the effectiveness of condoms to prevent HPV infection in women and men largely is unknown due to difficulties distinguishing new from pre-existing infections and the failure of most studies to analyze consistent and correct condom use. Since then, a well-designed prospective cohort study has documented that consistent and correct use of condoms was associated with 70% reduction in risk for incident cervical HPV infection in young women (85). In addition, literature reviews have concluded that condom use can reduce the risk of HPV-associated diseases including genital warts in men (71,78) and women (78) and cervical intraepithelial neoplasia and cervical cancer in women (71). Two recent randomized trials showed condom use was associated with higher rates of regression of HPV-associated penile lesions in men (86) and cervical intraepithelial neoplasia (CIN) in women (87) and higher clearance rates of HPV infection in women (87).

Systematic literature reviews have concluded that condom use reduces risk of genital HSV transmission in women (70,73) and men (70). The single study of discordant couples found that condom use was associated with a significant reduction in risk of acquiring HSV-2 for women but not for men (88). Recent prospective cohort studies also show that condom use reduces risk of HSV-2 acquisition for both men and women (89,90).

The body of literature examining condom effectiveness for the remaining STIs is sparse, by comparison. Clinical studies, however, have found condom use to be associated with reduced risk of pelvic inflammatory disease (PID) (91–93), sequelae of PID (91), and trichomoniasis (94–98) in women, and syphilis in men and women (94,97,99–101). One study showed that condoms reduced risk of hepatitis B in women (102). No studies have specifically addressed condom use and risk of chancroid.

Challenges to Measuring Condom Effectiveness

Measurement of condom effectiveness in clinical studies presents significant methodologic challenges for investigators. As a result, the exact magnitude of risk reduction from condom use has been difficult to quantify, even for individual STIs, because of limitations and variations in the measures, designs, and duration of observation across clinical studies. Two issues widely considered as critical remain how best to measure condom use and how best to identify study populations with documented exposure to infection (31,68).

The coitally dependent nature of condom use suggests that investigators should fully assess both the consistency and correctness of use when evaluating their effectiveness; however, such assessment rarely occurs in clinical studies. Because direct observation of condom use is not feasible, investigators must rely on self-reported measures of condom use. Such measures may be inaccurate (48,58,63,69,70,80–83,103,104) with over-reporting being of greater concern than under-reporting because of social desirability. Recent evaluations suggest that even reports of "consistent use" may not indicate use during every act of intercourse (91,103–105).

Assessment of self-reported condom use has improved in recent years. Condom use should be assessed during a time period appropriate for the population and STIs under study (e.g., last three or six months) (31,48,64,82) that also coincide with the period in which STI status is ascertained. Consistent use should be defined as use during *every* act of intercourse. Correctness of use and use problems should include assessment of condom-related behaviors that may result in exposure risk for STIs despite condom use, including breakage, slippage, and delayed application of condoms, and early removal of condoms (63). Additional research is needed to determine whether the most appropriate referent category for consistent and correct use is nonuse, as opposed to inconsistent/nonuse or the number of unprotected sex acts. Investigators should continue efforts to document the validity of self-reported use. Recent advances in data collection [such as use of audio computer-assisted self-interview (ACASI) and electronic diaries] may facilitate accurate reporting of condom use by increasing participant willingness to report less socially desirable behaviors and by facilitating recall of condom use and sexual behavior

(31,48,64,85). New biologic markers that detect the presence of semen or other male genital fluids in the vagina (68,106–108) or possibly the presence of latex markers of condom use also hold promise for documenting use or nonuse of condoms.

Documenting exposure to infection among study participants remains critical for improving the accuracy of condom effectiveness estimates (31). Limiting the study population to persons exposed to infection ensures that participants are at risk for STIs during the actual period of observation, regardless of condom use. A randomized controlled trial in which participants were assigned to use or nonuse of condoms with prospective sex partner(s) would generally be considered unethical (12,31), except under very limited conditions. Prospective cohort studies of uninfected persons in relationships with infected partners (i.e., discordant couples) also would reduce differences in exposure risk between condom users and nonusers. Although this design has been used to evaluate condom effectiveness against chronic, incurable STIs (74,75,88), it would be unethical for curable STIs because infected persons must be treated promptly upon diagnosis (12,31,32,62). Recent evaluations (60–62,65) suggest that populations exposed to infection during the period of condom use assessment can be identified for some curable STIs (e.g., gonorrhea and chlamydia) through existing mechanisms for partner notification and referral. Given that these and other design and measurement limitations generally result in bias toward the null, the magnitude of risk reduction associated with condom use is likely higher than that observed in clinical studies.

Targeting of Condom Use and Condom Promotion

Despite evidence that condom use can effectively reduce the risk of many STIs, the promotion of condoms remains controversial in many countries, including the United States. According to recent reviews (109–111), behavioral interventions featuring condom promotion have been associated with increases in reported condom use (112–118) and, to a lesser extent, decreases in STI incidence (112,113,118).

The appropriateness of condom use interventions depends on the population and setting of interest. Though there is generally widespread support for targeted interventions that encourage condom use (8), the mix of condom promotion versus other prevention strategies (e.g., abstinence and mutual monogamy) remains controversial in many countries, including the United States. This controversy is due in part to questions about the effectiveness of condoms for STI prevention as well as how rigorously, if at all, condoms should be recommended to specific populations (e.g., adolescents). Concerns also have been raised about the potential negative consequences of condom promotion (119), given that increased availability of condoms may not necessarily translate into sufficient use for effective STI prevention. For example, even among studies of couples discordant for HIV or genital herpes simplex virus (HSV), where there is known risk for infection, fewer than half of couples report regularly use of condoms (74,75,88). Of increasing interest is whether interventions promoting condom use may result in risk compensation (119,120) that facilitates the onset or frequency of high-risk sexual activity, as hypothesized in some studies (121,122). However, the most recent meta-analysis of 174 sexual risk reduction intervention studies concluded condom-related interventions do not "inadvertently undermine sexual risk reduction efforts by increasing the frequency of sexual behavior" (123).

Strategies for Increasing Effective Condom Use

Condom effectiveness depends heavily on the skill level and experience of the user (17). Studies have documented relatively high levels of problems with condom use that may reduce their effectiveness, many of which can be minimized with appropriate counseling and practice. Interventions promoting condom use should address user-related behaviors that result in exposure to STIs, including:

1. *Failure to use condoms with every act of intercourse.* Nonuse of condoms, rather than poor manufacturing quality or other condom-related problems, represents the largest barrier to effective use (124,125). The highest single priority for any STI prevention program should be to explore and address factors associated with nonuse of condoms among persons at risk, including lack of device acceptability, poor partner negotiation skills for use, and latex allergy or sensitivity. Where possible, persons at risk should be provided with an adequate supply of condoms at low or no cost. New strategies that emphasize condom use for contraception in addition to disease prevention (126) may help decrease nonuse.

2. *Failure to use condoms throughout intercourse.* Recent studies have documented that some men put condoms on after starting intercourse or remove condoms prior to ejaculation (59,63,66,79,127). These behaviors represent incorrect use and expose users and their partners to potential STI risk despite condom use. Individuals should be counseled to use condoms every time throughout intercourse, from beginning to end.

3. *Condom breakage and slippage.* Although users often fear that condoms will break or fall off during use, these events are rare with proper use and tend to be concentrated among a small proportion of users (128). The majority of studies show that, during vaginal sex, condoms break approximately 2% of the time during intercourse or withdrawal; a similar proportion slip off completely (17,21,129–133). However, rates of breakage and slippage vary widely across studies (21) (0–13% for breakage (129,134); 0–9% for slippage (129,135)). Reviews of studies evaluating breakage and slippage during anal intercourse suggest the rates may be slightly higher than that observed during vaginal intercourse; however, most studies were retrospective (136,137). While breakage and slippage have been associated with user behavior, it is unknown exactly what proportion of these events is attributable to failure of the product versus misuse.

4. *Improper lubricant use with latex condoms.* Unlike water-based lubricants (e.g., K-Y Jelly™), oil-based lubricants (e.g., petroleum jelly, baby oil, and hand lotions) reduce latex condom integrity (138) and may facilitate breakage. People may use oil-based products as condom lubricants, mistaking them for water-based lubricants because they readily wash off with water. Because certain vaginal medications (e.g., creams and suppositories for yeast infections and bacterial vaginosis) often contain oil-based ingredients that can damage latex condoms, clients who will be using these

medications should be advised to remain abstinent, use synthetic condoms, or use other risk-reduction measures until treatment is completed and the infection is cured.

Recommendations for Practice and Future Research

Numerous laboratory and clinical studies conducted during the last three decades have documented the association between condom use and reduced risk of STIs, including HIV. However, given recent questions regarding the degree of clinical effectiveness, additional research is needed on the amount of protection provided by consistent and correct condom use against individual STIs. Of particular importance is the extent to which proper condom use can prevent STIs that are transmitted by skin or mucosal contact in areas that may not be covered by the condom (e.g., HSV, HPV, syphilis, and chancroid). Further research to clearly document the anatomic distribution of infectious lesions and subclinical viral shedding in areas covered or protected by a condom would be a feasible and valuable complement to well-designed condom studies. For all STIs, improved study methodology is needed for evaluating condom effectiveness, particularly with respect to validation of self-reported use, ascertainment of exposure to infection, and measurement of incident infection.

Beyond studies of product effectiveness, additional information is needed on strategies to increase the consistency and correctness of condom use among sexually active persons at increased risk of STIs. Improved understanding of both barriers to condom use and solutions that address these barriers (such as new condom technologies) are also needed. Recent concerns about the potential adverse effects of condom promotion should be addressed through further study. Finally, more research is needed on how best to incorporate the role of condoms into comprehensive STI/HIV prevention strategies that may involve multiple prevention messages [e.g., "Abstinence, Be Faithful, Condoms" ("ABC")-oriented approach and also STI screening and treatment]. Such research is essential if the potential for condom use as a STI prevention intervention is to be fully realized.

Summary and Conclusions

When used properly, male latex condoms reduce the risk of many, if not most, STIs, including HIV, based on their barrier properties, biologic plausibility, and evidence from clinical and laboratory studies. Achieving consistent and correct use remains the largest problem influencing the "real world" effectiveness of condoms. Though condom-based interventions have shown increases in reported use, levels of nonuse remain substantial. To optimize use of male condoms in sexually active populations at risk for STIs, public health messages must reinforce and clearly communicate the scientific evidence on condom effectiveness.

References

1. Weinstock H, Berman S, Cates W. Sexually transmitted diseases among American youth: incidence and prevalence estimates, 2000. *Perspect Sex Repro Health.* 2004;36:6–10.

2. Centers for Disease Control and Prevention. Sexually transmitted diseases treatment guidelines 2006. *MMWR*. 2006;55(RR-11).

3. Chandra A, Martinez GM, Mosher WD, Abma JC, Jones J. Fertility, family planning, and reproductive health of U.S. women: data from the 2002 National Survey of Family Growth. *Vital Health Stat*. 2005;23:1–160.

4. Centers for Disease Control and Prevention. Youth risk behavior surveillance—United States, 2003. *MMWR*. 2004;53(SS-2):1–96.

5. Centers for Disease Control and Prevention. Trends in sexual risk behaviors among high school students—United States, 1991–2001. *MMWR*. 2002;51:856–859.

6. Anderson JE, Wilson R, Doll L, et al. Condom use and HIV risk behaviors among U.S. adults: data from a national survey. *Fam Plann Perspect*. 1999;31:24–28.

7. Abma JC, Chandra A, Mosher WD, et al. Fertility, family planning, and women's health: new data from the 1995 National Survey of Family Growth. *Vital Health Stat*. 1997;Series 23, Number 9.

8. Halperin DT, Steiner MJ, Cassell MM, et al. The time has come for common ground on preventing sexual transmission of HIV. *Lancet*. 2004;364:1913–1915.

9. Cates W Jr. The NIH condom report: the glass is 90% full. *Fam Plann Perspect*. 2001;33:231–233.

10. Boonstra H. Public health advocates say campaign to disparage condoms threatens STD prevention efforts. *The Guttmacher Report on Public Policy*. 2003;6:1–3.

11. Gilden D. Condom effectiveness, reviewed, revised, reduxed. *Community HIV/AIDS Mobilization Project (CHAMP) HHS Watch*; July 2005.

12. National Institute of Allergy and Infectious Diseases. Workshop Summary: Scientific Evidence on Condom Effectiveness for Sexually Transmitted Diseases (STD) Prevention. July 20, 2001. Available at http://www.niaid.nih.gov/dmid/stds/condomreport.pdf.

13. Carey RF, Lytle CD, Cyr WH. Implications of laboratory tests of condom integrity. *Sex Transm Dis*. 1999;26:216–220.

14. Lytle CD, Carney PG, Vohra S, et al. Virus leakage through natural membrane condoms. *Sex Transm Dis*. 1990;17:58–62.

15. Consumer Union: Condoms: Extra protection. *Consumer Reports* 2005;February.

16. Gallo M, Grimes D, Lopez L, Schulz K. Non-latex versus latex male condoms for contraception. *Cochrane Database Syst Rev*. 2006;CD003550.

17. Steiner MJ, Warner L, Stone KM, Cates W Jr. Condoms and other barrier methods for prevention of STD/HIV infection, and pregnancy. In: Holmes KK, Sparling PF, Mardh P-A, eds. *Sexually Transmitted Diseases*, 4th ed., McGraw-Hill, New York (in press).

18. Centers for Disease Control and Prevention. Nonoxynol-9 spermicide contraception use—United States, 1999. *MMWR*. 2002;51:389–392.

19. Centers for Disease Control and Prevention. CDC statement on study results of products containing nonoxynol-9. *MMWR*. 2000;49:717–718.

20. Fihn SD, Boyko EJ, Normand EH, et al. Association between use of spermicide-coated condoms and *Escherichia coli* urinary tract infection in young women. *Am J Epidemiol*. 1996;144:512–520.

21. Warner L, Hatcher RA, Steiner MJ. Male Condoms. In: Hatcher RA, Trussell J, Stewart F, Nelson AL, Cates Jr W, Guest F, et al, editors. *Contraceptive Technology*, 18th ed. New York: Ardent Media Inc., 2004, pp 331–353.

22. ASTM (American Society for Testing Materials). Annual book of ASTM standards: Easton MD: ASTM: section 9, rubber. Volume 09.02 Rubber products; standard specifications for rubber contraceptives (male condoms-D3492). West Conshohocken, PA: American Society for Testing Materials, 1996.

23. Carey RF, Herman WA, Retta SM, et al. Effectiveness of latex condoms as a barrier to human immunodeficiency virus-sized particles under conditions of simulated use. *Sex Transm Dis*. 1992;19:230–234.

24. Conant MA, Spicer DW, Smith CD. Herpes simplex virus transmission: condom studies. *Sex Transm Dis*. 1984;11:94–95.
25. Judson FN, Ehret JM, Bodin GF, et al. In vitro evaluations of condoms with and without nonoxynol 9 as physical and chemical barriers against *Chlamydia trachomatis*, herpes simplex virus type 2, and human immunodeficiency virus. *Sex Transm Dis*. 1989;16:51–56.
26. Katznelson S, Drew WL, Mintz L. Efficacy of the condom as a barrier to the transmission of cytomegalovirus. *J Infect Dis*. 1984;150:155–157.
27. Rietmeijer CA, Krebs JW, Feorina PM, et al. Condoms as physical and chemical barriers against human immunodeficiency virus. *JAMA*. 1988;259:1851–1853.
28. Van de Perre P, Jacobs D, Sprecher-Goldberger S. The latex condom, an efficient barrier against sexual transmission of AIDS-related viruses. *AIDS*. 1987;1:49–52.
29. Lytle CD, Routson LB, Seaborn GB, et al. An in vitro evaluation of condoms as barriers to a small virus. *Sex Transm Dis*. 1997;24:161–164.
30. Warner L, Steiner MJ. Male condoms. In: Hatcher RA, Trussell J, Stewart F, Nelson AL, Cates Jr W, Guest F, et al, eds. *Contraceptive Technology*, 19th ed. New York: Ardent Media Inc., 2007.
31. Warner L, Stone KM, Macaluso M, et al. A systematic review of design factors assessed in epidemiologic studies of condom effectiveness for preventing gonorrhea and chlamydia. *Sex Transm Dis*. 2006;33:36–51.
32. Stone KM, Thomas E, Timyan J. Barrier methods for the prevention of sexually transmitted diseases. In: Holmes KK, Sparling PF, Mardh P-A, eds. *Sexually Transmitted Diseases*, 3rd ed. New York: McGraw-Hill, 1998.
33. Ronald AL, Albritton W. Chancroid and *Haemophilus ducreyi*. In: Holmes KK, Sparling PF, March P-A, et al., eds. *Sexually Transmitted Diseases,* 3rd Ed. New York: McGraw-Hill, 1999, p. 518.
34. Musher DM. Early syphilis. In: Holmes KK, Sparling PF, March P-A, et al., eds. *Sexually Transmitted Diseases,* 3rd Ed. New York: McGraw-Hill, 1999, p. 479.
35. Corey L, Wald A. Genital herpes. In: Holmes KK, Sparling PF, March P-A, et al., eds. *Sexually Transmitted Diseases*, 3rd Ed. New York: McGraw-Hill, 1999, p. 295.
36. Barasso R, DeBrux J, Croissant O, Orth G. High prevalence of papillomavirus-associated penile intraepithelial neoplasia in sexual partners of women with cervical intraepithelial neoplasia. *N Engl J Med*. 1987;317:916–923.
37. Chuang TY, Perry HO, Kurland LT, et al. *Condyloma acuminatum* in Rochester, Minn, 1950–1978. *Arch Dermatol*. 1984;120:469–475.
38. Hippelainen M, Syrjanen S, Hippelainen M, et al. Prevalence and risk factors of genital human papillomavirus (HPV) infections in healthy males: a study on Finnish conscripts. *Sex Transm Dis*. 1993;20:321–328.
39. Kennedy L, Buntine DW, O'Connor D, et al. Human papillomavirus—a study of male sexual partners. *Med J Austr*. 1988;149:309–311.
40. Krebs HB, Schneider V. Human papillomavirus-associated lesions of the penis: colposcopy, cytology, and histology. *Obstet Gynecol*. 1987;70:299–304.
41. Schultz RE, Miller JW, MacDonald GR, et al. Clinical and molecular evaluation of acetowhite genital lesions in men. *J Urol*. 1990;143:920–923.
42. Weaver BA, Feng Q, Holmes KK, et al. Evaluation of genital sites and sampling techniques for detection of human papillomavirus DNA in men. *J Infect Dis*. 2004;189:677–678.
43. Nicolau SM, Camargo CG, Stavale JN, et al. Human papillomavirus DNA detection in male sexual partners of women with genital human papillomavirus infection. *Urology*. 2005;65:251–255.
44. Hernandez B, McDuffie K, Goodman M, et al. Comparison of physician- and self-collected genital specimens for detection of human papillomavirus in men. *J Clinic Micro*. 2006;44:513–517.
45. Cates W Jr. The condom forgiveness factor: the positive spin. *Sex Transm Dis*. 2002;29:350–352.

46. Cates W Jr. Contraception, contraceptive technology, and STDs. In: Holmes KK, Sparling PF, Mardh P-A, eds. *Sexually Transmitted Diseases*, 3rd ed., McGraw-Hill: New York, 1998.
47. Mann JR, Stine CC, Vessey J. The role of disease-specific infectivity and number of disease exposures on long-term effectiveness of the latex condom. *Sex Transm Dis*. 2002;29:344–349.
48. Aral SO, Peterman TA. Measuring outcomes of behavioural interventions for STD/HIV prevention. *Int J STD AIDS*. 1996;7(Suppl 2):30–38.
49. Gray R, Mawer MJ, Brookmeyer R, et al. Probability of HIV-1 transmission per coital act in monogamous, heterosexual, HIV-1 discordant couples in Rakai, Uganda. *Lancet*. 2001;357:1149–1153.
50. Mastro T, de Vincenzi I. Probabilities of sexual HIV-1 transmission. *AIDS*. 1996;10(suppl A):S75–S82.
51. Holmes KK, Johnson DW, Trostle HJ. An estimate of the risk of men acquiring gonorrhea by sexual contact with infected females. *Am J Epidemiol*. 1970;91:170–174.
52. Platt R, Rice PA, McCormack WM. Risk of acquiring gonorrhea and prevalence of abnormal adnexal findings among women recently exposed to gonorrhea. *JAMA*. 1983;250:3205–3209.
53. Lycke E, Lowhagen GB, Hallhagen G, et al. The risk of transmission of genital *Chlamydia trachomatis* infection is less than that of genital *Neisseria gonorrhoeae* infection. *Sex Transm Dis*. 1980;7:6–10.
54. Plummer FA, D'Costa LJ, Nsanze H, et al. Epidemiology of chancroid and haemophilus ducreyi in Nairobi, Kenya. *Lancet*. 1983;2:1293–1295.
55. Wasserheit JN. Epidemiologic synergy: interrelationships between human immunodeficiency virus infection and other sexually transmitted diseases. *Sex Transm Dis*. 1992;9:61–77.
56. Shlay JC, McClung MW, Patnaik JL, Douglas JM Jr. Comparison of sexually transmitted disease prevalence by reported condom use: errors among consistent condom users seen at an urban sexually transmitted disease clinic. *Sex Transm Dis*. 2004;31:526–532.
57. Shlay JC, McClung MW, Patnaik JL, Douglas JM Jr. Comparison of sexually transmitted disease prevalence by reported level of condom use among patients attending an urban sexually transmitted disease clinic. *Sex Transm Dis*. 2004;31:154–160.
58. Devine OJ, Aral SO. The impact of inaccurate reporting of condom use and imperfect diagnosis of sexually transmitted disease infection in studies of condom effectiveness: a simulation-based assessment. *Sex Transm Dis*. 2004;31:588–595.
59. Paz-Bailey G, Koumans EH, Sternberg M, et al. The effect of correct and consistent condom use on chlamydial and gonococcal infection among urban adolescents. *Arch Pediatr Adolesc Med*. 2005;159:536–542.
60. Warner L, Macaluso M, Newman DR, et al. Re: Condom effectiveness for prevention of *chlamydia trachomatis* infection. *Sex Transm Inf*. 2006;82:265.
61. Warner L, Macaluso M, Austin HD, et al. Application of the case-crossover design to reduce unmeasured confounding in studies of condom effectiveness. *Am J Epidemiol*. 2005;161:765–773.
62. Warner L, Newman DR, Austin HD, et al. Condom effectiveness for reducing transmission of gonorrhea and chlamydia: the importance of assessing partner infection status. *Am J Epidemiol*. 2004;159:242–251.
63. Warner L, Clay-Warner J, Boles J, Williamson J. Assessing condom use practices. Implications for evaluating method and user effectiveness. *Sex Transm Dis*. 1998;25:273–277.
64. Crosby R, DiClemente RJ, Holtgrave DR, Wingood GM. Design, measurement, and analytical considerations for testing hypotheses relative to condom effectiveness against non-viral STIs. *Sex Transm Inf*. 2002;78:228–231.

65. Niccolai L, Rowhani-Rahbar A, Jenkins H, et al. Condom effectiveness for prevention of *Chlamydia trachomatis* infection. *Sex Transm Inf*. 2005;81:323–325.
66. Fishbein M, Pequegnat W. Evaluating AIDS prevention interventions using behavioral and biological outcome measures. *Sex Transm Dis*. 2000;27:101–110.
67. Macaluso M, Kelaghan J, Artz L, et al. Mechanical failure of the latex condom in a cohort of women at high STD risk. *Sex Transm Dis*. 1999;26:450–458.
68. Steiner MJ, Feldblum PJ, Padian N. Invited commentary: condom effectiveness— will prostate specific antigen shed new light on this perplexing problem. *Am J Epidemiol*. 2003;157:298–300.
69. Zenilman JM, Weisman CS, Rompalo AM, et al. Condom use to prevent incident STDs: the validity of self-reported condom use. *Sex Transm Dis*. 1995;22:15–21.
70. Holmes KK, Levine R, Weaver M. Effectiveness of condom in preventing sexually transmitted infections. *Bull WHO*. 2004;84:454–461.
71. Manhart LE, Koutsky LA. Do condoms prevent genital HPV infection, external genital warts, or cervical neoplasia? A meta-analysis. *Sex Transm Dis*. 2002;29:725–735.
72. Aral SO, Peterman TA. A stratified approach to untangling the behavioral/biomedical outcomes conundrum. *Sex Transm Dis*. 2002;29:530–532.
73. Casper C, Wald A. Condom use and the prevention of genital herpes acquisition. *Herpes*. 2002;9:10–14.
74. Weller S, Davis K. Condom effectiveness in reducing heterosexual HIV transmission. *Cochrane Database Syst Rev*. 2001;3:CD003255.
75. Pinkerton SD, Abramson PR. Effectiveness of condoms in preventing HIV transmission. *Soc Sci Med*. 1997;44:1303–1312.
76. Alfonsi GA, Shlay J. The effectiveness of condoms for the prevention of sexually transmitted diseases. *Curr Wom Health Reviews*. 2005;1:151–159.
77. d'oro LC, Parazzini F, Naldi L, et al. Barrier methods of contraception, spermicides, and sexually transmitted diseases: a review. *Genitourin Med*. 1994;70:410–417.
78. Centers for Disease Control and Prevention. Report to Congress: Prevention of Genital Human Papillomavirus Infection, January 2004.
79. Calzavara L, Burchell AN, Remis RS, et al. Delayed application of condoms is a risk factor for human immunodeficiency virus infection among homosexual and bisexual men. *Am J Epidemiol*. 2003;157:210–217.
80. Rietmeijer CA, Bemmelen RV, Judson FN, et al. Incident and repeat infection rates of *chlamydia trachomatis* among male and female patients in an STD clinic. *Sex Transm Dis*. 2002;29:65–72.
81. Pequegnat W, Fishbein M, Celentano D, et al. NIMH/APPC workgroup on behavioral and biological outcomes in HIV/STD prevention studies. *Sex Transm Dis*. 2000;27:127–132.
82. Catania JA, Gibson DR, Chitwood DD, et al. Methodological problems in AIDS behavioral research: influences on measurement error and participation bias in studies of sexual behavior. *Psychol Bull*. 1990;108:339–362.
83. Turner CF, Miller HG. Zenilman's anomaly reconsidered: fallible reports, ceteris paribus, and other hypotheses. *Sex Transm Dis*. 1997;24:522–527.
84. Schachter J, Chow JM. The fallibility of diagnostic tests for sexually transmitted disease: the impact on behavioral and epidemiologic studies. *Sex Transm Dis*. 1995;22:191–196.
85. Winer RL, Hughes JP, Feng Q, et al. Condom use and the risk of genital human papillomavirus infection in young women. *New Engl J Med*. 2006;354:2645–2654.
86. Bleeker MC, Hogewoning CJ, Voorhorst FJ, et al. Condom use promotes regression of human papillomavirus-associated penile lesions in male sexual partners of women with cervical intraepithelial neoplasia. *Int J Cancer*. 2003;107:804–810.
87. Hogewoning CJ, Bleeker MC, van den Brule AJ, et al. Condom use promotes regression of cervical intraepithelial neoplasia and clearance of human papillomavirus: a randomized clinical trial. *Int J Cancer*. 2003;107:811–816.

88. Wald A, Langenberg AG, Link K, et al. Effect of condoms on reducing the transmission of herpes simplex virus type 2 from men to women. *JAMA*. 2001;285:3100–3106.

89. Gottlieb SL, Douglas JM Jr, Foster M, et al. Incidence of herpes simplex virus type 2 infection in 5 sexually transmitted disease (STD) clinics and the effect of HIV/STD risk-reduction counseling. *J Infect Dis*. 2004;190:1059–1067.

90. Wald A, Langenberg AG, Krantz, et al. The relationship between condom use and herpes simplex virus acquisition. *Ann Intern Med*. 2005;143:707–713.

91. Ness RB, Randall H, Richter HE, et al. Condom use and the risk of recurrent pelvic inflammatory disease, chronic pelvic pain, or infertility following an episode of pelvic inflammatory disease. *Am J Public Health*. 2004;94:1327–1329.

92. Baeten JM, Nyange PM, Richardson BA, et al. Hormonal contraception and risk of sexually transmitted disease acquisition: results from a prospective study. *Am J Obstet Gynecol*. 2001;185:380–365.

93. Kelaghan J, Rubin GL, Ory HW, Layde PM. Barrier-method contraceptives and pelvic inflammatory disease. *JAMA*. 1982;248:184–187.

94. Levine WC, Revollo R, Kaune V, et al. Decline in sexually transmitted disease prevalence in female Bolivian sex workers: impact of an HIV prevention project. *AIDS*. 1998;12:1899–1906.

95. Rosenberg MJ, Davidson AJ, Chen J-H, et al. Barrier contraceptives and sexually transmitted diseases in women: a comparison of female-dependent methods and condoms. *Am J Public Health*. 1992;82:669–674.

96. Sanchez J, Campos PE, Courtois B, et al. Prevention of sexually transmitted diseases (STDs) in female sex workers: prospective evaluation of condom promotion and strengthened STD services. *Sex Transm Dis*. 2003;30:273–279.

97. Joesoef MR, Linnan M, Barakbah Y, et al. Patterns of sexually transmitted diseases in female sex workers in Surabaya, Indonesia. *Int J STD AIDS*. 1997;8:576–580.

98. Fennema JSA, van Ameijden EJC, Coutinho RA, van Den Hoek A. Clinical sexually transmitted diseases among human immunodeficiency virus-infected and noninfected drug-using prostitutes. Associated factors and interpretation of trends, 1986 to 1994. *Sex Transm Dis*. 1997;24:363–371.

99. Ahmed S, Lutalo R, Wawer M, et al. HIV incidence and sexually transmitted disease prevalence associated with condom use: a population study in Rakai, Uganda. *AIDS*. 2001;16:2171–2179.

100. Finelli L, Budd J, Spitalny KC. Early syphilis. Relationship to sex, drugs, and changes in high-risk behavior from 1987–1990. *Sex Transm Dis*. 1993;20:89–95.

101. Gattari P, Speziale D, Grillo R, et al. Syphilis serology among transvestite prostitutes attending an HIV unit in Rome, Italy. *Eur J Epidemiol*. 1994;10:683–686.

102. Sanchez J, Gutuzzo E, Escamilla J. Sexually transmitted infections in female sex workers: reduced by condom use but not by a limited periodic examination program. *Sex Transm Dis*. 1998;25:82–89.

103. Thomas JC, Stratton S. Sexual transmission. In: Thomas JC, Weber DJ, eds. Epidemiologic Methods for the Study of Infectious Diseases. New York: Oxford University Press, 2001, pp 267–287.

104. Cecil H, Zimet GD. Meanings assigned by undergraduates to frequency statements of condom use. *Arch Sex Behav*. 1998;27:493–505.

105. van Duynhoven YTHP, van de Laar MJW, Schop WA, et al. Different demographic and sexual correlates for chlamydial infection and gonorrhoea in Rotterdam. *Int J Epidemiol*. 1997;26:1373–1385.

106. Walsh TL, Frezieres RG, Peacock K, et al. Use of prostate-specific antigen (PSA) to measure semen exposure resulting from male condom failures: implications for contraceptive efficacy and the prevention of sexually transmitted disease. *Contraception*. 2003;67:139–150.

107. Zenilman JM, Yuenger J, Gala N, et al. Polymerase chain reaction detection of Y chromosome sequences in vaginal fluid: preliminary studies of a potential biomarker for sexual behavior. *Sex Transm Dis.* 2005;32:90–94.
108. Macaluso M, Lawson L, Akers R, et al. Prostate-specific antigen in vaginal fluid as a biologic marker of condom failure. *Contraception.* 1999;59:195–201.
109. Golden MR, Manhart LE. Innovative approaches to the prevention and control of bacterial sexually infections. *Infect Dis Clin N Am.* 2005;19:513–540.
110. Ward DJ, Rowe B, Pattison H, et al. Reducing the risk of sexually transmitted infections in genitourinary medicine clinic patients: a systematic review and meta-analysis of behavioural interventions. *Sex Transm Infect.* 2005;81:386–393.
111. Manhart LE, Holmes KK. Randomized controlled trials of individual-level, population-level, and multilevel interventions for preventing sexually transmitted infections: what has worked? *J Infect Dis.* 2005;191(Suppl 1):S7–S24.
112. Kamb ML, Fishbein M, Douglas JM Jr, et al. Efficacy of risk-reduction counseling to prevent human immunodeficiency virus and sexually transmitted diseases: a randomized controlled trial. Project RESPECT Study Group. *JAMA.* 1998;280:1161–1167.
113. O'Donnell CR, O'Donnell L, San Doval A, Duran R, Labes K. Reductions in STD infections subsequent to an STD clinic visit. Using video-based patient education to supplement provider interactions. *Sex Transm Dis.* 1998;25:161–168.
114. The National Institute of Mental Health (NIMH) Multisite HIV Prevention Trial Group. The NIMH Multisite HIV Prevention Trial: reducing HIV sexual risk behavior. *Science.* 1998;280:1889–1894.
115. Boyer CB, Barrett DC, Peterman TA, Bolan G. Sexually transmitted disease (STD) and HIV risk in heterosexual adults attending a public STD clinic: evaluation of a randomized controlled behavioral risk-reduction intervention trial. *AIDS.* 1997;11:359–367.
116. DiClemente RJ, Wingood GM, Harrington KF, et al. Efficacy of an HIV prevention intervention for African American adolescent girls: a randomized controlled trial. *JAMA.* 2004;292:171–179.
117. Orr DP, Langefeld CD, Katz BP, Caine VA. Behavioral intervention to increase condom use among high-risk female adolescents. *J Pediatr.* 1996;128:288–295.
118. Shain RN, Piper JM, Newton ER, et al. A randomized, controlled trial of a behavioral intervention to prevent sexually transmitted disease among minority women. *N Engl J Med.* 1999;340:93–100.
119. Richens J, Imrie J, Copas A. Condoms and seat belts: the parallels and the lessons. *Lancet.* 2000;355:400–403.
120. Cassell MM, Halperin DT, Shelton JD, Stanton, D. Risk compensation: the Achilles' heel of innovations in HIV prevention? *BMJ.* 2006; 332:605–607.
121. Kajubi P, Kamya MR, Kamya S, et al. Increasing condom use without reducing HIV risk: results of a controlled community trial in Uganda. *J Acquir Immune Defic Syndr.* 2005;40:77–82.
122. Imrie J, Stephenson JM, Cowan FM, et al. A cognitive behavioural intervention to reduce sexually transmitted infections among gay men: randomised trial. *BMJ.* 2001;322:1451–1456.
123. Smoak ND, Scott-Sheldon LA, Johnson BT, Carey MP. Sexual risk reduction interventions do not inadvertently increase the overall frequency of sexual behavior: a meta-analysis of 174 studies with 116,735 participants. *J Acquir Immune Defic Syndr.* 2006;41:374–384.
124. Steiner MJ, Cates W Jr, Warner L. The real problem with male condoms is nonuse. *Sex Transm Dis.* 1999;26:459–462.
125. Warner L, Steiner MJ. Condom access does not ensure condom use: you've got to be putting me on. *Sex Transm Inf.* 2002;78:225.

126. Cates W Jr, Steiner MJ. Dual protection against unintended pregnancy and sexually transmitted infections: What is the best contraceptive approach? *Sex Transm Dis*. 2002;29:168–174.
127. Crosby RA, Sanders SA, Yarber WL, et al. Condom use errors and problems among college men. *Sex Transm Dis*. 2002;29:552–557.
128. Steiner M, Piedrahita C, Glover L, Joanis C. Can condom users likely to experience condom failure be identified? *Fam Plann Perspect*. 1993;25:220–223,226.
129. Albert AE, Warner DL, Hatcher RA, Trussell J, Bennett C. Condom use among female commercial sex workers in Nevada's legal brothels. *Am J Publ Health*. 1995;85:1514–1520.
130. Cook L, Nanda K, Taylor D. Randomized crossover trial comparing the eZ·on plastic condom and a latex condom. *Contraception*. 2001;63:25–31.
131. Valappil T, Kelaghan J, Macaluso M, et al. Female condom and male condom failure among women at high risk of sexually transmitted diseases. *Sex Transm Dis*. 2005;32:35–43.
132. Macaluso M, Kelaghan J, Artz L, et al. Mechanical failure of the latex condom in a cohort of women at high STD risk. *Sex Transm Dis*. 1999;26:450–458.
133. Walsh TL, Frezieres RG, Peacock K, et al. Effectiveness of the male latex condom: combined results for three popular condom brands used as controls in randomized clinical trials. *Contraception*. 2004;70:407–413.
134. Mukenge-Tshibaka L, Alary M, Geraldo N, Lowndes CM. Incorrect condom use and frequent breakage among female sex workers and their clients. *Int J STD AIDS*. 2005;16:345–347.
135. Russell-Brown P, Piedrahita C, Foldesy R, et al. Comparison of condom breakage during human use with performance in laboratory testing. *Contraception*. 1992;45:429–437.
136. Silverman BG, Gross TP. Use and effectiveness of condoms during anal intercourse. A review. *Sex Transm Dis*. 1997;24:11–17.
137. Richters J, Kippax S. Condoms for anal sex. In: Mindel A, ed. Condoms. London: BMJ Publishing Group, 2000, pp 132–146.
138. Voeller B, Coulson AH, Bernstein GS, Nakamura RM. Mineral oil lubricants cause rapid deterioration of latex condoms. *Contraception*. 1989;39:95–102.

11

STI Vaccines: Status of Development, Potential Impact, and Important Factors for Implementation

Nicole Liddon, Ph.D., Gregory D. Zimet, Ph.D., and Lawrence R. Stanberry, M.D.

Primary prevention efforts for sexually transmitted infections (STIs) have historically focused on behavioral strategies, including encouraging abstinence, the delay of sexual initiation, careful partner selection, condom use, and partner management. Several potential emerging technologies, including microbicides and prophylactic vaccines, could add an additional focus to efforts to change individual sexual risk, at least in the case of certain STIs (1). One of the difficulties associated with traditional behavioral primary prevention efforts is that they seek to modify contextually complex, socially imbedded behaviors, such as condom use. The requirement for sustained behavior change over time adds to the difficulty of achieving long-term success with these kinds of interventions. In contrast, vaccination typically involves no more than three discrete events, which may be amenable to brief targeted interventions. The contextual complexity of vaccination is substantially less than with condom use, and effective vaccines would have no requirement for sustained behavior change. Efforts to encourage vaccination may need to differentially target specific immunization behaviors, including original and follow-up dosages, and possible booster shots.

Although getting vaccinated against an STI is, in many ways, a simpler behavior than consistent use of condoms in a sexual relationship, vaccination certainly will be uniquely challenging, requiring different approaches than those used to encourage safer sexual behaviors. It has been suggested that to have maximal impact, STI vaccination should occur prior to initiation of sexual activity, which often occurs during young adulthood (1–4). This suggestion to vaccinate adolescents is based on several considerations, including vaccine safety and efficacy studies among adolescents, data on STI epidemiology and age of sexual initiation in the United States, cost effectiveness evaluations, and established and recommended adolescent health care visits. Based on such considerations, the Advisory Committee on Immunization Practices

Behavioral Interventions for Prevention and Control of Sexually Transmitted Diseases.
Aral SO, Douglas JM Jr, eds. Lipshutz JA, assoc ed. New York: Springer Science+
Business Media, LLC; 2007.

(ACIP) unanimously voted in June 2006 to recommend a newly licensed HPV vaccine for routine delivery to females 11–12 years of age and for females 13–26 years of age who have not previously been vaccinated.

Available vaccines will need to be accepted and administered effectively to impact the rates of STIs. Strategies to enhance coverage rates will need to promote widespread acceptance by health care providers, parents, and adolescents. As a result, issues of great importance include infrequent adolescent health care visits, parental consent, provider recommendation, universal reporting, and cost of vaccination (including insurance coverage and coverage by the "Vaccines for Children" program). STI vaccine implementation will be aided by the development of a number of vaccines to immediately target this specific age group, including new pertussis and updated meningococcal vaccines. While a new focus on adolescent vaccines could benefit implementation of STI vaccines, there are also several issues unique to STI vaccines.

The main objectives of the chapter are threefold: 1) to review the current state of STI vaccine development overall, and possible population-level impact for the specific case of HPV; 2) to discuss program and research implications, including special target populations; and 3) to suggest possible behavioral interventions to increase vaccine coverage rates. It should be noted that there is some difficulty in discussing vaccines in various stages of development and the unforeseen subsequent behavioral interventions. This chapter is written from the perspective of a need for an integrated understanding of issues to this point and offers a starting line from which public health experts can anticipate the needs of the public in response to these emerging technologies.

Status of STI Vaccine Development

The development of effective STI vaccines has been ongoing in some cases since the 1920s and has been difficult because STI pathogenesis generally does not involve hematogenous spread of the organism, a step targeted by many highly effective vaccines such as those for measles and hepatitis B virus. The pathogenesis of most STIs involves local replication with spread, when it occurs, along contiguous surfaces (e.g., spread from the vagina to the uterus and fallopian tubes) or by nonhematogenous routes (e.g., intraneuronal spread of HSV). Historically, vaccines have not been very effective at providing durable protection against mucosal infection, although new advances in immunology hold the promise of developing more effective vaccines against mucosal infection.

Clinical trial design issues have also plagued STI vaccine development. For instance, should a vaccine prevent HSV infection or disease? Bacterial infections like pelvic inflammatory disease (PID) are troubled by imprecise measurement of the primary outcome measures. Study generalizability is also threatened by trial samples, which often have consisted of discordant couples or "at risk" populations rather than the general public.

Despite particularly difficult disease etiologies and design and measurement problems, advances in immunobiology and recent exciting clinical trial results point to the real possibility of developing vaccines to control some STIs in the near future. What follows is a general review of individual STI vaccine development histories and a closer look at mathematical modeling of the impact of an HPV vaccine in particular.

Chlamydia Trachomatis

Chlamydia trachomatis is a mucosal pathogen that, depending on the biovar, is capable of causing urogenital infections, trachoma, conjunctivitis, pneumonia, and lymphogranuloma venereum (LGV). Early attempts to develop a chlamydia vaccine focused on ocular trachoma. These early trials established successful protection against the strain of chlamydia used to prepare the vaccine; however, human trials of whole-cell vaccines were halted because of limited protection and significant safety concerns (5). As knowledge of the organism has increased, other candidate antigens have been identified that may provide protection against the various strains of chlamydia (6–8). Immune response to some have been somewhat favorable, but at least one has been hypothesized to cause autoimmune inflammatory damage similar to that which is seen with some chlamydial infections (9). The recent completion of the sequencing of the chlamydia trachomatis genome provides new information that will undoubtedly lead to the discovery of new candidate vaccine antigens.

In addition to the search for new antigens, researchers have also explored new means of delivering these vaccines, including DNA vaccines and vector systems (7,10). No reported clinical trials of chlamydia vaccines are currently ongoing and only one of the major vaccine companies, Sanofi Pasteur, has publicly identified chlamydia for long-term vaccine development.

Neisseria Gonorrhoeae

Development of a vaccine against gonorrhea has been hampered by the lack of an animal model and a limited understanding of what constitutes protective immunity. As with chlamydia genital tract infection, many immunologically diverse strains of *Neisseria gonorrhoeae* are capable of causing genital tract infection and this diversity poses a challenge to the development of a broadly protective vaccine. In addition, an initial infection with *Neisseria gonorrhoeae* appears to provide little protection against re-infection making an analysis of responses to natural infection of limited value in understanding what constitutes protective immunity (11). Among the current research are a focus on identification of particular proteins, the discovery of new antigens, and development of strategies for delivering subunits that are free of a contaminating protein (12). There are no gonococcal vaccine candidates currently in clinical trials, although Sanofi Pasteur has identified *Neisseria gonorrhoeae* as a target for long-term vaccine development.

Herpes Simplex Virus

Genital herpes may be caused by either herpes simplex virus type 1 (HSV-1) or type 2 (HSV-2), and, although these viruses differ somewhat in their genetic make-up, it is believed that immune responses produced by HSV-2 will likely protect against infection or disease caused by either virus type. Because HSV establishes latent infection and causes periodic recurrent infections, the development of both prophylactic and therapeutic vaccines have been attempted. A potential benefit of an effective therapeutic HSV vaccine would be to prevent viral shedding and thus reduce viral transmission to sexual partners (13,14).

Therapeutic HSV Vaccines

The past 15 years of commercial therapeutic HSV vaccine development has focused on several types of vaccines, including subunit glycoprotein vaccines, replication-impaired mutants genetically modified live virus, and DNA-based products (15). Cantab (Xenova) developed a replication-impaired viral vaccine by deleting a gene that is required for viral replication (16). After early phase I success, the vaccine failed in a phase II trial involving 483 patients who had frequently recurring genital herpes (17), and further development of the Cantab vaccine for therapeutic use is not planned. The Theraherp vaccine is a genetically attenuated mutant that is less virulent.

Prophylactic HSV Vaccines

In terms of prophylactic vaccines, in the past 15 years only two recombinant subunit glycoprotein vaccines have advanced to phase III clinical evaluation. The first, developed by Chiron was tested in two phase III studies, including one that enrolled 531 discordant couples and another that recruited 1862 volunteers from STD clinics (i.e., high-risk persons). The vaccine failed to achieve its primary outcome, prevention of HSV infection. Post-hoc analysis suggested a weak trend toward efficacy in women compared with men (18). A second prophylactic glycoprotein vaccine was developed by GlaxoSmithKline Biologicals (GSK) and evaluated in two phase III trials involving more than 3300 discordant couples. The primary outcome of the trials was prevention of symptomatic genital herpes. Prevention of infection was a secondary outcome measure in these trials. Both studies demonstrated vaccine efficacy of about 73% against acquisition of genital HSV-2 disease and an efficacy of approximately 40% in prevention of HSV-2 infection in HSV seronegative women, but no protection in men or HSV-1–seropositive women (19). A double-blind, randomized, controlled trial (Herpevac) co-sponsored by the National Institutes of Health and GSK is currently evaluating this vaccine further at more than 40 trial sites in the United States and Canada (20).

The reasons for gender-specific protection seen with both the prophylactic vaccines are unclear. Two possible, nonexclusive explanations have been suggested. The first is that men and women respond immunologically differently to these vaccines because the vaccines each contained new experimental adjuvants for which there was limited information regarding how the adjuvants might work in men compared with women. The second possibility is that the pathogenesis of infection is different in male and female genital anatomy and that the vaccines may better protect against infection initiated at a mucosal site (e.g., the vagina) than when virus entry is through abrasions in keratinized epithelia (e.g., the circumcised penis).

Human Papillomavirus

There are more than 30 human papillomaviruses (HPVs) known to infect the human anogenital tracts and cause an array of deleterious health effects including anogenital warts, cervical and anal dysplasia, and associated cervical, vaginal, anal, and penile cancers. Cervical cancer is by far the greatest public health burden of HPV and is a leading cause of mortality among women in developing countries. Because HPV infections can be persistent, efforts are underway to develop therapeutic vaccines to treat chronically infected patients as well as prophylactic vaccines to protect individuals from becoming infected or establishing a persistent infection. Each type of vaccine apparently works in a unique way. Antibody-mediated immunity seems to be important in prophylaxis and robust cell-mediated immunity is probably required to ensure long-term therapeutic success (21).

Because only limited amounts of some types of HPV can be grown using specialized tissue culture systems, traditional methods of development could not be used in developing an HPV vaccine. However, advances of molecular biologic techniques have allowed for the development of HPV-subunit and -vectored vaccines.

Therapeutic HPV Vaccines

There is much current interest in developing therapeutic vaccines that target HPV-associated dysplasia and neoplasia and anogenital warts. Strategies have included subunit vaccines containing potent adjuvants, live vaccinia virus engineered to express HPV gene products, and novel approaches such as HSP–HPV peptide vaccines and autologous dendritic cell vaccines. A therapeutic vaccine developed by GSK consisting of a mutated HPV protein and combined with an adjuvant system showed no clinical response in women who had HPV-16–positive cervical intraepithelial neoplastic (CIN) lesions (22). Xenova developed two products focused on neoplasia, one of which showed immunity and reduction in lesion size in women who had vulvar and vaginal intraepithelial neoplasia (23,24). German investigators evaluated a vaccine in 15 patients who had stage IV cervical cancer (25). The vaccine induced T-cell responses in 4 of 11 subjects, but no objective clinical response was observed. Another phase I/II trial evaluated an HPV-16 L1E7 vaccine in patients who had CIN II/III and found histologic responses in 50% of the vaccine recipients and 15% of the placebo recipients (26). There have been two reported studies of therapeutic vaccines targeting the treatment of anogenital warts. Xenova developed a fusion protein that, when tested among 27 men with genital warts, showed some response in all subjects, with five men clearing their warts within 8 weeks of completing the immunization series (27). GSK developed a therapeutic vaccine composed of a HPV-6 L2E7 fusion protein and their AS02A adjuvant. A total of 320 participants with HPV-6 and/or HPV-11 anogenital warts were studied in a design that compared vaccine or placebo administered along with standard therapy (e.g., either ablative therapy or podophyllotoxin). Although a positive trend toward clearance was seen in patients infected with only HPV-6, the therapeutic vaccination failed to increase the efficacy of the conventional therapies (28).

In considering the development of therapeutic vaccines for the treatment of cervical neoplasia it will be necessary for these products to be highly efficacious because the current surgical approach to the management of early-stage HPV-associated CIN has high cure rates. An acceptable alternative needs to produce higher rates of cure than clinical trials have thus far and further development of this approach is necessary before therapeutic vaccines will be an acceptable alternative to surgery.

Prophylactic HPV Vaccines

At the present time, there is one FDA-approved prophylactic vaccine and one in the final stages of clinical development. Both vaccines contain HPV types 16 and 18 L1 virus like particles (VLP), and one also contains HPV types 6 and 11 VLP, which would target the prevention of the common causes of genital warts. GSK is developing the bivalent vaccine, which is currently in phase III clinical trial, and Merck has received licensure for the quadrivalent one.

Initial analyses of more than 10,000 women showed that Merck's quadrivalent vaccine protected against high-grade precancer or noninvasive cancer.

There were no CIN2/3 or AIS cases reported among women receiving three doses of the vaccine GARDASIL, compared with 21 cases among subjects receiving placebo doses. The initial analysis followed women an average of 17 months (29). A second analysis, which followed a larger cohort of subjects for two years, showed 97% efficacy against the same negative outcomes (30). In a trial involving 1113 women, GSK found a bivalent HPV-16/18 VLP vaccine highly efficacious (94%) in preventing incident and persistent infections and cytologic abnormalities in fully immunized volunteers (31).

A third HPV-16 vaccine, developed by the National Cancer Institute, has been most recently evaluated in a placebo-controlled phase II trial involving 220 healthy female volunteers in whom the vaccine was shown to induce robust B- and T-cell responses (32,33).

Population-Level Effects of an STI Vaccine: The Case of HPV

Mathematical modeling studies suggest that an efficacious HSV-2 vaccine with widespread and universal implementation could significantly impact the HSV epidemic and ultimately reduce health care costs (34–36). More modeling research has examined the epidemiological impact and cost-effectiveness of an HPV vaccine, perhaps because it is the only currently licensed STI vaccine. These studies have employed different modeling techniques (Markov model of HPV natural history and cervical cancer, disease transmission model, or both), which caution against making direct comparisons of the models. For instance, cost-effectiveness estimates in a transmission model may be more favorable than those produced in Markov models due to the ability of the former to include potential impact of herd immunity.

Overall, published models have found that HPV vaccines could decrease cervical cancer and increase life expectancy as well as reduce the need for costly colposcopy, biopsy, and treatment. These models generally assume between 75% and 90% efficacy to prevent high-risk HPV types; and either 10 years of protection duration and a booster at age 22 (37,38) or no waning immunity (39). Age of vaccination was often varied by the modelers. One model (40) looked at the cost effectiveness of vaccinating only girls vs. both genders to test for population-level differences depending on policy recommendations.

Taira et al. (40) showed a 61.8% reduction in cervical cancer compared with current screening and a cost of $14,583 per quality-adjusted life years (QALY). These modelers also showed a 55% decrease in cancer cases if vaccination were delayed to age 18. If vaccine efficacy wanes over 10 years and no booster is provided, vaccination of 18 year olds is more cost effective than vaccination of 12 year olds. Goldie et al. (39) found a 58.1% reduction in cervical cancer compared with current screening with a cost of $24,300 per QALY. Kulasingam and Myers saw a 36% reduction in cervical cancer and at a cost of $44,889 per life year saved, but assumed some changes in screening practices that the other models did not (38). Several studies have evaluated the impact of vaccinating both males and females. These conclude that inclusion of men in vaccination programs has a moderate impact on cervical cancer incidence (35,40) with greater benefits of vaccinating men if coverage rates among women are lower (40).

HPV vaccination cost effectiveness may exceed the above estimates because of the potential for changes in screening. Much of the potential economic benefit of such programs would be realized only if initiation of Papanicolaou screening for cervical cancer were delayed until an older age, the interval between screenings were increased, or both. Such changes in screening might make an HPV vaccination program cost-effective compared with current cervical cancer screening. However, Hughes et al. (35) stress that vaccination will not reduce the need for Pap testing programs. The two HPV types (e.g., 16 and 18) covered by the currently licensed vaccine and another close to licensure are implicated in only 70% of all cervical cancers. The HPV types related to almost one-third of cervical cancers, then, will not be covered by initial vaccines.

Modeling Limitations

A number of unknown factors yet to be considered in modeling attempts might affect the economic and disease transmission analyses of an HPV vaccination program. For instance, it is unclear whether a vaccination program would effectively reach Americans who are least likely to be protected from cervical cancer by conventional screening programs. The corollary of this observation is that vaccination programs may favor those women who are already protected through utilization of screening. Also, we do not know whether vaccine-induced type-specific immunity shifts the epidemiology of HPV infection toward other potentially oncogenic types. Other HPV types may become more prevalent if vaccination reduced transmission of HPV-16 and HPV-18. Overall population-level effects might be affected by a change in health behavior, sexual, health seeking, or otherwise. For instance, might a delay of Papanicolaou screening create a dearth in other beneficial health care areas such as counseling for other STI and pregnancy prevention compared to initiating regular screening at a younger age? A possible unintended impact via an increase in risky behavior has not been considered in HPV vaccine modeling discussions as it has in HIV vaccine models and comments (41,42).

It should be highlighted that models assuming between 70% (37) and 100% (38,39) coverage rates were the most impacting and that uptake is cited as one of the most important factors affecting model outcomes. Coverage rates in models also assume that full coverage is achieved including completion of an initial three-dose series and subsequent booster approximately 10 years later. Without reaching such coverage rates in the real world, mathematical models of vaccine impact on disease epidemiology and health care expenditures may mean little. The assumed uptake emphasizes the need for effective implementation of vaccination programs that stress broad acceptance to ensure full coverage.

Special Populations: What Available Research Tells Us

As illustrated above, prophylactic vaccines will need to be widely accepted if they are to impact rates of STI and their sequalae and to be maximally effective. Because of efficacy results, average age of sexual initiation, and the logistics of an existing preadolescent health care visit, it is thought that the initial vaccines should be administered in early adolescence. Strategies to enhance the needed uptake will include behavioral interventions and public health efforts to promote extensive acceptance among adolescents as well as significant players in the administration of health care to young people, namely parents and providers.

A unique potential barrier to vaccine acceptance may include the stigma associated with vaccination against a disease that is sexually transmitted and the possibility that acceptance of the vaccine may be seen as an admission of risky sexual behavior (43). For instance, although HPV vaccines may be presented to adolescents and their parents as a vaccine to prevent cervical cancer, thereby avoiding or diminishing the STI issue, any vaccine that protects against the HPV types responsible for both genital warts and cervical cancer would likely be categorized as an STI vaccine.

It should also be noted that there is a real possibility of "catch-up vaccinations" and public demand to vaccinate older individuals who will need to be targeted with different and specialized messages than the groups listed above. Also not addressed here is the possibility of a booster shot as many as 10 years after the initial dose. A booster shot itself poses unique challenges of follow-up, education, and administration of healthcare. For instance, will 12 year olds, whose parents made the decision regarding initial vaccination, be willing at age 22 to get a booster on their own? Will they even know their vaccination status?

Available Research/Data

Most data presented here include prelicensure data on acceptability of STI vaccines. The problem with these data is that they are likely limited by the hypothetical nature of the topic. Respondents to surveys and focus group participants may not be able to realistically anticipate their future reactions when faced with real-life decisions about vaccination. However, results from acceptability/intention research provide some understanding of the attitudes surrounding STI vaccinations prior to initiating a widespread immunization program and suggest that parents, providers, and adolescents already have definite attitudes that may shape their behavior once vaccines become available. This research, therefore, allows the development of information provision strategies, prelicensure, to help parents, providers, and adolescents make informed decisions when vaccines become widely available.

Adolescent and Young People

Overall, studies of adolescent and young people show that they would be accepting of STI vaccines under certain conditions (see Table 1). Namely, vaccine characteristics play into young people's decisions about acceptability. In in-depth interviews with adolescent women attending health clinics, subjects were more likely to favor vaccines with low or no cost, as well as high efficacy, and vaccines that come with a physician recommendation (44). A study of young women recruited from community and clinical sites, found that approximately 85% of participants indicated an intention to receive an HPV vaccine for cervical cancer prevention once it became available (45) and that these women had broadly positive attitudes about many aspects of HPV vaccination. Interestingly, concerns about the STI issue in HPV vaccine acceptability research have so far not been supported empirically. In a study of young adult and adolescent women attending health clinics, there seemed to be no preference for a vaccine that prevented genital warts and cancer vs. one that protected against just cancer alone (44).

Table 1 STI vaccine acceptability among adolescents/young adults.

Study	Disease(s)	Correlates of acceptance/intention
Rosenthal et al., 1995	HBV	1. Perceived parental acceptance
		2. Belief in universal recommendation
Rosenthal et al., 1999	HSV	1. Low cost
		2. Belief in universal recommendation
		3. Perceived risk
Zimet et al., 2000	HPV	1. Efficacy
		2. Physician recommendation
		3. Low cost
Boehner et al., 2003	HPV	1. Parents' attitudes
	HSV	2. Vaccine beliefs
		3. Universal recommendation
		4. Number of sex partners
		5. Cost
		6. Vaccine safety
		7. Concern about finding future sex partners (only for HSV)
Kahn et al., 2003	HPV	1. HPV knowledge
		2. Vaccination beliefs
		3. Normative beliefs (partners, parents, health care providers)
		4. Number of sex partners
Zimet et al., 2005	Gonorrhea	1. Parental intent to vaccinate
	HSV	2. Peer sexual behavior
Slomovitz et al., 2006	HPV	1. Unknown adverse events (negative association)
		2. Lack of sexual activity (negative association)

If HPV vaccines are safe and efficacious in men and modeling indicates it would significantly impact the spread of disease without being too costly, vaccinating men may be an important public health strategy for prevention of cervical cancer in women. As well, men can develop both genital warts and anogenital cancers as a result of an HPV infection and vaccination may therefore additionally benefit their health. Research shows similar rates of intended uptake among men and women. In a study of both male and female college students, there were no significant differences in acceptance by gender (46). Both males and females were more likely to accept an HPV vaccine if it was recommended for universal coverage, did not cost a lot, and was safe. This study suggests that young people would be more accepting of a vaccine that is not aimed at specific high-risk groups, perhaps because targeted vaccination attempts would stigmatize and alienate populations.

This study also revealed that students with greater number of sexual partners were more likely to say they would get an STI vaccine perhaps out of an increased perceived risk of contracting HPV. This finding suggests the need for interventions that highlight the high risk of acquisition, especially of HPV and HSV, which are prevalent among sexually active young people even with fewer partners. Such education may increase perceived risk and thereby increase the intention to get vaccinated.

Finally, Boehner et al. (46) showed that subjects who thought their parents would support the vaccine were more likely to say they intended to get one. Likewise, other studies show that parental influence is important to young people when deciding about STI vaccines. One study found that adolescents were more likely to accept hepatitis B vaccination if they perceived it as important to their parents (47) and to accept a hypothetical HSV-2 vaccination if they thought their parents would encourage it (48). Zimet et al. (49) found that the most important predictor of adolescent acceptance of STI vaccination was corresponding parental acceptance. All of these findings point to the need for an understanding of parental attitudes toward potential STI vaccines and their perceived roles within that decision making process.

Parents

Intention to Vaccinate

Studies suggest that parents of adolescents generally find STI vaccines acceptable (see Table 2) (3,50–53) and contrary to popular belief and media reports (54), research indicates that the sexual transmission of disease does not influence parental vaccine acceptability. Mays et al. (51) found that most parents reported that STI vaccination was a parental responsibility.

Overall, parental STI vaccine acceptance relates to concepts identified in behavioral and psychosocial theories, like the Health Belief Model. Parental acceptance is higher among those who perceived their children to be at greater risk for infection and perceive greater severity of disease. One study showed that parents were more likely to accept vaccination if there was no behavioral intervention to prevent the disease (53). Vaccine characteristics including cost, efficacy, and schedule are also related to vaccine acceptability for parents.

Among parents who disapprove of or are undecided about STI vaccines, low knowledge of disease etiology and prevalence help explain their apprehension (51,52). Research further shows that these parents may become more accepting after education. Davis et al. (50) found that among parents recruited from both medical and community sites, about 23% would not accept an HPV vaccine and an equal number of parents were undecided. After reading a one-page information sheet about HPV including information addressing prevalence of infection, mode of transmission, and severity of sequelae, 20% of those parents who initially rejected the vaccine changed their minds and said they would accept one. Likewise, 65% of the undecided parents said they would have their children vaccinated after reading the educational material (50).

This study illustrates that a simple educational intervention can initially and instantly impact vaccine acceptability, at least in the case of an STI for which there is generally low knowledge, like HPV. Providing disease information may not work for STIs for which there is greater awareness. Also, this educational intervention seems to have had a greater impact on parents who were initially undecided, indicating that parents who reject a vaccine outright may

Table 2 STI vaccine acceptability among parents

Study	Disease(s)	Correlates of acceptance/intention
Lazcano-Ponce et al., 2001	HPV	1. Having multiple partners.
		2. Vaccine knowledge
		3. General vaccine acceptance
Davis et al., 2004	HPV	1. Belief that vaccination would encourage earlier initiation (negative association).
Mays et al., 2004	HPV	1. STI history
	Gonorrhea	2. Specific disease characteristics
	HSV	3. Sense of protecting child
		4. Parents who decline perceived low risk.
Liddon et al., 2005	HSV	1. Child vaccinated against flu
		2. Being single
		3. Being female
Olshen et al., 2005	HPV	1. Perceived risk of child
		2. Older age
Zimet et al., 2005	STIs	1. Severity
		2. Vaccine efficacy
		3. No behavioral intervention
Zimet et al., 2005	Gonorrhea	1. STI history
	HSV	2. Perceived severity
		3. Perceived risk of child
		4. Belief that vaccination would encourage earlier initiation (negative association).
Short et al., 2004	HSV	1. Administration in a SBHC
Slomovitz et al., 2006	HPV	1. Unknown adverse events (negative association)
		2. Perceived lack of sexual activity (negative association)

have other motivations for doing so and that intervention efforts may need to identify and address these unique objections.

Age of Vaccination
Published literature has identified another parental belief issue for public health practitioners to contend with; it is unclear whether parents will accept vaccination for the age groups for which recommendations are likely to be made. Although one study found that almost 70% of parents in the South would accept an HSV-2 vaccine for their child, more than half of those thought vaccination should take place later in adolescence (3). Zimet et al. (49) found a parental preference for HPV vaccination of adolescents age 17 and older. Likewise, focus groups on HPV vaccine showed some concern about vaccinating younger adolescents (52). These results highlight the need for public health efforts that not only encourage vaccination against STIs, but seek to

change parental attitudes about appropriate timing of the vaccination. Such efforts need to include messages for both parents and providers about the importance of early vaccination. In the case of the HSV-2 vaccine and in light of efficacy among double negative individuals, parents may feel more comfortable hearing that there is a need for patients to be seronegative for HSV-1, which is more likely at a younger age. This strategy could serve as a practical communication option for providers dealing with parents who may be influenced by the stigma of STIs.

Perceptions of Sexual Activity

One possible explanation for parental beliefs about appropriateness of STI vaccination at older ages is a general misperception about adolescent sexual activity. One study of urban African American adolescents and their mothers found that parents tended to underestimate the sexual activity of their teens (54). This finding was replicated in analyses of nationally representative data gathered from the National Longitudinal Study of Adolescent Health (55). In this study of 2006 14 and 15 year olds, a majority of mothers were unaware of their child's sexual activity. All adolescents in the study had never had sexual intercourse at the beginning of the study period. Researchers evaluated the associations between initiation of sexual intercourse and mothers' perception of whether their children were sexually active. Among students in 8th through 11th grades who had had sexual intercourse, 50% of the mothers of these students were not aware that their children were sexually active.

A telephone interview sponsored by a major television network of 1000 teens between 13 and 18 and their parents found that parents were unaware of their child's anticipation of sexual activity in general (56). The divergence continues when it comes to teens' actual behavior, with 27% of teens reporting sexual activity and only about half of their parents (15%) believing their teens had gone beyond kissing. One in-home intervention with parents, the IMPACT study, was effective in increasing parental monitoring (parental supervision and communication with their adolescents) and also of changing parent perceptions of their child's sexual activity (57). The intervention showed an initial baseline misperception by parents of their adolescent's risk including sexual activity. Six months after the intervention, report rates between both parent and child were more concordant. It is not clear, however, whether the increase in congruency of sexual report was a change in the child's behavior with increased monitoring (e.g., a decrease in sexual activity because parents were more involved with their child and supervised them more) or whether parents actually became more realistic about their child's sexual activity.

It is also unclear whether an intervention like the one mentioned above is necessary for changing perceptions about age of appropriate STI vaccination. Parental involvement interventions that increase specific knowledge of their child's sexual activity may be appropriate for parents of adolescents and for situations where sustained parental involvement is necessary because their children are making continual decisions about sex, such as whether or not to use a condom. They may not, however, be right for parents of preadolescents who need encouragement for one-time behavior modification like getting their child vaccinated. General information about average age of sexual initiation and the overall landscape of influences they can expect their child to experience in adolescence may be more helpful here. That is, a description of how teens encounter messages about sex daily in the media, school, and through interactions with peers, may be helpful in encouraging parents to become involved at an earlier age, including protecting them through vaccination. For vaccination purposes, it may not be necessary to address sexual activity of their particular child, but to perhaps educate parents about child development and average age of sexual initiation in general.

Parental Consent Issues

Another implementation issue pertaining to parents is obtaining consent/assent. This poses few problems in situations where parents and their preadolescent or adolescent children are both present. But, if adolescents are vaccinated in health care settings where they are not with a parent or guardian, then obtaining a signed consent form may prove difficult (58). Passive consent policies in school programs have helped resolve missed opportunities resulting from forgotten or lost signed consent forms for the provision of other health care, including condom availability programs. It is not clear, however, whether STI vaccinations will be, or can be, provided in schools under passive consent conditions.

Other policies will be necessary for settings where adolescents may seek care without their parents' awareness. In some situations, state laws allow minors to consent themselves for certain types of care including emergency services, reproductive health services, counseling and testing for substance use or drug and alcohol treatment, and outpatient mental health services. Every state has a law allowing minors to consent for diagnosis and treatment of STIs, although these laws vary based on the age and/or disease. Some include provisions covering services for prevention of STIs, which may allow administration of STI vaccination. Research shows that requiring parental consent for health care in some settings would discourage adolescents from seeking health care (59).

Provider Influence

Provider recommendation is one of the strongest predictors of parental acceptance of STI vaccines (50). This fact points to the importance of concurrent public health campaigns to increase STI vaccine acceptability targeting both providers and parents.

Providers

As evidenced above, health care providers are important sources of health information and parents respect physician recommendations about their child's health, including vaccines. Therefore, the success of HPV vaccination programs will depend largely on health care providers' (including nurses, pediatricians, family physicians, and others) willingness and ability to recommend STI vaccines to both the parents and patients. Vaccine recommendations should focus on providing disease and vaccine information as well as effectively communicating the advantages of vaccination (4).

Intent to Recommend

Previous studies of physician records demonstrated that factors associated with immunization practices for hepatitis B and in general include provider characteristics, knowledge and attitudes about vaccination (60,61). Although previous research on physician immunization practices can inform provider interventions, it may be limited by the nature of the immunization itself. Physician attitudes about recommending STI vaccines may differ from their attitudes about routine childhood vaccines. For example, providers may anticipate specific barriers to immunizing children vs. adolescents. They may also be more reluctant to suggest vaccination against STI that stem from a personal reluctance to discuss sexual activity with preadolescents or perceived parental resistance to STI vaccines.

Research supports this latter suggestion. A national study of pediatricians found that half (50.1%) perceived parental reluctance to have children immunized against a sexually transmitted infection as a potential barrier to vaccinating 10–15-year-old patients. Additionally, 26% of pediatricians surveyed feared that parents would think that their child was being singled out for vaccination because they were at risk for an STI (2).

Four research studies have been published on health care providers' attitudes about STI vaccination and others have thus far been presented at professional conferences or meetings (see Table 3). In one study, 224 nurses (predominantly pediatric nurse practitioners) rated their willingness to recommend the several different vaccines to parents of adolescents (62). In all, 13 vaccine scenarios were presented and varied according to patient age (11, 14, or 17 years old); infection prevented by the vaccine (mononucleosis, genital herpes, human immunodeficiency virus); gender of the patient; and whether the vaccine had been endorsed by the American Academy of Pediatrics (AAP). All vaccine scenarios were well received and overall attitudes towards recommending vaccination were positive. Nurses were more receptive to recommending a vaccine to older patients and with AAP endorsement. The disease and patient gender did not substantially influence likelihood to recommend.

Another study examined how 207 members of the American College of Obstetricians and Gynecologists (ACOG) rated willingness to recommend vaccine scenarios, but focused specifically on HPV vaccine alone (63). Each scenario was uniquely defined according to patient's age (13, 17, or 22 years old); vaccine efficacy (50% or 80%); ACOG recommendation (yes or no); and disease targeted (genital warts, cervical cancer, or both). Overall, mean willingness to vaccinate was high across all scenarios, but physicians rated vaccines with ACOG approval and higher efficacy most favorably. They were relatively less inclined to recommend a vaccine that only prevented genital warts or vaccination for younger patients (i.e., 13 year olds).

Data on pediatricians showed that those who were female and younger are more likely to recommend a vaccine to all ages and both genders (2). The researchers surveyed 513 members of the AAP by mail about intention to recommend each of two types of HPV vaccine (a cervical cancer/genital wart vaccine and a cervical cancer vaccine) to girls and boys of three different ages (11, 14, and 17). Results showed that pediatrician recommendation was positively associated with higher estimate of the percentage of sexually active adolescents in one's practice, number of adolescent patients seen in their practice, higher HPV knowledge, and AAP endorsement. On the contrary, pediatricians who perceived more barriers, including parental reluctance and concern, were less likely to recommend vaccinations. Another study by the same research team used a similar methodology and survey to examine family physicians' attitudes about adolescent HPV vaccine (64). Participants were

Table 3 STI vaccine acceptability among healthcare providers.

Study	Disease (s)	Correlates of acceptance/intention
Raley et al., 2004 (Gynecologists)	HPV	1. Older age of adolescent
		2. Vaccine type (cervical cancer and genital wart vs. single)
		3. Vaccine efficacy
		4. Professional organization endorsement (ACOG)
Mays and Zimet, 2004 (Nurse practitioners)	HSV	1. Professional organization (AAP)
		2. Older age of adolescent patient (17 vs. 14 and 11)
		3. More clinical involvement with adolescents
Riedesel et al., 2005 (Family practice physicians)	HPV	1. Patient gender (acceptance higher for girls)
		2. Patient age (acceptance higher for older adolescents)
		3. Vaccine type (acceptance higher for cervical cancer and genital wart vs. either one alone)
		4. Provider gender (females more likely to recommend)
		5. HPV knowledge
		6. Professional organization endorsement
		7. Perceived barriers
Kahn et al., 2005 (Pediatricians)	HPV	1. Older age of adolescent
		2. Estimate of patients who are sexually active
		3. Number of adolescent patients seen
		4. HPV knowledge
		5. Professional organization endorsement
		6. Perceived barriers
		7. Patient gender (acceptance higher for girls regardless of vaccine type)

significantly more willing to consider vaccinating older adolescents and female patients. Endorsement by professional organizations, such as the American Academy of Family Physicians (AAFP), also was important in determining recommendation.

There are several common findings across these studies that point to important areas of focus for public health professionals. First, approval by professional organizations is important, suggesting that endorsements by these organizations may be necessary for widespread utilization of STI vaccines by health care providers. It should be cautioned, however, that endorsement alone may not be sufficient for widespread adoption by providers. For instance, one study found that only 21% of pediatricians in one city were immunizing infants against hepatitis B virus (HBV) despite the recommendation of the AAP for universal infant HBV immunization (65).

There also may be a relative reluctance to vaccinate younger adolescents. As with parents, there appears to be a need for interventions that not only encourage vaccination, but also provide information to health care providers about the ideal age of vaccination. Since vaccination at younger ages was more accepted by providers who perceived a higher percentage of sexually active patients, intervention efforts should educate providers about the average age of sexual initiation and stress the need for immunization prior to such initiation.

In addition, research suggests that providers who believe that a discussion of adolescent sexuality will have to accompany a recommendation are less likely to recommend an HPV vaccine to their patients. Other research over the years has also documented the reluctance of health care providers to discuss the topic of sex with adolescent patients or parents (66,67). HPV vaccine campaigns targeted at providers will surely have to address how to encourage providers to broach the issue as well as increase their comfort with doing so.

Research suggests that age of adolescent was also important to this group, with preference for vaccinating at age 17 or 22 vs. age 13. This older age preference may result not from perceived age of sexual initiation, but from patient characteristics. It may be that obstetricians see fewer younger adolescents and thusly answered the age of delivery question in realistic terms, based on their daily practices.

Nurse practitioners (largely from pediatric practices) were also more likely to favor STI vaccines if they were recommended by the American Academy of Pediatrics (AAP) and for older adolescents (62). There was particular resistance to vaccinating younger adolescents without the professional endorsement. It is not clear from the research whether there is an interaction in these two significant findings and whether a professional recommendation could sway nurse practitioners to suggest vaccination for their younger patients.

Possible Public Health Efforts

Considering the only recent approval of an HPV vaccine, the hypothetical nature of others to prevent STIs and the lack of information on immunization in adolescents, the following are part of an emerging and ongoing discussion about strategies for vaccine implementation.

Lessons Learned

Several new vaccines are currently recommended for administration to the adolescent population and more are expected in the near future. All of these have some common issues such as poor health care utilization among adolescents and problems with parental consent. Each vaccine program and especially the case of STI vaccines, also has unique issues which makes identical implementation strategies impossible. Past experience can, however, suggest potential pitfalls and shed light on solutions that may be applied to STI vaccines. For instance, Varicella vaccine implementation suffered from variable "buy-in" among health care providers who were reluctant to suggest it for their patients amidst many competing health priorities. This history points to the need for upfront strategies such as professional organization endorsement, education aimed at increasing providers' awareness of STI vaccination as a health care visit priority, and limitation of clinic-level barriers such as vaccine supply and reimbursement. Perhaps the vaccine most suggested as a template for examining new STI vaccine implementation is that of the hepatitis B virus vaccine. During the 1980s, a risk-based strategy was suggested, which proved challenging on a number of levels. Traditional providers such as family practitioners and pediatricians found it difficult to implement without tools to determine risk status of adolescents that frequented these types of providers. It was suggested that a venue-based approach targeting the places frequented by high-risk youth frequent, such as STI clinics, was a better approach, but this approach resulted in little improvement in overall vaccination coverage rates. The overall failures of risk-based strategies led to a consensus that universal vaccination policies are likely to be more effective.

Although targeted venues may not work within a risk-based strategy, it may prove effective under a universal recommendation. Schools are obvious vaccination sites and junior high and middle schools in particular may provide an opportunity to reach all adolescents prior to the increasing drop-out rates that accompany transition to high school. Students who quit school at this point are likely to also be at greater health risk, including STI acquisition, and might not otherwise benefit from the new vaccines. Although resources are increasingly limited across the country, every school has the potential to at least promote adolescent immunization, if not administer it directly. One survey indicated that parental acceptance of an HSV-2 vaccine would increase if the vaccine were to be offered in a school-based health clinic (SBHC) (66).

School-based hepatitis B vaccine demonstration projects proved this point. These programs included special vaccine education for students, parents and teachers as well as reminders, recalls, and incentives for vaccination. These programs were evaluated and showed that high coverage rates are possible with well-organized, school based programs that subsidize vaccination and with concerted combined efforts of school administrators and employees, local, state, and federal health departments, parents, and community providers (67,68). Provision of free vaccine was essential to success: in one study of young adults in college and in which vaccine was promoted but not subsidized, only 1.9% of students were vaccinated (69).

State-enacted mandatory vaccination policies clearly would have the greatest public health impact for STI vaccination. Such laws are largely responsible for the dramatic increase in hepatitis B coverage among children and adolescents in a number of states (70,71). It is unclear, however, if laws mandating STI vaccination at middle school entry are likely to be passed. Given that such laws would have to be passed by legislatures on a state-by-state basis, it is unlikely that there will be significant mandates enacted in the near future.

Modifying Behavior

Some public health efforts for effective vaccine delivery programs will focus on modifiable factors associated with intention to recommend STI vaccination. Theories of health behavior including the Theory of Planned Behavior posit that specific factors like attitudes about a behavior and perceived risk and control, are causally associated with behaviors and may be changed via education or other behavioral intervention. Although some factors are not modifiable (e.g., provider age and gender, parents' STI history), others potentially can be changed and could be targeted in interventions to increase intention to recommend STI vaccines. For instance, interventions for providers that aim to lessen perceptions of parental refusal may lead to behavioral change around recommending a vaccine.

Increasing/Changing Knowledge and Attitudes About STIs

High acceptability of an STI vaccine depends somewhat on public perceptions of need, which hinges on knowledge about the specific STI, something that varies in U.S. samples. For instance, among university students, only 37% had ever heard of HPV (72) yet patients attending health clinics had higher rates of knowledge (67%) (73). Even among persons who have heard about HPV, studies show that misconceptions about the disease persist, including a lack of knowledge about the links between genital HPV infection, abnormal Pap smear results, and cervical cancer (73–76).

Overall, these findings suggest a need for education among young women and the parents of adolescents about HPV and HPV vaccination prior or simultaneous to vaccination attempts. It appears that more HPV information would be welcome as studies show that women are interested in learning about the transmission and prevention of HPV. Furthermore, a vast majority think that such information should be given to individuals prior to the initiation of sexual activity (73). Anhang et al. (77) similarly reported that the women in their study wanted more information about HPV transmission, prevention, treatment, and the risks associated with HPV infection.

Other findings are particularly relevant for physicians and emphasize the value of physician-provided education. Women who identified physicians as their primary source of information about HPV had higher HPV knowledge than those who identified other sources. Also, providers have been identified as important sources of education more frequently than health education classes, the Internet, friends, or family.

The conclusions suggested by the findings above are that women and young people need HPV information and are eager to hear it from their health care providers. But research on some providers points to additional public health needs. If, as stated earlier, vaccines are targeted at adolescents and young people prior to sexual initiation, pediatrician offices may be called upon to administer a majority of vaccines. Research shows that pediatricians know less about the sexually transmitted virus, perhaps as a result of less exposure in clinical practice to HPV-related disease compared with other providers who are more likely to see adult, sexually active patients.

Kahn et al. (2) found that HPV knowledge among a sample of 513 pediatricians was fair, with less than half correctly distinguishing the types associated with cervical cancer and genital warts and about one-third correctly approximating the prevalence of HPV infection in sexually active adolescents. Early results from another study show varying pediatrician HPV knowledge, with only one in five providers surveyed knowing the difference between types associated with genital warts and cervical cancer, but four in five identifying HPV infection as often asymptomatic (78).

Adolescent and adult women clearly want more information about infection, transmission, screening, and prevention of STIs, and they look to their providers for such education. However, this desire for information does not automatically imply that an STI vaccine will be widely accepted by women for themselves or for their children. We can logically expect, however, that, at a minimum, patients and parents will expect health care providers to offer information and guidance as vaccines to prevent STIs become available.

The Media and HPV Knowledge

With the availability of an HPV vaccine, there has been and it is expected that there will continue to be extensive media coverage, including information and discussions on the Internet. It also is predictable that some of the information will be misinformation. Recent news media coverage of HPV has been incomplete and, at times, misleading (77). There is reason to believe that the same will be true for information about an HPV vaccine. Rosenthal remarked that a 2005 newspaper article highlighted parents' caution about the HPV vaccine even though most scientific research suggested parental interest in HPV and other STI vaccines (79). Press coverage of vaccination programs in general often have an anti-immunization slant and patients who research vaccines on the Internet often come across anti-vaccination web sites (80).

Because accurate and balanced media reporting on medical issues can be a source of corrective education (81), efforts should focus on identifying accurate news and web-based information for patients, parents, and providers. Simple public health interventions could include brochures listing appropriate and up-to-date web sites for patients or communication to providers about HPV, the vaccine, and recommended guidelines for administration. One study by Gilbert et al. (82) identified frequently asked questions about HPV and developed brief and accurate answers to each. Such health communication projects, like answers to common questions, could readily be integrated into provider training or incorporated into written material and web sites. Concerted media campaigns could provide journalists with accurate disease and vaccine information as well as access to experts who can provide regular information.

Provider Recommendations

Research described here should reassure health care providers who might be concerned about offering or recommending STI vaccination to their preadolescent and adolescent patients. Women want more information on HPV and value information provided by health care providers. Also, most young women and parents hold positive views about STI vaccination for themselves and their children and the sexual transmissibility of a disease does not apparently present a significant barrier to vaccine acceptability for a majority of parents. The overriding concern for parents appears to be the protection of their children. Parents overwhelmingly look to physicians for recommendations regarding vaccination in general and this can be expected to remain true for any new STI vaccines. Health care providers should anticipate that parents will have varying attitudes about vaccination against an STI, including opposition that may come from either anti-vaccine attitudes in general or particular concerns about STI vaccines (4).

Several authors have suggested approaches clinicians can use to initiate and guide discussion with parents who are against or undecided about vaccination (83,84), including asking parents about what questions or concerns they have about vaccination. Any counseling efforts made by providers should take seriously parents' and adolescents' opinions about vaccination, even if the opinions are based on misinformation. People who feel respected and that their perspectives are considered may be more open to corrective information provided by the physician.

Ball (83) suggests a process of elicitation, listening, and respectful response. Diekema (85) emphasizes the importance of respectful discussion and includes excellent suggestions for responding to parents who oppose immunization.

Strategies suggested by Spigener and Mayeaux (86) for developing multiple approaches to deliver HPV-related information in busy office settings can be adopted for providing vaccine information. These include involvement of nurse educators to follow up and expand information provided by physicians. Also, the provision of clear and accurate written materials is important and should be the focus of health communication specialists. Anhang et al. (77) discuss health communication strategies and the importance of a "shared decision-making" approach between health care provider and patient. During this process, the health care provider offers information and asks for feedback from the patient so that, ultimately, an informed collaborative decision can be made regarding health care.

Important Cross-Cutting Intervention Components

Research and popular media reports indicate that some parental opposition to HPV vaccine acceptance is linked to the belief that vaccination against an STI will increase sexual risk among adolescents (49,52,87,88). Although at present it is not possible to assess whether vaccinated individuals will engage in more risky behavior, other adolescent research suggests against it. This belief is based on an assumption that the fear of HPV infection is motivation for safer sex or abstinence and removing that fear via vaccination will encourage sexual activity. However, research indicates that knowledge of HPV is low across populations (89,90) and nationally representative data show that fear of STIs (including other STIs and HIV) is not a major motivation for abstinence among young people (91). As well, other adolescent sexual behavior interventions like school-based condom availability programs and emergency contraception show no evidence of increased sexual risk among similar populations (92–95). Perhaps most importantly, there are multiple other factors associated with adolescent sexual behavior including parental, school, and community influences (96–100), and the decision for adolescents to have sex or not are rarely based on a single factor like fear of HPV.

Concerns about disinhibition in response to HPV vaccination can readily be addressed and do not diminish the tremendous promise of HPV vaccine and other STI vaccines. In fact, public health professionals and other interested groups can use implementation of STI vaccines as an opportunity to significantly improve adolescent and long-term adult health. The disinhibition hypothesis needs to be explored on a number of levels. Theoretically, beliefs about disinhibition affect all realms of public health and multiple types of intervention from new technology to policy changes. In terms specific to STI vaccines, we have the responsibility to monitor cohorts of immunized individuals post-licensure to ensure negative behavior change does not emerge in the population or subgroups to gauge changes in sexual risk and sexual health care seeking that may accompany an HPV vaccine. Monitoring unintended changes in sexual or health care–seeking behavior possibly resulting from availability of STI vaccines is necessary to allow for development of interventions to curb such changes before they lead to other negative health consequences.

Interventions to encourage STI vaccination should address the above-mentioned concerns as well as emphasize the risks associated with particular STIs (e.g., persistent infection with high-risk HPV types), but should be careful not to increase confusion or psychological stress (4). In addition, because STI vaccines will only offer protection against particular STIs (and in some cases only particular strains of STIs), vaccination will not preclude the need for regular sexual or reproductive health care and for continued risk behavior counseling. Franco and Harper (101) stress that it will be essential to ensure that recipients of an HPV vaccine know this and are encouraged to continue to get regular Pap testing because the vaccine will only provide protection against certain types of cancer-causing HPV strains and not all of them. Likewise, to counter-effect any possible reduced perception of acquiring an STI after being vaccinated, recipients should be counseled about the limitations of the vaccine to prevent all STIs and unintended pregnancies and about the merits of abstaining from sex or otherwise reducing the risk of other STIs via condom use.

Summary and Conclusions, Future Directions for Research

The recent and future development of STI vaccines presents a unique opportunity to provide adolescents with a package of preventive interventions that should be considered within the context of an overall health promotion approach. New or improved vaccines, including meningitis and pertussis, recommended for administration at preadolescence may help establish a standardized well-child health care visit at that age. A young adolescent health care visit at 11–12 years of age is currently recommended by professional organizations such as the American Academy of Pediatrics and the American Medical Association. Ultimately the success of prophylactic STI vaccines will depend on widespread implementation of such a visit.

If a well-adolescent visit is widely implemented, ensuring acceptance of STI vaccines will require concerted public health efforts aimed at adolescents, parents, and health care providers at all levels. An important component of such efforts should be providing groups with accurate and pertinent information on both the risks of disease and the benefits of a vaccine. This may take the form of educating providers and building skills to facilitate recommendations. Also needed at this level is adequate administrative support including sufficient reimbursement and vaccine supplies. Humiston and Rosenthal (102) propose methods to promote higher vaccination rates among adolescents, like the use of nontraditional settings for vaccine delivery and provider-based interventions (e.g., the use of standing orders).

Overall, numerous and simultaneous efforts are needed for all populations involved. Communication among all interested parties (including public health experts, policy makers, advocacy groups, and vaccine manufacturers) is key. These groups can learn some general operating guidelines from the implementation of upcoming HPV vaccines. However, unique disease-specific issues will still exist for other potential STI vaccines and will call for specific public health and research efforts.

References

1. Rupp RE, Stanberry LR, Rosenthal SL. Vaccines for sexually transmitted infections. *Pediatr Ann.* 2005;34:818–814.
2. Kahn JA, Zimet GD, Bernstein DI, Riedesel JM, Lan D, Huang B, et al. Pediatricians' intention to administer human papillomavirus vaccine: the role of practice characteristics, knowledge, and attitudes. *J Adolesc Health.* 2005;37:502–510.

3. Liddon N, Pulley L, Cockerham WC, Lueschen G, Vermund SH, Hook EW. Parents'/guardians' willingness to vaccinate their children against genital herpes. *J Adolesc Health*. 2005;37:187–193.

4. Zimet GD. Improving adolescent health: focus on HPV vaccine acceptance. *J Adolesc Health*. 2005;37:S17–S23.

5. Brunham RC, Zhang DJ, Yang X, McClarty GM. The potential for vaccine development against chlamydial infection and disease. *J Infect Dis*. 2000;181(Suppl 3):S538–S543.

6. Batteiger BE, Rank RG, Bavoil PM, Soderberg LS. Partial protection against genital reinfection by immunization of guinea-pigs with isolated outer-membrane proteins of the chlamydial agent of guinea-pig inclusion conjunctivitis. *J Gen Microbiol*. 1993;139:2965–2972.

7. Eko FO, He Q, Brown T, McMillan L, Ifere GO, Ananaba GA, et al. (). A novel recombinant multisubunit vaccine against Chlamydia. *J Immunol*. 2004;173:3375–3382.

8. Starnbach MN, Loomis WP, Ovendale P, Regan D, Hess B, Alderson MR, et al. An inclusion membrane protein from *Chlamydia trachomatis* enters the MHC class I pathway and stimulates a CD8+ T cell response. *J Immunol*. 2003;171:4742–4749.

9. Beagley KW, Timms P. *Chlamydia trachomatis* infection: incidence, health costs and prospects for vaccine development. *J Reprod Immunol*. 2000;48:47–68.

10. Turner MS, Giffard PM. Expression of *Chlamydia psittaci-* and human immunodeficiency virus-derived antigens on the cell surface of *Lactobacillus fermentum* BR11 as fusions to bspA. *Infect Immun*. 1999;67:5486–5489.

11. McKnew DL, Lynn F, Zenilman JM, Bash, MC. Porin variation among clinical isolates of *Neisseria gonorrhoeae* over a 10-year period, as determined by Por variable region typing. *J Infect Dis*. 2003;187:1213–1222.

12. Rokbi B, Renauld-Mongenie G, Mignon M, Danve B, Poncet D, Chabanel C, et al. Allelic diversity of the two transferrin binding protein B gene isotypes among a collection of *Neisseria meningitidis* strains representative of serogroup B disease: implication for the composition of a recombinant TbpB-based vaccine. *Infect Immun*. 2000;68:4938–4947.

13. Jones CA, Cunningham AL. Development of prophylactic vaccines for genital and neonatal herpes. *Expert Rev Vaccines*. 2003;2:541–549.

14. Jones CA, Cunningham AL. Vaccination strategies to prevent genital herpes and neonatal herpes simplex virus (HSV) disease. *Herpes*. 2004;11:12–17.

15. Stanberry LR, Cunningham AL, Mindel A, Scott LL, Spruance SL, Aoki FY, et al. Prospects for control of herpes simplex virus disease through immunization. *Clin Infect Dis*. 2000;30:549–566.

16. McLean CS, Erturk M, Jennings R, Challanain DN, Minson AC, Duncan I, et al. Protective vaccination against primary and recurrent disease caused by herpes simplex virus (HSV) type 2 using a genetically disabled HSV-1. *J Infect Dis*. 1994;170:1100–1109.

17. Stanberry LR. Clinical trials of prophylactic and therapeutic herpes simplex virus vaccines. *Herpes*. 2004;11(Suppl 3):161A–169A.

18. Corey L, Langenberg AG, Ashley R, Sekulovich RE, Izu AE, Douglas JM Jr, et al. Recombinant glycoprotein vaccine for the prevention of genital HSV-2 infection: two randomized controlled trials. Chiron HSV Vaccine Study Group. *JAMA*. 1999;282:331–340.

19. Stanberry LR, Spruance SL, Cunningham AL, Bernstein DI, Mindel A, Sacks S, et al. Glycoprotein-D-adjuvant vaccine to prevent genital herpes. *N Engl J Med*. 2002;347:1652–1661.

20. www.niaid.nih.gov website

21. Stern AM, Markel H. The history of vaccines and immunization: familiar patterns, new challenges. *Health Aff (Millwood)*. 2005;24:611–621.

22. Hallez S, Simon P, Maudoux F, Doyen J, Noel JC, Beliard A, et al. Phase I/II trial of immunogenicity of a human papillomavirus (HPV) type 16 E7 protein-based vaccine in women with oncogenic HPV-positive cervical intraepithelial neoplasia. *Cancer Immunol Immunother*. 2004;53:642–650.
23. Davidson EJ, Sehr P, Faulkner RL, Parish JL, Gaston K, Moore RA, et al. Human papillomavirus type 16 E2- and L1-specific serological and T-cell responses in women with vulval intraepithelial neoplasia. *J Gen Virol*. 2003;84:2089–2097.
24. Baldwin PJ, van der Burg SH, Boswell CM, Offringa R, Hickling JK, Dobson J, et al. Vaccinia-expressed human papillomavirus 16 and 18 e6 and e7 as a therapeutic vaccination for vulval and vaginal intraepithelial neoplasia. *Clin Cancer Res*. 2003;9:5205–5213.
25. Ferrara A, Nonn M, Sehr P, Schreckenberger C, Pawlita M, Durst M, et al. Dendritic cell-based tumor vaccine for cervical cancer II: results of a clinical pilot study in 15 individual patients. *J Cancer Res Clin Oncol*. 2003;129:521–530.
26. Schreckenberger C, Kaufmann AM. Vaccination strategies for the treatment and prevention of cervical cancer. *Curr Opin Oncol*. 2004;16:485–491.
27. Lacey CJ, Thompson HS, Monteiro EF, O'Neill T, Davies ML, Holding FP, et al. Phase IIa safety and immunogenicity of a therapeutic vaccine, TA-GW, in persons with genital warts. *J Infect Dis*. 1999;179:612–618.
28. Vandepapeliere P, Barrasso R, Meijer CJ, Walboomers JM, Wettendorff M, Stanberry LR, et al. Randomized controlled trial of an adjuvanted human papillomavirus (HPV) type 6 L2E7 vaccine: infection of external anogenital warts with multiple HPV types and failure of therapeutic vaccination. *J Infect Dis*. 2005; 192:2099–2107.
29. Koutsky LA, Ault KA, Wheeler CM, Brown DR, Barr E, Alvarez FB, et al. A controlled trial of a human papillomavirus type 16 vaccine. *N Engl J Med*. 2002; 347:1645–1651.
30. Skjeldestad FE. Prophylactic Quadrivalent Human Papillomavirus (HPV (Types 6,11,16,18) L1 Virus Like Particle (VLP) vaccine (Gardisil™) Reduces Cervical Intraepilthelial Neoplasia (CIN) 2/3 Risk. Presentation to the Infectious Disease Society of America meeting. October 2005; San Francisco.
31. Harper DM, Franco EL, Wheeler C, Ferris DG, Jenkins D, Schuind A, et al. Efficacy of a bivalent L1 virus-like particle vaccine in prevention of infection with human papillomavirus types 16 and 18 in young women: a randomised controlled trial. *Lancet*. 2004;364:1757–1765.
32. Harro CD, Pang YY, Roden RB, Hildesheim A, Wang Z, Reynolds MJ, et al. Safety and immunogenicity trial in adult volunteers of a human papillomavirus 16 L1 virus-like particle vaccine. *J Natl Cancer Inst*. 2001;93:284–292.
33. Pinto LA, Edwards J, Castle PE, Harro CD, Lowy DR, Schiller JT, et al. Cellular immune responses to human papillomavirus (HPV)-16 L1 in healthy volunteers immunized with recombinant HPV-16 L1 virus-like particles. *J Infect Dis*. 2003; 188:327–338.
34. Garnett GP, Dubin G, Slaoui M, Darcis T. The potential epidemiological impact of a genital herpes vaccine for women. *Sex Transm Infect*. 2004;80:24–29.
35. Hughes JP, Garnett GP, Koutsky L. The theoretical population-level impact of a prophylactic human papilloma virus vaccine. *Epidemiology*. 2002;13:631–639.
36. Schwartz E J, Blower S. Predicting the potential individual- and population-level effects of imperfect herpes simplex virus type 2 vaccines. *J Infect Dis*. 2005; 191:1734–1746.
37. Sanders GD, Taira AV. Cost-effectiveness of a potential vaccine for human papillomavirus. *Emerg Infect Dis*. 2003;9:37–48.
38. Kulasingam SL, Myers ER. Potential health and economic impact of adding a human papillomavirus vaccine to screening programs. *JAMA*. 2003;290:781–789.

39. Goldie SJ, Kohli M, Grima D, Weinstein MC, Wright TC, Bosch FX, et al. Projected clinical benefits and cost-effectiveness of a human papillomavirus 16/18 vaccine. *J Natl Cancer Inst.* 2004;96:604–615.

40. Taira AV, Neukermans CP, Sanders GD. Evaluating human papillomavirus vaccination programs. *Emerg Infect Dis.* 2004;10:1915–1923.

41. Smith RJ, Blower SM. Could disease-modifying HIV vaccines cause population-level perversity? *Lancet Infect Dis.* 2004;4:636–639.

42. Blower SM, McLean AR. Prophylactic vaccines, risk behavior change, and the probability of eradicating HIV in San Francisco. *Science.* 1994;265:1451–1454.

43. Zimet GD, Mays RM, Fortenberry JD. Vaccines against sexually transmitted infections: promise and problems of the magic bullets for prevention and control. *Sex Transm Dis.* 2000;27:49–52.

44. Zimet GD, Mays RM, Winston Y, Kee R, Dickes J, Su L. Acceptability of human papillomavirus immunization. *J Womens Health Gend Based Med.* 2000;9:47–50.

45. Kahn JA, Rosenthal SL, Hamann T, Bernstein DI. Attitudes about human papillomavirus vaccine in young women. *Int J STD AIDS.* 2003;14:300–306.

46. Boehner CW, Howe SR, Bernstein DI, Rosenthal SL. Viral sexually transmitted disease vaccine acceptability among college students. *Sex Transm Dis.* 2003;30:774–778.

47. Rosenthal SL, Kottenhahn RK, Biro FM, Succop PA. Hepatitis B vaccine acceptance among adolescents and their parents. *J Adolesc Health.* 1995;17:248–254.

48. Rosenthal SL, Lewis LM, Succop PA, Bernstein DI, Stanberry LR. College students' attitudes regarding vaccination to prevent genital herpes. *Sex Transm Dis.* 1999;26:438–443.

49. Zimet GD, Perkins SM, Sturm LA, Bair RM, Juliar BE, Mays RM. Predictors of STI vaccine acceptability among parents and their adolescent children. *J Adolesc Health.* 2005;37:179–186.

50. Davis K, Dickman ED, Ferris D, Dias JK. Human papillomavirus vaccine acceptability among parents of 10- to 15-year-old adolescents. *J Low Genit Tract Dis.* 2004;8:188–194.

51. Mays RM, Sturm LA, Zimet GD. Parental perspectives on vaccinating children against sexually transmitted infections. *Soc Sci Med.* 2004;58:1405–1413.

52. Olshen E, Woods ER, Austin SB, Luskin M, Bauchner H. Parental acceptance of the human papillomavirus vaccine. *J Adolesc Health.* 2005;37:248–251.

53. Zimet GD, Mays RM, Sturm LA, Ravert AA, Perkins SM, Juliar BE. Parental attitudes about sexually transmitted infection vaccination for their adolescent children. *Arch Pediatr Adolesc Med.* 2005;159:132–137.

54. Jaccard J, Dittus PJ, Gordon VV. Parent-adolescent congruency in reports of adolescent sexual behavior and in communications about sexual behavior. *Child Dev.* 1998;69:247–261.

55. McNeely C, Shew ML, Beuhring T, Sieving R, Miller BC, Blum RW. Mothers' influence on the timing of first sex among 14- and 15-year-olds. *J Adolesc Health.* 2002;31:256–265.

56. The 411 about Teens and Sex web site. Available at http://www.msnbc.msn.com/id/6872269 (accessed March 20, 2006).

57. Stanton BF, Li X, Galbraith J, Cornick G, Feigelman S, Kaljee L, Zhou Y. Parental underestimates of adolescent risk behavior: a randomized, controlled trial of a parental monitoring intervention. *J Adolesc Health.* 2000;26:18–26.

58. Deeks SL, Johnson IL. Vaccine coverage during a school-based hepatitis B immunization program. *Can J Public Health.* 1998;89:98–101.

59. Jones RK, Boonstra H. Confidential reproductive health services for minors: the potential impact of mandated parental involvement for contraception. *Perspect Sex Reprod Health.* 2004;36:182–191.

60. Freed GL, Bordley WC, Clark SJ, Konrad TR. Universal hepatitis B immunization of infants: reactions of pediatricians and family physicians over time. *Pediatrics*. 1994;93:747–751.
61. Loewenson PR, White KE, Osterholm MT, MacDonald KL. Physician attitudes and practices regarding universal infant vaccination against hepatitis B infection in Minnesota: implications for public health policy. *Pediatr Infect Dis J*. 1994;13:373–378.
62. Mays RM, Zimet GD. Recommending STI vaccination to parents of adolescents: the attitudes of nurse practitioners. *Sex Transm Dis*. 2004;31:428–432.
63. Raley JC, Followwill KA, Zimet GD, Ault KA. Gynecologists' attitudes regarding human papilloma virus vaccination: a survey of Fellows of the American College of Obstetricians and Gynecologists. *Infect Dis Obstet Gynecol*. 2004; 12:127–133.
64. Riedesel JM, Rosenthal SL, Zimet GD, Bernstein DI, Huang B, Lan D, et al. Attitudes about human papillomavirus vaccine among family physicians. *J Pediatr Adolesc Gynecol*. 2005;18:391–398.
65. Siegel RM, Baker RC, Kotagal UR, Balistreri WF. Hepatitis B vaccine use in Cincinnati: a community's response to the AAP recommendation of universal hepatitis B immunization. *J Natl Med Assoc*. 1994;86:444–448.
66. Short MB, Rupp R, Stanberry LR, Rosenthal SL. Parental acceptance of adolescent vaccines within school-based health centres. *Herpes*. 2005;12:23–27.
67. Molliconi SA, Zink T. Managed care organizations and public health: exploring collaboration on adolescent immunizations. *J Sch Health*. 1997;67:286–289.
68. Harris PA, Kerr J, Steffen D. A state-based immunization campaign: the New Mexico experience. *J Sch Health*. 1997;67:273–276.
69. Marron RL, Lanphear BP, Kouides R, Dudman L, Manchester RA, Christy C. Efficacy of informational letters on hepatitis B immunization rates in university students. *J Am Coll Health*. 1998;47:123–127.
70. Fogarty KJ, Massoudi MS, Gallo W, Averhoff FM, Yusuf H, Fishbein D. Vaccine coverage levels after implementation of a middle school vaccination requirement, Florida, 1997–2000. *Public Health Rep*. 2004;119:163–169.
71. Averhoff F, Linton L, Peddecord KM, Edwards C, Wang W, Fishbein D. A middle school immunization law rapidly and substantially increases immunization coverage among adolescents. *Am J Public Health*. 2004;94:978–984.
72. Yacobi E, Tennant C, Ferrante J, Pal N, Roetzheim R. University students' knowledge and awareness of HPV. *Prev Med*. 1999;28:535–541.
73. Holcomb B, Bailey JM, Crawford K, Ruffin MT. Adults' knowledge and behaviors related to human papillomavirus infection. *J Am Board Fam Pract*. 2004;17:26–31.
74. Dell DL, Chen H, Ahmad F, Stewart DE. Knowledge about human papillomavirus among adolescents. *Obstet Gynecol*. 2000;96:653–656.
75. Pitts M, Clarke T. Human papillomavirus infections and risks of cervical cancer: what do women know? *Health Educ Res*. 2002;17:706–714.
76. Waller J, McCaffery K, Forrest S, Szarewski A, Cadman L, Wardle J. Awareness of human papillomavirus among women attending a well woman clinic. *Sex Transm Infect*. 2003;79:320–322.
77. Anhang R, Stryker JE, Wright TC Jr, Goldie SJ. News media coverage of human papillomavirus. *Cancer*. 2004;100:308–314.
78. Daley MF, Liddon N, Crane LA, Beaty BL, Barrow J, Babbel C, Markowitz L, Dunne EF, Stokley S, Dickinson LM, Berman S, Kempe A. A National Survey of Pediatrician Knowledge and Attitudes Regarding Human Papillomavirus Vaccination. *Pediatrics*. 2006;188(6):2280–2289.
79. Rosenthal SL, Stanberry LR. Parental acceptability of vaccines for sexually transmitted infections. *Arch Pediatr Adolesc Med*. 2005;159:190–192.
80. Davies P. Anti-vaccination websites. *JAMA*. 2002;288:1717.

81. Lashuay N, Tjoa T, Zuniga de Nuncio ML, Franklin M, Elder J, Jones M. Exposure to immunization media messages among African American parents. *Prev Med*. 2000;5:522–528.
82. Gilbert LK, Alexander L, Grosshans JF, Jolley L. Answering frequently asked questions about HPV. *Sex Transm Dis*. 2003;30:193–194.
83. Ball LK, Evans G, Bostrom A. Risky business: challenges in vaccine risk communication. *Pediatrics*. 1998;101:453–458.
84. Sturm LA, Mays RM, Zimet GD. Parental beliefs and decision making about child and adolescent immunization: from polio to sexually transmitted infections. *J Dev Behav Pediatr*. 2005;26:441–452.
85. Diekema DS. Responding to parental refusals of immunization of children. *Pediatrics,* 2005;115:1428–1431.
86. Spigener SD, Mayeaux EJ. Patient education and issues of HPV infection. *Hosp Pract*. 1998;33:133–135.
87. Washam C. Targeting teens and adolescents for HPV vaccine could draw fire. *J Natl Cancer Inst*. 2005;97:1030–1031.
88. Stanberry LR, Rosenthal SL. Progress in vaccines for sexually transmitted diseases. *Infect Dis Clin North Am*. 2005;19:477–490, xi.
89. Dell DL, Chen H, Ahmad F, Stewart DE. Knowledge about human papillomavirus among adolescents. *Obstet Gynecol*. 2000;96:653–656.
90. Pitts M, Clarke T. Human papillomavirus infections and risks of cervical cancer: What do women know? *Health Education Research* 2002;17:706–714.
91. Abma JC, Martinez GM, Mosher WD, Dawsom BS. Teenagers in the United States: sexual activity, condom use and childbearing, 2002. *Vital and Health Statistics*. 2004; Series 23, No. 24.
92. Kirby D. The impact of schools and school programs upon adolescent sexual behavior. *J Sex Res* 2002;39:27–33.
93. Raine T, Harper C, Leon K, Darney P. Emergency contraception: advance provision in a young, high-risk clinic population. *Obstet Gynecol*. 2000;96:1–7.
94. Raine TR, Harper CC, Rocca CH, Fischer R, Padian N, Klausner JD, Darney PD. Direct access to emergency contraception through pharmacies and effect on unintended pregnancy and STIs: a randomized controlled trial. *JAMA*. 2005;293:54.
95. Schuster MA, Bell RM, Berry SH, Kanouse DE. Impact of a high school condom availability program on sexual attitudes and behaviors. *Fam Plann Perspect*. 1998;30:67–72.
96. Averett SL, Rees DI, Argys LM. The impact of government policies and neighborhood characteristics on teenage sexual activity and contraceptive use. *Am J Public Health*. 2002;92:1773–1778.
97. Stanton B, Li X, Pack R, Cottrel L, Harris, C, Burns JM. Longitudinal influence of perceptions of peer and parental factors on African American adolescent risk involvement. *J Urban Health* 2002;79:536–548.
98. Whitaker DJ, Miller KS, May DC, Levin ML. Teenage partners' communication about sexual risk and condom use: the importance of parent-teenager discussions. *Fam Plann Perspect* 1999;31:117–121.
99. Cohen DA, Farley TA, Taylor SN, Martin DH, Schuster MA. When and where do youth have sex? The potential role of adult supervision. *Pediatrics*. 2002;110:e66.
100. Lonczak HS, Abbott RD, Hawkins JD, Kosterman R, Catalano RF. Effects of the Seattle social development project on sexual behavior, pregnancy, birth, and sexually transmitted disease outcomes by age 21 years. *Arch Pediatr Adolesc Med*. 2002;156:438–447.
101. Franco EL, Harper DM. Vaccination against human papillomavirus infection: a new paradigm in cervical cancer control. *Vaccine*. 2005;23:2388–2394.
102. Humiston SG, Rosenthal SL. Challenges to vaccinating adolescents: vaccine implementation issues. *Pediatr Infect Dis J*. 2005;24:S134–S140.

Part 3

Interventions by Population

12

Behavioral Interventions for Prevention and Control of STDs Among Adolescents

Kathleen A. Ethier, Ph.D., and Donald P. Orr, M.D.

For the last several decades, public health professionals have increasingly recognized that the burden of sexually transmitted infections (STIs) is disproportionately high among adolescents and young adults. *The Hidden Epidemic*, the 1997 seminal report of the Institute of Medicine, clearly identified adolescents as a population at high risk for STIs (1). There has been a concerted effort to track rates of STI in this population, investigate its causes, and develop interventions to reduce risk and associated disease. In this chapter, we will define the burden of STI among youth, review behavioral and biological risk for STI, and discuss the current literature on effective adolescent risk reduction interventions.

We will take an ecological or social context approach that acknowledges the impact of social environmental factors on health and, therefore, intervention strategy (2). By social context, we mean the important people (e.g., peers, parents), places (e.g., neighborhoods), institutions (e.g., schools, health care organizations), and societal processes (e.g., culture, policy) that can influence adolescent behavior and health. As a period of biologic, cognitive, and psychosocial transitions, adolescence may be more sensitive to contextual influences than other periods. Biologic, cognitive, and social changes during adolescence can affect behaviors and relationships and require guidance from important others and institutions that may not be prepared for their roles. For example, peers share information that may not be correct, parents may not recognize adolescent risk behavior, and schools may be too politically or financially challenged to provide effective prevention programming. In our review, we will identify the social context influences on adolescent risk for STIs and intervention strategies designed to address those influences.

The difficulties in determining burden, risk, and intervention strategies for adolescents are numerous. First, the age range that constitutes adolescence is ill defined. Risks for STI may start before puberty, especially when familial, biologic, and environmental factors are taken into account. The average age of puberty has decreased, with at least the physical aspect of adolescence starting earlier. The implications of teenage risk factors for young adulthood suggest that we must look further into the future to examine the impact of prevention strategies (3). There also appear to be distinct periods and transition points within adolescence that may lead to increased risk behavior, such as the move

Behavioral Interventions for Prevention and Control of Sexually Transmitted Diseases. Aral SO, Douglas JM Jr, eds. Lipshutz JA, assoc ed. New York: Springer Science+ Business Media, LLC; 2007.

from middle school to high school or when a teenager gets a driver's license. Surveillance studies, etiologic studies, and intervention studies may define adolescence differently or may focus on a particular age range within adolescence. Looking across these different approaches to summarize the findings is difficult.

The nature of the adolescent's sexual experience within the context of US society is also a challenge for STI prevention. The vast majority of research on adolescent sexuality in the biomedical literature relates to coitus as a risk factor for STIs and pregnancy. The context of coitus as related to adolescent psychosocial development and the positive aspects such as pleasure, enhancement of interpersonal relationships, desire for parenthood, and rehearsal for adult roles is often left out of attempts to prevent the biomedical consequences of adolescent sexuality. In contrast to public perceptions of the positive aspects of adult sexuality, there is a general lack of awareness and understanding that adolescent sexual behaviors serve these multiple functions and that they have multiple determinants (4). Although sexual activity among American adolescents is an important public health and social concern, with the exception of HPV, most adolescents do not acquire an STI despite being sexually active. Viewing sexual activity as solely a risk behavior may lead to the development of overly simplified (largely ineffective) interventions to control coitus and STIs. Such interventions are costly in terms of financial resources and may have both negative developmental and biological outcomes (3). U.S. attitudes about sexuality make research on adolescent sexuality difficult and tend to impede the development and implementation of potentially effective interventions to prevent STI. As we will discuss in this chapter, the majority of adolescents initiate sexual activity before they leave high school. The early high school years appear to be a transition point for most. The factors that underlie early versus later sexual debut and the risks associated with that sexual activity differ. Prevention techniques appear to be ineffective if they fail to address where an adolescent is in that process.

Finally, we are challenged by the fact that most of our models for understanding STI risk and prevention have been developed with and for adults. Evidence suggests that adolescents are not "little adults." The nature of their risk, the underlying factors associated with that risk, and effective modes of prevention may be relatively unique to this life-stage. At the same time, the health behaviors developed during this time have long-term implications for health in the following stages, making intervention during this period essential. As public health professionals, this is our challenge—to reduce disease and to promote health so that our youth can become healthy adults.

The Burden of STDs Among Adolescents

We can examine the burden of STI among youth through several sources of data: Centers for Disease Control and Prevention (CDC) data on reportable STDs (chlamydia, gonorrhea and syphilis), data collected as part of the CDC Prevalence Monitoring Project, and school-based screening studies. Each of these sources of data is imperfect on its own, and the limits of each will be discussed. However, taken together they give us an idea of how much disease is likely to be present and where it resides.

Centers for Disease Control and Prevention Surveillance Data

The CDC collects reports on chlamydia, gonorrhea, syphilis, chancroid, and hepatitis B and C. In 2002, STDs were reported at the highest rates of any reportable disease. In 2004, 929,462 cases of chlamydia and 330,132 cases of gonorrhea were reported, translating into an overall rate of 319.6 per 100,000 for chlamydia and 113.5 per 100,000 of gonorrhea. The Healthy People 2010 goal for gonorrhea is 19 per 100,000. Of the reported cases in 2004, 35% of chlamydia cases and 27% of gonorrhea cases were reported among adolescents ages 15–19. Rates of chlamydia and gonorrhea are higher among 15–19-year-old females than any age or gender group representing rates of 2,761.5 per 100,000 for chlamydia and 610.9 per 100,000 for gonorrhea. Chlamydia and gonorrhea rates are higher among female adolescents as compared with males, and higher among black youth as compared with whites or Hispanic youth. While case report data provide excellent information regarding infection rates, they require that individuals be diagnosed and do not address prevalence of disease or the burden of STIs other than those that are currently reportable. A major concern with adolescents is that they may not get regularly screened for STIs and are probably less likely to get screened than adults, leading to an underestimate of the actual presence of STI in this population. Also, roughly half of teenagers ages 15–19 have initiated sex while a much higher proportion of adults are sexually experienced. Although rates can be corrected for sexual activity (5), surveillance reports do not take sexual activity into account and so the rates of STI among sexually active youth—those at risk for infection and transmission—are substantially higher than those in adults.

Prevalence Monitoring Studies

Chlamydia screening programs among women in family planning clinics in the 10 HHS regions, entrants to Job Corps programs and among female adolescents in juvenile detention centers provide prevalence estimates for this organism. In 2003, positivity rates in family planning regions among 15–19-year-old females ranged from 5.9% to 13.9%. The Healthy People 2010 goal for chlamydia positivity among 15–24-year-old women in family planning clinics is 3.0%. In general, rates in the HHS regions have held steady and rates were highest in the south (13.9% in Region VI and 11.8% in Region IV) and in Region 2 (12.9%), which includes New York. Similar regional patterns are evident in data collected among Job Corps entrants and young women in juvenile detention.

These data provide excellent information on prevalence in higher risk populations, particularly sexually active females. They are not representative of the general population of youth and may not include the highest risk women, such as those with no access to health care, since screening occurred through their health care provider in most cases.

School-Based Screening

Screening high school populations for chlamydia provides insight into the prevalence of disease in school-based populations, which likely best represents the general population of adolescents. Several reports provide data on screening in public high schools. In a Louisiana study, 6.5% of students screened (without regard to the presence of symptoms) tested positive for *C. trachomatis*, including 9.7% of females and 4.0% of males (6). In San Francisco, 0.8% of asymptomatic males and 3.9% of asymptomatic females were infected with *C. trachomatis* (7). In Philadelphia, 5.3% of all students screened were found to be infected with *C. trachomatis* including 7.9% of females and 2.6% of males (8).

School screening attempts to reach the majority of youth and thus provides one snapshot of the prevalence of STI in a general population. However, it has limitations. It may miss the youth at highest risk because they are not in school, parents may differentially consent to their adolescent's participation, and some youth may refuse to provide biological samples. As discussed later in this chapter, many adolescents become sexually experienced during high school and the percentage of high school students who are sexually active ranges from 32.8% in 9th grade to 63.5% in 12th grade (9). Any over-sampling of younger or older students can dramatically impact the results. Further, we know very little about the biases inherent in willingness to provide samples for testing.

Summary of Epidemiologic Data

Taken together, these data indicate that the burden of STIs in youth is high. Youth ages 15–24 years (and 15–19-year-old females in particular) have highest rates of bacterial genitourinary infections of any age group. Prevalence estimates range depending on disease, population and geographic region with the highest rates in the southeast and among urban, poor populations, especially African-Americans. It is estimated that between 6% and 16% of adolescent/young adult females are infected with *C. trachomatis*, with lower estimates for males. Weinstock et al. (10) estimate that, of the approximately 18.9 million new cases of STI that occurred in 2000, 9.1 million (48%) were among youth 15–24 years old.

Risk for STI Among Adolescents

Biological Risk for STI Among Adolescents

Epidemiological data demonstrating that high rates of STI decline with age suggest the existence of a biological vulnerability unique to adolescents (11,12). Proposed mechanisms include developmental changes in the cervix (such as ectopy), an immature immunological response, and the influence of fluctuating sex hormone levels and behaviors on the vaginal environment.

The immune protective system of the reproductive tract is poorly understood; recent research is beginning to reveal some of the mechanisms that will lead to an understanding of the immune responses to sexually transmitted pathogens (13–16). At present there are insufficient data to support directly the hypothesis that there is something unique about the adolescent immune system that explains the increased risk for STI in this age group. Exposure to sexually transmissible pathogens as individuals become sexually active presents the risk for acquisition. It is not clear whether the risk for adolescents is greater than for individuals who defer sexual activity until they are older. However, a recent study by Brunham and colleagues (17) demonstrated that the relative risk of a second infection with *C. trachomatis* was greater among adolescent women and men compared with adults. The investigators did not control for sexual behaviors thus differences in sexual practices between adolescents and adults might also explain the elevated risk among the youngest.

Developmental changes in the female reproductive tract (ectopy and alterations of the normal vaginal microflora) related to puberty might increase risk for STI. The columnar epithelium of the lower genital tract regresses into the endocervical canal during puberty. Persistence of columnar epithelia on the ectocervix (cervical ectopy or ectropion) is more common among adolescents and during pregnancy. It is unclear whether it is more common in women using oral contraceptives (OC). Cervical ectopy has been thought to increase the risk for acquisition of some STIs that infect the columnar epithelia cells especially *C. trachomatis* (Ct) and *N. gonorrhoeae* (Ng). Extension of endocervical columnar epithelium onto the ectocervix might increase the likelihood of infection by increasing the number of cells exposed to these organisms. However, data are conflicting. Some cross-sectional studies have reported associations between cervical ectopy and infection with Ct and Ng (18–21).

The results from prospective studies also do not support ectopy as a risk factor for Ct or Ng. However, most do not specifically target adolescents. One early prospective study of British adolescent women did not find an increased risk for Ct among adolescents with ectopy compared with those without (22). However, this study did not quantify the amount of ectopy using colposcopy or photography. Morrison and colleagues (23) prospectively followed women attending Planned Parenthood clinics to examine risk factors for incident STI. They speculate that ectopy could represent an independent risk factor for cervicitis from Ct infections independent of the effects of hormonal contraception, although the hazard ratio (HR) was not significant (HR, 2.3; 95% confidence interval, 0.9–6.0).

Ectopy has been found to be associated with other STIs. One study reports an association of HPV 16 and18 and cervical ectopy (24). Data linking HIV to ectopy are conflicting. In a retrospective study of U.S. adolescents and young adults, Moscicki and colleagues (25) did not find an association of HIV and ectopy when other risk factors were controlled. Other data, however, suggest that ectopy may be important as a risk factor for HIV. Moss (26) reported increased risk of transmission for HIV among serodiscordant African couples in the presence of cervical ectopy. Another cross-sectional study implicated ectopy as a risk for HSV (19). Additional prospective research is required to clarify whether ectopy is a risk for STIs.

The microorganisms normally resident in the vagina are thought to serve an important protective function against colonization by genitourinary pathogens. The microorganisms and the vagina compromise an ecosystem in which there is interaction of the flora and the vaginal environment (27). The ecosystem is influenced by many factors such as changing levels of sex steroids during puberty, menstrual cycle variation, and with hormonal contraceptives, sexual activity, infection, and practices such as douching and use of vaginal microbicides and sexual behaviors (28–34). The concentration of various species of microorganisms is lower and lactobacilli are absent among prepubertal girls (35). In response to rising levels of estrogen during puberty, vaginal epithelial cells mature and pH decreases to normal adult levels. Lactobacilli appear but are not necessarily associated with the changing pH. It is believed that

H_2O_2-producing lactobacilli and lower pH are important in protecting the vagina from pathogens (36). Thus, factors that alter the normal flora may influence the risk for STI primarily by increasing the risk for bacterial vaginosis.

The majority of adolescent women have irregular menstrual cycles due to anovulation during the first two years following menarche. A cross-sectional study of adolescent women attending found that abnormal menstrual cycles increased the odds ratio for elevated vaginal pH, a risk factor for bacterial vaginosis (37). Bacterial vaginosis (BV) is associated with risk for other STIs.

Exogenous sex hormones, such as hormonal contraceptives, influence the vaginal ecosystem. Hormonal contraceptives have been linked to STI risk in multiple studies. Estrogens and progesterone influence the female reproductive epithelia in ways that could increase risk. Increased cervical ectopy, thinning of the epithelia with changes of underlying vascularity, and alteration of cell surface characteristics might underlie risk associated with the use of hormonal contraceptives. If hormonal contraceptives increase risk for STI, it is especially relevant for adolescents. Hormonal contraception remains the mainstay for pregnancy prevention in this age group. They have been estimated to be responsible for approximately 50% of the reduction in U.S. adolescent pregnancy rates in this age group over the past decade (38).

Although there are several cross-sectional studies supporting increased risk linking oral contraceptives (OC) with *C. trachomatis*, the data are not without controversy. A review of 29 cross-sectional studies examining OC use and chlamydial infection calculated a pooled unadjusted odds ratio of 1.9 (95% confidence interval [CI], 1.7–2.1) (39). However, the results from prospective studies are somewhat conflicting. In an older study of adolescents, Rahm et al. (22) did not find increased risk for Ct among OC users. Baeten and colleagues (40), in a study of Kenyan commercial sex workers, demonstrated increased risk for Ct and candida and decreased risk for BV among users of OC. Depot medroxyhydroprogesterone acetate (DMPA) increased the risk for chlamydia and decreased the risk for BV and Trichomonas vaginalis (TV).

Another prospective study of women attending Planned Parenthood clinics in the United States found that the use of OCs did not increase the risk for cervical infection with *N. gonorrhoeae* and/or *C. trachomatis* (23). In contrast, the use of DMPA increased the risk for cervical infection over three-fold. After adjusting for other risk factors, including having multiple sex partners and condom use, the risk remained significant for incident Ct infection (HR, 4.3; 95% CI, 1.7–11.1) but not for cervical infection with Ng. Cervical ectopy was not a significant mediator of infection.

Research examining hormonal contraceptives and risk for HIV suggests little or no increased risk. A meta-analysis by Wang et al. (41) reported an increased risk, with an odds ratio (OR) of 1.19 (95% CI, 0.99–1.42) for 28 studies. The OR increased when the analysis was limited to the eight most rigorous studies (OR, 1.60; CI, 1.05–2.44). Using a case-control design Mati and colleagues (42) did not identify a risk between HIV and use of OC in Kenyan family planning clients and concluded that if such a risk exists it would not be very large. A prospective study of Tanzanian women found no significant risk for HIV seroconversion and the use of OC, DMPA, or intrauterine devices (43). However, a recent study demonstrated that the short-term use of hormonal contraceptives among HIV-1 positive women in Kenya modestly increased shedding of HIV-1 infected cells, but not of the concentration of

HIV-1 RNA; the implications for transmission are unclear (44). Another study among HIV-infected women demonstrated that short-term use of OC did not increase shedding of HSV (45). A recent prospective longitudinal study of 18–35-year-old women at high risk for HIV in Uganda and Zimbabwe found no association between hormonal contraceptive use and HIV acquisition including women with STIs (46).

Douching is common among adolescent populations at high risk for STI, especially African-Americans, approximately 50% of whom douche at least once a month (47). A review by Martio and colleagues (48) reported prevalence and frequency of douching increased with age and was more common among African-American women Although cross-sectional studies have identified douching as a risk factor for STIs, two recent prospective studies demonstrate no increased risk for pelvic inflammatory disease (PID) or cervicitis with *C. trachomatis* or *N. gonorrhoeae* among women who douched (32,49). Depending on the frequency of douching and the specific composition used, douching may alter the normal vaginal flora. Beigi and colleagues (50) have demonstrated that douching two or more times during the past month and having three or more sex partners in the past year predicted an absence of H_2O_2-producing lactobacillus colonization among women with BV. H_2O_2-producing lactobacillus is believed to be protective against STI. Thus, reduction or absence of these organisms may be responsible for the association of frequent douching and BV. BV has been demonstrated to increase the risk for HIV and TV among Kenyan commercial sex workers (51). It has also been found to be an independent risk factor for the acquisition of HSV2, Ct and Ng among women exposed to these organisms (52,53).

Male circumcision has been implicated as a risk factor for the transmission of HIV in cross-sectional studies conducted in developing countries (54–56). Two prospective studies among African men engaging in sex with prostitutes also found that uncircumcised status independently increased the risk for incident HIV-1 infection four-fold (57,58). Several prospective randomized clinical trials examining the effect of circumcision of adult African men on HIV transmission are currently underway. Although presence of a foreskin is not unique to adolescents and does not explain their elevated risk for STI, if the prospective studies demonstrate that prophylactic circumcision is protective, adolescents would almost certainly become one focus of intervention.

Multiple studies have demonstrated strong associations among HIV transmission and various STIs (syphilis, Ct, Ng, TV, BV, HSV, chancroid) (59). Since adolescents have elevated rates of STI, they may be at elevated risk for HIV. Decreasing prevalent and incident STIs in at-risk populations has been suggested as a way to reduce incident HIV. Evidence that treating STIs reduces the incidence of HIV has been conflicting. Unfortunately, no studies have targeted adolescent populations. One randomized controlled trial (RCT) of improved STI diagnosis and treatment for rural Tanzanian adult populations with a relatively low seroprevalence of HIV (3.8–4.4%) significantly reduced the risk of incident HIV infection by 40% (60). Another RCT conducted in Africa provided periodic mass treatment with azithromycin, ciprofloxacin, and metronidazole to adolescents and adults. This treatment resulted in significant reductions of incident STIs, but did not reduce incident HIV-1 infection (61). The prevalence of HIV in these communities was much higher (15.9%), which may have accounted for the differences.

In summary, at the present time we could find no data to indicate that there are biologic factors unique to adolescents that increase the risk for STI. However, the association of concurrent STI with increased risk for HIV transmission and the association of DMPA with acquisition for Ct suggest that biological factors may explain a portion of the increased STI risk during adolescence.

Behavioral Risk for STI Among Adolescents

A number of behaviors have been associated with increased STIs among adolescents, including early initiation of sexual activity, having multiple sexual partners and new partners, and having unprotected sex, and these behaviors have been the primary focus of behavioral interventions for adolescents. Although there are other behaviors that contribute to STI risk (e.g., exchange of sex for money or drugs), these likely occur in small numbers, there is no data on a national scale to assess behavioral prevalence, and no interventions have yet been designed to address them. In describing prevalence of risk behavior, we present data from the Youth Risk Behavior Surveillance System (YRBS) as well as the National Survey of Family Growth (NFSG) regarding the prevalence of risk behaviors among youth. The YRBS is a biannual survey of high school youth started in 1991, conducted in school systems throughout the country by the CDC to monitor six categories of priority health behaviors among high school youth (9,62). It is currently our broadest and most consistent source of adolescent health data representative of U.S. adolescents attending high school. The NSFG is a multi-wave (1988, 1995, 2002), nationally representative, cross-sectional study of males and females ages 15–44 conducted via in-person interviews using laptop computers. The 2002 wave includes data on sexual activity and contraceptive use of 1,150 females and 1,121 males aged 15–19 years (63). The NSFG is a valuable source of data on adolescents outside of the school setting and the methodology provides the opportunity for greater depth in inquiry. Taken together, these studies provide an important picture of behavioral prevalence in the general population of adolescents in the United States.

Early Initiation of Sexual Activity

Younger age at sexual initiation has been associated with greater numbers of partners, less condom use, pregnancy risk, and STIs (12,64,65). The effect of age at initiation on bacterial infection does appear to diminish as adolescents move into young adulthood, however. Results from the National Longitudinal Study of Adolescent Health indicate that 18 year olds who had sex before the age of 13 were more than twice as likely to test positive for *C. trachomatis*, *N. gonorrhoeae*, or *T. vaginalis* than 18 year olds who had sex at 17, whereas 24 year olds who had sex before the age of 13 were no more likely to test positive for an STI than 24 year olds who had sex at age 17 (12). These data suggest that interventions to delay the onset of sexual activity, although protective for adolescents, would not provide protection against bacterial infections into young adulthood.

According to most recent YRBS data (9), nearly 47% of high school students reported having had sexual intercourse, a decline from 54.1% of high school students who reported having had sexual intercourse in 1991. Among 9th graders, 34.3% have had sexual intercourse and this percentage increases by close to 10% with each grade; 63.1% of 12th graders have had sexual intercourse. Males are more likely than females to be sexually experienced in earlier grades (e.g., 39.3% vs. 29.3% in 9th grade) but percentages are the same by 11th grade. In terms of race/ethnicity, 41.8% of white students, 67.6% of black students, and 51.0% of Hispanic students were sexually experienced. Differences between racial/ethnic groups and increases in percentage of students who are sexually active within each group are similar from 9th grade to 12th grade. According to the 2002 results from the NSFG (63), 46.8% of females and 46.0% of males ages 15–19 have had sex. Rates do not vary by gender overall, but do differ by gender and race/ethnicity. Among 15–19 year olds, 40.4% of Hispanic females compared with 55.5 % of Hispanic males had sex, 46.1% of white females compared with 41.1% of white males had sex, and 57.0% of black females compared with 63.4% of black males had sex.

The YRBS also documents the proportion of adolescents who have had sex before the age of 13. Although the percentages are small, indicating that the majority of sexually experienced adolescents transition to sexual activity in the high school years, the youth who initiate sexual activity at such an early age are at even higher risk for STI. Overall, 62% of high school students had sexual intercourse before the age of 13, a decrease from 1991. Males are more likely to initiate sex early and 4.0% of white students, 16.5% of black students, and 7.3% of Hispanic students had sex before the age of 13. These results are supported by results from the NSFG. In 2002, 5.7% of never married females and 7.9% of never married males had sex before the age of 14. These proportions have decreased since 1995 for both males (from 11.0%) and females (from 8.0%), suggesting that adolescents may be delaying intercourse until older ages more than they were 7 years prior (63).

These numbers suggest that the majority of individuals transition into sexual activity during the high school years. In terms of designing interventions to delay sexual activity among youth, the transition point to sexual experience for most adolescents is important. Unpublished data from the YRBS indicate that, among students who were sexually experienced, 56.6% initiated sexual activity between the ages of 13 and 15. These data suggest that the transition from middle school to high school is important as are the early high school years.

Multiple Partners and New Partners

Having multiple sexual partners or even having a new partner puts adolescents at risk for STI (66). This may occur primarily because of a higher chance of exposure to an infected individual, but also because prevention behavior (e.g., condom use) changes with new or different partners (4). According to the YRBS (9), 14.3% of students have had four or more lifetime partners. This percentage increases by grade from 9.4% in 9th grade to 21.4% in 12th grade. Males (16.5%) are more likely than females (12.0%) to have four or more lifetime partners and 11.4% of white students, 28.2% of black students, and 15.9% of Hispanic fall into this category.

No nationally representative data exist regarding the prevalence of new partner acquisition, however, the NSFG measures numbers of partners in the past

12 months; more than one partner in the past 12 months could serve as a proxy for having had a new partner. Among all 15–19 year olds, 13.9% of females and 18.1% of males had more than one partner in the previous 12 months. Given that 57.4% of females and 60.3% of males had either never had sex or did not have sex in the previous 12 months, these figures represent a substantial proportion of the sexually active youth in the survey.

Unprotected Sex

There has been a great deal of controversy regarding the degree of protection from HIV and STIs that is provided by condoms. Although there are few studies on condom effectiveness specific to adolescents, the scientific data on the effectiveness of consistent and correct use of condoms to reduce the risk of transmission of STIs are increasingly supportive of benefit for a variety of STIs (67). By necessity, measures of consistent and correct use are self-reported and fraught with the potential for error regardless of the age of the subject (reporter). Compared with adult's report, adolescent's reports may be subject to greater error because of age or lack of experience. However, there is no reason to believe that the biological plausibility that a barrier reduces the risk of STI transmission is not valid for adolescents. One study, in fact, has demonstrated that condoms are effective in preventing chlamydia and gonorrhea among adolescents when used consistently and correctly (68).

Because of these issues, studies often measure condom use at last intercourse as a proxy measure for behavior over time. Although this measure is, of course, imperfect, it does allow investigators to examine the portion of youth who at least know about condoms and their use. The YRBS data indicate that the majority of students (62.9%) who have been sexually active in the past three months used a condom the last time they had sexual intercourse. This percentage has increased steadily from 46.2% in 1991. Older students, particularly females, are less likely to use condoms, which may be due to increased use of hormonal contraceptives. Further, in 2005, 62.6% of white students, 68.9% of black students, and 57.7% of Hispanic students who were currently sexually active used a condom the last time they has sex. According to the 2002 NSFG, 54.3% of currently sexually active females and 70.7% of currently sexually active males used a condom the last time they had sex. In 2002, 47.5% of recently sexually active males and 31.4% of sexually active females used a condom every time they had sex in the prior four weeks.

In terms of patterns of condom use, adolescents who use condoms from the time they start having sex appear to be more likely to use them subsequently. Analyses from AddHealth suggest that adolescents who used a condom the first time they had sex were twice as likely to have used a condom the last time they had sex (69).

Summary

Because of the range of behaviors that are related to STI acquisition among youth, including sexual initiation, condom use, and number and type of partner, behavioral prevention for adolescents is particularly challenging. For youth who have not yet initiated sexual activity, strategies to delay sexual experience may be most important, with prevention strategies related to partner factors and condom use most essential for sexually active youth. Given that the majority of adolescents transition to sexual activity at some point during high school, a comprehensive approach is necessary to reach the highest proportion of youth. The challenge is to develop effective interventions to increase the proportion of sexually active adolescent who use condoms consistently and correctly, to decrease numbers of partners, and to increase STI screening. In the following sections, we will examine the factors that impact these behaviors and the available effective interventions to prevent risk behavior among youth.

Effective Behavioral Interventions to Reduce Risk for STI Among Adolescents

In this section, we will discuss effective behavioral interventions to delay initiation of sexual activity, decrease numbers of partners, and increase condom use. We present effective interventions at each social context level, where available, and suggest approaches that might be useful in future research where effective approaches do not currently exist.

Individual-Level Interventions

Individual-level behavioral interventions are the primary methodology associated with STI prevention among youth. They include most school-based curricula as well as programs evaluated in other venues. Comprehensive behavioral interventions, including messages about abstinence and condom/contraceptive use, have been extensively evaluated and a number have been shown to be effective (70). In a review of intervention studies published in the 1990s to reduce sexual risk behavior among adolescents, which were evaluated with appropriate scientific methods, 10 were shown to have positive effects on some aspect of sexual risk behaviors. The individual-level interventions included in this review are: *Be Proud Be Responsible* (71), *Making a Difference* (72), *Focus on Kids* (73), *Reach for Health* (74,75), *Reducing the Risk* (76), *Teen Incentives Program* (77), *Teen Outreach Program* (78,79), *Youth AIDS Prevention Project* (80–82), *Becoming a Responsible Teen* (83), and a skills-based AIDS risk reduction intervention (84). Since 2000, several of these have been replicated and additional reports on effective programs have been published (85–87).

In terms of risk behavior for STI, programs have had varying impact on different behaviors. Relatively few have scientifically demonstrated an effect on sexual initiation, and those that are effective have often not been abstinence-based or abstinence-only. Only one abstinence-based study published in the 1990s, *Making a Difference*, had positive effects without also producing negative effects. *Postponing Sexual Involvement*, in two studies, found some positive effects on sexual initiation but negative effects on recent sexual activity, pregnancy rates, and STI rates. *Draw the line/Respect the line*, an intervention for middle school students that was not specifically abstinence-based or abstinence-only was effective in delaying intercourse for boys but not for girls (87). *Reach for Health*, a community youth service program combined with a comprehensive health curriculum among middle school students, demonstrated short-term (six months) and long-term (two year) effects on sexual initiation. Among those who were sexually inexperienced youth at baseline, 80% of males and 65.2% of females in the curriculum-only condition had initiated sex, compared with 61.5% of males and 48.3% of females who participated in the community service program for one year and 50.0% of males and 39.6% of females who participated in the community service program for two years. Most other studies designed to impact sexual initiation, including evaluations of "abstinence-only-until-marriage" programs, have either been too poorly designed to rely on the results, have demonstrated null effects on the target behaviors, or have negatively affected other risk behaviors.

Studies that have targeted other risk behaviors, like condom use, have been more successful. *Be Proud, Be Responsible* had a positive effect (that is, the intervention group had more positive outcomes than the comparison group) on intentions to engage in risky behavior, a risk behavior index, frequency of sex, number of partners, occasions of sex without a condom, and having anal sex. Another study by Jemmott et al. (72) examined the effectiveness of *Making Proud Choices*, a comprehensive/safer sex curriculum, and *Making a Difference*, an abstinence-based approach. They found that, among sexually experienced youth, both curricula were effective in decreasing frequency of intercourse and the safer sex curricula was effective at decreasing unprotected sex. Sexually experienced youth receiving the abstinence-based curricula, however, were more likely to have unprotected sex and used condoms less frequently. *Focus on Kids* also demonstrated a positive effect on unprotected sex over the course of 24 months (73). A skills-based risk reduction intervention by Jemmott et al. (85) implemented among sexually experienced African-American and Latino adolescent females demonstrated effectiveness in reducing unprotected intercourse and numbers of partners.

A few studies have included biomarkers in their outcome measures and examined the impact of an individual-level intervention on disease rates. DeClimente and his colleagues (88) conducted a randomized controlled trial of an intervention consisting of four 4-hour sessions for sexually experienced African-American girls recruited from community health care centers in an urban area. They found positive effects of the intervention on a variety of measures important in the prevention of STIs, including condom use (e.g., consistency, demonstration of correct use, number of protected intercourse occasions) and new partner acquisition. They also demonstrated a reduction in incident infection with *C. trachomatis*. The power of the study to detect a reduction in *N. gonorrhoeae* and *T. vaginalis* was limited because of the small sample size and low incidence of these infections. Jemmott et al. (85) demonstrated that, compared with adolescents in the control group, sexually experienced adolescent females who received a skills-based risk reduction intervention had lower rates of unprotected intercourse; they had lower incident infection with *C. trachomatis*, *N. gonorrhoeae*, or *T. vaginalis* only at 12 months. Several other studies have demonstrated significant reductions in risk behaviors and trends toward a reduction in subsequent STIs (89,90). These studies suggest the importance of continuing to examine the impact of behavioral interventions for adolescents on disease. STI, obviously, has multiple determinants, only some of which may be impacted by a particular intervention. An intervention that impacts behavior without an accompanying decrease in disease should be reconsidered. However, studies that include biomarker measurement must do so with sufficient power to detect changes in these outcomes, which can be prohibitive.

Effective individual-level interventions have a number of factors in common (70). First, effective programs tend to focus on specific skills (e.g., condom use, negotiation, problem-solving) for reducing sexual risk rather than broad-based approaches. Recent research comparing skills-based approaches with informational approaches reinforces the need to provide youth, particularly those at highest risk, with the means to prevent risk behavior (85,86). Second, the duration and intensity of the intervention are important. The shortest programs are least likely to be effective. Further, some studies have shown that when the number of session or the length of sessions is reduced, even when the content remains the same, interventions are less likely to be effective (83,91,92). It also appears that programs should be targeted to the level of sexual experience of youth. Programs to prevent sexual activity appear only to be effective among younger adolescents who have not yet initiated sexual activity and do not appear to have long-term effects.

There are a number of practical considerations for health professionals when choosing an intervention curriculum and in the implementation of these programs. The effective interventions are of long duration and generally involve repeated delivery, making implementation in most clinical settings difficult to impossible. Shorter interventions will be required if they are to be feasible in clinical encounters with adolescents in health care settings.

Fidelity with which the intervention is implemented is a second concern. The impact of number of sessions and the length of sessions on intervention effectiveness has problematic implications for implementation. Schools and community-based organizations face serious time and resource constraints that may make it impossible to fully implement programs with fidelity.

Third, programs may have unexpected or unclear effects if they are combined, either purposely or accidentally, with other programs. For instance, in two separate evaluations, the *Postponing Sexual Involvement* (PSI) program was combined with two different supplemental curricula. The two studies demonstrated some positive (e.g., less sexual initiation, less frequent sex among intervention participants) and negative (e.g., increased pregnancy and STI rates) effects. The effects were different in the two studies and it is unclear whether this was due to the PSI intervention or to the programs with which it was combined. Thus, it is important for health professionals to track other programs being offered in their communities and to make sure they do not implement conflicting programs.

An additional consideration for program implementation is facilitator training. There have been questions in the implementation and evaluation of interventions for adolescents regarding appropriate facilitators. Some programs have attempted to match facilitators and program participants on the basis of demographic characteristics and others have examined the use of trained peer educators as facilitators. Looking across intervention studies, it appears that the race, ethnicity, gender, or age of the facilitator is less important than the training that the facilitators receive. If facilitators are well trained, they should be effective, regardless of demographics.

Finally, programs with demonstrated effectiveness have been evaluated in a variety of venues. A number of interventions have been designed using very general samples recruited from schools (74,76–80) while others have been tested using community samples (71–73). Other studies, however, have demonstrated the effectiveness of interventions for higher risk youth in very specific settings like juvenile detention centers (91, 93), drug treatment programs (86), or adolescent medicine clinics (85,90). Little is known about whether programs evaluated in one venue are equally effective when implemented in other settings. Since most programs have not been evaluated in a variety of settings, we know little about how a change in venue can impact effectiveness.

Most effective programs for adolescent sexual risk reduction have been replicated and disseminated through structured efforts that encourage fidelity in implementation as well as continued program evaluation but which also often encourage tailoring of interventions to target populations (94–99). Few studies have examined the impact of adapting an effective intervention for a new population or venue. An interesting and important exception to this is a recent study by Stanton and her colleagues (100), who examined the effectiveness of *Focus on Kids* when implemented in a very different setting with a very different population (community and school settings in 12 rural counties in West Virginia), than the original (inner-city, African-American youth). They implemented both an unaltered version of *Focus on Kids* and a modified version tailored to the new target population. Neither version was as effective in the new population as the original program had been with urban youth. Further, the original version of *Focus on Kids* was more effective than the tailored version. Finally, logistic issues impacted the delivery of both versions, which may have had an unquantifiable detrimental effect on the effectiveness of the programs. This study has important implications for dissemination and implementation of individual-level interventions and the need for additional work on how best to translate research into program.

Social Relationships: Parents, Partners, and Social Networks

For adults, the relationship with a romantic or sexual partner has the most impact on sexual behavior. For adolescents, however, parents play an important role in the timing of initiation of sexual activity as well as protective behaviors. Peer networks and norms are also influential and recent research has demonstrated the importance of social and sexual networks—with the accompanying behavioral rules and norms—on the sexual behavior and STI risk of youth. In this section, we will present the evidence for these relationships, currently available effective interventions, and suggestions for further work in these emerging areas.

The Role of Parents in Adolescent Sexual Behavior and Interventions to Improve Parental Monitoring and Communication

The impact of parents on adolescent sexual behavior has gained increasing attention in recent years and has lead to a new focus on interventions for parents. Family bonds, parent-child relationship satisfaction, parental monitoring, supervision and involvement, and communication about sex have all been shown to be related to aspects of adolescent sexual behavior and risk for STI. In general, the results in this area have been strong and consistent.

Family cohesion and positive family relationships have predicted delayed coital debut and a greater likelihood of contraceptive use (101). Greater parental monitoring has been related to a decreased likelihood of coital debut and less risky sexual behavior (102–105). Monitoring appears to be most effective when it concerns a cluster of behaviors, for example, when parents know where their kids are, who they are with, and what they are doing (104,106–112).

Parental communication about sex, including sexual risk and protection against STI, HIV, and pregnancy, has had a positive influence on delay in coital debut and has increased consistent condom and contraceptive use (104,113–118). Parental messages regarding sex should be comprehensive and begin before sexual debut. There is some evidence that parents should focus on encouraging their children to delay sexual activity (107), however, this strategy has not been tested as an intervention to prevent sexual initiation. Analyses from AddHealth indicate that adolescents who perceive that their parents more strongly disapproved of their having sex were less likely to have an STI six years later than those whose parents did not express disapproval (119).

There is also evidence that a combination of these factors—having a good parent-child relationship, monitoring, and communication—are related to decreased sexual risk behavior. For instance, among adolescent females in AddHealth who were not sexually experienced at baseline, relationship satisfaction, mother's disapproval of her daughter having sex, and frequency of the mother's communication with the parents of her daughters friends were associated with later sexual initiation (120).

Given the strength and consistency of the impact of parental factors, they represent a key level of intervention to prevent sexual risk behavior, particularly initiation of sexual activity, among adolescents. However, there are only a few studies that examine parent interventions targeting adolescent sexual risk behaviors or health care utilization. Most published studies that have evaluated parent interventions have combined them with other intervention activities (e.g., *Safer Choices, Focus on Kids*). Some of the new parent-focused interventions currently being evaluated by the Centers for Disease Control and Prevention are also combination interventions (121,122) while others are being investigated as stand-alone interventions (123).

Parent interventions have generally focused on increasing parental communication about sex, increasing parental monitoring, or increasing family cohesion through improving family relationships. They have worked with a variety of methods to try to reach parents and provide them with information and skills. *Safer Choices*, a multi-component intervention to decrease sexual risk behavior, included a parent intervention along with other school-based activities (124). Parents in intervention schools received newsletters that provided information about the program and information about STI/HIV and pregnancy prevention. The school-based curriculum used in the study also included student-parent homework assignments to increase communication about STI/HIV and pregnancy prevention. Although the parent intervention was not evaluated independently from the other activities, students in the intervention schools reported more communication with parents about sex at follow-up than those in comparison schools (124). The *ImPACT* program (*Informed Parents and Children Together*) (125) was a parental monitoring intervention administered to parents and adolescents. All of the youth had previously participated in the *Focus on Kids* program and half received booster sessions as part of the *ImPACT* program. The intervention consisted of a videotape and discussion. The intervention resulted in significantly reduced risk behavior in adolescents. Both studies indicate that intervening with parents can contribute to reduction of adolescent risk.

Traditionally, parent interventions have been plagued by problems with recruitment and retention. Parent education programs are typically held at schools at times not chosen by parents. Parents may miss these programs, not because they are uninterested or do not see such programs as useful or necessary, but because of scheduling difficulties due to work conflicts, child care, or other family responsibilities. Future parent interventions must address these issues and be creative and innovative in how they engage and involve parents especially those whose children/adolescents are at highest risk for STI.

Partner Factors that Impact Sexual Risk Behavior and STI and Interventions to Address These Factors

There are a number of factors regarding romantic partners that impact the initiation of intercourse and condom and contraceptive use within relationships and likelihood of infection. These include partner- and relationship-specific characteristics and the extent to which there are concurrent or sequential partnerships.

Similarity between partners can be defined by demographic characteristics, age, or area of residence or school. As adolescents get older, their partners become more heterogeneous (126). Partner differences have an impact on sexual behavior, condom and contraceptive use, and STI, but often in different ways. For instance, age difference between partners is associated with early sexual debut. Adolescent females, particularly younger adolescents, with older partners are more likely to have sexual intercourse with that partner than those with same age partners (127). There is no evidence to suggest that other types of partner differences have a similar impact on initiation of sexual activity. On the other hand, condom use is higher in partnerships with dissimilar race or ethnicity or neighborhood, although the less similar partners are in either age, grade, or school, the less likely they are to use condoms (126). These findings suggest that adolescents may perceive the need to use protection with partners who are "culturally" different from themselves, as represented by race/ethnicity and neighborhood, but do not perceive the same need with partners who are separated by age or school. Interestingly, these choices may translate into STI risk, since having an older partner or one who does not attend the same school is related to a higher likelihood of self-reported STI, although other differences between partners were not (128).

First sexual relationships are important because patterns of behavior at first sex predict subsequent behavior (69). Manlove et al. (98) used data from the first two waves of AddHealth to examine the characteristics of first sexual partnerships and their association with contraceptive use and consistency during those relationships. They found that adolescents who waited longer to have sex with their first partner and who discussed contraception with that partner before having sex were more likely to use contraceptives and to use them consistently. Those who had taken a virginity pledge or who had an older partner were less likely to use contraception. Adolescents who characterized their relationship as somewhere between romantic and nonromantic (affectionate and physical but not committed) were less likely to use contraception.

In terms of relationship length, number, and timing, several factors have been shown to have an impact on STI risk among adolescents. Those reporting concurrent (overlapping in time) or sequential (nonoverlapping in time) part-nerships also reported less condom use and were more likely to report an STI than single-relationship teens (129). Adolescent females who report past STD diagnoses also report shorter gaps between partners (130).

To date, no published interventions have effectively addressed issues like partner similarity, age differences between partners, or relationship length. Although some individual-level interventions have been effective in reducing numbers of partners and influencing partner interactions by teaching negotia-tion or communication skills to adolescents, these typically only influence one half of the partnership. Dyadic interventions would include programs aimed at romantic/sexual partners to change the partners' behavior. Several studies have examined sexual risk reduction interventions for adult couples (131–133), however, effective behavioral interventions at this level do not exist for ado-lescents. Many barriers to dyadic interventions with adolescents exist. These include the short-term (at times noncommitted) nature of most adolescent rela-tionships, particularly among younger youth and the fact most adolescents, even if they receive health care from the same provider or system do not make a joint visit.

Peer Groups, Social and Sexual Networks, and STI Prevention

Peer relationships have implications for STI risk and infection among adoles-cents. The study of social and sexual networks has also contributed substan-tially to our understanding of adolescent risk. Adolescents are generally members of peer groups, networks of similarly aged adolescents, and the cohe-siveness of these peer groups can be based on friendship ties, perceived simi-larity, shared interests, membership in similar social categories, or geographic location. Peer groups have norms regarding a variety of behaviors, including sexual and health care seeking behavior, and can provide information (or mis-information) in these areas. For instance, perceptions of peer sexual activity have a strong impact on the sexual activity of adolescents (134).

Peer-level interventions that are directed at social networks can be aimed at changing the norms and skills regarding STI prevention behavior within peer groups, or can attempt to change interactions within peer groups regarding prevention behavior. These programs can intervene directly with individual peer groups (73) or can take a more systemic approach targeting particular peer group members (e.g., popular opinion leaders or peer role models) to change peer group norms, skills, and behavior (135).

One emerging area of study has potential implications for STI risk among adolescents. Bearman et al. (136), using AddHealth data, described the net-work structure of 477 sexual partnerships linking 573 youth in a single Midwestern town. They found that 52% of the romantically involved students were linked in a single network over the course of 18 months. This is signifi-cant in the context of the duration of infectiousness, estimated as approxi-mately 15 months for chlamydia (137). The network structure demonstrated by Bearman and colleagues differs significantly from adult networks (see Chapter 4 in this volume) and has important implications for STI transmission. Although a large proportion of adolescents in the network only had one part-ner, they were linked to the others in the network by chains of partnerships that would allow STI to be transmitted throughout a large proportion of the popu-lation. Interestingly, gap length between partners may be less a factor on the individual level for adolescents; that is, an individual is less at risk because of a short gap between his/her own sexual partners than because of a short gap between a string of partners in the network. In addition to having strong implications for disease transmission, the structure of the network described by Bearman and colleagues has implications for prevention. They describe a network of this nature as "fragile" such that breaks in one part of the network prevent transmission to other parts of the network.

At this time, sexual network interventions do not currently exist for adolescents, but they could be a valuable tool in STI prevention. Interventions of this kind must take into account the uniqueness of adolescent sexual networks beyond just their structure. First, adolescents lack the mobility of adults and their networks often occur in "enclosed settings" like schools or neighborhoods. New members are continually being added to the network from within the setting as they become sexually active; thus, they are known to the other members of the network. Third, there are "dating rules" that are unique to adolescents that involve previous partnerships and status. For instance, Bearman et al. (136) use the example of a prohibition on dating "your ex-partner's current partner's ex-partner" because of the low status nature of that type of partnership and demonstrate that a rule of this sort can partially explain the spanning tree network they found among adolescents. All of these issues must be taken into account in the examination of adolescent networks.

Important Systems and Institutions: Schools, Communities, and Health Care Settings

Adolescents are deeply embedded in their neighborhoods, schools, and communities and are affected by the accessibility of these settings. In terms of risk for STI, the availability and accessibility of health care and STI services may have an important impact on disease risk.

School Interventions

A large number of interventions for adolescents are "school-based," that is, they use schools as the venue through which to access the population of interest. However, these school-based interventions are not generally aimed at changing the way the school interacts with the adolescents nor do they make services more available or more likely to be utilized. A number of factors about schools and their interactions with students are associated with adolescent sexual behavior and risk for STI. Being in school is protective against sexual risk behavior; adolescents who drop out of school are more likely to initiate sex at younger ages and are more likely to have unprotected sex (138). School bonding, also defined as involvement, investment, and attachment to school, has been related to decreased sexual risk behavior (139–142) as has after-school supervision (143). In addition, schools can be a point of access to health care through the implementation of school-based preventative services and health care clinics, and several studies have examined the utility of these approaches.

Although most studies designed to impact school bonding have not included measures of sexual behavior (144), a few intervention studies have demonstrated such an effect. One study that has examined the impact of a school bonding intervention on risk behavior has shown significant impact on a variety of adolescent risk behaviors over many years (145). The Seattle Social

Development Project was designed to increase attachment to school, beginning in elementary school, and participants were followed into young adulthood. The investigators increased school bonding through inclusive teaching methods that involved students in the implementation of their curriculum. Long-term follow-up indicates that the program was successful in reducing sexual risk behavior (as well as a variety of other behaviors including violence and delinquency), pregnancy, and STIs into the participants' early 20s. Studies of service learning programs, including Reach for Health and Teen Outreach Program, where students are involved in community service through school programs, have also demonstrated effectiveness in reducing sexual risk behavior (75,78).

Adult supervision in the after-school hours has emerged as an important factor in adolescent risk behavior. Recent research has shown that the likelihood of initiating sexual activity increased with the number of unsupervised hours that adolescents have during the week (143). Some evidence indicates that after-school activity can help decrease this risk. For instance, adolescent girls who play sports are less likely to initiate sexual behavior and have fewer sexual partners than those who do not (106,115). Although no studies have examined the effect of increasing participation in after-school activities on initiating sexual activity, given the importance of supervision in reducing sexual risk behavior, activities that keep adolescents engaged and supervised in the after-school hours should be an important aspect of preventing sexual initiation. It is also unclear whether supervision decreases sexual activity or numbers of partners among adolescents who are already sexually active. A study of sexually active adolescent females indicates that those who are more closely supervised have sex at other times of day (e.g., later in the 24 hour period) (146).

Preventative services implemented in schools can include school health centers and the inclusion of reproductive health care within schools (147). School health centers have emerged as one approach to providing accessible comprehensive acute and preventative adolescent health services (149,150). School health centers have varied in the degree to which they provide reproductive health services for adolescents. Most studies have demonstrated that the presence of a school-based health center does not increase sexual activity among students (144), and several studies have demonstrated increased use of contraceptives among students with access to a school-based health center compared with those without a school-based health clinic (76,150).

Some schools have included condom availability programs (CAPs) as a way to make barrier methods more accessible to sexually active adolescents (151). These programs are also used to provide educational information. They have been controversial, although they have not been found to increase sexual activity among students (152), and parents in urban areas (e.g., New York city) support condom availability in high schools (153). Evidence regarding the effects of these programs on condom use is mixed (151,154,155). All studies have demonstrated that sexual activity does not increase as a result of CAPs. Although several studies did not find an increase in condom use among students with access to a CAP, several studies have demonstrated that these programs have a positive effect on condom use among students (156–158).

The goal of school STI screening and treatment programs is to increase adolescents' access to STI screening and treatment services. Screening programs within schools have not been widely implemented. However, there is some evidence that programs of this type can reduce prevalence of STI within the school setting (159). Unfortunately, the majority of school-based health clinics do not provide reproductive health care. Moreover, there is concern that programs delivering abstinence-only education actually provide inaccurate information about contraception and prevention of STI (160). Including reproductive health care in school-based clinics and condoms at school is so politically charged that they may be unlikely to become effective interventions.

Neighborhoods and Communities

Communities are typically defined as groups of individuals and their organizations and resources, brought together by common interest, lifestyle, characteristics, or residence within a particular geographic area. Adolescents learn norms and standards regarding sexual behavior and health care seeking from interactions with and observation of community members or organizations (e.g., community leaders or role models, faith-based organizations, youth programs, etc.). Neighborhood characteristics can have an impact on sexual behavior among youth (161). Adolescents also typically access services provided from within their community, and the availability of those services may determine whether an adolescent receives prevention messages or health care services at all.

As with other contextual levels, it is important to distinguish between "community-based" and "community-level" interventions for STI, including HIV and teen pregnancy prevention. The former utilizes a particular community to access high-risk adolescents in order to provide them with an intervention. Community-level interventions, however, have the goal of changing the community in some structural way. Community-level interventions have included community or neighborhood mobilization and outreach to increase awareness and norms regarding prevention messages and services or increase utilization of community-based services or activities, including faith-based organizations (e.g., Seattle Minority Youth Health Project) (162). Cross-sectional data suggests that involvement in a religious institution is associated with delays in sexual initiation (163,164). Systematic evaluation of these types of interventions has been lacking and could contribute significantly to our array of available prevention tools.

Health Care Interventions

Medical institutions, in general, and health care providers, in particular, are necessary in diagnosing and treating infection and can play an important role in providing sexual behavior messages to adolescents. Various approaches have been taken with providers to increase attention to guidelines more generally and risk assessment and STI screening specifically for adolescents. These approaches have included information transfer to health care providers in individual or group settings, learning through social influence (training, outreach to offices, quality improvement in small groups, and use of local opinion leaders), feedback, and reminders, (165–169). More systems-level approaches have attempted to increase the availability, utilization, and provision of reproductive health services for adolescents, including organizational interventions, financial interventions, and/or regulatory interventions. Organizational interventions are directed at changing the organization of services (teamwork, process of care), structure of care (initiation and follow-up), and care content (care flow sheets, screening and charting tools). Financial and regulatory interventions include broadening of the range of reimbursable activities to include screening asymptomatic adolescents for STI and the provision of financial rewards or penalties for specific activities. Regulatory interventions include the provision of guidelines to screen all sexually active women ages 16–24 for chlamydia or confidentiality around the provision of services (e.g., billing statements that do not indicate an adolescent's utilization of sexual health services to the parents of adolescents) (170). Shafer and colleagues (171) demonstrated that a systemic intervention to managed care providers significantly increased the rate of screening adolescents for *C. trachomatis*. Ozer et al. (165) examined a combination of individual-level training of primary care providers to counsel adolescents about a variety of health risk behaviors, including sexual behavior, and organizational changes, including screening and charting tools integrated into the clinics, on the rates of screening and counseling among adolescents in the practice. They found that screening and counseling rates increased following provider training and were supported by the organizational changes.

Societal Impact: Media, Culture, and Policy

The broader culture, media, and government policy have an impact on adolescent sexual behavior. Sociodemographic variables, like race and socioeconomic status, are not risk factors for STI themselves. However, they can be markers for societal factors that have an impact on sexual behavior and STI, including population size and spread, cultural beliefs about sexual activity, contraceptive use and childbearing, and the lack of health care coverage and access. Singh et al. (172) examined the relationship between socioeconomic disadvantage and sexual behavior among adolescent females in five developed countries (United States, Canada, France, Great Britain, and Sweden). They found consistent patterns of relationships between socio-disadvantage and sexual risk behavior across all five countries. They found that early sexual activity was associated with education but not income. At all socioeconomic levels, U.S. adolescents were less likely to use contraceptives and were also more likely to be disadvantaged.

One way that society imparts cultural beliefs about sexual activity and risk prevention occurs through the media, which appears to have an influence on adolescent behavior. A recent review of the literature on the effects of media exposure on adolescent sexual behavior reports that youth between the ages of 8 and 18 are exposed to almost eight hours of a combination of TV, videos, movies, video games, radio, audio, and computer per day (173). Sexual content in media is pervasive (173). A recent longitudinal study demonstrated that adolescents who view more sexual content on television are more likely to initiate sexual activity (174). Interventions could either use the media to influence adolescent behavior or could limit media content or media exposure. More work is necessary to examine whether these approaches would be successful in reducing adolescent risk behavior and STI.

Public policy, whether it is guidelines, laws, or funding streams for programs, may have important impact on the sexual behavior of adolescents and resulting STI, particularly as it affects the availability of health care services. Recent examples, including increased funding for abstinence-only-until-marriage education (175) and implementation of parental notification and consent laws for contraception and abortion (176), may not be in the best interests of adolescents. Policy can also have an impact on the availability of important preventative services and thus on the use of those services (161). Although randomized controlled trials to examine the impact of policy interventions are impossible, some evaluation of the intended and unintended consequences of policy interventions have been conducted.

Minor consent laws regarding contraception and abortion, although not directly related to STI, are intended to regulate the sexual activity of youth and therefore can present an interesting means by which to examine the consequences of these types of policies. Zavodny (176) examined the effect of an Illinois county law requiring parental consent for minors to receive contraception on birth and abortion rates in that county as compared with nearby counties for the year prior to and two years following the enactment of the new law. She found that the relative proportion of births and abortions to women under 19 years of age in the county with the consent law increased significantly compared with the nearby counties with no consent law. This increase was not due to a decrease in abortions, which did not decline significantly during those years. Based on these findings, Zavodny concluded that the parental consent law increased the frequency of teenage pregnancy and birth without decreasing sexual intercourse in this age group, which was the likely intention of the policy. Jones et al. (177) surveyed 1526 adolescent females regarding their response to parental notification laws and found that only 7% would stop having sex as a result and that many would switch to no contraception or an unreliable method. Santelli and colleagues (178), taking a broader approach, used national data to explain drops in teen pregnancy rates in the 1990s and found that these changes were equally explained by increased use of contraceptives and decreased rates of sexual activity. These results suggest that policies should promote both approaches to pregnancy prevention, which has direct implications for STI prevention as well because the majority of screening for STI among adolescent women occurs within the context of receipt of contraceptive services.

Abstinence-only-until-marriage programs have been promoted as a means of preventing STI and pregnancy among youth. Government support for abstinence education has increased since first being introduced in the 1996 reauthorization of the Social Security Act. At that time, funds were made available to state and local departments of education to implement abstinence education programs in schools through Title V, Section 501(b) of the act. Since 2000, emphasis has shifted from providing funds to school systems for programming to providing funds to community and faith-based organizations to develop and provide programs in both schools and communities. Organizations that receive funds must provide programs that meet eight criteria: programs must 1) exclusively teach the social, psychological, and health gains from abstinence; 2) teach abstinence outside of marriage as the expected standard; 3) teach that abstinence is the only effective prevention for pregnancy and STIs; 4) teach that mutual monogamy within marriage is the expected standard; 5) teach that sexual activity outside of marriage is likely to have harmful psychological and physical effects; 6) teach that unwed childbearing is harmful for children and parents; 7) teach adolescents how to reject sexual advances; and 8) teach the importance of self-sufficiency before engaging in sexual activity. Although a full-scale evaluation is currently ongoing, some evidence has become available regarding the effectiveness of these policies and the resulting programs.

Evaluations conducted in several states, including Texas, Arizona, and Minnesota, have indicated that rates of sexual behavior have not significantly declined in response to increased abstinence-only education. A report from Representative Henry Waxman's office reviewing the 13 most often used curricula supported by federal funding finds that 11 of these include extensive inaccuracies and misinformation. Three states, California, Pennsylvania, and Maine, now do not accept Title V funding.

Multi-Level Interventions

Although research on social-context level interventions is continuing to emerge, their promise is clear. Because adolescents are embedded and entwined in their social world, no single level can be expected to be fully successful if the risk and potential of other areas of the environment are not included. Ultimately, the goal would be to create a complete environment that supported health and reduced risk. The next step in that effort is to examine how to address multiple contextual levels in an integrated way. A few studies have examined the impact of intervening with multiple coordinated interventions at different levels to reduce drug and alcohol use (Project Northland) (179), improve youth development (Seattle Social Development Project) (145), and decrease sexual risk behavior (Safer Choices) (124) and have shown that it is feasible and effective to intervene in this manner.

Safer Choices implemented intervention activities to address school organization, sex education curriculum and staff development, peer resources and school environment, parent education regarding communication, and school–community linkages. These activities were implemented yearly for two years in 10 high schools with matched comparison schools. They examined the impact of the set of intervention activities on initiation of sexual activity, unprotected intercourse, and number of sex partners. Participants were followed for a total of three years. Although there was no significant difference between students in the intervention and comparison schools in initiation of sexual activity, intervention school students were less likely to have unprotected sex, had fewer partners, and were more likely to use condoms and effective methods of birth control.

Summary

The existing literature on behavioral interventions for adolescents suggests that there are a variety of effective interventions to reduce risk behavior and prevent disease although the reductions in incident infections are modest and the time required for the interventions high. Effective individual-level interventions have been available for over a decade. That rates of risk behavior and STI remain high suggests that they are not being effectively translated and disseminated. More work must be done in this area to study replication of effective adolescent programs, to disseminate them more widely, and to continue to evaluate their effectiveness in the field.

In addition, individual approaches for adolescents may not be sufficient. The etiologic literature indicates that ecological factors have important effects on adolescent risk behavior and resulting STIs. Public health professionals have acknowledged the importance of taking a more ecological approach and some interventions exist for most social context levels. Clearly, more work must be done to develop interventions in these areas, particularly at multiple levels, and then translate and disseminate them for use.

References

1. Institute of Medicine. *The hidden Epidemic: Confronting Sexually Transmitted Diseases.* Washington, DC: National Academy Press; 1997.
2. Revenson TA. All other things are not equal: an ecological approach to personality and disease. In: Friedman HS, ed. *Personality and Disease.* New York: John Wiley & Sons; 1990.
3. Bruckner H, Bearman P. After the promise: the STI consequences of adolescent virginity pledges. *Journal of Adolescent Health.* 2005;36:271–278.
4. Fortenberry JD, Temkit M, Tu W, Graham CA, Katz BP, Orr DP. Daily mood, partner support, sexual interest and sexual activity among adolescent women. *Health Psychology.* 2005;24:252–257.
5. Kassler WJ, Tanfer K, Aral SO. Gonorrhea rates among US men adjusted for sexual activity. *American Journal of Public Health.* 1994;84:1524–1525.
6. Cohen DA, Nsuami M, Martin DH, Farley T. Repeated school-based screening for sexually transmitted diseases: a feasible strategy for reaching adolescents. *Pediatrics.* 1998;101:96.
7. Kent CK, Branzuela A, Fischer L, Bascom T. Chlamydia and gonorrhea screening in San Francisco high schools. *Sexually Transmitted Diseases.* 2003;29:373–375.
8. Centers for Disease Control and Prevention, Division of STD Prevention, Program Development and Support Branch. *Monthly Report.* January 20, 2004.
9. Centers for Disease Control and Prevention. Youth Risk Behavior Surveillance— United States, 2005. *Morbidity and Mortality Weekly Report.* 2005;55:1–108.
10. Weinstock H, Berman S, Cates W. Sexually transmitted diseases among American youth: incidence and prevalence estimates, 2000. *Perspectives on Sexual and Reproductive Health.* 2004;36:6–10.
11. Clay JC, Bowman CA. Controlling chlamydial infection. *Genitourinary Medicine.* 1996;72:145.
12. Kaestle CE, Halpern CT, Miller WC, Ford CA. Young age at first sexual intercourse and sexually transmitted infections in adolescents and young adults. *American Journal of Epidemiology.* 2005;161:8:774–780.
13. Wira CR, Fahey JV. The innate immune system: gatekeeper to the female reproductive tract. *Immunology.* 2004;111:13–15.
14. Geisler WM, Tang J, Wang C, Wilson CM, Kaslow RA. Epidemiological and genetic correlates of incident *Chlamydia trachomatis* infection in North American adolescents. *Journal of Infectious Diseases.* 2004;190:1723–1729.
15. Johansson M, Lycke NY. Immunology of the human genital tract. *Current Opinion in Infectious Diseases.* 2003;16:43–49.
16. Morton RS, Kinghorn GR. Genitourinary chlamydial infection: a reappraisal and hypothesis. *International Journal of STD & AIDS.* 1999;10:765–775.
17. Brunham RC, Pourbohloul B, Mak S, White R, Rekart JL. The unexpected impacts of a *Chlamydia trachomatis* infection control program on susceptibility to reinfection. *Journal of Infectious Diseases.* 2005;192:1836–1844.
18. Quinn TC, Gaydos C, Shepherd M, Bobo L, et al. Epidemiologic and microbiologic correlates of *Chlamydia trachomatis* infection in sexual partnerships. *Journal of the American Medical Association.* 1996;276:21:1737–1742.
19. Critchlow CW, Wolner-Hanssen P, Eschenbach DA, et al. Determinants of cervical ectopia and of cervicitis: age, oral contraception, specific cervical infection, smoking, and douching. *American Journal of Obstetrics and Gynecology.* 1995;173:534–543.
20. Chacko MR, Lovchik JC. *Chlamydia trachomatis* infection in sexually active adolescents: prevalence and risk factors. *Pediatrics,* 1984;73:836–840.

21. Louv WC, Austin H, Perlman J, Alexander WJ. Oral contraceptive use and the risk of chlamydial and gonococcal infections. *American Journal of Obstetrics and Gynecology*. 1989;160:396–402.

22. Rahm VA, Odlind V, Pettersson R. *Chlamydia trachomatis* in sexually active teenage girls. Factors related to genital chlamydial infection: a prospective study. *Genitourinary Medicine*. 1991;67:317–321.

23. Morrison CS, Bright P, Wong EL, Kwok C, Yacobson I, Gaydos CA, Tucker HT, Blumenthal PD. Hormonal contraceptive use, cervical ectopy, and the acquisition of cervical infections. *Sexually Transmitted Diseases*. 2004;31:561–567.

24. Rocha-Zavaleta L, Yescas G, Cruz RM, Cruz-Talonia F. Human papillomavirus infection and cervical ectopy. *International Journal of Gynaecology & Obstetrics*. 2004;85:259–266.

25. Moscicki AB, Ma Y, Holland C, Vermund SH. Cervical ectopy in adolescent girls with and without human immunodeficiency virus infection. *Journal of Infectious Diseases*. 2001;183:865–870.

26. Moss GB, Clemetson D, D'Costa L, et al. Association of cervical ectopy with heterosexual transmission of human immunodeficiency virus: results of a study of couples in Nairobi, Kenya. *Journal of Infectious Diseases*. 1991;164:588–591.

27. Pybus V, Onderdonk AB. Microbial interactions in the vaginal ecosystem, with emphasis on the pathogenesis of bacterial vaginosis. *Microbes & Infection*. 1999;1:285–292.

28. Brabin L. Interactions of the female hormonal environment, susceptibility to viral infections, and disease progression. *AIDS Patient Care and STDs*. 2002;16:211–221.

29. Burton JP, Reid G. Evaluation of the bacterial vaginal flora of 20 postmenopausal women by direct (Nugent score) and molecular (polymerase chain reaction and denaturing gradient gel electrophoresis) techniques. *Journal of Infectious Diseases*. 2002;186:1770–1780.

30. Clarke JG, Peipert JF, Hillier SL, Heber W, Boardman L, Moench TR, Mayer K. Microflora changes with the use of a vaginal microbicide. *Sexually Transmitted Diseases*. 2002;29:288–293.

31. Eschenbach DA, Thwin SS, Patton DL, et al. Influence of the normal menstrual cycle on vaginal tissue, discharge, and microflora. *Clinical Infectious Diseases*. 2000;30:901–907.

32. Ness RB, Hillier SL, Richter HE, et al. Douching in relation to bacterial vaginosis, lactobacilli, and facultative bacteria in the vagina. *Obstetrics & Gynecology*. 2002;100:765–772.

33. Schwebke JR, Richey CM, Weiss HL. Correlation of behaviors with microbiological changes in vaginal flora. *Journal of Infectious Diseases*. 1999;180:1632–1636.

34. Vallor AC, Antonio MA, Hawes SE, Hillier SL. Factors associated with acquisition of, or persistent colonization by, vaginal lactobacilli: role of hydrogen peroxide production. *Journal of Infectious Diseases*. 2001;184:1431–1436.

35. Hill GB, St. Clari KK, Gutman LT. Anaerobes predominate among the vaginal microflora of prepubertal girls and lactobacilli are absent. *Clinical Infectious Disease*. 1995;20(Suppl 2):S269–S270.

36. Redondo-Lopez V, Cook RL, Sobel JD. Emerging role of lactobacilli in the control and maintenance of the vaginal bacterial microflora. *Review of Infectious Diseases*. 1990;12:856–872.

37. Brabin L, Roberts SA, Fairbrother E, et al. Factors affecting vaginal pH levels among female adolescents attending genitourinary medicine clinics. *Sexually Transmitted Infections*. 2005;81:483–487.

38. Santelli JS, Kaiser J, Hirsch L, Radosh A, Simkin L, Middlestadt S. Initiation of sexual intercourse among middle school adolescents: the influence of psychosocial factors. *Journal of Adolescent Health*. 2004;34:200–208.

39. Cottingham J, Hunter D. *Chlamydia trachomatis* and oral contraceptive use: a quantitative review. *Genitourinary Medicine.* 1992;68:209–216.

40. Baeten JM, Nyange PM, Richardson BA, et al. Hormonal contraception and risk of sexually transmitted disease acquisition: results from a prospective study. *American Journal of Obstetrics and Gynecology.* 2001;185:380–385.

41. Wang CC, Reilly M, Kreiss JK. Risk of HIV infection in oral contraceptive pill users: a meta-analysis. *Journal of Acquired Immune Deficiency Syndromes.* 1999;21:51–58.

42. Mati JK, Hunter DJ, Maggwa BN, Tukei PM. Contraceptive use and the risk of HIV infection in Nairobi, Kenya. *International Journal of Gynaecology & Obstetrics.* 1995;48:61–67.

43. Kapiga SH, Lyamuya EF, Lwihula GK, Hunter DJ. The incidence of HIV infection among women using family planning methods in Dar es Salaam, Tanzania. *AIDS.* 1998;12:75–84.

44. Wang CC, McClelland RS, Overbaugh J, et al. The effect of hormonal contraception on genital tract shedding of HIV-1. *AIDS.* 2004;18:205–209.

45. McClelland RS, Wang CC, Richardson BA, et al. A prospective study of hormonal contraceptive use and cervical shedding of herpes simplex virus in human immunodeficiency virus type 1-seropositive women. *Journal of Infectious Diseases.* 2002;185:1822–1825.

46. Morrison CS, Richardson BA, Celentano DD, et al. The hormonal contraception and risk of HIV-1 acquisition (HC-HIV) study. Presented at the International Society for Sexually Transmitted Disease Research. 2005 July 10–13; Amsterdam, The Netherlands.

47. Oh MK, Merchant JS, Brown P. Douching behavioral in high-risk adolescents. What do they use, when and why do they douche? *Journal of Pediatric and Adolescent Gynecology.* 2002;15:83–88.

48. Martino JL, Youngpairoj S, Vermund SH. Vaginal douching: personal practices and public policies. *Journal of Women's Health.* 2004;131048–1065.

49. Rothman KJ, Funch DP, Alfredson T, Brady J, Dreyer NA. Randomized field trial of vaginal douching, pelvic inflammatory disease and pregnancy. *Epidemiology.* 2003;14:340–348.

50. Beigi RH, Wiesenfeld HC, Hillier SL, Straw T, Krohn MA. Factors associated with absence of H_2O_2-producing Lactobacillus among women with bacterial vaginosis. *Journal of Infectious Diseases.* 2005;191:924–1292.

51. Martin HL, Richardson BA, Nyange PM, et al. Vaginal lactobacilli, microbial flora, and risk of human immunodeficiency virus type 1 and sexually transmitted disease acquisition. *Journal of Infectious Diseases.* 1999;180:1863–1868.

52. Cherpes TL, Meyn LA, Krohn MA, Lurie JG, Hillier SL. Association between acquisition of herpes simplex virus type 2 in women and bacterial vaginosis. *Clinical Infectious Diseases.* 2003;37:319–325.

53. Wiesenfield HC, Hillier SL, Krohn MA, Landers DV, Sweet RL. Bacterial vaginosis is a strong predictor of *Neisseria gonorrhoeae* and *Chlamydia trachomatis* infection. *Clinical Infectious Diseases.* 2003;36:663–668.

54. Agot KE, Ndinya-Achola JO, Kreiss JK, Weiss NS. Risk of HIV-1 in rural Kenya: a comparison of circumcised and uncircumcised men. *Epidemiology.* 2004;15:157–163.

55. Reynolds SJ, Shepherd ME, Risbud AR, et al. Male circumcision and risk of HIV-1 and other sexually transmitted infections in India *Lancet.* 2004;363:1039–1040.

56. Siegfried N, Muller M, Deeks J, et al. HIV and male circumcision—a systematic review with assessment of the quality of studies. *The Lancet Infectious Diseases.* 2005;5:165–173.

57. Lavreys L, Rakwar JP, Thompson ML, et al. Effect of circumcision on incidence of human immunodeficiency virus type 1 and other sexually transmitted diseases:

a prospective cohort study of trucking company employees in Kenya. *Journal of Infectious Diseases*. 1999;180:330–336.

58. Cameron DW, D'Costa LJ, Maitha GM, et al. Female to male transmission of human immunodeficiency virus type 1: risk factors for seroconversion in men. *Lancet*. 1989;334:403–407.

59. Fleming DT, Wasserheit JN. From epidemiological synergy to public health policy and practice: the contribution of other sexually transmitted diseases to sexual transmission of HIV infection. *Sexually Transmitted Infections*. 1999;75:3–17.

60. Grosskurth H, Todd J, Mwijarubi E, et al. Impact of improved treatment of sexually transmitted diseases on HIV infection in rural Tanzania: randomised controlled trial. *Lancet*. 1995;346:530–536.

61. Wawer MJ, Sewankambo NK, Serwadda D, et al. Control of sexually transmitted diseases for AIDS prevention in Uganda: a randomised community trial. *Lancet*. 1999;353:525–535.

62. Brener ND, Kann L, Kinchen SA, et al. Methodology of the Youth Risk Behavior Surveillance System. *Morbidity and Mortality Weekly Report*. 2004;53(RR-12):1–16.

63. Abma JC, Martinez GM, Mosher WD, Dawson BS. Teenagers in the US: sexual activity, contraceptive use and childbearing. *Vital Health Statistics*. 2004;24:1–48.

64. Coker AL, Richter DL, Valois RF, McKeown RE, Garrison CZ, Vincent ML. Correlates and consequences of early initiation of sexual intercourse. *Journal of School Health*. 1994;64:372–377.

65. Van Ranson K, Rosenthal S, Biro F, Lewis L, Succop P. Longitudinal risk of STD acquisition in adolescent girls using a generalized estimating equations model. *Journal of Pediatric and Adolescent Gynecology*. 2000;13:87.

66. Niccolai LM, Ethier KA, Kershaw TS, Lewis JB, Meade CS, Ickovics JR. New sexual partner acquisition and sexually transmitted disease risk among adolescent females. *Journal of Adolescent Health*. 2004;34:216–223.

67. Warner L, Stone KM. Male Condoms. In: SO Aral and JM Douglas, eds. *Behavioral Interventions for Prevention and Control of Sexually Transmitted Diseases, Including HIV*. New York: Springer-SBM; 2007.

68. Paz-Bailey G, Koumans EH, Sternberg M, et al. The effect of correct and consistent condom use on chlamydial and gonococcal infection among urban adolescents. *Archives of Pediatrics and Adolescent Medicine*. 2005;159:536–542.

69. Shaffi T, Stovel K, Davis R, Holmes K. Is condom use habit forming?: Condom use at sexual debut and subsequent condom use. *Sexually Transmitted Diseases*. 2004;31:366–372.

70. Robin L, Dittus P, Whitaker D, et al. Behavioral interventions to reduce incidence of HIV, STD and pregnancy among adolescents: a decade in review. *Journal of Adolescent Health*. 2004;34:3–26.

71. Jemmott JB, Jemmott LS, Fong GT. Reductions in HIV risk-associated sexual behaviors among black male adolescents: effects of an AIDS prevention intervention. *American Journal of Public Health*. 1992;82:372–377.

72. Jemmott JB, Jemmott LS, Fong GT. Abstinence and safer sex HIV risk reduction interventions for African American adolescents: a randomized controlled trial. *Journal of the American Medical Association*. 1998;279:1529–1536.

73. Stanton BF, Li X, Ricardo I, Galbraith J, Feigelman S, Kaljee L. A randomized, controlled effectiveness trial of an AIDS prevention program for low-income African-American youths. *Archives of Pediatrics and Adolescent Medicine*. 1996;150:363–372.

74. O'Donnell L, Stueve A, Doval AS. The effectiveness of the Reach for Health Community Youth Service Learning Program in reducing early and unprotected sex among urban middle school students. *American Journal of Public Health*. 1999;89:176–181.

75. O'Donnell L, Stueve A, O'Donnell C, et al. Long-term reductions in sexual inhibition and sexual activity among urban middle schoolers in the Reach for Health Service Learning Program. *Journal of Adolescent Health.* 2002;31:93–100.

76. Kirby D, Waszak C, Ziegler J. Six school-based clinics: their reproductive health services and impact on sexual behavior. *Family Planning Perspectives.* 1991;23:6–16.

77. Bayne Smith MA. Teen Incentives Program: evaluation of a health promotion model for adolescent pregnancy prevention. *Journal of Health Education.* 1994;25:24–29.

78. Allen JP, Philliber S, Herling S, et al. Preventing teen pregnancy and academic failure: experimental evaluation of a developmentally based approach. *Child Development.* 1997;64:729–742.

79. Walter HJ, Vaughan RD. AIDS risk reduction among a multi-ethnic sample of urban high school students. *Journal of the American Medical Association.* 1993;27:725–730.

80. Weeks K, Levy SR, Zhu C, et al. Impact of a school-based AIDS prevention program on young adolescents' self-efficacy skills. *Health Education Research.* 1995;10:329–344.

81. Levy SR, Perhats C, Weeks K, et al. Impact of a school-based AIDS prevention program on risk and protective behavior for newly sexually active students. *Journal of School Health.* 1995;65:145–151.

82. Weeks K, Levy SR, Gordon AK, et al. Does parent involvement make a difference? The impact of parent interactive activities on students in a school-based AIDS prevention program. *AIDS Education and Prevention.* 1997;9(Suppl 1):90–106.

83. St. Lawrence JS, Brasfield TL, Jefferson KW, et al. Cognitive-behavioral intervention to reduce African American adolescents' risk for HIV infection. *Journal of Consulting and Clinical Psychology.* 1995;63:221–237.

84. Walter HJ, Vaughan RD. AIDS risk reduction among a multiethnic sample of urban high school students. *JAMA.* 1993;270:725–730.

85. Jemmott JB, Jemmott LS, Braverman PK, Fong GT. HIV/STI risk reduction interventions for African American and Latino adolescent girls at an adolescent medicine clinic: a randomized controlled trial. *Archives of Pediatrics and Adolescent Medicine.* 2005;159:440–449.

86. St. Lawrence JS, Crosby RA, Brasfield TL, O'Bannon RE 3rd. Reducing STD and HIV risk behavior of substance-dependent adolescents: a randomized controlled trial. *Journal of Consulting and Clinical Psychology.* 2002;70:1010–1021.

87. Coyle KK, Kirby DB, Marin BV, Gomez CA, Gregorich SE. Draw the line/respect the line: a randomized trial of a middle school intervention to reduce sexual risk behaviors. *American Journal of Public Health.* 2004;94:843–851.

88. DiClemente RJ, Wingood GM, Harrington KF, et al. Efficacy of and HIV prevention intervention for African American adolescent girls: a randomized controlled trial. *Journal of the American Medical Association.* 2005;292:171–179.

89. Downs JS, Murray PJ, Bruine de Bruin W, Penrose J, Palmgren C, Fischoff B. Interactive video behavioral intervention to reduce adolescent females' STI risk: a randomized controlled trial. *Social Science and Medicine.* 2004;59:1561–1572.

90. Shrier LA, Ancheta R, Goodman E, Chiou VM, Lyden MR, Emans SJ. Randomized controlled trial of a safer sex intervention for high-risk adolescent girls. *Archives of Pediatrics and Adolescent Medicine.* 2001;155:73–79.

91. St. Lawrence JS, Crosby RA, Belcher L, et al. Sexual risk reduction and anger management interventions for incarcerated male adolescents: a randomized controlled trial of two interventions. *Journal of sex Education Therapy.* 1999;24:9–17.

92. Rotheram-Borus MJ, Gwadz M, Fernandez MI, et al. Timing of HIV interventions on reductions in sexual risk among adolescents. *American Journal of Community Psychology.* 1998;26:73–96.

93. Magura S, Kang SY, Shapiro JL. Outcomes of intensive AIDS education for male adolescent drug users in jail. *Journal of Adolescent Health.* 1994;15:457–463.

94. Neumann MS, Sogolow ED. Replicating effective programs: HIV/AIDS prevention technology transfer. *AIDS Education and Prevention.* 2000;12:35–48.

95. Kegeles SM, Rebchook GM, Hays RB, et al. From science to application: the development of an intervention package. *AIDS Education Prevention.* 2000;12(5 Suppl):62–74.

96. Collins J, Robin L, Wooley S, et al. Programs-that-work: CDC's guide to effective programs that reduce health-risk behavior of youth. *Journal of School Health.* 2002;72:93–98.

97. Solomon J, Card JJ. Making the list: understanding, selecting, replicating effective teen pregnancy prevention programs, National Campaign to Prevent Teen Pregnancy. Washington DC. 2004.

98. Manlove J, Ryan S, Franzetta K. Patterns of contraceptive use within teenagers' first sexual relationships. *Perspectives on Sexual & Reproductive Health.* 2003;35: 246–255.

99. Sogolow ED, Kay LS, Doll LS, et al. Strengthening HIV prevention: application of a research-to-practice framework. *AIDS Education and Prevention.* 2000; 12(5 Suppl):21–32.

100. Stanton B, Guo J, Cottrell L, et al. The complex business of adapting effective interventions to new populations: an urban to rural transfer. *Journal of Adolescent Health.* 2005;37:163.

101. McNeely C, Shew ML, Beuhring T, Sieving R, Miller BC, Blum RW. Mothers' influence on the timing of first sex among 14- and 15-year-olds. *Journal of Adolescent Health.* 2002;31:256–265.

102. Forehand R, Miller KS, Dutra R, Chance MW. Role of parenting in adolescent deviant behavior: replication across and within two ethnic groups. *Journal of Consulting and Clinical Psychology.* 1997;65:1036–1041.

103. Miller KS, Kotchick BA, Dorsey S, Forehand R, Ham AY. Family communication about sex: what are parents saying and are their adolescents listening? *Family Planning Perspectives.* 1999;30:218–222.

104. Romer D, Stanton B, Galbraith J, Feigleman S, Black MM, Li X. Parental influence on adolescent sexual behavior in high poverty settings. *Archives of Pediatric and Adolescent Medicine.* 1999;153:1055–1062.

105. Baker JG, Rosenthal SL, Leonhardt D, et al. Relationship between perceived parental monitoring and young adolescent girls' sexual and substance use behaviors. *Journal of Pediatric and Adolescent Gynecology.* 1999;12:17–22.

106. Sabo DF, Miller KE, Farrell MP, Melnick MJ, Barnes GM. High school athletic participation, sexual behavior and adolescent pregnancy: a regional study. *Journal of Adolescent Health.* 1999;25:207–216.

107. Dittus PJ, Jaccard J. Adolescents' perceptions of maternal disapproval of sex: relationship to sexual outcomes. *Journal of Adolescent Health.* 2000;26:268–278.

108. Stanton B, Li X, Pack R, Cottrell L, Harris C, Burns JM. Longitudinal influence of perceptions of peer and parental factors on African American adolescent risk involvement. *Journal of Urban Health.* 2002;79:536–548.

109. Huebner AJ, Howell LW. Examining the relationship between adolescent sexual risk-taking and perceptions of monitoring, communication, and parenting styles. *Journal of Adolescent Health.* 2003;33:71–78.

110. Bettinger JA, Celentano DD, Curriero FC, Adler NE, Millstein SG, Ellen JM. Does parental involvement predict new sexually transmitted disease in female adolescents? *Archives of Pediatrics and Adolescent Medicine.* 2004;158: 666–710.

111. Borawski EA, Ievers-Landis CE, Lovegreen LD, Trapl ES. Parental monitoring, negotiated unsupervised time, and parental trust: the role of perceived parenting

practices in adolescent health risk behaviors. *Journal of Adolescent Health.* 2003;33:60–70.

112. Rosenthal SL, Von Ranson KM, Cotton S, Biro FM, Mills L, Succop PA. Sexual initiation: predictors and developmental trends. *Sexually Transmitted Diseases.* 2001;28:527–532.

113. Dittus PJ, Jaccard J, Gordon VV. Direct and nondirect communication of maternal beliefs to adolescents: adolescent motivations for premarital sexual activity. *Journal of Applied Social Psychology.* 1999;29:1927–1963.

114. Holtzman D, Rubinson R. Parent and peer communication effects on AIDS-related behavior among U.S. high school students. *Family Planning Perspectives.* 1995;27:235–240.

115. Miller KS, Levin ML, Whitaker DJ, Xu X. Patterns of condom use among adolescents: the impact of mother-adolescent communication. *American Journal of Public Health.* 1998;88:1542–1544.

116. Whitaker DJ, Miller KS, May DC, Levin ML. Teenage partners' communication about sexual risk and condom use: the importance of parent-teenager discussions. *Family Planning Perspectives.* 1999;31:117–121.

117. Karofsky PS, Zeng L, Kosorok MR. Relationship between adolescent-parental communication and initiation of first intercourse by adolescents. *Journal of Adolescent Health.* 2001;28:41–45.

118. Hutchinson MK, Jemmott JB 3rd, Jemmott LS, Braverman P, Fong GT. The role of mother-daughter sexual risk communication in reducing sexual risk behaviors among urban adolescent females: a prospective study. *Journal of Adolescent Health.* 2003;33:98–107.

119. Ford CA, Pence BW, Miller WC, et al. Predicting adolescents' longitudinal risk for sexually transmitted infection: results from the National Longitudinal Study of Adolescent Health. *Archives of Pediatrics and Adolescent Medicine.* 2005;159:657–664.

120. McNeely CA, Nonnemaker JM, Blum RW. Promoting school connectedness: evidence from the National Longitudinal Study of Adolescent Health. *Journal of School Health.* 2002;72:138–146.

121. Dittus PJ, Jaccard J, Guillamo-Ramos V. Linking Lives. *Presentation to the Division of Reproductive Health, Centers for Disease Control and Prevention.* 2005; Atlanta, GA.

122. Ethier KA, DeRosa CJ, Kim DH, Anderson-Mahoney P, Kerndt PR. *Project Connect. Presentation to the Division of Reproductive Health, Centers for Disease Control and Prevention.* 2005; Atlanta, GA.

123. Long N, Austin BJ, Gound MM, et al. The Parents Matter! Program Interventions: content and the facilitation process. *Journal of Child and Family Studies.* 2004;13:47–65.

124. Coyle K, Basen-Engquist K, Kirby D, et al. Safer choices: reducing teen pregnancy, HIV, and STDs. *Public Health Reports.* 2001;116(Suppl 1):82–93.

125. Stanton B, Cole M, Galbraith J, et al. Randomized trial of a parent intervention: parents can make a difference in long-term adolescent risk behaviors, perceptions, and knowledge. *Archives of Pediatrics and Adolescent Medicine.* 2004;158:947–955.

126. Ford K, Sohn W, Lepkowski J. Characteristics of adolescents' sexual partners and their association with use of condoms and other contraceptive methods. *Family Planning Perspectives.* 2001;33:100–105.

127. Kaestle CE, Morisky DE, Wiley DJ. Sexual intercourse and the age difference between adolescent females and their romantic partners. *Perspectives on Sexual & Reproductive Health.* 2002;34:304–309.

128. Ford K, Lepkowski JM. Characteristics of sexual partners and STD infection among American adolescents. *International Journal of STD & AIDS.* 2004;15:260–265.

129. Kelley SS, Borawski EA, Flocke SA, Keen KJ. The role of sequential and con-current sexual relationships in the risk of sexually transmitted diseases among adolescents. *Journal of Adolescent Health*. 2003;32:296–305.
130. Kraut-Becher JR, Aral SO. Gap length: an important factor in sexually transmit-ted disease transmission. *Sexually Transmitted Diseases*. 2003;30:221–225.
131. El-Bassel N, Witte SS, Gilbert L, Wu E, Chang K, Hill J, Steinglass P. The effi-cacy of a relationship-based HIV/STD prevention program for heterosexual couples. *American Journal of Public Health*. 2003;93:963–969.
132. El-Bassell N, Witte SS, Gilbert L, et al. Long-term effects of an HIV/STI sexual risk reduction intervention for heterosexual couples. *AIDS and Behavior*. 2005;9:1–13.
133. Harvey SM, Henderson JT, Thorburn S, et al. A randomized study of a pregnancy and disease prevention intervention for Hispanic couples. *Perspectives on Sexual and Reproductive Health*. 2004;36:162–169.
134. Romer D, Black M, Ricardo I, et al. Social influences on the sexual behavior of youth at risk for HIV exposure. *American Journal of Public Health*. 1994;84:977–985.
135. Smith MU, Dane FC, Archer ME, Devereaux RS, Katner HP. Students together against negative decisions (STAND): evaluation of a school-based sexual risk reduction intervention in the rural south. *AIDS Education and Prevention*. 2000;12:49–70.
136. Bearman PS, Moody J, Stovel K. Chains of affection: the structure of adolescent romantic and sexual networks. *American Journal of Sociology*. 2004;110:44–91.
137. Brunham RC, Plummer FA. A general model of sexually transmitted epidemiol-ogy and its implications for control. *Medical Clinics of North America*. 1990;74:1339–1352.
138. Darroch JE, Landry DJ, Oslak S. Age difference between sexual partners. *Family Planning Perspectives*. 1999;31:160–167.
139. Billy JOG, Brewster KL, Grady WR. Contextual effects on the sexual behavior of adolescent women. *Journal of Marriage and the Family*. 1994;56:387–404.
140. Lammers C, Ireland M, Resnick M, Blum R. Influences on adolescents' decision to postpone onset of sexual intercourse: a survival analysis of virginity among youths aged 13 to 18 years. *Journal of Adolescent Health*. 2000;26:42–48.
141. Manlove J. The influence of high school dropout and school disengagement on the risk of school-age pregnancy. *Journal of Research on Adolescence*. 1998;8:187–220.
142. Bonny AE, Britto MT, Klostermann BK, Hornung RW, Slap GB. School discon-nectedness: identifying adolescents at risk. *Pediatrics*. 2000;106:1017–1021.
143. Cohen DA, Farley TA, Taylor SN, Martin DH, Schuster MA. When and where do youths have sex? The potential role of adult supervision. *Pediatrics*. 2002;110:66.
144. Kirby D. The impact of schools and school programs upon adolescent sexual behavior. *Journal Sex Research*. 2002;39:27–33.
145. Lonczak HS, Abbott RD, Hawkins JD, Kosterman R, Catalano RF. Effects of the Seattle social development project on sexual behavior, pregnancy, birth, and sex-ually transmitted disease outcomes by age 21 years. *Archives of Pediatrics & Adolescent Medicine*. 2002;156:438–447.
146. Fortenberry JD, Blythe MJ, Katz BP, Juliar BA, Tu W, Orr DP. Factors associated with time of day of sexual activity among adolescent women. *Journal of Adolescent Health*. 2006;38:275–281.
147. Kirby D. Antecedents of adolescent initiation of sex, contraceptive use, and preg-nancy. *American Journal of Health Behavior*. 2002;26:473–485.
148. Kaplan DW, Calonge BN, Guernsey BP, Hanrahan MB. Managed care and school-based health centers: use of health services. *Archives of Pediatrics and Adolescent Medicine*. 1998;152:25–33.
149. Burstein GR, Waterfield G, Joffe A, Zenilman JM, Quinn TC, Gaydos CA. Screening for gonorrhea and chlamydia by DNA amplification in adolescents

attending middle school health centers. Opportunity for early intervention. *Sexually Transmitted Disease*. 1998; 25:395–402.

150. Zabin LS, Emerson MR, Ringers PA, Sedivy V. Adolescents with negative pregnancy test results. An accessible at-risk group. *Journal of the American Medical Association*. 1996;275:113–117.

151. Kirby DB, Brown NL. Condom availability programs in U.S. schools. *Family Planning Perspectives*. 1996;28:196–202.

152. Wolk LI, Rosenbaum R. The benefits of school-based condom availability: cross-sectional analysis of a comprehensive high school-based program. *Journal of Adolescent Health*. 1995;17:184–188.

153. Guttmacher S, Lieberman L, Wai HC, Ward D, Radosh A, Rafferty Y, Freudenberg N. Gender differences in attitudes and use of condom availability programs among sexually active students in New York City public high schools. *Journal of the American Medical Women's Association*. 1995;50:99–102.

154. Kirby D. Making condoms available in schools. The evidence is not conclusive. *Western Journal of Medicine*. 2000;172:149–151.

155. Kirby D. Reflections on two decades of research on teen sexual behavior and pregnancy. *Journal of School Health*. 1999;69:89–94.

156. Furstenberg FF Jr, Geitz LM, Teitler JO, Weiss CC. Does condom availability make a difference? An evaluation of Philadelphia's health resource centers. *Family Planning Perspectives*. 1997;29:123–127.

157. Guttmacher S, Lieberman L, Ward D, Freudenberg N, Radosh A, Des Jarlais D. Condom availability in New York City public high schools: relationships to condom use and sexual behavior. *American Journal of Public Health*. 1997;87:1427–1433.

158. Schuster MA, Bell RM, Berry SH, Kanouse DE. Impact of a high school condom availability program on sexual attitudes and behaviors. *Family Planning Perspectives*. 1998;30:67–72.

159. Cohen DA, Nsuami M, Martin DH, Farley TA. Repeated school based screening for sexually transmitted diseases: a feasible strategy for reaching adolescents. *Pediatrics*. 1999;104:1281–1285.

160. Connolly C. Some abstinence programs mislead teens, report says. *Washington Post*. December 2, 2004; p A01.

161. Averett SL, Rees DI, Argys LM. The impact of government policies and neighborhood characteristics on teenage sexual activity and contraceptive use. *American Journal of Public Health*. 2002;92:1773–1778.

162. Cheadle A, Wagner E, Walls M, Diehr P, Bell M, Anderman C, McBride C, Catalano RF, Pettigrew E, Simmons R, Neckerman H. The effect of neighborhood-based community organizing: results from the Seattle Minority Youth Health Project. *Health Services Research*. 2001;36:671–689.

163. Mott FL, Fondell MM, Hu PN, Kowaleski-Jones L, Menaghan EG. The determinants of first sex by age 14 in a high-risk adolescent population. *Family Planning Perspectives*. 1996;28:13–18.

164. Marsiglio W, Mott FL. The impact of sex education on sexual activity, contraceptive use and premarital pregnancy among American teenagers. *Family Planning Perspectives*. 1986;18:151–162.

165. Ozer EM, Adams SH, Lustig JL, et al. Increasing the screening and counseling of adolescents for risky health behaviors: a primary care intervention. *Pediatrics*. 2005;115:960–968.

166. Balas EA, Weingarten S, Garb CT, Blumenthal D, Boren SA, Brown GD. Improving preventive care by prompting physicians. *Archives of Internal Medicine*. 2000;160:301–308.

167. Hulscher ME, Wensing M, Grol RP, van der Weijden T, van Weel C. Interventions to improve the delivery of preventive services in primary care. *American Journal of Public Health*. 1999;89:737–746.

168. Anderson LA, Janes GR, Jenkins C. Implementing preventive services: to what extent can we change provider performance in ambulatory care? A review of the screening, immunization, and counseling literature. *Annals of Behavioral Medicine.* 1998;20:161–167.
169. Rabin DL, Boekeloo BO, Marx ES, Bowman MA, Russell NK, Willis AG. Improving office-based physician's prevention practices for sexually transmitted diseases. *Annals of Internal Medicine.* 1994;121:513–519.
170. Scholes D, Stergachis A, Heidrich FE, Andrilla H, Holmes KK, StammWE. Prevention of pelvic inflammatory disease by screening for cervical chlamydial infection. *New England Journal of Medicine.* 1996;334:1362–1366.
171. Shafer MB, Tebb KP, Partell RH, et al. Effect of a clinical practice improvement intervention on chlamydia screening among adolescent girls. *Journal of the American Medical Association.* 2002;288:2846–2852.
172. Singh S, Darroch JE, Frost JJ. Socioeconomic disadvantage and adolescent women's sexual and reproductive behavior: the case of five developed countries. *Family Planning Perspectives.* 2001;33:251–259.
173. Escobar-Chaves SL, Tortolero SR, Markham CM, Low BJ, Eitel P, Thickstun. Impact of the media on adolescent sexual attitudes and behaviors. *Pediatrics.* 2005;116:303–326.
174. Collins RL, Elliott MN, Berry SH, et al. Watching sex on television predicts adolescent initiation of sexual behavior. *Pediatrics.* 2004;114:280–289.
175. Landry DJ, Kaeser L, Richards CL. Abstinence promotion and the provision of information about contraception in public school district sexuality education policies. *Family Planning Perspectives.* 1999;31:280–286.
176. Zavodny M. Fertility and parental consent for minors to receive contraceptives. *American Journal of Public Health.* 2004;94:1347–1351.
177. Jones RK, Purcell A, Singh S, Finer LB. Adolescent reports of parental knowledge of adolescents' use of sexual health services and their reactions to mandated parental notification for prescription contraception. *Journal of the American Medical Association.* 2005;293:340–348.
178. Santelli JS, Abma J, Ventura S, et al. Can changes in sexual behaviors among high school students explain the decline in teen pregnancy rates in the 1990's? *Journal of Adolescent Health.* 2004;35:80–90.
179. Perry CL, Williams CL, Komoro KA, et al. Project Northland high school interventions: community action to reduce adolescent alcohol use. *Health Education and Behavior.* 2000;1:29–49.

13

Biological and Behavioral Risk Factors Associated with STDs/HIV in Women: Implications for Behavioral Interventions

Donna Hubbard McCree, Ph.D., M.P.H., R.Ph., and Anne M. Rompalo, M.D.

Women are disproportionately affected by the burden and consequences of STDs, including human immunodeficiency virus (HIV). Of the estimated 19 million cases of STDs that occur annually in the United States (1), about two-thirds are in women (2). Further, both bacterial and viral STDs are associated with negative sequelae in women. Untreated gonococcal and chlamydial infections can produce significant and disproportionate reproductive system morbidity in women, including pelvic inflammatory disease, infertility, ectopic pregnancy, and chronic pelvic pain (2,3). Additionally, about 70% of chlamydia infections and 50% of gonococcal infections are asymptomatic in women, causing a delay in seeking care and an increase in the risk for negative sequelae (3,4).

Genital human papillomavirus (HPV) infection, the most common sexually transmitted viral infection worldwide, can also produce negative sequelae for women. Although most genital HPV infections are transient (i.e., are cleared by a healthy immune system), persistent infection with oncogenic or high-risk types are associated with cervical abnormalities and cervical cancer, while infection with other types can produce genital warts (5). Further, infection with herpes simplex virus, also common in women, can produce painful outbreaks, and in pregnant women, can result in perinatal transmission and serous neonatal infection (3).

HIV/acquired immunodeficiency syndrome (AIDS) has become a significant public health concern for women. An estimated 14 million women are infected with HIV worldwide (2). Further, women between the ages of 18 and 44 years represent the fastest growing population with HIV/AIDS in the United States (6). In 2004, women represented 30% of the 33,132 reported cases of HIV infection and 23% of the 415,195 persons living with AIDS in the United States (7). African-American women are disproportionately affected by STDs, including HIV/AIDS, compared with women in all other ethnic/racial groups. The rate of AIDS diagnosis in African-American women is about 25 times the rate for Caucasian women and four times the rate for Hispanic women (8). In 2001, HIV infection was the leading cause of death for 25–34-year-old African-American women and the third leading cause of death for 35–44-year-old African-American women (8,9).

Behavioral Interventions for Prevention and Control of Sexually Transmitted Diseases.
Aral SO, Douglas JM Jr, eds. Lipshutz JA, assoc ed. New York: Springer Science+ Business Media, LLC; 2007.

Given the statistics and negative sequelae, preventing STDs/HIV in women is an important public health goal (10). A myriad of biological, behavioral, and contextual factors are associated with the burden of STDs in women. This chapter will review the unique biological and behavioral factors associated with the acquisition and transmission of STDs, including HIV, in women and will provide examples of published interventions that target women and focus on these factors.

Unique Factors Related to STD/HIV Risks in Women

Biological Risk Factors

The female reproductive system is susceptible to STDs in several unique ways. Anatomically, it is composed of an array of epithelial cell types, several communicating compartments, and a unique microbiological balance all of which are physiologically influenced by hormonal flux. Furthermore, biological factors that may increase female susceptibility to STDs vary with age.

The cellular morphology of the cervix and vagina vary over a woman's lifetime and are directly influenced by hormonal changes. At birth, maternal estrogen stimulates a stratified squamous epithelial lining in the neonatal vagina, which is susceptible to trichomonas and candidal infections but resistant to chlamydial and gonococcal infections (11). When this maternal estrogen wanes, the stratified squamous epithelium is replaced by a thin, atrophic columnar epithelium, which remains until menarche and which will support the growth of both *Chlamydia trachomatis* and *Neisseria gonorrhea*. At puberty, estrogen stimulation returns to stimulate a thicker, glycogen-containing stratified squamous epithelium that covers the vaginal vault to the squamocolumnar junction on the cervix and also that is less susceptible to chlamydial and gonococcal infections (12).

The cervix consists primarily of dense collagenous connective tissue. The cervical canal consists of columnar epithelium, but the part of the ectocervix that projects into the vagina is covered by stratified squamous, nonkeratinizing epithelium. The columnar epithelium of the cervical canal, or endocervix, may extend out beyond the external os where it forms small patches known as physiological eversion, or ectopy. Cervical ectopy is a common physiological process in adolescence, as well as during pregnancy and in response to hormonal contraceptive use. A larger surface area of columnar epithelium is exposed to potential infectious inoculum when ectopy is present, and so the size of ectopy is believed to correlate with the risk of cervical chlamydial and gonococcal infections (13–15).

With age, the uterus elongates and the squamocolumnar junction migrates into the cervical canal (16). At menopause, a sharp decline in estrogen levels effects atrophic changes in the vagina, with thinning of the epithelium, decreased lubrication, and narrowing and shortening of the vaginal canal. Sexually active postmenopausal women experience less pronounced changes (17).

The estrogen stimulation associated with puberty also affects the vaginal flora. Prepubescent girls have vaginal flora predominately composed of anaerobic rods and cocci and low levels of lactobacilli (12). At puberty, glycogen is deposited on the vaginal epithelium under estrogenic control. The vaginal epithelial cells metabolize the glycogen to form glucose. Lactobacilli that are part of the normal vaginal flora use the glucose for nutrients and produce lactic acid, which keeps the vagina at an acidic pH. In addition to producing acid, some species of lactobacilli produce hydrogen peroxide (H_2O_2), which may play a crucial role in protecting against overgrowth of pathogens in the vagina, leading to bacterial vaginosis, and which also acts as a natural microbicide with the vaginal ecosystem, especially important in killing HIV. As estrogen declines during menopause, there is also a decline in glycogen production and vascularity in the vagina.

Physiological hormonal changes throughout a woman's lifespan also affect the production and consistency of cervical mucus, which also may serve as a defense against infection (18). Cervical mucus is abundant through the first month of life, becomes scant with loss of maternal estrogen, and becomes copious around puberty. The mucus secreted at adolescence, unlike that of older adolescents or adult women, is easily penetrated by organisms and sperm. Once monthly menstrual cycles are established, maximal secretion and minimal viscosity occurs during midcycle or the periovulatory phase. A thick, viscous cervical mucus acts as a functional barrier against attachment of pathogens to epithelial surfaces and against the ascent of organisms into the uterus and fallopian tubes. It may also provide a substrate for antibacterial enzymes, antibodies, and leukocytes (11). Adolescent girls also experience opening of the endocervical canal at 9 or 10 years of age. Given their immunological naïveté, their easily penetrable cervical mucus, and the opening of the cervical canal, sexually active adolescent girls have major biological predisposition for ascent of pathogens into the upper reproductive tract and a higher incidence of pelvic inflammatory disease (11,18).

Additional biological risk factors associated with risk for STDs in women are related to the type of sexual intercourse and the often asymptomatic nature of STDs in women. Receptive anal intercourse and penile-vaginal intercourse have higher risks for discharge-related STDs and HIV than does oral sex. Additionally, as previously stated, women infected with many STDs as compared with men have minimal or nonspecific symptoms or no symptoms. Symptoms of vaginal discharge that can be associated with gonorrhea, trichomonas, or chlamydial infections are often misinterpreted by women and their health care providers as being caused by yeast infections. Additionally, incorrect treatment with vaginal yeast medications, over-the-counter preparations, or home remedies and douches often delay or confound diagnosis (19). Further, genital ulcer diseases caused by syphilis or genital herpes infections are also not recognized early in many women, either due to lack of symptoms or by the inability to detect lesions on the female genitalia or cervix. Syphilis is more commonly diagnosed in its secondary stage among women, whereas men report more frequently with visible primary stage lesions (20). Finally, women with primary or recurrent genital herpes infections often misinterpret symptoms as being caused by urinary tract infections or by yeast (20).

Since symptoms do not always herald STDs in women, screening should be based on risk. For example, the Centers for Disease Control and Prevention (CDC) (4) recommends yearly screening for *Chlamydia trachomatis* in all sexually active women who are 25 years of age or younger and in all older women with risk factors (e.g., a new partner or multiple partners). Further, since a high prevalence of chlamydia is found in women following treatment due to reinfection either from an untreated sexual partner or from a new partner, women with chlamydial infection should be retested three months after treatment (4). Ensuring that all sexual partners are treated before resuming sexual activity is difficult if the male partner has no symptoms or if the threat of violence with disclosure of infection is an issue. Without treatment of all partners, recurrent infection often occurs. Patient-delivered partner therapy recently has been evaluated and can be very effective in decreasing reinfection with gonorrhea and chlamydia, especially among women (21). This is particularly important since symptoms may not be associated with infection and because repeat infections confer an elevated risk of pelvic inflammatory disease (PID) and its sequelae. Similarly, since gonococcal infections among women often are asymptomatic, the U.S. Preventive Services Task Force (22) recommends routine screening of all sexually active women who are at risk. Risk factors include a previous gonorrhea infection, other STDs, new or multiple sex partners, inconsistent condom use, commercial sex work, and drug use.

In addition to the asymptomatic nature of many STDs in women, another factor that contributes to underdiagnoses or delayed diagnoses of STDs in women relates to STD diagnostic test sensitivity. Until the development of very sensitive nucleic acid amplification tests (NAATs), women were at a technical diagnostic disadvantage because available diagnostics for cervical STDs were not extremely sensitive, possibly due to contamination by resident nonpathogenic organisms, or to the presence of cervical mucus or blood (23).

Because women are more biologically susceptible to STDs if exposed than men and are more likely to have unrecognized and untreated infections, short-term and long-term health consequences often result. With inadequate treatment, an estimated 10–45% of women with gonorrhea and 10–30% of women with chlamydia infections may develop PID (24).

Behavioral Risk Factors

Behavioral risk factors that place women at risk for STDs/HIV include early sexual debut and partner characteristics, e.g., multiple partners, concurrent partners, and risky partners. In fact, it is more often the behavior of the male partner than that of the woman that affects a woman's risk (25,26), as most women acquire STDs, including HIV, from heterosexual contact with an infected male partner (25). Additionally, because STDs are often asymptomatic in women and transmission of some STDs, particularly HIV, from men to women is more efficient (10), women who engage in less risky behavior may be at greater risk of becoming infected than men (26). Therefore, the behavioral risk factors for STDs/HIV in women must be discussed with regard to the social and contextual factors that affect women's sexual behavior. Social factors are defined as external factors that impact groups of people similarly, e.g., social and cultural norms, social status, and incarceration history (27). Contextual factors form the environment in which individuals exist and include relationships, victimization, drug abuse, and the exchange of drugs and/or money for sex (27).

Social and cultural norms within groups often influence their behavior in relationships. Gender dynamics (i.e., traditional gender roles for women that allow men to make decisions about sexual behavior) limit the ability of women to protect themselves from and increase their vulnerability to STDs and

HIV (26). Additionally, a sex-ratio imbalance in which women outnumber men (i.e., among African-Americans in the United States) may limit the bargaining advantage of women in male-female relationships and hamper their ability to negotiate protective behaviors like condom use (27). Further, cultural norms that support involvement in subcultures like the exchange of sex and/or money for drugs may increase risky sexual behavior and hinder safe sex practices (28). Women involved in the sex exchange subculture are subject to violence; victimization; and higher risk sexual behaviors like multiple and risky sexual partners, and a higher frequency of unprotected sex (27).

Poverty plays a significant role in the susceptibility of women to STDs and HIV. Poverty is associated with poorer health status, substance use, increased levels of and chronic stress, violence, and limited access to health care (29–32). The available literature also suggests that lower income couples hold more traditional values about gender roles (33,34), increasing a woman's dependence on her male partner and limiting her ability to protect herself (27).

Sexual networks, sets of individuals who are linked directly or indirectly through sexual behavior (35), can influence a woman's STD and HIV risk. Within sexual networks, partner concurrency (i.e., overlapping sexual relationships) fosters the transmission of STDs. Therefore, women who are in sexual networks that have high concurrent sexual partnerships are at greater risk for STDs, including HIV (35). Differences in sexual networks have been used to explain differences in the STD/HIV rates between African-American and Caucasian women (36). African-American women tend to be in racially segregated sexual networks with higher partner concurrency rates due to lower marriage rates and younger age at sexual debut (35).

Incarceration history is also a factor in the STD/HIV rates in women. Women with a history of incarceration also report engaging in more high-risk behavior such as injecting drug use and unprotected sex prior to their incarceration (37–39). Further, women with a history of incarceration may turn to substance abuse to mute the trauma of incarceration (27).

The meaning and nature of the relationship in which sex occurs affects a woman's risk for STDs/HIV. Research (26,40,41) has shown that gender roles within a relationship can influence sexual behavior and risk for STDs. Gender roles for women are often related to connection and caring for other (27). Therefore, women may engage in risky behaviors like drug use to strengthen the bond between them and their partners (42), and/or to create or maintain relationships (43). Further, relationship power, i.e., relationship control and decision-making power (44) can significantly affect sexual protective behaviors like the ability to negotiate condom use and actual condom use in relationships. More often men have decision power over sexual behavior issues and control over condom use. Women are often unable to make an independent decision to use condoms (26).

Research has also shown that past victimization, e.g., history of child sexual abuse (45); substance abuse, including injection drug use (46–48); alcohol and crack cocaine use (49,50); and mental health problems, e.g., depression (51,52), are related to STD/HIV risk behavior in women. Past victimization can influence a women's decision to engage in high-risk sexual behavior (27). Further, these factors are often interrelated and more prevalent in populations that are disproportionately affected by STDs like African-American and Hispanic women (27).

Behavioral Risk Factors in Lesbians

Sexual orientation is characterized by behavior (gender of sex partners), affective (attraction or desire), and cognitive (identify) dimensions (53). Women use terms like heterosexual, bisexual, or lesbian to describe their sexual orientation, while researchers use terms like women who have sex with women (WSW), women who have sex with men (WSM), or women who have sex with both men and women (MSMW) to describe the sexual behavior of women (53). Approximately 2.3 million women in the United States describe themselves, i.e., their sexual orientation, as lesbian (54). There are few studies on the prevalence of STDs/HIV in lesbians and fewer on the STD/HIV risk behaviors of this population. Results from studies on the prevalence of STDs/HIV in lesbians show that lesbians have an unusually high prevalence of bacterial vaginosis and that the transmission of STDs like trichomoniasis, genital herpes, HPV, and HIV has been reported in this population (53–55). The available literature on STD/HIV risk behaviors in lesbians suggest that sexual practices like digital-vaginal or digital-anal contact with shared penetrative sex toys between women provide an environment for STD transmission to occur (54). These studies also show limited knowledge of the potential for STD transmission between lesbians (54).

Despite the evidence on STDs/HIV among lesbians, there is a paucity of literature on prevention interventions in this population. Given the statistics, however, prevention interventions are necessary for women who describe themselves as lesbians. Based on results from the literature, interventions targeting this population should include education of risk for STD transmission between women, incorporate themes of personal responsibility, target the range of sexual practices (i.e., digital-vaginal penetration and use of vaginally insertive sex toys in lesbians), be framed in terms of sexual enjoyment and healthy sexuality, and emphasize respect for one's body and sexual choices (54).

STD/HIV Prevention Interventions that Target Women

Behavioral interventions seek to increase knowledge, change attitudes, and promote the adoption of safer behaviors, and develop environmental conditions that support positive behavior change (56). Successful STD/HIV interventions, then, have a multifactor approach at different social and structural levels, target behaviors that involve contact with core group members or high-risk activity, include a condom promotion component, develop and implement structural and ecologic changes that foster the adoption of STD/HIV prevention practices, and have strong leadership at political and public health levels that affect the targeted community (56). Published STD/HIV prevention interventions for women have focused on improving knowledge, self-efficacy, and risk-reduction behavior (57). While individual-level constructs like knowledge, self-efficacy, and risk perception are important, STD/HIV prevention efforts that focus on women must also include a recognition of the unique biological and behavioral risk factors that make women more susceptible to STDs (57) and the social and contextual factors that affect women's sexual behavior (58). Further, because of the rates and unique issues related to STD/HIV acquisition and transmission in ethnic minority women, interventions targeting these populations should also be culturally specific (40,

57,59–61). There is debate in the literature about the meaning of "culturally specific"; definitions range from incorporating discussions on cultural values, customs, traditions, racial/ethnic pride, and/or cultural barriers to adopting safer sex behaviors into interventions (25,57,61), to providing ethnicity-specific educational resources, and having ethnically matched facilitators (57).

Based on the available literature, the most efficacious prevention interventions specifically targeting women have involved theory-based skills training strategies, e.g., Social Learning Theory (62); focused on relationship and negotiation skills, and included multiple contacts (63). Almost all of the published STD/HIV prevention interventions have promoted consistent use of male condoms as the desired prevention strategy (25). Effective interventions for promoting condom use have used a randomized control study design; emphasized gender-power dynamics; been peer-led; and presented in multiple sessions (40).

The following section will outline the evidence on the effectiveness of and provide examples of published interventions to reduce risk factors for STDs/HIV in women. These examples do not include studies that have male participants. The discussion is organized by the level of the intervention (i.e., individual, group, or community).

Individual Level

Most of the published interventions targeting individual women are brief and single-session, have focused on risk-reduction education including activities to strengthen risk-reduction behavior skills (e.g., correct condom use, sexual communication training, problem solving skills); and included exercises to promote the development of positive attitudes, beliefs, and intentions about positive behavioral change and reinforcement of support for behavioral change efforts (58). While these types of interventions offer brevity, they are often limited in the amount of individualized skill-building they provide (25).

Scholes et al. (64) developed a theory-based tailored minimal self-help intervention to increase condom use among young women. The intervention was based on social science theory and included individually tailored materials (i.e., a self-help magazine-style booklet, *Insights*; a tailored booster feedback newsletter, *Extra Insights;* and a safe sex kit with male and female condoms, a condom carrying case, and condom-use instructions). The control condition was usual care. The primary study outcomes were proportion of sexually active women who used condoms with any partner, proportion of sexually active women who used condoms with a nonprimary partner, and the average percentage of total episodes of intercourse during which condoms were used; all measured for the prior three months. Women in the intervention group reported significantly greater condom use overall with recent primary partners, higher proportion of intercourse episodes in which condoms were used, more condom use discussions with a partner, and higher condom use self-efficacy with primary partners than women in the control condition.

Additionally, Bryan and colleagues (65) developed a multicomponent, one-session condom promotion intervention targeting sexually active college women. The intervention consisted of videotaped segments, lectures and audience participation, and skill-building exercise intervention; and addressed women's perceptions about sexuality, beliefs about STDs, and self-efficacy for condom use. The control group received a stress management session. The intervention produced increased intentions among participants to use condoms immediately post-intervention, and reported increased condom use at last intercourse six weeks and six months post-intervention.

Schilling et al. (38) report on an individual level intervention for decreasing STD transmission. This study examined the use of patient-delivered partner treatment with azithromycin to prevent repeat chlamydia infection in women. The goal was to determine whether repeat infection with *Chlamydia trachomatis* could be reduced by providing women with doses of azithromycin for their male sex partners. This randomized, multicenter controlled trial included two study conditions: patient-delivered partner treatment (women asked to deliver azithromycin to their male sex partners) or self-referral (women asked to refer their sex partners for treatment). Results showed that the risk of reinfection was lower among women in the patient-delivered partner treatment condition but the difference was not statistically significant.

Group Level

There are many published small-group interventions targeting women. These interventions typically involve a substantial amount of contact with participants, usually draw on constructs of social-cognitive and reasoned-action theories; attempt to increase participants' knowledge about STD/HIV prevention, strengthen behavior-change motivation, and teach STD/HIV risk-reduction skills (58). They are also typically tailored to address the needs of the targeted group.

Shain et al. (66,67) describe two different trials of a behavioral intervention to prevent gonorrhea and chlamydia in minority women. Project SAFE (66) was a theory-based, culture-specific, behavioral, risk-reduction intervention designed to reduce chlamydia and gonorrhea infection in low-income African-American and Mexican-American women. The intervention consisted of three small-group, multicomponent, three to four hour sessions delivered to five or six participants by a race- and gender-matched trained facilitator. The intervention condition was adapted from the AIDS Risk Reduction Model (68), and included elements of the several social and psychological theories including the Health Belief Model (69), self-efficacy theory (62), decision-making models (70), and diffusion theory (71). The control condition was standard STD counseling. The main outcome variable was chlamydial or gonorrheal infection. Results showed that the rates of subsequent chlamydial or gonorrheal infection in the intervention group were significantly lower than in the control group at both the 6- and 12-month follow-up periods.

Project Safe 2 (67) included a second intervention arm, five optional monthly support groups following the standard intervention, and additional follow-up at 1 year, 18 months, and 2 years post-intervention. With Project Safe 2, investigators sought to confirm results from the original study, examine long-term efficacy of the new intervention by including a two-year follow-up period, determine whether the efficacy changes over time, and determine the additional benefits of the optional support groups. The main outcome was subsequent chlamydia or gonorrhea infection. Results showed that adjusted subsequent chlamydial or gonorrhea infection rates were higher in the control condition than in the other two conditions. Additionally, women who participated in the support groups had the lowest adjusted infection rates in year 1 and cumulatively. Further, women in the intervention conditions were significantly less likely to have repeat infection than women in the control condition.

Eldridge et al. (72) developed an intervention targeting women entering court-ordered inpatient substance abuse treatment. The intervention was a four-session behavioral skills training condition that provided skill-building training for sexual negotiation and condom use; the control condition was a three-hour HIV education session (25,72). Women in the intervention group had significantly improved prevention attitudes, more positive expected partner reaction, and improved sexual communication and condom use skills as compared with women in the control condition. There was improvement with regard to the number of partners, frequency of risky acts, and number of drugs used in both the intervention and control groups. Results from the study, however, should be interpreted with regard to the attrition rate at follow-up; the follow-up assessment response rate was 49%.

Baker et al. (2003) compared the effectiveness of two different intervention, skills treatment (ST) and health education (HE), for reducing new STD infections in heterosexual women. The ST condition was based on the relapse prevention model (73), a model that includes traditional approaches to skills training and skills to support the initiation and long-term maintenance of safer sex behavior change. This condition included didactic presentations, discussion, and role-play group exercises to practice safer sex skills. The HE condition included didactic presentations on women's health with a focus on sexual health and nonstructured discussion sessions. Both conditions were delivered in 16 weekly two-hour group sessions with 5 to 10 participants per group. The main outcomes were new STD acquisition and self-reports of sexual behavior. Study results showed that participants in the ST condition were significantly less likely to be diagnosed with an STD and demonstrated superior risk reduction skills at 12-month follow-up compared with participants in the HE condition. Further, participants in both conditions had a significant reduction in self reports of risky sexual behavior immediately following the intervention and at 12-month follow-up. Based on study results, the ST intervention was superior to the HE intervention in reducing new STD acquisition.

Van Devanter et al. (2) assessed the effectiveness of a STD/HIV behavior change intervention on increasing use of the female condom. The WINGS (Women in Group Support) project was a randomized trial of an education, skills-training, and support-group intervention for women at high risk for STD/HIV infection. The intervention was composed of six weekly group sessions in which women received information about STDs/HIV; skills training in communication, goal setting, and use of the male condom; and information about the female condom, a video demonstration on its use, live demonstration of female condom use, and the opportunity to practice using the condoms. The control condition was a one-hour session that included a nutrition video on healthy food choices. Women in the intervention group had more positive attitudes toward the female condom, demonstrated increased skills in female condom use, and were more likely to use the female condom and say that they intended to use it than women in the control group. Women in the control group also increased their use of the female condom from baseline.

Community Level

Community-level interventions targeting women include a focus on structural/policy interventions to assist women in reducing their STD/HIV risks (25,74). These types of interventions may be more cost-effective than individual or group level interventions because they reach a large number of women (25). Additionally, they may produce a generalization of empowerment among participants to other community issues (25).

Lauby et al. (75) describe a community-level HIV prevention intervention for inner-city women. The goal of the intervention was to modify community norms, attitudes, and behaviors concerning condom use among community women. The intervention was based on the Transtheoretical Model of Behavior Change (75) and included three components: a media campaign, outreach, and community mobilization. The media campaign involved the use of flyers, brochures, posters, and newsletters to relay role-model stories of women in different degrees of readiness to use condoms; these stories described how women overcame barriers to condom use and progressed to more consistent condom use. The outreach was stage-based and included one-on-one or group-level contact to provide prevention messages, encourage and reinforce behavior change, and distribute condoms and role model stories. The community mobilization component involved the recruitment of peers as volunteers to provide HIV information, referral, condoms, and role model stories. The comparison condition was the usual HIV prevention programs available in the matched communities. Results showed that women in the intervention communities were more likely to report ever using condoms post-intervention with main partners than women in the comparison communities.

Sikemma et al (76) developed a multi-site community level intervention for women living in 18 low-income housing developments in five U.S. cities. Participants from housing developments randomized to the intervention condition received peer-led small-group workshops and community events while participants from housing developments in the comparison condition received HIV informational brochures, free condoms, and order forms to obtain additional condoms. The major outcome was assessment of HIV risk behavior in the housing developments at baseline and one-year post-intervention. The proportion of women reporting unprotected intercourse declined and the percentage of intercourse occasions for which condoms were used increased for women in the intervention condition as compared to women in the control condition (76). Additionally, women in the intervention condition scored higher on the AIDS knowledge measure and were more likely to report having a condom at home or on her person than women in the comparison condition.

Conclusion

This chapter highlights the unique biological and behavioral factors related to the acquisition and transmission of STDs/HIV in women and provides examples of published interventions that target women. Additional research is needed to determine the most effective gender- and race/ethnicity-appropriate theories and interventions for STD/HIV prevention in women (26). This research should continue to examine the role of social and contextual factors (e.g., mental health issues, past childhood sexual abuse, incarceration history, and substance abuse associated with women's sexual behavior), how these factors are associated with STD/HIV acquisition and transmission, and appropriate methods for addressing these factors in STD/HIV prevention. Additional research is also needed on barriers and facilitators of early testing for STDs/HIV (26) so that the negative sequelae associated with these infections in women may be avoided. Further, additional research is needed on specific populations of women who remain disproportionately affected by STDs/HIV (i.e., high-risk ethnic minority women, despite the plethora of interventions conducted in this group). Women in these populations may have complicated life experiences associated with their ability to practice safer sex that may require additional support and different types of interventions (10). Effective interventions in this population may include structural level interventions like incarceration reform and organized substance abuse treatment and support.

Further research should be conducted on successful interventions to determine in which populations of women they are most successful, if they can be shortened and adapted for different populations of women and women in different environments and still maintain their effectiveness, and whether they will maintain their effectiveness over longer periods of time. Interventions are also needed for pregnant women, as research (77) has shown that pregnant women remain sexually active and therefore at risk for STDs/HIV throughout their pregnancy. These women, however, are often excluded from behavioral intervention trials, and few interventions have been developed for this population (66,78). Further, because the behavior of the male partner is usually the significant factor in STD/HIV risk for women, interventions targeting heterosexual men are needed. There is a paucity of published interventions and a general lack of attention to STD/HIV interventions for heterosexual men (10). This oversight might reinforce traditional gender roles that sexual safety is a woman's concern (10), and put men at risk and increase women's risk for STDs/HIV. Finally, there is a clear need to translate and disseminate research on effective interventions for women into practice. Few effective interventions have been translated into practice, as effective translation is often impeded by lack of funding for implementation and lack of field-based support (56). In order to have a significant impact on STD/HIV rates in women, effective interventions must be developed that are sustainable, cost-effective, and translatable within the current public health infrastructure (79).

References

1. Weinstock H, Berman S, Cates W. Sexually transmitted diseases among American youth: incidence and prevalence estimates, 2000. *Perspectives on Sexual & Reproductive Health.* 2004;36:6–10.
2. Van Devanter N, Gonzales V, Merzel C, Parikh NS, Celantano D, Greenberg J. Effect of an STD/HIV behavioral intervention on women's use of the female condom. *American Journal of Public Health.* 2002;92:109–115.
3. Centers for Disease Control and Prevention. STDs in women and infants. In: *Sexually Transmitted Disease Surveillance, 2004.* Atlanta, GA: U.S. Department of Health and Human Services; September 2005.
4. Centers for Disease Control and Prevention. STD Treatment Guidelines 2002. *MMWR.* 2002;51(No. RR-6).
5. Castle PE, Solomon D, Schiffman M, Wheeler CM. Human papillomavirus type 16 infections and 2-year absolute risk of cervical precancer in women with equiv-

ocal or mild cytologic abnormalities. *Journal of the National Cancer Institute*. 2005;97:1066–1071.

6. Robinson BB, Uhl G, Miner M, et al. Evaluation of a sexual health approach to prevent HIV among low income, urban, primarily African American women: results of a randomized controlled trial. *AIDS Education and Prevention*. 2002; 14(Suppl A):81–96.

7. Centers for Disease Control and Prevention. *HIV/AIDS Surveillance Report, 2004*. Volume 16. Atlanta, GA: U.S. Department of Health and Human Services, Centers for Disease Control; 2005.

8. Centers for Disease Control and Prevention. *HIV/AIDS Surveillance Report, 2003*. Volume 15. Atlanta, GA: U.S. Department of Health and Human Services, Centers for Disease Control; 2004.

9. Anderson RN, Smith BL. Deaths: leading causes for 2001. *National Vital Statistics Reports*. 2003;52:32–33, 53–54.

10. Baker SA, Beadnell B, Stoner S, et al. Skills training versus health education to prevent STDs/HIV in heterosexual women: a randomized controlled trail utilizing biological outcomes. *AIDS Education and Prevention*. 2003;15:1–14.

11. Bolan G, Ehrhardt AA, Wasserheit JN. Gender perspectives and STDs. In: Holmes KK, Sparling PF, Mardh PA, et al., eds. *Sexually Transmitted Diseases*, 3rd Ed. New York: McGraw-Hill; 1998; pp 117–127.

12. Hammerschlag MR, Alpert S, Rosner I, Thurston P, Semine D, McComb D, McCormack WM. Microbiology of the vagina in children: normal and potentially pathogenic organisms. *Pediatrics*. 1978;62:57–62.

13. Draper DL, Donegan EA, James JF, Sweet RL, Brooks GF. Scanning electron microscopy of attachment of *Neisseria gonorrhoeae* colony phenotypes to surfaces of human genital epithelia. *American Journal of Obstetrics and Gynecology*. 1980;138:818–826.

14. Harrison HR, Costin M, Meder JB, et al. Cervical *Chlamydia trachomatis* infection in university women: relationships to history, contraception, ectopy, and cervicitis. *American Journal of Obstetrics and Gynecology*. 1985;153: 244–251.

15. Jacobson DL, Peralta L, Farmer M, Graham N, Gaydos C, Zenilman J. Relationship of hormonal contraception and cervical ectopy as measured by computerized planimetry to chlamydial infection in adolescents. *Sexually Transmitted Diseases*, 2000;27:313–319.

16. Singer A. The uterine cervix from adolescence to menopause. *British Journal of Obstetrics and Gynecology*. 1975;82:81–99.

17. Mooradian AD Greiff V. Sexuality in older women. *Archives of Internal Medicine*. 1990;150:1033–1038.

18. Cohen M, Black JR, Proctor RA, Sparling PF. Host defenses and the vaginal mucosa: a re-evaluation. *Scandinavian Journal of Urology Nephrology Supplement*. 1984;86:13–22.

19. Irwin DE, Thomas JS, Spitters CE, et al. Self-treatment among clients attending sexually transmitted diseases clinics and the effect of self-treatment on STD symptom duration. *Sexually Transmitted Diseases*. 1997;24:372–377.

20. Rompalo AM, Joesoef MR, O'Donnel JA, et al. Clinical manifestations of early syphilis by HIV status and gender: results of the syphilis and HIV study. *Sexually Transmitted Diseases*. 2001;28:158–165.

21. Golden MR. Expedited partner therapy for sexually transmitted diseases. *Clinics in Infectious Diseases*. 2005;41:630–633.

22. U.S. Preventive Services Task Force. Screening for gonorrhea. May 2005. Available at: www.ahcpr.gov/clinic/uspstf/uspsgono.htm.

23. Gaydos CA. Nucleic acid amplification tests for gonorrhea and chlamydia: practice and applications. *Infectious Disease Clinics of North American*. 2005;19: 367–386.

24. Platt R, Rice PA, McCormack WM. Risk of acquiring gonorrhea and prevalence of abnormal annexal findings among women recently exposed to gonorrhea. *Journal of the American Medical Association*. 1983;250:3205.
25. O'Leary A. Women at risk for HIV from a primary partner; balancing risk and intimacy. *Annual Review of Sex Research*. 2000;11:191–234.
26. Pequegnat W, Stover E. Considering women's contextual and cultural issues in HIV/STD prevention research. *Cultural Diversity and Ethnic Minority Psychology*. 1999;5:287–291.
27. Logan TK, Cole J, Leukefeld C. Women, sex, and HIV: social and contextual factors, meta-analysis of published interventions, and implications for practice and research. *Psychological Bulletin*. 2002;128:851–885.
28. Windle M. The trading of sex for money or drugs, sexually transmitted diseases (STDs), and HIV-related risk behaviors among multisubstance using alcohol inpatients. *Drug and Alcohol Dependence*, 1997;49:33–38.
29. Institute of Medicine. *The Hidden Epidemic: Confronting Sexually Transmitted Diseases*. Washington, DC: National Academy Press; 1997.
30. Nyamathi A, Wayment H, Dunkel-Schetter C. Psychosocial correlates of emotional distress and risk behavior in African-American women at risk for HIV infection. *Anxiety, Stress, and Coping: An International Journal*. 1993;6:133–148.
31. Sikkema K, Heckman T, Kelly J, et al. HIV risk behaviors among women living in low-income, inner-city housing developments. *American Journal of Public Health*. 1996;86:1123–1128.
32. Staveteig S, Wigton A. *Racial and Ethnic Disparities: Key Findings from the National Survey of American's Families*. Washington, DC: Urban Institute; February 2000. Report No. B-5.
33. Brownridge D, Halli S. "Living in sin" and sinful living: toward filing a gap in the explanation of violence against women. *Aggression and Violent Behavior*. 2000;5:565–583.
34. Lenton R. Power versus feminine theories of wife abuse. *Canadian Journal of Criminology*. 1995;37:305–330.
35. Adimora AA, Schoenbach VJ. Social context, sexual networks, and racial disparities in rates of sexually transmitted infections. *The Journal of Infectious Diseases*. 2005;191:S115–S122.
36. Yoom Y, Laumann EO. Social network effects on the transmission of sexually transmitted diseases. *Sexually Transmitted Diseases*. 2002;29:689–697.
37. El-Bassel N, Gilbert L, Schilling R, Ivanoff A, Borne D, Safyer S. Correlates of crack abuse among drug-using incarcerated women: psychological trauma, social support, and coping behavior. *American Journal of Drug and Alcohol Abuse*. 1996;22:41–57.
38. Schilling R, El-Bassel N, Ivanoff A, Gilbert L, Su K, Safyer S. Sexual risk behavior of incarcerated, drug-using women, 1992. *Public Health Reports*. 1994;109:539–547.
39. Templer D, Walker S. Self-reported high-risk behavioral history of HIV positive prison inmates. *Psychological Reports*. 1995;76:237–238.
40. DiClemente R, Wingood G. A randomized controlled trial of an HIV sexual risk-reduction intervention for young African-American women. *Journal of the American Medical Association*. 1995;274:1271–1276.
41. Ehrhardt A, Wasserheit J. Age, gender, and sexual risk behaviors for sexually transmitted diseases in the United States. In: Wasserheit JN, Aral SO, Holmes KK, Hitchcock P, eds. *Research Issues in Human Behavior and Sexually Transmitted Diseases in the AIDS Era*. Washington, DC: American Society of Microbiology; 1991:97–121.
42. Covington S, Surry J. The relational model of women's psychological development: implications for substance abuse. In: Wilsnack R, Wilsnack S, eds. *Gender*

and Alcohol: Individual and Social Perspectives. New Brunswick, NJ: Rutgers Center of Alcohol Studies; 1997; pp 335–351.

43. Regan P, Dreyer C. Lust? Love? Status? Young adults' motives for engaging in casual sex. *Journal of Psychology & Human Sexuality.* 1999;11:1–25.

44. Pulerwitz J, Gortmaker S, DeJong W. Measuring sexual relationship power in HIV/STD research. *Sex Roles.* 2000;42:637–660.

45. Bensley L, Van Eenwyk J, Simmons K. Self-reported childhood sexual and physical abuse and adult HIV-risk behaviors and heavy drinking. *American Journal of Preventive Medicine.* 2000;18:151–158.

46. El-Bassel N, Gilbert L, Rajah V, Foleno A, Frye V. Fear and violence: raising the HIV stakes. *AIDS Education and Prevention.* 2000;12:154–170.

47. Kalichman S, Williams E, Cherry C, Belcher L, Nachimson D. Sexual coercion, domestic violence and negotiating condom use among low-income African American women. *Journal of Women's Health.* 1998;7:371–378.

48. The NIMH Multisite HIV Prevention Trial Group. The NIMH Multisite HIV Prevention Trial: reducing HIV sexual risk behavior. *Science.* 1998;280:1889–1894.

49. Rees V, Saitz R, Horton N, Samet J. Association of alcohol consumption with HIV sex- and drug-risk behaviors among drug users. *Journal of Substance Abuse Treatment.* 2001;21:129–134.

50. Wingood G, DiClemente R. The influence of psychosocial factors, alcohol, and drug use on African-American women's high risk sexual behavior. *American Journal of Preventative Medicine.* 1998;15:54–59.

51. Orr S, Celentano D, Santelli J, Burwell L. Depressive symptoms and risk factors for HIV acquisition among black women attending urban health centers in Baltimore. *AIDS Education and Prevention.* 1994;6:230–236.

52. Simon P, Thometz E, Bunch J, Sorvillo F, Detels R, Kerndt P. Prevalence of unprotected sex among men with AIDS in Los Angeles county, California, 1995–1997. *AIDS.* 1999;14:987–990.

53. Koh AJ, Gomez CA, Shade S, Rowley E. Sexual risk factors among self-identified lesbians, bisexual women, and heterosexual women accessing primary care settings. *Sexually Transmitted Diseases.* 2005;32:563–569.

54. Marrazzo JD, Coffey P, Bingham A. Sexual practices, risk perception and knowledge of sexually transmitted disease risk among lesbian and bisexual women. *Perspectives on Sexual and Reproductive Health.* 2005;37:6–12.

55. Marrazzo JD. Dangerous assumptions: lesbians and sexual death. *Sexually Transmitted Diseases.* 2005;32:570–571.

56. Zenilman JM. Behavioral interventions—rationale, measurement, and effectiveness. *Infectious Disease Clinics of North American.* 2005;19:541–562.

57. Mize SJS, Robinson BE, Bockting WO, Scheltema KE. Meta-analysis of the effectiveness of HIV prevention interventions for women. *AIDS Care.* 2002;14: 163–180.

58. Kelley JA, Kalichman SC. Behavioral research in HIV/AIDS primary and secondary prevention: recent advances and future directions. *Journal of Consulting and Clinical Psychology.* 2002;70:626–639.

59. Ickovics J, Rodin J. Women and AIDS in the United States: epidemiology, natural history, and mediating mechanisms. *Health Psychology.* 1992;11:1–16.

60. Jemmott J, Jemmott L, Spears H, Hewitt N, Cruz-Collins M. Self-efficacy, hedonistic expectancies, and condom-use intentions among inner-city black adolescent women: a social cognitive approach to AIDS risk behavior. *Journal of Adolescent Health.* 1992;13:512–519.

61. Mays VM, Cochran S. Issues in the perception of AIDS risk and risk reduction activities by Black and Hispanic/Latina women. *American Psychologist.* 1988;43:949–957.

62. Bandura A. *Self-efficacy: The Exercise of Control.* New York: Freeman; 1997.

63. Exner MT, Seal DW, Ehrhardt AA. A review of HIV Interventions for at-risk women. *AIDS and Behavior*. 1997;1:93–124.

64. Scholes D, McBride CM, Grothaus L, et al. A tailored minimal self-help intervention to promote condom use in young women: results from a randomized trial. *AIDS*. 2003;17:1547–1556.

65. Bryan AD, Aiken LS, West SG. Increasing condom use: evaluation of a theory-based intervention to prevent sexually transmitted disease in young women. *Health Psychology*. 1996;15:371–382.

66. Shain RN, Piper JM, Newton ER et al. A randomized, controlled trial of a behavioral intervention to prevent sexually transmitted disease among minority women. *The New England Journal of Medicine*. 1999;340:93–100.

67. Shain RN, Piper JM, Holden AEC, et al. Prevention of gonorrhea and chlamydia through behavioral intervention results of a two-year controlled randomized trial in minority women. *Sexually Transmitted Diseases*, 2004;31:401–408.

68. Cantania JA, Kegeles SM, Coates TJ. Towards an understanding of risk behavior: an AIDS risk reduction model (ARRM). *Health Education Quarterly*. 1990;17:53–72.

69. Becker MH, Joseph JG. AIDS and behavioral change to reduce risk: a review. *American Journal of Public Health*. 1988;78:394–410.

70. Fishbein M, Ajzen I. *Belief, Attitude, Intention and Behavior: An Introduction to Theory and Research*. Reading, MA: Addison-Wesley; 1975.

71. Rogers EM. *Diffusion of Innovations*. New York: Free Press; 1983.

72. Eldridge GD, St. Lawrence JS, Little CE, et al. Evaluation of an HIV risk reduction intervention for women entering inpatient substance abuse treatment. *AIDS Education and Prevention*. 1997;9(A):62–76.

73. Marlett GA, Gordon JR. *Relapse Prevention: Maintenance Strategies in the Treatment of Addictive Behaviors*. New York: Guilford; 1995.

74. O'Leary A, Martins P. Structural factors affecting women's HIV risk: a life-course example. *AIDS*. 2000;14(Suppl 1):68–72.

75. Lauby JL, Smith PJ, Stark M, Person B, Adams J. A community-level prevention intervention for inner-city women: results of the women and infants demonstration trial. *American Journal of Public Health*. 2000;90:216–222.

76. Sikkema K, Kelly JS, Winett RA, et al. Outcome of a randomized community-level HIV prevention intervention for women living in 18 low-income housing developments. *American Journal of Public Health*. 2000;90:57–63.

77. Hobfall SE, Jackson AP, Lavin J, Britton PR, Shepherd JB. Safer sex knowledge, behavior, and attitudes of inner-city women. *Health Psychology*. 1993;12:481–488.

78. Hobfoll SE, Jackson AP, Lavin J, Johnson RJ, Schroder KEE. Effects and generalizability of communally oriented HIV-AIDS prevention versus general health promotion groups for single, inner-city women in urban clinics. *Journal of Consulting and Clinical Psychology*. 2002;70:950–960.

79. Golden MR, Manhart LE. Innovative approaches to the prevention and control of bacterial sexually transmitted infections. *Infectious Disease Clinics of North America*. 2005;19:513–540.

STD Prevention with Men Who Have Sex with Men in the United States

Kevin A. Fenton, M.D., Ph.D., and Frederick R. Bloom, R.N., Ph.D.

Men who have sex with men (MSM) have assumed particular importance in the epidemiology of STDs in many western industrialized countries (1,2). In part, this is driven by the higher prevalence of sexual risk behaviors within this population subgroup and the consequent increased probability of STD transmission and acquisition. Other factors, for example, patterns and distribution of sexual networks, background disease prevalence, and the effectiveness of targeted prevention interventions, also contribute to the observed and evolving epidemiology. In this chapter, we overview the recent increases in reported STDs among MSM in the United States, explore the behavioral and psychosocial determinants of STD transmission, and consider the evidence regarding effective STD and HIV behavioral interventions for improving sexual health outcomes within this group.

A wide-ranging set of search strategies was used in an attempt to identify as many types of recent data sources relevant to the subject. The topic search was developed using a combination of specific STD prevention terms, terms for interventions specific to the topic area, and general health promotion/health education/public health terms combined with topic terms such as STD or sexual behavior, and limited to the United States. MEDLINE, EMBASE, PsycINFO, Sociofile, and CINAHL databases were searched from January 1999 to October 2005 for references published in the English language. The search strategies were as similar as possible for the different databases, however, index terms differed across some databases. Review of the published literature was supplemented with data obtained from relevant STD surveillance and prevention reports. Attempts were made to obtain all papers, including journal articles, reports and book chapters, with prioritization of review articles.

Male Homosexual Behavior in the United States:
Changing Demographic Contexts

Population-based probability sample surveys provide some of the most up-to-date information on the patterns and distribution of male homosexual behavior in the United States (3,4). While data from the United Kingdom suggest that the prevalence of male homosexual behavior and sexual risk behavior in

Behavioral Interventions for Prevention and Control of Sexually Transmitted Diseases. Aral SO, Douglas JM Jr, eds. Lipshutz JA, assoc ed. New York: Springer Science+ Business Media, LLC; 2007.

MSM are increasing (5), comparable trend data from serial probability sample surveys in the United States are lacking. Data from the 2002 National Survey of Family Growth (NSFG) (6) indicates that 2.9% of U.S. males reported having had a male sexual partner in the last 12 months, equating to approximately 1.77 million men, with 1.6% or men reporting having had only a male sex partner in the last 12 months. Substantially more men reported some homosexual contact during their lifetime. Among males, 15–44 years of age, 5.7% had oral sex with another male at some time in their lives, and 3.7% had anal sex with another male—overall, 6.0% of U.S. men aged 15–44 years reported having had oral or anal sex with another male. There was marked heterogeneity across ethnic groups in the reporting of homosexual sexual orientation, with 2.6% of white, 2.1% of Hispanic, and 1.6% of black men in the United States describing their orientation as homosexual. However, Hispanic and black men were significantly more likely to describe their orientation as "something else" compared with white men (7.3% and 7.5% compared with 2.3%, respectively).

Another major demographic trend occurring within the homosexually active male population in the United States is the growing prevalent pool of MSM with diagnosed HIV infection, in part a reflection of the success of the highly active antiretroviral therapies (HAART) for HIV infection (7). This is of public health importance given the emerging evidence of the higher prevalence of sexual risk behaviors, greater propensity toward serodiscordant sexual mixing, and increasing STD incidence among HIV-positive compared with HIV-negative MSM (1,2). In one study, 22% of HIV positive MSM reported that they had engaged in unprotected insertive anal intercourse in the previous three months with a partner who was HIV-seronegative or whose serostatus was unknown (8). Both of these demographic features—increasing proportion of males reporting homosexual sexual behavior and the growing prevalent pool of HIV positive homosexual men—have a tremendous impact on the sexual health outcomes within this population subgroup, as will be discussed later in this chapter.

The Nature, Causes, and Burden of STDs Among MSM

Characteristics of the Burden

National Surveillance Data

In concert with other western industrialized settings, data from national surveillance data sources suggest that numbers and rates of STDs among MSM have been increasing in recent years. However, the United States is somewhat unique among developed countries (9) in that national notifiable STD surveillance data reported to the Centers for Disease Control (CDC) do not currently contain information regarding sexual orientation or gender of sex partners. This severely limits our understanding of national trends in reported STDs in MSM.

Some understanding of the excess burden of disease borne by MSM may, however, be inferred by examining the male:female (M:F) ratio of reported STDs. For example, the overall M:F syphilis rate ratio has been steadily increasing since 1996, when it was 1.2:1, to 5.2:1 in 2003, with a rate of 4.7 per 100,000 among men and 0.9 per 100,000 among women (10). Sentinel surveillance studies and special research projects have also been established to characterize the incidence and prevalence of STDs among MSM. Nine U.S.

cities (the study sites include STD clinics in six areas as well as three STD clinics in community-based gay men's health clinics) currently participate in the MSM Prevalence Monitoring Project (10), and submit data on syphilis gonorrhea, chlamydia, and HIV testing activities from MSM attendees. Between 1999 and 2003, overall median syphilis seroreactivity among MSM increased from 4.1% to 10.5%; median gonorrhea positivity in MSM was 13.7% (range, 12.9–16.5%) in 1999 and 15.3% (range, 13.7–17.2%) in 2003 (10). Gonorrhea positivity was higher in HIV-positive MSM compared with MSM who were HIV-negative or of unknown HIV status. Other key findings related to the prevalence of STDs among HIV-positive individuals. Rectal gonorrhea positivity was 11% in HIV-positive MSM and 6.1% in MSM who were HIV negative or of unknown HIV status; and the median positivity of chlamydia in STD clinics was 7.9% (range, 3.8–17.0%) in HIV-positive MSM and 6.7% (range, 3.9–10.0%) in MSM who were HIV negative or of unknown HIV status (10). Another national surveillance project, the Gonococcal Isolate Surveillance Project (GISP), monitors trends in antimicrobial susceptibilities of strains of *Neisseria gonorrhoeae* in the United States, and provides some data on STD trends in MSM. Overall, the proportion of isolates from MSM increased from 4% in 1988 to 19.6% in 2003, with more of the increase occurring after 1993 (10).

STD Clinic-Based Studies

STD clinics in the United States remain a major focus for the diagnosis and management of STDs in MSM. Studies undertaken within this setting may help to provide more detailed understanding of STD trends, prevalence, and incidence in a behaviorally high-risk group of MSM, and give some insights into the behavioral and social determinants of disease incidence. Tabet et al. (11) followed a cohort of 578 HIV-negative MSM over 12 months in Seattle and found: 31 men (5.7/100 person-years) had 34 episodes of a symptomatic bacterial STD syndrome (urethritis, epididymitis, or proctitis); five seroconverted to HIV-1 (1.3/100 p-y), four to HSV-2 (1.0/100 p-y), and seven to HSV-1 (4.3/100 p-y). Unprotected insertive anal sex and nitrite inhalant ("poppers") use were independently associated with incident STD. Wong et al. (12) studied factors for early syphilis infection among 1318 MSM attending the San Francisco STD clinic in a cross-sectional, self-administered, behavioral survey between November 2002 and March 2003. Fifty-three (4.0%) were diagnosed with early syphilis. Factors independently associated with syphilis included nonwhite race, HIV-infection, using both methamphetamine and sildenafil, using methamphetamine without sildenafil, using sildenafil without methamphetamines, stronger gay community affiliation, and having recent Internet partners. Fox et al. (13) compared gonococcal urethritis cases among MSM with those among heterosexual men from 29 STD clinics. Of 34,942 cases, the proportion represented by MSM increased from 4.5% in 1992 to 13.2% in 1999 ($p < 0.001$). Compared with heterosexuals, MSM were older, more often white, and were more likely to be diagnosed with gonorrhea previously. MSM now account for an increasing proportion of diagnoses in STD clinics, and these studies draw attention to the need for primary and secondary prevention interventions with this group.

STD clinic studies also provide an excellent venue for studying the interaction between STD and HIV infection among high-risk MSM. Weinstock et al. (14)

estimated HIV incidence and trends in incidence among MSM and heterosexual men and women in 13 STD clinics in nine cities in the United States from 1991 through 1997. Of 129,774 specimens tested, 362 (0.28%) were from persons estimated to be recently infected. HIV incidence among MSM was 7.1%, 14 times higher than that among heterosexuals, which was 0.5%. However, HIV incidence among MSM and heterosexuals remained unchanged during the time studied. Similarly, Torian et al. (15) measured trends in HIV seroprevalence among 4076 MSM presenting to New York City STD clinics between 1990 and 1999 using remnant serum originally drawn for routine serologic tests for syphilis. Overall, HIV seroprevalence declined from 47% in 1990 to 18% in 1999 ($p < 0.01$). Seroprevalence declined from 34% to 11% among white men, from 47% to 19% among Hispanic men, and from 56% to 28% among black men. Seroprevalence among MSM with gonorrhea declined but remained high. This study highlighted the burden of STDs among HIV-positive MSM. Two thirds of the known HIV-positive men had a new STD diagnosed at the survey visit, and gonorrhea was diagnosed almost twice as frequently among seropositive versus seronegative MSM (19% versus 10%; $p < 0.05$). Some caution is required when interpreting findings from STD clinics, however, as MSM with a higher prevalence of risky sexual behaviors are more likely to be seen in this setting, and the findings of clinic-based studies are unlikely to be representative of MSM in the wider community.

Community, Population-Based, and Internet Surveys

Population-based, convenience sample surveys have grown in popularity over the past two decades and are now a major source of information on behavioral trends among MSM. These studies have demonstrated increasing risk behaviors among MSM, and have provided valuable information on the factors associated with prevalent diagnosed and undiagnosed STDs. For example, Harawa et al. (16) surveyed 3316 ethnically diverse MSM aged 15 to 22 years, and found that HIV prevalence was 16% for both black and multiethnic black participants, 6.9% for Latinos, and 3.3% for whites. However, potentially risky sex and drug-using behaviors were generally reported most frequently by whites and least so by blacks. In a multiple logistic regression analysis, positive associations with HIV included older age, being out of school or work, sex while on crack cocaine, and anal sex with another male regardless of reported condom use level.

Population-based surveys are also useful in monitoring attitudes and beliefs, which influence risk behaviors, within MSM populations. Stockman et al. (17) analyzed data from 303 HIV-negative or untested participants (including 105 MSM from gay bars) who had been interviewed at different recruiting venues in the 2001 cross-sectional, anonymous, HIV Testing Survey (HITS) in San Francisco. Participants were asked questions about their attitudes and beliefs about HIV prevention fatigue. The researchers found a mean HIV prevention fatigue score of 2.02 (range, 3.67–1.00) with no significant difference by age, gender, race, or monthly income. HIV prevention fatigue varied significantly by risk population, and was not associated with unprotected anal intercourse at last sex among MSM. There was no direct association between HIV prevention fatigue and high-risk sexual behavior among HIV-negative gay men. Similarly, Reimen et al. (18) in a cross-sectional survey of 456 sexually active, culturally diverse, HIV-positive MSM showed that less than 25% engaged in unprotected anal sex (with any partner) within the past three months. Most men believed there was significant health risk (to partner or self) associated with unprotected sex when on HAART. There was no increased risk behavior associated with being on HAART, although the perception of negative health consequences, including HIV transmission, when on HAART was significantly lower for the relatively small subset of men who reported unprotected sex.

Over the past decade, the Internet has become an increasingly important tool for acquiring new sexual partners; promoting disease awareness, prevention, and control; and accessing sex partners of STD infected patients to conduct appropriate partner notification, evaluation, and management (19). Comparisons of the social, demographic, and behavioral characteristics of online and offline samples must, however, take into account the confounding effects of HIV status and seeking sex on the Internet. Studies within the U.S. and Europe (20) have consistently shown that MSM respondents who use the Internet are more likely to be young, geographically more isolated, and more behaviorally and self-identified as bisexual than those who complete conventionally distributed written questionnaires (21,22). The Internet offers valuable opportunities for conducting behavioral surveillance among MSM because it reaches some men who may not be easily accessed in the community yet who are at high risk for HIV and STDs. Collaboration between public health departments, community partners, and other jurisdictions have enabled the examination of online social/sexual networks that are used commonly in their gay and bisexual communities and develop more effective means of communicating prevention and control messages online (23).

Summary

In the United States, evidence from clinic, community, and surveillance sources confirm the disproportionate disease burden being borne by MSM, and the worsening of sexual health outcomes (risk behavior, reported, and incident HIV/STDs) in many areas. However, it is important to bear in mind that the various STDs are in different epidemic phases, and a one-size-fits-all approach to STD prevention and interventions may not be appropriate. For example, although HIV incidence appears to be relatively stable or increasing slightly (24,25), prevalence continues to increase with attendant implications for providing tailored and culturally competent prevention interventions for MSM. This, however, contrasts with the recent dramatic rises in syphilis and antimicrobial-resistant gonorrhea, and also with the reemergence of rare pathogens such as *Lymphogranuloma venereum* (LGV) (26,27), which may have medium- and long-term implications for HIV transmission and MSM's sexual health outcomes.

Biological, Behavioral, and Social Determinants of Disease Incidence Among MSM

The epidemiology of acute STDs in MSM reflects a dynamic interplay between biological characteristics of the organisms, host factors including sexual behavior, and the effectiveness of STD prevention and control interventions. In this section, we outline some of the key biological, behavioral, and social factors that influence the changing patterns and distribution of STDs in MSM, and provide a context for the nature and range of recent trends.

Biological Factors Influencing STD Acquisition Risk in MSM

A number of biological factors may influence STD acquisition risk in MSM, but research aimed at separating the mode of transmission from other biological and behavioral factors can be difficult. The infectivity of STDs in one potential donor may differ from that in another because of differences in organism subtypes or specific subspecies that are more or less well adapted to the biological individuality of that donor (28). Organism and host biological characteristics are also strong predictors of transmission and acquisition of STDs, including HIV infection. For example, Grassly et al. (29) demonstrated that density-dependent "endogenous" biological factors, e.g., the nonlinear dynamics of the parasite population, may provide a strong influence on population ecology for STDs, thereby explaining epidemics of syphilis in the *United States* as an example of unforced, endogenous oscillations in disease incidence.

A variety of host factors influence HIV/ STD transmission dynamics. The age of the recipient may be a surrogate for maturation senescence in the host cellular immune processes involved in defending against viral penetration and integration (28). Various sex practices determine the nature and intensity of the physical contact of microbe-containing donor cells or secretions with tissues of the susceptible recipient. Another critical factor is the condition of immune activation in both donors and recipients, especially in areas of close contact; the absence of circumcision, ulceration, and other causes of mucosal disruption may increase access to or activates cells targeted by HIV-1 and other pathogens (28). In recent years, evidence from observational studies in sub-Saharan Africa has shown that circumcised men have a lower risk of acquiring HIV infection than uncircumcised men (30,31). However the relationship between circumcision and STD risk has rarely been examined in homosexual men. A cross-sectional study (32) found that uncircumcised homosexual men in the United States were more likely to have prevalent HIV infection, but it was not known whether these men had been infected by insertive or receptive intercourse. Buchbinder et al. (33) enrolled 3257 MSM in six U.S. cities from 1995 to 1997 as part of the HIV Network for Prevention Trials Vaccine Preparedness Study and found lack of circumcision, nitrite inhalant use, and receptive oral sex to ejaculation with an HIV-positive partner to be independent risk factors for HIV seroconversion.

Behavioral Risk for STD Among MSM

Assessing trends in risk behavior among MSM is extremely difficult, because only limited longitudinal data have been collected on the sexual practices of this population (2). Nevertheless, the available data suggest that, similar to other developed countries, risk behavior among MSM appears to be increasing. In one San Francisco study, the percentage of young MSM who reported engaging in unprotected anal intercourse increased from 37% in 1993–1994 to 50% in 1996–1997 (34). In 1996–1997, 46% of MSM who reported having had unprotected anal intercourse had engaged in this behavior with a partner whose HIV serostatus was unknown or different from their own. A similar trend toward increased risk behavior was observed in community surveys that were also conducted in San Francisco from 1994 through 1997 (35).

Initiation of Sexual Activity

Data from the U.S. National Survey of Family Growth (6) suggest that, although 77.4% of all males aged 15–24 years had ever had any opposite-sex sexual contact, 5.0% reported having any oral or anal sex with a male, increasing from 3.9% among 15–17 year olds to 7.4% among 22–24 year olds. There was little variation across ethnic groups, with 5.4% of Hispanic or Latino, 4.6% of white, and 5.7% of black or African-American males aged 15–24 years reporting any oral or anal sexual contact with another male. Somewhat higher proportions reported any same-sex sexual contact, with 4.5% of 15–19 and 5.5% of 20–24 year old males reporting. With respect to reported sexual orientation, among 18–19 year olds, 1.7% reported being homosexual, 1.4% bisexual, and 3.5% something else, whereas among 20–24 year olds this increased to 2.3%, 2.0%, and 3.5%, respectively. Behavioral trend data are difficult to obtain, for previously discussed reasons, however, data from the 1991 National Survey of Men (36,37) found 3.0% of men aged 20–24 years reported any same-sex sexual contact, whereas this figure had increased to 5.5% in 2002.

Lifetime Sexual Behavior Trajectory

Relatively little research has mapped the lifetime trajectory of sexual risk behavior among MSM. STD surveillance data would suggest that, unlike heterosexuals, where sexual risk behavior is most prevalent between 16–25 years (corresponding to the peak ages for reported STDs), risk behavior persists for longer periods among MSM, with reported acute STDs and HIV peaking in the 25–35 year and older age groups (10). Recent outbreaks of syphilis and LGV have occurred among a somewhat older demographic of MSM, many of whom are HIV positive (10). The reasons for the persistence of sexual risk behavior among MSM may reflect opportunistic as well as social factors. Among heterosexual males, transition to cohabiting and married marital status is uniformly associated with reductions in sex partner acquisition rates (6,38), whereas among homosexual men, cohabiting status may not exert as powerful a behavioral risk deterrent as in heterosexuals (39). Alternative sexual risk practices (e.g., fisting, sadomasochism, fetishes) and lifestyles are more prevalent with increasing age and HIV-positive status (40,41) and may help to explain the patterns and distribution of some STDs in older MSM. Although relatively little work has been done on social and economic status and high-risk behavior among MSM in the *United States*, studies from Western Europe suggest risk associations exist with lower socioeconomic and educational attainment (1) and form part of the social determinants of risk behavior among MSM.

Young gay and bisexual men in the United States are more likely than older MSM to engage in risky sexual practices (42). HIV prevalence is also high, underscoring the need to evaluate and intensify prevention efforts for young MSM, particularly MSM of color. Waldo et al. (43) surveyed 719 15–22-year-old MSM in commercial venues and found an HIV seroprevalence of 2.0% among those aged 15–17 years and 6.8% among those aged 18–22 years. Men aged 15–17 years used alcohol, ecstasy, and heroin less frequently than those aged 18–22 years. However, in both age groups, use of amphetamines, ecstasy, and amyl nitrate was associated with unprotected anal intercourse. Valleroy et al. (44) interviewed 3492 15–22-year-old MSM in the Young

Men's Survey and found 7.2% HIV prevalence, increasing from 0% among 15 year olds to 9.7% among 22 year olds. Prevalent HIV infection was independently associated with nonwhite ethnicity, having ever had anal sex with a man, and having had sex with 20 or more men.

Sexual Practices and MSM

Penetrative sex (anal, oral) prevalence and associated factors. As the number of persons living with HIV has increased in recent years, more attention has been paid to the sexual practices of MSM in general and HIV positive MSM in particular (45). Although many HIV-seropositive MSM believe they have a responsibility to protect their sex partners from HIV infection (46), a notable minority participate in behaviors that can transmit HIV to uninfected partners (47,48). Behavioral surveillance and ad hoc research studies have confirmed that MSM are reporting more anal intercourse (protected and unprotected) with partners of known and unknown HIV serostatus, and between a third and 50% of MSM report a recent history of unprotected anal intercourse. Guenther-Grey (49) surveyed 15–25-year-old young MSM between 1999 and 2002 and found a prevalence of unprotected anal intercourse ranging between 27–35% in 1999, compared with 14–39% in 2002. Denning et al. (50) analyzed behavioral surveillance data from 970 HIV-positive MSM who had a single, steady male sex partner with negative or unknown serostatus in 12 states between 1995 and 2000. Two hundred seventy-eight (29%) reported unprotected anal intercourse during the previous year. Among the men who were aware of their infection, factors found to be predictive of unprotected anal intercourse in multivariate modeling were heterosexual self-identification, crack cocaine use, no education beyond high school, and a partner with unknown serostatus.

Whereas some unprotected anal intercourse is occurring within the context of negotiated safety (NS) and serosorting, numerous studies have demonstrated the vulnerability of those using this practice (51). NS is commonly practiced among HIV-negative men in seroconcordant relationships, however, men often violate NS-defining rules, placing themselves and potentially their primary partners at risk for HIV infection. Guzman et al. (52) in a community-based survey of San Francisco MSM found that 38 (50%) of 76 HIV negative men in a long-term relationship had NS relationships. Among those practicing NS, 29% had violated their NS-defining rule in the prior three months, including 18% who reported UAI with others and 18% who reported an STD in the prior year. Only 61% of NS men adhered fully to rules and agreed to disclose rule breaking. The authors concluded that prevention efforts regarding NS should emphasize the importance of agreement adherence, disclosure of rule breaking, and routine sexually transmitted infection (STI) testing (52).

Many studies have underscored the difficulty of maintaining safer sexual practices for an extended period, and investigators have pointed out the potential for a return to riskier sexual practices (53,54). Data from the Multicenter AIDS Cohort Study show that over a two-year period, 47% of men returned to unprotected receptive anal intercourse and 44% returned to unprotected insertive anal intercourse (55). According to a recent report from the San Francisco Men's Health Study, most of the men (68%) who were followed from 1993 through 1997 reported on one or more occasions that they had engaged in unprotected anal intercourse (56).

Fisting, use of toys, and other esoteric sex practices. More recent attention has been paid to the role of diversity in sexual practices and their relationship to STD acquisition. Oral sex is a highly prevalent behavior among MSM, and there is ample evidence of the transmission of STDs via this route, especially syphilis (57). The role of both fisting and the use of sexual toys have been implicated in recent outbreaks of LGV in Western European countries (27,58). Fisting has also been identified as a risk factor for hepatitis C seroconversion, particularly among HIV-positive MSM (59,60). Relatively few studies have been undertaken to assess the prevalence and distribution of fisting among MSM in the United States. However, studies in the United Kingdom suggest that this behavior is quite prevalent among HIV-positive and older MSM (40,41). These studies also suggest an overlapping of risk behaviors, with MSM who practice fisting being more likely to report higher rates of sex partner acquisition, higher prevalence of unprotected anal intercourse, greater use of recreational drugs, including alcohol, ecstasy, and crystal methamphetamine, and more recent reported STDs than men who do not practice fisting (40,41).

Men Who Have Sex with Men and Women

Some men and women who reported that they had sexual experiences with members of their own sex may also have had opposite-sex partners in their lives. Approximately 1% of men aged 15–44 years of age in the NSFG reported having both male and female sexual partners in the last 12 months (6). In response to a question that asked, "Do you think of yourself as heterosexual, homosexual, bisexual, or something else?," about 2.3% of men answered homosexual, 1.8% bisexual, 3.9% "something else," and 1.8% did not give an answer (6). Marked variations in the reporting of sexual orientation were observed. Although 1.7% of white, Hispanic, and black men described themselves as bisexual, 7.3% of Hispanic, and 7.5% of black men identified their orientation as "something else" compared with 2.3% of white men (6). The higher prevalence of alternative designation of sexual orientation among ethnic minority men has been described in other socioanthropologic studies (61,62) and may have implications for sexual risk behaviors within this group, as well as STD transmission risk among women their female sex partners due to "bridging" between behaviorally exclusive heterosexual and homosexual networks. Behaviorally bisexual youth are also at increased risk. Goodenow et al. (63) examined the prevalence of AIDS-related risk behaviors among male high school students with female, male, and both-sex sexual partners and showed that bisexual experience predicted multiple sexual partners, unprotected intercourse, STDs, and injection drug use; school AIDS education and condom instruction predicted less AIDS-related risk.

MSM Who Inject Drugs

Studies of MSM who are current or recovering substance users, particularly those who inject drugs, have documented high levels of risk for HIV infection (64,65). MSM who inject drugs (MSM/IDU) pose unique challenges for HIV risk reduction efforts because they have multiple risks for STD/HIV acquisition and transmission. In addition, MSM/IDU often do not identify strongly with either MSM, because they may not gay identify, or IDU, because they do not use heroin. Therefore, targeted HIV prevention strategies for this group are urgently needed. Findings from CDC surveillance data suggest that, currently, over half of MSM/IDU with AIDS were Hispanics and non-Hispanic blacks, and most MSM/IDU with AIDS were reported from large metropolitan statistical areas (66). Bull et al. (67), in a study of 100 MSM/IDU, found high-risk sexual behaviors with multiple partners of both genders. Condom use was inconsistent and infrequent for all types of sex. Forty-five percent of the sample were HIV infected. The injection drugs of choice for this sample were cocaine (90%) and methamphetamine (59%). Semple et al. (68) studied 194 methamphetamine (meth)-using HIV-positive MSM enrolled in a sexual risk reduction intervention. Men who injected meth were significantly more likely to be Caucasian, bisexual, homeless, divorced/separated, with lower educational attainment as compared with noninjectors. Injectors also reported more years of meth use, greater frequency and amount of meth use, more social and health problems, including higher prevalence of STDs and hepatitis C, and more sexual risk behaviors.

The Psychosocial Context of Behavioral Risk for STD Among MSM

Individual Factors

Psychological factors (e.g., self-esteem, emotional distress, self-efficacy) and mental health. Rates of distress, depression, anxiety, mood, substance use disorders, and suicidal thoughts are high in MSM, which in turn have important public health ramifications (69,70). Mills et al. (71) in a household-based probability sample of 2,881 MSM interviewed between 1996 and 1998 in four large American cities found that the seven-day prevalence of depression in MSM was 17.2%, higher than in adult U.S. men in general. Both distress and depression were associated with lack of a domestic partner; not identifying as gay, queer, or homosexual; experiencing multiple episodes of antigay violence in the previous five years; and very high levels of community alienation. Distress was also associated with experiencing early antigay harassment. Depression was also associated with histories of attempted suicide, child abuse, and recent sexual dysfunction. Being HIV positive was correlated with distress and depression but not significantly when demographic characteristics, developmental history, substance use, sexual behavior, and current social context were controlled by logistic regression. Gilman et al. (72) examined data from the National Comorbidity Survey and found that 2.1% of men reported one or more same-sex sexual partners in the past five years. These respondents had higher 12-month prevalences of anxiety, mood, and substance use disorders and of suicidal thoughts and plans than did respondents with opposite-sex partners only. Further research is needed to replicate and explore the causal mechanisms underlying these associations.

Increased depression, suicide, substance use, homelessness, and school dropout have also been reported gay, lesbian, and bisexual (GLB) youth and HIV-positive individuals. Lock et al. (73) conducted a community school-based health survey that included an opportunity to self-identify as GLB. They identified significantly increased health risks for self-identified GLB youth in mental health, sexual risk-taking, and general health risks compared with self-identified heterosexuals. HIV-positive men had significantly higher levels of psychiatric symptomatology and syndromal depression than HIV-negative men. Dickey et al. (74) examined 174 HIV-positive and 760 HIV-negative MSM enrolled in the Pittsburgh site of the Multicenter AIDS Cohort Study (MACS). They found that HIV-positive men who were younger, lacked full-time employment, claimed relatively high support from their relatives, and demonstrated high use of active behavioral coping strategies were at greater risk for psychiatric symptomatology and/or syndromal depression.

Childhood sexual abuse is associated with high-risk sexual behavior in men who have sex with men, although relatively few studies have sought to quantify the prevalence, distribution, and associated factors with childhood sexual abuse in MSM and its relationship to adverse mental health outcome. However, the evidence is beginning to accrue and suggest that MSM of color (especially Latino MSM) may be at especial disadvantage (75). Kalichman et al. (76), in a study of 647 MSM attending a large gay pride event, found that men who have a history of childhood sexual abuse were more likely to: engage in high-risk sexual behavior (i.e., unprotected receptive anal intercourse), trade sex for money or drugs, report being HIV positive, and experience nonsexual relationship violence. Data from population-based prevalence studies are currently scant and should be an area for future development in this field.

Attitudes. In response to the onset of the U.S. HIV epidemic during the early 1980s, gay men, as individuals or members of communities, reduced sexual risk by changing their behaviors and often expecting those changes to be adopted by others, resulting in an emergent sexual norm (77). This normative change set a moral standard applauding those who were "safer" while exerting social pressure on others who were not (78). At present, there is an apparent shift toward unsafe behavior for MSM in the United States (79). Increasing morbidity has been documented for MSM during the past five to seven years in the incidence of HIV (80), syphilis (81), and gonorrhea (82). A number of studies have also examined whether MSM who intentionally engage in unprotected anal sex may be influenced by perceptions that medical advances have mitigated the threat of HIV and the intimate relationship between illicit drug use and sexual risk taking. Three prevailing beliefs have been explored related to sexual risk taking with MSM: medication treatment advances, the low probability related to HIV transmission, and a healthy immune system, capable of resisting infection (83,84).

Recreational drug use and MSM. Sexual behavior in drug users varies in association with the drug used, the drug subculture and setting, and the need to maintain the drug addiction. For example, among MDMA (3,4-methylene-dioxymethamphetamine) users, higher frequency of MDMA use was associated with being younger, having more visits to bars or clubs, more gay/bisexual friends, and having an HIV-negative test result or never having been tested (85,86). Viagra use appears to have become a stable fixture of the sexual culture of MSM, crossing age, race, and socioeconomic subgroups for primary and secondary (e.g., due to drugs, HIV disease, psychological problems) erectile dysfunction (87,88). Viagra appears to be an emerging contributing factor to unsafe sex, potentially increasing HIV transmission (89). The recent phenomenon of the circuit party has led to investigation of the context in which drug use and sex have become the focus of large, gay-oriented parties over long weekends. Mansergh et al. (90) surveyed 295 San Francisco MSM who had attended a circuit party in the previous year. Nearly all respondents reported use of drugs during circuit party weekends, including ecstasy (75%), ketamine (58%), crystal methamphetamine (36%), gamma hydroxybutyrate or gamma butyrolactone (25%), and Viagra (12%). Two thirds of the men reported having sex (oral or anal), 49% reported having anal sex, and 28% reported having unprotected anal sex during the three-day period.

Substance use is associated with increased risk for HIV transmission by HIV-positive people to uninfected partners through sexual contact. Alcohol use may increase HIV sexual risk behavior, although findings have varied across study populations and methods (91,92). Previous research has documented an association between meth use and high-risk sex among HIV-negative MSM, however, as yet, relatively little is known about the sexual risk behaviors of HIV positive meth-using MSM.

Beckett et al. (92) found that substance use was most prevalent among MSM and predicted high-risk sex. Substance use and current dependence were associated with being sexually active among MSM but not IDUs; marijuana, alcohol, and hard drug use were most strongly associated with being sexually active among MSM. Crystal methamphetamine use was associated with high rates of anal sex, low rates of condom use, multiple sex partners, sexual marathons, and anonymous sex. Other studies confirm that the personal motivations associated with meth use include sexual enhancement and self-medication of negative affect associated with HIV-positive serostatus (93), whereas MDMA use is associated with being more "out," which may be advantageous in helping gay men deal with harmful psychological effects of stigma, but may place individuals in settings that expose them to MDMA (94).

Viagra use and abuse by MSM have been studied recently (87,88). Chu et al. (95) conducted a community-based anonymous survey of 837 MSM and found that 32% had ever used Viagra. Significant independent predictors of Viagra use were white race, older age, HIV positivity, illicit drug use, and having had unprotected anal sex with potentially serodiscordant partners. Paul et al. (88) in a population-based telephone sample of MSM in San Francisco found that recent Viagra use was reported by 29% of the sample and was associated with HIV serostatus, greater numbers of male sexual partners, higher levels of unprotected anal sex, and higher levels of illicit recreational drug use. Other studies have shown that over one third of Viagra users had combined Viagra with other drugs, 18% with amyl nitrate (95). Only a minority (44%) obtained Viagra under the care of a physician.

Cultural and Ethnic Factors

In addition to the demographic, psychosocial, and situational factors that have repeatedly been associated with HIV risk, (96,97), several newly emerging factors may partially account for recent trends toward increased sexual risk taking. Of these, the association between beliefs about HAART and increased sexual risk taking has received the most attention (98,99). Some researchers have speculated that pharmaceutical advertisements that minimize the negative aspects of HIV infection and HAART with unrealistically upbeat portrayals of HIV-seropositive persons may also lead to increased risk behavior (100). Although few data are available, other medical advances, such as the testing of vaccine candidates, the availability of postexposure therapy, and viral load monitoring, have the potential to affect the sexual practices of MSM by influencing their perceptions of the risk and consequences of HIV infection (101,102).

Other emerging factors might also lead to increased risk behaviors among MSM. A four-city study indicates that "AIDS burnout," which results from years of exposure to prevention messages and long-term efforts to maintain safer sex practices, is an independent predictor of unprotected anal intercourse among HIV-seropositive MSM (103). As HIV prevention efforts have been expanded to meet the needs of other populations, decreased visibility and gaps in prevention services for MSM may have reduced the relevance of HIV infection among gay men in some communities.

Labeling and identity. Black men who have sex with men and women but who do not identify as gay or disclose their bisexual activities to main female partners, also known as men "on the down-low," have been cited as the main reason for the increase in HIV infections in black women (61). The risks of bisexuality among black men are exacerbated by incarceration, homophobia, and drug use. Millet et al. (61) reviewed scientific articles related to men on the "down-low." They found low agreement between professed sexual identity and corresponding sexual behavior among black and other MSM. Black MSM are more likely than MSM of other racial or ethnic groups to be bisexually active or identified, and, compared with white MSM, are less likely to disclose their bisexual or homosexual activities to others. However, black MSM who do not disclose their homosexual or bisexual activities engage in a lower prevalence of HIV risks than black MSM who do disclose; and black men who are currently bisexually active account for a very small proportion of the overall population of black men (2%). Other studies (104) have found contrasting results in that covert and unprotected sex among bisexually active black men was commonplace for reasons that included prostitution, habituation to same-sex relations during incarceration, and the desire to maintain a facade of heterosexuality in homophobic communities.

Effects of the AIDS pandemic. After 20 or more years since the onset of the HIV/AIDS epidemic in the United States, some argue that increasing risk is a result of complacency on the part of MSM. Complacency has been attributed to minimization of the risk of HIV in gay and mainstream popular culture due to advances in treatment and increased survival for those with HIV (105). Others suggest that alternative reasons for complacency include the fact that younger MSM did not see the worst effects of HIV during the early 1980s (106), or that, among older men, long-term exposure to prevention messages has lead to messages being disregarded as background noise (107). Still others argue that substance use has led to an increase in sexual risk and contributes to an increasing incidence of sexual risk for MSM (108,109).

Alternatively, social determinates have also been suggested as playing an elemental role in changing risk behaviors for MSM. Bloom et al. (77) argue that the AIDS epidemic's devastating effect on gay communities contributed to present-day risk increases. AIDS deaths, and the effect of those losses on community fragmentation and damaged social networks, took a great toll on gay communities in many urban areas of North America (110,111). Rather than offering a protective effect for their members, providing social structures, maintaining a system of values, and offering a haven from stigmatization (112,113), gay communities lost the capacity to maintain healthy norms and support friendship networks as a result of the disability and death of community members (78,114,115). An increase in risk behaviors can occur as a response to stressors such as community loss, uncertainty, disease, and stigmatization (116,117). Bloom et al. (77) hypothesize that increased drug use and sexual risk behaviors are part of an overall response to these stressors, thus contributing to the growing incidence of STD morbidity in gay men.

Policy, Media, and Sociopolitical Factors

Media representations of MSM in the United States are both positive and negative. Openly gay entertainment figures are often treated in a positive light, however, this does not necessarily translate to acceptance of same-sex sexuality or open displays of affection (118). Signorile (118) contrasts acceptance of Al and Tipper Gore's affectionate displays during his presidential campaign and media criticism of Ellen DeGeneres' displays of affection with Anne Heche at a Clinton White House event. Alternatively, gay men who are experiencing increases in STDs or HIV have been presented as complacent with the risk of contracting or spreading HIV (119,120). The *Los Angeles Times* went even further, implicating gay men as intentionally spreading disease when it reported that HIV-positive gay men "were knowingly engaging in unprotected sex although they could pass on the AIDS virus" (121). In contrast, an alternative view was simply that knowing one's HIV status was not sufficient to influence sexual risk behavior.

The situation for same-sex media coverage when combined with ethnic minority status is also fodder for blame. Press coverage of nonidentified gay men has seen an increase in attention to African-American men, or men on the down-low (122). In the recent focus on men on the down-low, wives or female partners are the innocent victims of the men who deceive them (123,124), independent of social processes that influence behavior and without distinguishing between sexual desire and sexual transmission of disease. Thus, men who maintain families and marriages to women while engaging in sex with other men are portrayed as vectors of disease, recalling earlier days of the HIV/AIDS epidemic in the United States, with its discourse on "innocent victims" as distinguished from those who were not innocent and therefore deserved the punishment of disease.

A more subtle influence, but equally important to our understanding of the context of sexual risk, is press coverage of gay marriage issues. In an era where debate over rights of ethnic minorities or interracial marriage would no longer be tolerated, where the views of those opposed to equal rights of women, African Americans, or any other U.S. citizen would be seen as bigotry and not be privileged with publication in mainstream press, newspapers across America publish pro and con views of gay marriage. The acceptance that criticism of equal marriage rights is a valid point of debate only serves to further discrimination and prejudice. Such macro-level influences fostering discrimination and marginalization have been shown to increase sexual risk (125,126).

Social Policy: Gay Marriage, Antidiscrimination, and Equality Legislation

While there have been some strides in national, state, and local legislation and policy regarding equal rights for persons regardless of sexual identity, there has been increasing effort in the United States to move policy toward greater restrictions to the rights of those who do not identify with mainstream heterosexual culture (with the rare exception of several North Eastern U.S. states) (125,127,128). Several European countries and Canada recognize same-sex marriage, and South Africa's courts recognized same-sex marriage in 2006, and alternative legal recognition, such as civil union is recognized in 14 additional countries (127,129). Communities in the United States, however, have overwhelmingly sought to limit the influence of the few states, such as Massachusetts, that have approved gay marriage or domestic partnership. On a national level, the Defense of Marriage Act and the proposed Federal Marriage Amendment have brought to a federal level attempts to limit the rights of same-sex couples (130,131).

Homophobia and sexual risk behavior. Sociocultural factors, including homophobia and its consequent increase in psychological distress, have been correlated to increased sexual risk behaviors in general and, more specifically, in African-American and Latino MSM (126,132–155,135). Some note homophobia as an influence on addictions and drug use for gay men (133). Thus, homophobia serves as a social stressor for Latino men similar to community fragmentation resulting from the AIDS pandemic. Others, recognizing the causal relationship between homophobia (and other social issues) and risk behavior, posit that increased community involvement can help to ameliorate this adverse relationship (134). Importantly, the persistence of community fragmentation resulting from the impact of HIV/AIDS makes involvement all the more difficult for those living in such conditions.

Differences in health risks among GLB youth are mediated by victimization at school. Bontempo et al. (135) examined the 1995 Youth Risk Behavior Survey taken in Massachusetts and Vermont and found that GLB youths reporting high levels of at-school victimization reported higher levels of substance use, suicidality, and sexual risk behaviors than heterosexual peers reporting high levels of at-school victimization. Also, GLB youths reporting low levels of at-school victimization reported levels of substance use, suicidality, and sexual-risk behaviors that were similar to heterosexual peers who reported low at-school victimization.

The importance of multicausal factors for STD infection came to the forefront early in the HIV/AIDS pandemic and has continued to be an important area of inquiry. Most recently, the concept of syndemics, including the broad concept of oppression, has been used by medical anthropologists and others in public health to indicate the synergistic relationship between disease and social influences and conditions (136).

Summary

In examining the social determinants of STD acquisition risk among MSM, it is vitally important that the psychological and social determinants are considered alongside behavioral influences. The data suggest that there is a paucity of information on the mental health needs of MSM and their impact on risk behaviors. There also remains a dearth of information on the role that recreational drug use and abuse play in the lives of MSM. Taken together, the data suggest that many of these risks are overlapping and are found as part of a constellation of factors affecting the lives of MSM that lead to increased morbidity and mortality.

Effective Interventions

This section summarizes the evidence on the effectiveness of the set of individual interventions or combinations of interventions currently available to reduce risk factors for STD among MSM. It highlights interventions for which there is evidence of effectiveness. In collating the evidence, particular attention was paid to systematic reviews and reviews of reviews rather than primary studies. Two recent reviews of reviews were particularly useful in summarizing the state of the evidence regarding effective interventions for STD and HIV prevention among MSM (137,138). The interventions are organized by intervention level, that is, the target of the intervention with the intention of ultimately leading to behavior change and disease reduction.

Individual Level

Individual-level interventions interact directly with MSM to change behavior and/or reduce disease. Individual-level interventions are defined as any one-to-one or face-to-face, interactive interventions and include the following: voluntary counseling and testing (VCT); one-to-one counseling on its own (i.e., no HIV testing); individual cognitive behavioral therapy; face-to-face detached or outreach work; couple counseling; telephone help lines; and some Internet-based work. Testing and counseling is the most frequently cited intervention delivered individually/one-to-one, however, there is insufficient evidence either to support or discount the effectiveness of HIV VCT in influencing the sexual risk behaviors of MSM, regardless of whether they test seropositive or seronegative. Two reviews, Wolitski et al. (139), and Oakley et al. (140), specifically discuss HIV VCT interventions with MSM, covering nine different studies between them. The studies in Wolitski and colleagues' review provide inconsistent and in some cases conflicting results, however, the authors conclude that the studies "document substantial risk related behavior change among MSM but do not provide consistent evidence regarding the effects of HIV VCT on different sexual risk practices."

Individual risk counseling can be effective. Peersman et al. (141) found two "partially effective" counseling interventions, which resulted in changes in only some of the stated outcome measures that related to the aims of the intervention; and one ineffective intervention. Of the two studies with clear evidence of effectiveness in a review by Stephenson et al. (142), one was a one-to-one counseling intervention. However, two other risk counseling interventions were ineffective in achieving STI outcomes, although all three did report some improved behavioral outcomes (e.g.. increased condom use).

Dyadic Interventions

Systematic reviews have concluded that partner notification can be an effective means of newly detecting infections; that provider referral is more effective than patient referral; and that patient referral can be improved by simple forms of patient assistance (138). There is insufficient review-level evidence to conclude that contract referral is more effective than patient referral; or to make any conclusions about the potential harms of partner notification (138). Finally, there is tentative review-level evidence to conclude that patient referral can be improved by patient education and counseling, that partner notification is cost effective, and that patient referral is more cost effective than contract or provider referral (138). Although there is robust evidence of the effectiveness of partner notification, relatively few studies have specifically examined the effectiveness among MSM populations.

Peer Interventions

Small Group Sessions

Group-level interventions are delivered to small groups of individuals, usually from the same peer group, and are facilitated in some way. Sessions can be one-off or multiple, of varying length and intensity, and either didactic or interactive (or a mixture of both). They include school-based sex education and small group work, including cognitive behavioral therapy (CBT). Small group sessions, providing a mixture of risk education, training in self-management, and assertiveness skills and health problem solving, are effective in reducing unprotected anal intercourse. Choi (143) implemented a three-hour intervention targeted at Asians and Pacific Islanders in the United States and designed to increase positive ethnic and sexual identity, to enhance AIDS knowledge and attitudes toward safer sex, and to increase sexual negotiation skills and eroticize safer sex. The authors judged the intervention effective in reducing the number of sex partners at three-month follow-up (by 46%). Kelly et al. (144) showed that twelve 70–90-minute weekly group sessions that included AIDS education, cognitive behavioral self-management, sexual assertion training, and affirmation of social support was effective in reducing the frequency of anal intercourse and in increasing the use of refusal skills. Other studies have found the use of day-long workshops focusing on relationship goals and risk reduction or skills training promoting safer sex and risk reduction (145) to be effective in increasing condom use for insertive anal intercourse. Peterson et al. (146) tested a nine-hour intervention delivered in three 3-hour segments focusing on cognitive behavioral skills training to African-American MSM, including an emphasis on safer sex negotiation skills, self-management skills, and developing a positive self-identity. They found a reduction in the proportion reporting any UAI (from 45% to 20% at 18-month follow-up).

Multi-Component Small-Group Work

Multi-component small-group work consists of a number of elements drawn together, usually to impart information and to build safer sex skills (137). Building a range of components into group-level interventions contributes to their effectiveness in influencing the sexual risk behaviors of MSM (140). For example, Oakley (140) concluded that "there is some support for the importance and potential effectiveness of ... intensive sessions which include roleplay, assertiveness training, or other interactive approaches: skills training of this type seems to improve the possibility for the negotiation of safer sex among MSM." Kegeles and Hart (147) suggest that "addressing the wider health and psychosocial needs of gay men is of equal or greater importance in preventing HIV in a well-informed population as work with an exclusive focus on condom use or safer sex." They also suggest that interventions that encourage individuals to take pride in themselves and that seem to reinforce a positive sense of self-identity are more likely to be effective (146,148).

Multi-Session Small-Group Work

There is good evidence that cognitive behavioral group work, focusing on risk reduction, sexual negotiation, and communication skills training (and rehearsal, for instance, through role-play), can be effective in influencing the sexual risk behaviors of MSM (137,138). Small-group sessions providing a mixture of risk education, training in self-management and assertiveness skills, and health problem solving are effective in reducing unprotected anal intercourse. Many multi-session, small-group interventions have been shown to be effective (144,146). However, there is some uncertainty as to whether it is the "multi-session" nature of these interventions that makes them effective or whether it reflects their content, since cognitive behavioral skill building interventions are likely to be delivered through a number of sessions. Consequently, there is insufficient review-level evidence either to support or discount the conclusion that multi-session interventions are, in themselves, more effective than single-session interventions in influencing sexual risk behaviors of MSM (137,138).

Community Interventions

Community-level interventions are delivered by or within a defined "community"—i.e., an "at risk" population in a specific geographical region (149)—or target population and include a wide variety of approaches. They can be aimed at both the population at risk and organizations and professionals working with these populations. Interventions can include small media (e.g., leaflet/booklet), mass media (e.g., gay press advertising), condom and lubrication provision, peer education and social diffusion, community empowerment and development (including building infrastructures), some Internet interventions (e.g., chat rooms), and some organizational/institutional interventions influencing the practice of organizations (e.g., training, technical advice).

Changing Community Systems or Norms to Prevent Community Members Risk Behavior

A number of studies have shown the effectiveness of using peers, opinion leaders, and role models from the relevant community in influencing the sexual risk behaviors of MSM either via changing norms regarding safer sex and/or providing credible sources of information to increase knowledge of HIV risk and risk reduction among MSM (140,150,151). Other studies using opinion leaders in the community (152,153) have been shown to be effective. For example, Kelly et al. (154) used bartenders to identify popular patrons to receive five two-hour training sessions in which they were taught how to deliver safer sex messages, and then to have on average 10 conversations with friends and acquaintances in which they encouraged the adoption or maintenance of safer sex. The intervention was effective at 12-month follow-up (among men who attended the bars and who were not in exclusive relationships), in reducing the mean number of occasions of unprotected anal intercourse, increasing condom use, and reducing the proportion of men reporting unprotected anal intercourseduring the previous two months.

Media Campaigns

Media campaigns can have substantial impact on raising awareness about HIV- and STD-related issues and may have some influence on sexual attitudes and risk behaviors. In response to sharp increases in syphilis in San Francisco between 1999 and 2002, the local public health department launched a social marketing campaign to increase testing for syphilis and awareness and knowledge about syphilis among gay and bisexual men. Montoya et al. (155) undertook a convenience sample of 244 gay and bisexual men (18–60 years of age) to evaluate the effectiveness of the campaign. After controlling for other potential confounders, unaided campaign awareness was a significant correlate of having a syphilis test in the last 6 months (odds ratio, 3.21; 95% confidence interval, 1.30–7.97) compared with no awareness of the campaign. A comparison of respondents aware of the campaign with those not aware also revealed significant increases in awareness and knowledge about syphilis. More generally, there have been no systematic reviews of the impact of media interventions for improving sexual health outcomes among MSM.

Multi-Level Interventions

A number of authors have argued that behavioral interventions are most likely to be effective if they operate at several levels to affect several modifying factors at once (156,157). Some interventions may be effective at changing one or two modifying factors, but may have little or no impact on sexual behavior unless there are simultaneous complementary interventions to change other personal or structural modifying factors influencing the sexual risk of HIV transmission.

Sociopolitical-level interventions include legislation, including antidiscrimination laws and laws about age of consent to sex; equality work (activities to reduce discrimination and social exclusion by influencing local and national policies); facilitation interventions (research and development, program planning, communication and collaboration between agencies); resource allocation; and regulation (e.g., labeling of condoms). While different studies have explored the impact of individual factors, there has been no systematic review of evidence either to support or discount the effectiveness of any sociopolitical interventions in influencing the sexual risk behaviors of MSM. Similarly, no review studies have examined the effectiveness of these kinds of interventions in changing health, intermediate health or health promotion outcomes/intervention impact measures.

Summary

Reviews of evidence suggest that cognitive behavioral group work, focusing on risk reduction, sexual negotiation, and communication skills training and rehearsal, can be effective in influencing the sexual risk behaviors for MSM (137,138). However, it is questionable how transferable such training is to ethnic minority and lesser-educated MSM. Community-level interventions, involving peers and popular opinion leaders, can also be effective in influencing the sexual risk behaviors for MSM. Evidence exists to both support and discount the effectiveness of "brief" interventions in influencing the sexual risk behaviors of MSM. Interventions with MSM are more likely to be effective if they are targeted and tailored to the specific community and, ideally, if implementation follows a degree of formative research. This is particularly important if interventions are to overcome the difficulties of accessing MSM who do not identify as gay or bisexual, are not part of any identifiable gay community, or have cultural or other inhibitions to recognizing safer sex messages as being relevant to their personal sexual activity (140). This underscores the importance of undertaking prior ethnographic research to identify the cultural context, values, beliefs, social mores, and community norms of the targeted group, in order to provide the basis for the content and design of the intervention.

Conclusions

Although the literature contains more evidence relating to interventions with MSM compared with the other priority populations, there remains substantial gaps in our knowledge as far as STD prevention interventions are concerned. In general, the literature is replete with evaluations of small-group work interventions for MSM. However, from the public health point of view, and taking into consideration the need for scaling up and disseminating interventions, small-group work is highly resource-intensive to be of great immediate benefit. Small-group work may also not be acceptable to a large number of men, as it requires a certain degree of interest, commitment, and recognition that one is at risk (147). Community-level interventions are much less common and there is a paucity of interventions pitched at the sociopolitical level. This is worrying, as the reviewed studies repeatedly emphasize that interventions do need to be placed within the broader context of men's lives and address wider determinants of health (i.e., structural modifying factors). Aggleton (158) argues that there are sound reasons to believe from health education research that, without a supportive environment and public policy for sexual risk reduction, the effects of more individualistically focused prevention efforts are likely to be short lived. Community-level interventions involving peers and popular opinion leaders can be effective in influencing the sexual risk behaviors of MSM.

Recent demographic changes, unsupportive psychosocial contexts, and evolutions of STD epidemics present challenges for the improving sexual health among MSM. Although considerable advances have been made in developing and evaluating behavioral and structural interventions, however, much of this has been in the pre-HAART era and a new vision for prevention interventions in the context of HAART are now required. Whichever direction is chosen, practitioners must strive to place interventions within the broader context of men's lives, addressing the range of factors that influence risk at both the personal and at the structural level. Recent sociopolitical challenges would suggest that efforts to actively tackle discrimination toward MSM and to change gay community norms toward improved condom use should be an urgent priority. Work with MSM of color remains in its infancy and more needs to be done to help tailor and target interventions that have been shown to be effective. Finally, the review underscores the need for a holistic approach to prevention that incorporates HIV and other STDs as part of wider efforts to improve sexual health among MSM. The interactions and interconnectedness of these epidemics behooves us to continue ongoing collaboration of efforts to achieve added value and seek greater efficiencies in our prevention efforts.

References

1. Fenton KA, Imrie J. Increasing rates of sexually transmitted diseases in homosexual men in Western Europe and the United States: why? *Infect Dis Clin North Am.* 2005;19:311–331.
2. Wolitski RJ, Valdiserri RO, Denning PH, Levine WC. Are we headed for a resurgence of the HIV epidemic among men who have sex with men? *Am J Public Health.* 2001;91:883–888.
3. Black D, Gates G, Sanders S, Taylor L. Demographics of the gay and lesbian population in the United States: evidence from available systematic data sources. *Demography.* 2000;37:139–154.

4. Anderson JE, Stall R. Increased reporting of male-to-male sexual activity in a national survey. *Sexually Transmitted Diseases*. 2002;29:643–646.

5. Mercer CH, Fenton KA, Copas AJ, Wellings K, Erens B, McManus S, Nanchahal K, MacDowall W, Johnson AM. Increasing prevalence of male homosexual partnerships and practices in Britain 1990-2000: evidence from national probability surveys. *AIDS*. 2004;18:1453–1458.

6. Advance Data 362. Sexual Behavior and Selected Health Measures: Men and Women 15-44 Years of Age, United States, 2002. 56 pp. (PHS) 2003-1250.

7. Janssen RS, Valdiserri RO. HIV prevention in the United States: increasing emphasis on working with those living with HIV. *J Acquir Immune Defic Syndr*. 2004;37(Suppl 2):S119–S121.

8. Gomez CA; The Seropositive Urban Men's Study Team. Sexual HIV transmission risk behaviors among HIV-seropositive (HIV+) injection drug users and HIV+ men who have sex with men: implications for interventions. In: Program and Abstracts of the National HIV Prevention Conference; August 29–September 1, 1999; Atlanta, GA. Abstract 180.

9. Lowndes CM, Fenton KA; European Surveillance of STI's Network. Surveillance systems for STIs in the European Union: facing a changing epidemiology. *Sex Transm Infect*. 2004;80:264–271.

10. Centers for Disease Control and Prevention. Sexually Transmitted Disease Surveillance, 2003. Atlanta GA: U.S. Department of Health and Human Services; September 2004.

11. Tabet SR, Krone MR, Paradise MA, Corey L, Stamm WE, Celum CL. Incidence of HIV and sexually transmitted diseases (STD) in a cohort of HIV-negative men who have sex with men (MSM). *AIDS*. 1998;12:2041–2048.

12. Wong W, Chaw JK, Kent CK, Klausner JD. Risk factors for early syphilis among gay and bisexual men seen in an STD clinic: San Francisco, 2002-2003. *Sexually Transmitted Diseases*. 2005;32:458–463.

13. Fox KK, del Rio C, Holmes KK, Hook EW 3rd, Judson FN, Knapp JS, Procop GW, Wang SA, Whittington WL, Levine WC. Gonorrhea in the HIV era: a reversal in trends among men who have sex with men. *American Journal of Public Health*. 2001;91:959–964.

14. Weinstock H, Dale M, Gwinn M, Satten GA, Kothe D, Mei J, Royalty J, Linley L, Fridlund C, Parekh B, Rawal BD, Busch MP, Janssen RS. HIV seroincidence among patients at clinics for sexually transmitted diseases in nine cities in the United States. *Journal of Acquired Immune Deficiency Syndromes: JAIDS*. 2002;29:478–483.

15. Torian LV, Makki HA, Menzies IB, Murrill CS, Weisfuse IB. HIV infection in men who have sex with men, New York City Department of Health sexually transmitted disease clinics, 1990-1999: a decade of serosurveillance finds that racial disparities and associations between HIV and gonorrhea persist. *Sexually Transmitted Diseases*. 2002;29:73–78.

16. Harawa NT, Greenland S, Bingham TA, Johnson DF, Cochran SD, Cunningham WE, Celentano DD, Koblin BA, LaLota M, MacKellar DA, McFarland W, Shehan D, Stoyanoff S, Thiede H, Torian L, Valleroy LA. Associations of race/ethnicity with HIV prevalence and HIV-related behaviors among young men who have sex with men in 7 urban centers in the United States. Journal *of Acquired Immune Deficiency Syndromes: JAIDS*. 2004;35:526–536.

17. Stockman JK, Schwarcz SK, Butler LM, de Jong B, Chen SY, Delgado V, McFarland W. HIV prevention fatigue among high-risk populations in San Francisco. *Journal of Acquired Immune Deficiency Syndromes: JAIDS*. 2004;35:432–434.

18. Remien RH, Halkitis PN, O'Leary A, Wolitski RJ, Gomez CA. Risk perception and sexual risk behaviors among HIV-positive men on antiretroviral therapy. *AIDS & Behavior*. 2005;9:167–176.

19. Centers for Disease Control and Prevention (CDC). Internet use and early syphilis infection among men who have sex with men–San Francisco, California, 1999-2003. *MMWR. Morbidity & Mortality Weekly Report.* 2003;52:1229–1232.

20. Elford J, Bolding G, Davis M, Sherr L, Hart G. Web-based behavioral surveillance among men who have sex with men: a comparison of online and offline samples in London, UK. *Journal of Acquired Immune Deficiency Syndromes: JAIDS.* 2004;35:421–426.

21. Ross MW, Mansson SA, Daneback K, Tikkanen R. Characteristics of men who have sex with men on the internet but identify as heterosexual, compared with heterosexually identified men who have sex with women. *Cyberpsychol Behav.* 2005;8:131–139.

22. Ross MW, Mansson SA, Daneback K, Cooper A, Tikkanen R. Biases in internet sexual health samples: comparison of an internet sexuality survey and a national sexual health survey in Sweden. *Soc Sci Med.* 2005;61:245–252.

23. Ross MW, Tikkanen R, Mansson SA. Differences between Internet samples and conventional samples of men who have sex with men: implications for research and HIV interventions. *Social Science & Medicine.* 2000;51:749–758.

24. Centers for Disease Control and Prevention (CDC). HIV incidence among young men who have sex with men–seven U.S. cities, 1994-2000. *MMWR Morb Mortal Wkly Rep.* 2001;50:440–444.

25. Catania JA, Osmond D, Stall RD, Pollack L, Paul JP, Blower S, Binson D, Canchola JA, Mills TC, Fisher L, Choi KH, Porco T, Turner C, Blair J, Henne J, Bye LL, Coates TJ. The continuing HIV epidemic among men who have sex with men. *Am J Public Health.* 2001;91:907–914.

26. LGV reported in Europe and the U.S. *AIDS Clin Care.* 2005;17:77.

27. Centers for Disease Control and Prevention (CDC). Lymphogranuloma venereum among men who have sex with men–Netherlands, 2003-2004. *MMWR Morb Mortal Wkly Rep.* 2004;53:985–988.

28. Kaslow RA, Dorak T, Tang JJ. Influence of host genetic variation on susceptibility to HIV type 1 infection. *J Infect Dis.* 2005;191(Suppl 1):S68–S77.

29. Grassly NC, Fraser C, Garnett GP. Host immunity and synchronized epidemics of syphilis across the United States. *Nature.* 2005 ;433:417–421.

30. Weiss HA, Quigley MA, Hayes RJ. Male circumcision and risk of HIV infection in sub-Saharan Africa: a systematic review and meta-analysis. *AIDS.* 2000;14:2361–2370.

31. Van Dam J, Anastasi MC. Male circumcision and HIV prevention. Directions for future research. Report of a meeting, Washington, DC, 7–8 February 2000, The Population Council Inc.

32. Kreiss JK, Hopkins SG. The association between circumcision status and HIV infection among homosexual men. *J Infect Dis.* 1993;168:1404–1408.

33. Buchbinder SP, Vittinghoff E, Heagerty PJ, Celum CL, Seage GR 3rd, Judson FN, McKirnan D, Mayer KH, Koblin BA. Sexual risk, nitrite inhalant use, and lack of circumcision associated with HIV seroconversion in men who have sex with men in the United States. *Journal of Acquired Immune Deficiency Syndromes: JAIDS.* 2005;39:82–89.

34. Ekstrand ML, Stall RS, Paul JP, Osmond DH, Coates TJ. Gay men report high rates of unprotected anal sex with partners of unknown or discordant HIV status. *AIDS.* 1999;13:1525–1533.

35. Centers for Disease Control and Prevention. Increases in unsafe sex and rectal gonorrhea among men who have sex with men-San Francisco, California, 1994-1997. *MMWR Morb Mortal Wkly Rep.* 1999;48:45–48.

36. Billy JOG, Tanfer K, Grady WR, Klepinger DH. The sexual behavior of men in the United States. *Fam Plann Perspect.* 1993;25:52–60.

37. Tanfer K. National Survey of Men: design and execution. *Fam Plann Perspect.* 1993;25:83–86.

38. Johnson AM, Mercer CH, Erens B, Copas AJ, McManus S, Wellings K, Fenton KA, Korovessis C, MacDowall W, Nanchahal K, Purdon S, Field J. Sexual behaviour in Britain: partnerships, practices, and HIV risk behaviours. *Lancet.* 2001;358:1835–1842.

39. Fenton KA, Mercer CM, Johnson AM. Evolution of sexual risk behaviours and STD transmission risk among MSM. Oral presentation at the 16th Biennial Meeting of The International Society for Sexually Transmitted Diseases Research (ISSTDR). Amsterdam. 10–13 July 2005, Amsterdam, The Netherlands. Abstract available at http://www.isstdr.nl/0605%20ISSTDR%20Program%20Book%20DEF.pdf.

40. Imrie J, Mercer CH, Davis MDM, Stephenson JM, Hart GJ, Williams IG, Davidson OR, FentonKA. MP-185 prevalence and correlates of `fisting' in a UK clinic sample of HIV positive men who have sex with men (MSM). 16th Biennial Meeting of the International Society For Sexually Transmitted Diseases Research (ISSTDR). Amsterdam. 10–13 July 2005, Amsterdam, The Netherlands. Available at http://www.isstdr.nl/0605%20ISSTDR%20Program%20Book%20DEF.pdf.

41. Mercer CH, Imrie J, Davis MDM, Stephenson JM, Hart GJ, Williams IG, Davidson OR, Fenton KA. MP-105 'the core within the core': ultra-high risk sexual behaviour and STI/HIV transmission risk in a UK sample of HIV-positive men who have sex with men (MSM). 16th Biennial Meeting of the International Society for Sexually Transmitted Diseases Research (ISSTDR). Amsterdam. 10–13 July 2005, Amsterdam, The Netherlands. Available at http://www.isstdr.nl/0605%20ISSTDR%20Program%20Book%20DEF.pdf

42. Mansergh G, Marks G. Age and risk of HIV infection in men who have sex with men. *AIDS.* 1998;12:1119–1128.

43. Waldo CR, McFarland W, Katz MH, MacKellar D, Valleroy LA. Very young gay and bisexual men are at risk for HIV infection: the San Francisco Bay Area Young Men's Survey II. *Journal of Acquired Immune Deficiency Syndromes: JAIDS.* 2002;4:168–174.

44. Valleroy LA, MacKellar DA, Karon JM, Rosen DH, McFarland W, Shehan DA, Stoyanoff SR, LaLota M, Celentano DD, Koblin BA, Thiede H, Katz MH, Torian LV, Janssen RS. HIV prevalence and associated risks in young men who have sex with men. Young Men's Survey Study Group. *JAMA.* 2000;284:198–204.

45. Janssen R. Serostatus approach to fighting the HIV epidemic (SAFE): a new prevention strategy to reduce transmission. In: Program and abstracts of the 8th Conference on Retroviruses and Opportunistic Infections; February 2001; Chicago, IL. Abstract S20.

46. Wolitski RJ, Gomez C, Parsons J, Ambrose T, Remien R. HIV-seropositive men's perceived responsibility for preventing HIV transmission of HIV to others. In: Program and abstracts of the XII International Conference on AIDS; July 1998; Geneva, Switzerland. Abstract 23361.

47. Marks G, Burris S, Peterman TA. Reducing sexual transmission of HIV from those who know they are infected: the need for personal and collective responsibility. *AIDS.* 1999;13:297–306.

48. Denning P, Nakashima AK, Wortley P. Increasing rates of unprotected anal intercourse among HIV-infected men who have sex with men in the United States. In: Program and Abstracts of the XIII International Conference on AIDS; July 9-14, 2000; Durban, South Africa. Abstract ThOrC714.

49. Guenther-Grey CA, Varnell S, Weiser JI, Mathy RM, O'Donnell L, Stueve A, Remafedi G; Community Intervention Trial for Youth Study Team. Trends in sexual risk-taking among urban young men who have sex with men, 1999-2002. *Journal of the National Medical Association.* 97(7 Suppl):38S–43S.

50. Denning PH, Campsmith ML. Unprotected anal intercourse among HIV-positive men who have a steady male sex partner with negative or unknown HIV serostatus. *American Journal of Public Health.* 2005;95:152–158.

51. Semple SJ, Patterson TL, Grant I. The sexual negotiation behavior of HIV-positive gay and bisexual men. *Journal of Consulting & Clinical Psychology.* 2000;68: 934–937.
52. Guzman R, Colfax GN, Wheeler S, Mansergh G, Marks G, Rader M, Buchbinder S. Negotiated safety relationships and sexual behavior among a diverse sample of HIV-negative men who have sex with men. *Journal of Acquired Immune Deficiency Syndromes: JAIDS.* 2005;38:82–86.
53. Ekstrand ML, Coates TJ. Maintenance of safer sexual behaviors and predictors of risky sex: the San Francisco Men's Health Study. *Am J Public Health.* 1990;80:973–977.
54. Graham RP, Kirscht JP, Kessler RC, Graham S. Longitudinal study of relapse from AIDS-preventive behavior among homosexual men. *Health Educ Behav.* 1998;25:625–639.
55. Adib SM, Joseph JG, Ostrow DG, Tal M, Schwartz SA. Relapse in sexual behavior among homosexual men: a 2-year follow-up from the Chicago MACS/CCS. *AIDS.* 1991;5:757–760.
56. Ekstrand ML, Stall RS, Paul JP, Osmond DH, Coates TJ. Gay men report high rates of unprotected anal sex with partners of unknown or discordant HIV status. *AIDS.* 1999;13:1525–1533.
57. Ciesielski CA. Sexually transmitted diseases in men who have sex with men: an epidemiologic review. *Curr Infect Dis Rep.* 2003;5:145–152.
58. Elam G, MacDonald N, Fenton K, Gilbart V, Hickson H, Imrie J, McGarrigle CA, Power R, Evans B. In: TO-004 the role of HIV testing in risk perceptions and safer sex: qualitative results from an investigation into risk factors for seroconversion among gay men who HIV test. 16th Biennial Meeting of the International Society for Sexually Transmitted Diseases Research (ISSTDR). Amsterdam. 10-13 July 2005, Amsterdam, The Netherlands. Available at http://www.isstdr.nl/0605%20ISSTDR%20Program%20Book%20DEF.pdf.
59. Gambotti L, Batisse D, Colin-de-Verdiere N, Delaroque-Astagneau E, Desenclos JC, Dominguez S, Dupont C, Duval X, Gervais A, Ghosn J, Larsen C, Pol S, Serpaggi J, Simon A, Valantin MA, Velter A; Acute Hepatitis C Collaborating Group. Acute hepatitis C infection in HIV positive men who have sex with men in Paris, France, 2001-2004. *Euro Surveill.* 2005;10:115–117.
60. Bodsworth NJ, Cunningham P, Kaldor J, Donovan B. Hepatitis C virus infection in a large cohort of homosexually active men: independent associations with HIV-1 infection and injecting drug use but not sexual behaviour. *Genitourin Med.* 1996;72:118–122.
61. Millett G, Malebranche D, Mason B, Spikes P. Focusing "down low": bisexual black men, HIV risk and heterosexual transmission. *J Natl Med Assoc.* 2005;97 (7 Suppl):52S–59S.
62. Miller M, Serner M, Wagner M. Sexual diversity among black men who have sex with men in an inner-city community. *J Urban Health.* 2005;82(1 Suppl):i26–i34.
63. Goodenow C, Netherland J, Szalacha L. AIDS-related risk among adolescent males who have sex with males, females, or both: evidence from a statewide survey. *American Journal of Public Health.* 2002;92:203–210.
64. Fuller CM, Absalon J, Ompad DC, Nash D, Koblin B, Blaney S, Galea S, Vlahov D. A comparison of HIV seropositive and seronegative young adult heroin- and cocaine-using men who have sex with men in New York City, 2000-2003. *Journal of Urban Health.* 2005;82(1 Suppl):i51–i61.
65. Paul JP, Stall R, Davis F. Sexual risk for HIV transmission among gay/bisexual men in substance-abuse treatment. *AIDS Educ Prev.* 1993;5:11–24.
66. Anonymous. HIV/AIDS among men who have sex with men and inject drugs–United States, 1985-1998. *MMWR Morbidity & Mortality Weekly Report.* 2000;49:465–470.

67. Bull SS, Piper P, Rietmeijer C. Men who have sex with men and also inject drugs-profiles of risk related to the synergy of sex and drug injection behaviors. *Journal of Homosexuality.* 2002;42:31–51.
68. Semple SJ, Patterson TL, Grant I. A comparison of injection and non-injection methamphetamine-using HIV positive men who have sex with men. *Drug & Alcohol Dependence.* 2004;76:203–212.
69. Ryan CM, Huggins J, Beatty R. Substance use disorders and the risk of HIV infection in gay men. *Journal of Studies on Alcohol.* 1999;60:70-77.
70. Cochran SD, Mays VM. Lifetime prevalence of suicide symptoms and affective disorders among men reporting same-sex sexual partners: results from NHANES III. *American Journal of Public Health.* 2000;90:573–578.
71. Mills TC, Paul J, Stall R, Pollack L, Canchola J, Chang YJ, Moskowitz JT, Catania JA. Distress and depression in men who have sex with men: the Urban Men's Health Study. [erratum appears in *Am J Psychiatry.* 2004 Apr;161(4):776]. *American Journal of Psychiatry.* 2004;161:278–285.
72. Gilman SE, Cochran SD, Mays VM, Hughes M, Ostrow D, Kessler RC. Risk of psychiatric disorders among individuals reporting same-sex sexual partners in the National Comorbidity Survey. *American Journal of Public Health.* 2001;91:933-939.
73. Lock J, Steiner H. Gay, lesbian, and bisexual youth risks for emotional, physical, and social problems: results from a community-based survey. *Journal of the American Academy of Child & Adolescent Psychiatry.* 1999;38:297–304.
74. Dickey WC, Dew MA, Becker JT, Kingsley L. Combined effects of HIV-infection status and psychosocial vulnerability on mental health in homosexual men. *Social Psychiatry & Psychiatric Epidemiology.* 1999;34:4–11.
75. Arreola SG, Neilands TB, Pollack LM, Paul JP, Catania JA. Higher prevalence of childhood sexual abuse among Latino men who have sex with men than non-Latino men who have sex with men: data from the Urban Men's Health Study. *Child Abuse & Neglect.* 2005;29:285–290.
76. Kalichman SC, Gore-Felton C, Benotsch E, Cage M, Rompa D. Trauma symptoms, sexual behaviors, and substance abuse: correlates of childhood sexual abuse and HIV risks among men who have sex with men. *J Child Sex Abus.* 2004;13:1–15.
77. Bloom FR, Leichliter JS, Whittier DK, McGrath JW. Syphilis and gay men: the biological impact of social stress. In: Feldman D, ed. *AIDS, Culture, and Gay Men.* Gainesville, FL: University of Florida Press; (in press).
78. Odets W. In the Shadow of the Epidemic: Being HIV-Negative in the Age of AIDS. Chapel Hill, NC: Duke University;. 1995.
79. Stall R, Hays R, Waldo C, Ekstrand M, McFarland W. The gay '90s: A review of research in the 1990s on sexual behavior and HI risk among men who have sex with men. *AIDS.* 2000;13:S1–S4.
80. Centers for Disease Control and Prevention (CDC). HIV prevalence, unrecognized infection, and HIV testing among men who have sex with men–five U.S. cities, June 2004-April 2005. *MMWR Morb Mortal Wkly Rep.* 2005;54:597–601.
81. Kahn RH, Heffelfinger JD, Berman SM. Syphilis outbreaks among men who have sex with men: a public health trend of concern. *Sex Transm Dis.* 2002;29:285–287.
82. Fox KK, del Rio C, Holmes K, et al. Gonorrhea in the HIV era: a reversal of trends among men who have sex with men. *American Journal of Public Health.* 2001;91:959–964.
83. Halkitis PN, Zade DD, Shrem M, Marmor M. Beliefs about HIV non-infection and risky sexual behavior among MSM. *AIDS Education & Prevention.* 2004;16:448–458.
84. Koblin BA, Perdue T, Ren L, Thiede H, Guilin V, MacKellar DA, Valleroy LA, Torian LV. Attitudes about combination HIV therapies: the next generation of gay men at risk. *Journal of Urban Health.* 2003;80:510–519.

85. McElrath K. MDMA and sexual behavior: ecstasy users' perceptions about sexuality and sexual risk. *Subst Use Misuse.* 2005;40:1461–1477.

86. Romanelli F, Smith KM, Pomeroy C. Use of club drugs by HIV-seropositive and HIV-seronegative gay and bisexual men. *Top HIV Med.* 2003;11:25–32.

87. Swearingen SG, Klausner JD. Sildenafil use, sexual risk behavior, and risk for sexually transmitted diseases, including HIV infection. *Am J Med.* 2005;118:571–577.

88. Paul JP, Pollack L, Osmond D, Catania JA. Viagra (sildenafil) use in a population-based sample of U.S. men who have sex with men. *Sex Transm Dis.* 2005;32:531–533.

89. Wong W, Chaw JK, Kent CK, Klausner JD. Risk factors for early syphilis among gay and bisexual men seen in an STD clinic: San Francisco, 2002-2003. *Sex Transm Dis.* 2005;32:458–463.

90. Mansergh G, Colfax GN, Marks G, Rader M, Guzman R, Buchbinder S. The Circuit Party Men's Health Survey: findings and implications for gay and bisexual men. *American Journal of Public Health.* 2001;91:953–958.

91. Vanable PA, McKirnan DJ, Buchbinder SP, Bartholow BN, Douglas JM Jr, Judson FN, MacQueen KM. Alcohol use and high-risk sexual behavior among men who have sex with men: the effects of consumption level and partner type. *Health Psychology.* 2004;23:525–532.

92. Beckett M, Burnam A, Collins RL, Kanouse DE, Beckman R. Substance use and high-risk sex among people with HIV: a comparison across exposure groups. *AIDS & Behavior.* 2003;7:209–219.

93. Semple SJ, Patterson TL, Grant I. Motivations associated with methamphetamine use among HIV+ men who have sex with men. *Journal of Substance Abuse Treatment.* 2002;22:149–156.

94. Klitzman RL, Greenberg JD, Pollack LM, Dolezal C. MDMA ('ecstasy') use, and its association with high risk behaviors, mental health, and other factors among gay/bisexual men in New York City. *Drug & Alcohol Dependence.* 2002;66:115–125.

95. Chu PL, McFarland W, Gibson S, Weide D, Henne J, Miller P, Partridge T, Schwarcz S. Viagra use in a community-recruited sample of men who have sex with men, San Francisco. *Journal of Acquired Immune Deficiency Syndromes: JAIDS.* 2003;33:191–193.

96. Fisher JD, Fisher WA, Williams SS, Malloy TE. Empirical tests of an information-motivation-behavioral skills model of AIDS-preventive behavior with gay men and heterosexual university students. *Health Psychol.* 1994;13:238–250.

97. Stall RD, Hays RB, Waldo CR, Ekstrand M, McFarland W. The Gay '90s: a review of research in the 1990's on sexual behavior and HIV risk among men who have sex with men. *AIDS.* 2000;14(suppl 3):S101–S114.

98. Kelly JA, Hoffmann RG, Rompa D, Gray M. Protease inhibitor combination therapies and perceptions of gay men regarding AIDS severity and the need to maintain safer sex. *AIDS.* 1998;12:F91–F95.

99. Vanable PA, Ostrow DG, McKirnan DJ, Taywaditep KJ, Hope BA. Impact of combination therapies on HIV risk perceptions and sexual risk among HIV-positive and HIV-negative gay and bisexual men. *Health Psychol.* 2000;19:134–145.

100. Suarez T, Miller J. Negotiating risks in context: a perspective on unprotected anal intercourse and barebacking among men who have sex with men-where do we go from here? *Arch Sex Behav.* 2001;30:287–300.

101. Chesney MA, Chambers DB, Kahn JO. Risk behavior for HIV infection in participants in preventive HIV vaccine trials: a cautionary note. *J Acquir Immune Defic Syndr Hum Retrovirol.* 1997;16:266–271.

102. Remien RH, Smith RA. HIV prevention in the era of HAART: implications for providers. *AIDS Reader.* 2000;10:247–251.

103. Ostrow DG, Fox K, Chmiel JS, et al. Attitudes toward highly active retroviral therapy predict sexual risk-taking among HIV-infected and uninfected gay men in the Multicenter AIDS Cohort Study (MACS). In: Program and Abstracts of the XIII International Conference on AIDS; July 9-14, 2000; Durban, South Africa. Abstract ThOrC719.

104. Lichtenstein B. Secret encounters: black men, bisexuality, and AIDS in Alabama. *Medical Anthropology Quarterly*. 2000;14:374–393.

105. Kelly J, Hoffman R, Rompa D, Gray M. Protease inhibitor combination therapies and perceptions of gay men regarding AIDS severity and the need to maintain safer sex. *AIDS*. 1998;12:F91–F95.

106. Mansergh G, Marks G. Age and risk of HIV infection in men who have sex with men. *AIDS*. 1998;12:1119–1128.

107. McAullife T, Kelly J, Sikkema K. Sexual HIV risk behavior levels among young and older gay men outside of AIDS epicenters: findings of a 16 city sample. *AIDS and Behavior*. 1999;3:111–119.

108. Mansergh G, Colfax GN, Marks G, et al. The circuit party men's health survey: Findings and implications for gay and bisexual men. *American Journal of Public Health*. 2001;91:953–958.

109. Purcell DW, Parsons JT, Halkitis PN, Mizuno Y, Woods WJ. Substance use and sexual transmission risk behavior of HIV-positive men who have sex with men. *Journal of Substance Abuse Treatment*. 2001;13(1–2):185–200.

110. Berube A. Caught in the storm: AIDS and the meaning of social disaster. *Out/Look*. 1988;1:8–19.

111. Rubin G. Elegy for the Valley of Kings: AIDS and the leather community in San Francisco, 1981-1996. In: Levine MP, Nardi PM, Gagnon JH, eds. *In Changing Times: Gay Men and Lesbians Encounter HIV/AIDS*. Chicago: University of Chicago; 1997;101–144.

112. Crocker J, Major B. Social stigma and self esteem: self-protective properties of stigma. *Psychological Review*. 1989;96:608–630.

113. Peterson JL, Folkman L, Bakeman R. Stress, coping, HIV status, psychosocial resources and depressive mood in African American, gay, bisexual and heterosexual men. *American Journal of Community Psychology*. 1996;24: 461–487.

114. Bloom FR. Searching for meaning in everyday life: negotiating selves in the HIV spectrum. *Ethos: Journal of the Society for Psychological Anthropology*. 1998;25:454–479.

115. Weiss R. Uncertainty and the lives of persons with AIDS. *Journal of Health and Social Behavior*. 1989;30:270–281.

116. Albee GW. Prologue: a model for classifying prevention programs. In: Joffe JM, Albee GW, Kelly LD, eds. *Readings in Primary Prevention of Psychopathology*. Hanover, NH: University Press of New England; 1984;ix–xviii.

117. McGrath JW. The biological impact of social responses to the AIDS epidemic. *Medical Anthropology*. 1992;15:63–79.

118. Signorile M. *Hitting Hard*. New York: Carol and Graf; 2005.

119. Savage D. I'm complacent, you're complacent. September 19, 2002. Available at: http://www.thestranger.com.

120. Rogers G, Cuny M, Oddy J, Pratt N., Beilby J, Wilkinson D. Depressive disorders and unprotected casual anal sex among Australian homosexually active men in primary care. *HIV Medicine*. 2003;4:271–275.

121. Bernstein S. Anti-syphilis campaign has impact, but worries remain. *Los Angeles Times*. January 19, 2001: B4.

122. Millett G, Malebranche D, Mason B, Spikes P. Focusing: "down low": bisexual black men, HIV risk and heterosexual transmission. *JAMA*. 2005;97:52S–59S.

123. Dodd DA. Black journalists' group debates 'down low' coverage. *Atlanta Journal-Constitution*, August 6, 2005.

124. Anderson, L. The demons behind the down low. *POZ* 2004 Sept;(105). Accessible at: http://www.poz.com/articles/158_399.shtml.
125. APA Council of Representatives. Resolution of sexual orientation and marriage. The American Psychological Association, 2004.
126. Meyer IH. Prejudice, social stress, and mental health in lesbian, gay, and bisexual populations: conceptual issues and research evidence. *Psychological Bulletin.* 2003;129:674–697.
127. Chauncey G. *Why Marriage? The History Shaping Today's Debate Over Gay Equality.*Cambridge, MA: Basic Books; 2004.
128. Axel-Lute P. Same-sex marriage: a selective bibliography of the legal literature. *Rutgers School of Law Newark, On-line Resources.* Available at: http://law-library.rutgers.edu/SSM.html.
129. CBC News. Same sex marriage law passes 158-133. Available at: http://www.cbc.ca/story/canada/national/2005/06/28/samesex050628.html%20Same-sex%20marriage%20law%20passes%20158-133.
130. Kersch KI. Full faith and credit for same-sex marriages?" *Political Science Quarterly.* 1997;112:117–136.
131. Perry MJ. Why the Federal Marriage Amendment is not only not necessary, but a bad idea. *San Diego Law Review.* 2005;42:925–934.
132. Meyers HF, Javanbakht M, Martinez M, Obediah S. Psychosocial predictors of risky sexual behaviors in African American men: Implications for prevention. *AIDS Education and Prevention.* 2003;15(Suppl A):66–79.
133. Guss JR, Drescher J. *Addictions in the Gay and Lesbian Community.* New York: Haworth Press; 2000.
134. Ramirez-Valles J. The protective effects of community involvement for HIV risk behavior: a conceptual framework. *Health Education Research.* 2002;17:389–403.
135. Bontempo DE. D'Augelli AR. Effects of at-school victimization and sexual orientation on lesbian, gay, or bisexual youths' health risk behavior. *Journal of Adolescent Health.* 2002;30:364–374.
136. Singer M, Clair S. Syndemics and public health: reconceptualizing disease in biosocial context. *Medical Anthropology Quarterly.* 2003;17:423–441.
137. Ellis S, Barnett-Page E, Morgan A, Taylor L, Walters R, Goodrich J. HIV prevention: a review of reviews assessing the effectiveness of interventions to reduce the risk of sexual transmission. Evidence briefing. London: Health Development Agency; March 2003.
138. Ellis S, Grey A. STI Prevention: A Review of Reviews Assessing the Effectiveness of Non-Clinical Interventions to Reduce the Risk of Sexually Transmitted Infections. London: Health Development Agency; 2003.
139. Wolitski RJ, MacGowan RJ, Higgins DL et al. The effects of HIV counseling and testing on risk- related practices and help-seeking behavior. *AIDS Education and Prevention.* 1997;(Suppl. B):S52–S67.
140. Oakley A, Oliver S, Peersman G, et al. Review of Effectiveness of Health Promotion Interventions for Men Who Have Sex with Men. London: Institute of Education, Social Science Research Unit. EPPI-Centre; 1996.
141. Peersman G, Harden A, Oliver S. Effectiveness Reviews in Health Promotion. London: Institute of Education, Social Science Research Unit, EPPI-Centre; 1999.
142. Stephenson JM, Imrie J, Sutton SR. Rigorous trials of sexual behaviour interventions in STD/HIV prevention: what can we learn from them? *AIDS.* 2000;14(Suppl 3):S115–S124.
143. Choi KH, Lew S, Vittinghoff E, Catania JA, Barrett DC, Coates TJ. The efficacy of brief group counseling in HIV risk reduction among homosexual Asian and Pacific Islander men. *AIDS.* 1996;10(1):81–87.
144. Kelly JA, St Lawrence JS, Hood HV, Brasfield TL. Behavioral intervention to reduce AIDS risk activities. *J Consult Clin Psychol.* 1989;57:60–67.

145. Valdiserri RO, Lyter DW, Leviton LC, Callahan CM, Kingsley LA, Rinaldo CR. AIDS prevention in homosexual and bisexual men: results of a randomized trial evaluating two risk reduction interventions, *AIDS*. 1989;3(1):21–26.

146. Peterson JL, Coates TJ, Catania J, Hauck WW, Acree M, Daigle D, Hillard B, Middleton L, Hearst N. Evaluation of an HIV risk reduction intervention among African-American homosexual and bisexual men. *AIDS*. 1996;10:319–325.

147. Kegeles SM, Hart GJ. Recent HIV prevention interventions for gay men: individual, small group and community-based studies. *AIDS*. 1998;12(Suppl): S209–S215.

148. Choi KH, Coates TJ. Prevention of HIV infection. *AIDS*. 1994;8:1371–1389.

149. Exner TM, Seal DW, Ehrhardt AA. A review of HIV interventions for at-risk women. *AIDS and Behavior*. 1997;1:93–124.

150. Honnen TJ, Kleinke CL. Prompting bar patrons with signs to take free condoms. *J Appl Behav Anal*. 1990;23:215–217.

151. Kegeles SM, Hays RB, Coates TJ. The Mpowerment Project: a community-level HIV prevention intervention for young gay men. *Am J Public Health*. 1996;86 (8 Pt 1):1129–1136.

152. Kelly JA, St Lawrence JS, Diaz YE, Stevenson LY, Hauth AC, Brasfield TL, Kalichman SC, Smith JE, Andrew ME. HIV risk behavior reduction following intervention with key opinion leaders of population: an experimental analysis. *Am J Public Health*. 1991;81:168–171.

153. St Lawrence JS, Brasfield TL, Diaz YE, Jefferson KW, Reynolds MT, Leonard MO. Three-year follow-up of an HIV risk-reduction intervention that used popular peers. *Am J Public Health*. 1994;84:2027–2028.

154. Kelly JA, Murphy DA, Sikkema KJ, McAuliffe TL, Roffman RA, Solomon LJ, Winett RA, Kalichman SC. Randomised, controlled, community-level HIV-prevention intervention for sexual-risk behaviour among homosexual men in US cities. Community HIV Prevention Research Collaborative. *Lancet*. 1997;350: 1500–1505.

155. Montoya JA, Kent CK, Rotblatt H, McCright J, Kerndt PR, Klausner JD. Social marketing campaign significantly associated with increases in syphilis testing among gay and bisexual men in San Francisco. *Sexually Transmitted Diseases*. 2006;32:395–399.

156. Kelly JA. Advances in HIV/AIDS education and prevention. *Family Relations*. 1995;4:345–352.

157. Shepherd J, Peersman G, Weston R, et al. Cervical cancer and sexual lifestyle: a systematic review of health education interventions targeted at women. *Health Education Research*. 2000;15:681–694.

158. Aggleton P. Sexual Behaviour and HIV/AIDS. A Review of the Effectiveness of Health Education and Health Promotion. Utrecht: Dutch Centre for Health Promotion and Health Education and IUHPE/EURO; 1994.

15

STD Repeaters: Implications for the Individual and STD Transmission in a Population

Jami S. Leichliter, Ph.D., Jonathan M. Ellen, M.D., and Robert A. Gunn, M.D., M.P.H.

Defining STD "Repeaters"

STD repeaters are important as a population of study for two primary reasons: 1) repeat infections may lead to an increased risk in STD sequelae, and 2) persons with repeat infections represent a disproportionate share of STD morbidity and may be members of the core group or core transmitters. We argue that it is likely that there are two different groups of repeaters. First, there are women who are the recipients of repeat infection as a result of the risky behaviors of their sex partners. Second, there are heterosexual and homosexual men and some women who engage in behavior that is more typical of core transmission patterns. These groups will require different interventions. We discuss these issues further later in the chapter.

Time Frame and Diseases

It is worth delineating what we mean when we talk about "STD repeaters" or "repeat infections with STDs." Generally, when used in the research literature, "repeaters" are individuals who acquire more than one nonviral STD infection in a specified period of time. Some studies focus solely on repeat episodes of gonorrhea (1–6); some focus exclusively on two or more infections with chlamydia (7–11). Other studies consider several different STDs when defining repeaters (12–15). What appears to be most important is that, regardless of specific disease, repeaters are an important population and are at an increased risk for STD acquisition and sequelae. Furthermore, some repeaters may be largely responsible for maintaining core transmission groups that spread disease throughout the community.

The time frame for inclusion as a "repeat" infection with an STD varies from study to study. The bulk of research on STD repeaters attempts to eliminate persistent infections that are due to treatment failure. Situations such as this do not represent a longer-term continued risk behavior or new risk behavior. One study limited repeat infections to those where a test of cure was conducted after the first infection or the patient was asymptomatic for at least two weeks before the "repeat" infection (1). Other studies also have included a test of cure for the initial infection (12,16,17).

Behavioral Interventions for Prevention and Control of Sexually Transmitted Diseases. Aral SO, Douglas JM Jr, eds. Lipshutz JA, assoc ed. New York: Springer Science+Business Media, LLC; 2007.

While a test of cure may be ideal for determining repeat infection, it has not been used in many studies for various reasons. A test of cure for gonorrhea or chlamydia is not commonplace in the United States. In fact, CDC treatment guidelines do not recommend a test of cure for chlamydia or gonorrhea, given that treatments are highly efficacious and that most positive follow-up tests are due to reinfection (18). Additionally, most public STD clinics provide directly observed single-dose therapy (e.g., azithromycin for chlamydia and ceftriaxone or a single-dose antibiotic for gonorrhea) to infected clients. However, some clinics disseminate a seven-day course of therapy (e.g., doxycycline). Although treatment compliance with a longer-term therapy is a concern, two studies have indicated that both therapies are effective (19,20).

Given these complexities, some researchers have limited the definition of subsequent infections to those that occur a set number of days after the initial infection in an attempt to eliminate as many unresolved or persistent infections as possible. Probably the most common time frame for consideration as a repeat infection is an infection that is diagnosed 30 days or more after an initial STD (6,8,10,15,21). Shorter gaps between infections have been used including 14 or more days (22) and 10 or more days (23). Some studies have not reported the use of a minimum time between test results (13).

The outer time frame for consideration as a "repeat" infection has varied in the literature. Most researchers use a cutoff that ranges from one to two years when defining a "repeat" infection (2,6,8,12–15,17,24–31). Other studies appear to select an arbitrary cutoff based on the data that are available at time of data analysis (5,7,10,21,32–34). In some studies, the outer window for determining a repeat infection has been extended to the individual's lifetime (35).

Parameters for Review of Literature

Standard literature search engines (Ovid and PubMed) were used to search for relevant articles in the following databases: Medline, PsycINFO, SocioFile, and AIDSline. Given the lack of a standardized language denoting individuals who acquire repeated infections with STDs, various key words were used as search terms. Used in combination with "sexually transmitted diseases" or "sexually transmitted infections" and names of specific diseases (e.g., gonorrhea, chlamydia, trichomonas vaginalis), these key words included repeater, repeat, subsequent, reinfection, recidivists, recurrent, and recurrence. Additionally, reference lists from more recent studies were used to identify some of the earlier studies on STD repeaters. Articles that did not exclusively focus on repeaters but primarily focused on intervention effectiveness in other populations while using reinfection as a main outcome were not included for two reasons: 1) there are numerous intervention studies that use reinfection as a main outcome and it would be difficult to include all of them in our review, and 2) reinfection as measured in intervention research studies may be biased by research methodology and not reflect the characteristics of repeat infection seen in the usual care settings.

The Nature, Causes, and Burden of Repeat STDs

Importance of Repeaters as a Population

Repeaters and the Sequelae of STDs

One reason that STD repeaters are a concern of clinicians, public health practitioners, and researchers is that STDs have been found to be related to complications such as infertility, ectopic pregnancy, and pelvic inflammatory disease (PID). Specifically, infections with *Chlamydia trachomatis* or *Neisseria gonorrhoeae* are known to cause PID (36). *C. trachomatis* also has been associated with ectopic pregnancy (37–39). It has been estimated that two-thirds to three-fourths of PID cases have mild to moderate symptoms or are asymptomatic and may go unrecognized (36,40). Additionally, a lack of accepted criteria for diagnosing PID has resulted in difficulties estimating the incidence of PID (36). Estimates of PID occurrence in the United States range from 800,000 to over one million episodes (41,42), with 189,662 cases diagnosed in emergency rooms in 2002 (18). PID is important to public health, given its high costs. The estimated costs associated with PID range from $1060 to $1410 per case (43,44).

Repeated infections with *C. trachomatis* are of special importance to public health, given their relationship to PID and tubal infertility (33,40). It appears as though a dose-response relationship between repeated infections and PID may exist (45). A retrospective cohort study of women in Wisconsin found that women with repeated chlamydial infections were more likely to be hospitalized for sequelae (33). Specifically, women with two infections and three or more infections were four and six times more likely to be hospitalized for PID than women with only one infection (33). The risk of ectopic pregnancy was also significantly higher for women with two infections (odds ratio [OR] = 2.1) and three or more infections (OR=4.5) (33).

Role of Repeaters in Maintaining/Transmitting STDs

Repeat infections with STDs are also important to public health professionals due to the role repeaters appear to play in sustaining the transmission of STDs within a community. Recent studies have shown that repeat infections are relatively common and account for a disproportionate share of STD morbidity, especially for gonorrhea (6,46,47). During a five-year period in Alaska, 16.9% of persons infected with gonorrhea were repeaters, and this group accounted for 33.5% of all gonorrhea infections (46). A study of those attending a clinic in London found similar results. Of those with gonorrhea, 18.8% were repeaters and accounted for 35.8% of gonorrhea infections (47) These results are similar to a study conducted in the 1970s (1). More recently, a study of all gonorrhea cases reported in San Diego, California, from 1995 to 2001 showed a lower proportion of repeat gonorrhea infections—4.5% of infections were repeat infections and gonorrhea repeaters accounted for 9.6% of all infections (6). The authors of several studies have proposed that intervening with STD repeaters may reduce morbidity in the overall community (3,23,48).

In 1978, Yorke and colleagues (49) first suggested that "core" group members may also be STD repeaters. Since that time, other researchers have suggested that STD repeaters represent a core group (4). Findings from other studies lend some support to the idea of repeaters as members of a core group (6,15,23). A thorough review of core group theory has already been published (50), but it is thought that core groups aid in the transmission of STDs by maintaining a reservoir of infection (51). Repeaters are just one of the many ways in which the notion of an STD core has been conceptualized (50). Whether or not all STD repeaters are core transmitters remains to be seen; however, we do know that repeaters account for a disproportionate number of clinic visits and resources (4,52).

Characteristics of the Burden

Estimates of Repeat STDs

Since the last decade of the 20th century, the proportion of STD cases that are attributable to repeat infections has been examined in various populations through recruitment at medical clinics and the use of surveillance systems for reportable diseases. Using state or local surveillance systems in the United States, it has been estimated that 4.5% to 24.4% of select reportable STDs are due to repeat infections (6,23,26,32,33). Studies of public STD clinic clients have found that 8.9% to 38% experience a repeat sexually transmitted infection (5,12,12,46,47,52–54). It is likely that these estimates vary for several reasons, including 1) local morbidity, 2) fluctuations in morbidity over time, 3) the use of different time frames and diseases when categorizing repeaters, and 4) the likelihood of those with repeat infections seeking health care, being tested for STDs, and having their diagnosis reported to the local health department. Despite the range in estimates, these studies demonstrate the extent of the problem of repeat infections.

Recent studies also have examined the extent of repeat STDs in other clinic populations, including adolescent or reproductive health clinics and other community-based clinics. In a prospective longitudinal study of females recruited from adolescent health clinics and who had an STD at enrollment, 38.4% had a subsequent infection with chlamydia within three years (16). The majority of these repeat infections occurred within nine months of the initial infection. Given that all participants were treated and had a test of cure for their initial infection, it is likely that all subsequent infections can be attributed to a new infection rather than a persistent infection. Another study of 216 females attending an adolescent clinic identified recurrent cervicitis due to chlamydia or gonorrhea in 9.3% (31). Studies conducted in multiple, diverse clinics focusing on STDs, reproductive health, and adolescent medicine have also found high rates of repeaters among those with an STD. Repeat STDs ranged from 11% in men with chlamydia to 41.1% of female adolescents (15–19 years) who had an initial infection with chlamydia, gonorrhea, or *Trichomonas vaginalis* when recruited from STD, adolescent, or reproductive health clinics (8,9,12,16,31,55). Interestingly, participants in the study with the highest percentage of repeat STDs all had a test of cure performed after they were treated for the initial STD (12).

Finally, studies estimating the rate of STD repeaters in other populations also have been conducted in the United States. Of 180 adolescents who had an STD at first admission to a juvenile detention facility, 10% of males and 28.9% of females became reinfected with gonorrhea or chlamydia (25). A cohort study of active duty soldiers in the U.S. army found that 7.5% had a repeat diagnosis of chlamydia (7). Another study of male soldiers found that 5% had a repeat infection (56).

Recent international studies also have found substantial repeat STDs among clinic clients. A study of patients attending one of three STD clinics in England found that 14% of participants had a repeat infection. Similar to the U.S. studies, repeat infections seemed to vary in different geographic and clinic populations—ranging from 8% at a Sheffield clinic to 17.3% and 19% at two London clinics (13). In a Belgrade STD clinic, 29% of men had acquired a repeat infection in their lifetime (57). Two African studies also have highlighted the importance of STD repeaters. One study found that nearly 40% ($n = 52$) of 138 STD clinic clients in Uganda experienced repeat STDs (58). Finally, a study of 60 STD patients in a city clinic in Zimbabwe found that 87% of men and 47% of women had repeat infections (59).

Time (Speed) to Repeat Infection

A few studies have investigated the time it takes a repeater to acquire a subsequent infection. Although time to reinfection is likely influenced by factors such as seeking health care and an individual's sexual behavior, it is important to examine the average time (mean or median) it takes to become reinfected with an STD. Of women with repeat chlamydia, 54.4% acquired the subsequent infection within nine months of the initial infection (16). Similarly, Burstein and colleagues found a median time to repeat chlamydial infection of 6.3 months (60) and 7.6 months (8) among adolescent females in Baltimore. Other studies identified a longer time period for acquiring a subsequent infection. In Uganda, 39% of STD repeaters had a repeat infection within 6 months of the initial infection and 64% had the subsequent infection within a year (58). One American study that included both men and women found the mean time to repeat chlamydial infection was 318 days (10.5 months) for those who were coinfected with gonorrhea and 258 days (8.5 months) for those who did not have gonorrhea at followup; however, these time periods were not significantly different (61). Another study of gonorrhea repeaters demonstrated a mean time to repeat infection of 405 days (13.3 months) (34).

Demographic and Behavioral Risk for Repeat STDs

Demographic Risk Factors

A large portion of the research focusing on repeat STDs has examined the epidemiologic factors associated with the acquisition of a subsequent infection. Of these factors, the most common demographics that were studied include sex, age, and race or ethnicity; however, much of the repeaters literature is focused on specific subpopulations. Findings from the majority of studies suggest that adolescents and young adults are at the highest risk for repeat STDs (5,8,10,23,32,48,52,62). Given that adolescents and young adults have the highest burden for STDs in the United States, these results are not surprising.

Research has also examined the relationship between race or ethnicity, sex, and repeat infections. Perhaps the most consistent finding across studies is that African Americans or blacks have a higher burden of repeat infections (3,4,12,23,26,32,33,47,48,63). Similar to findings regarding age, these results are not surprising given the significant racial disparities that exist for many STDs. Most studies that compare men and women have found that men are more likely to become repeaters than women (5,48,52).

It is worth noting that there have been some inconsistent findings with respect to age and sex. For instance, two international studies of male repeaters found that repeaters were more likely to be older than their nonrepeater counterparts (35,47). One of these studies examined men age 20 to 50 years and covered a range of STDs (35), while the other study investigated repeated gonorrhea and found that the mean age of repeaters was 27.8 years as compared with 24.7 years for nonrepeaters (47). Additionally, research suggests that men are at a higher risk for repeat infections, yet a longitudinal study of repeated gonorrhea found no differences between men and women in the proportion of repeaters (4). Studies that have focused exclusively on women have found substantial numbers of repeat STDs (12,16,17,60). Furthermore, one study found that adolescent and young adult women were more likely to acquire a subsequent infection and have a shorter time to reinfection (140 vs. 209 days, $p < 0.05$) than men (63).

Behavioral Risk Factors

General studies. The relationship between sexual behaviors and repeated infections with STDs has been examined in several studies. Findings from the literature have been mixed, and in many instances it appears as though risk factors are often sex-specific. In the past 20 years, several studies that include both men and women have examined the relationship between sexual behaviors and repeat STDs (3,5,13,21,58,62,63). A few of these studies have suggested that multiple sex partners are a risk factor for repeat infection (5,13,58); however, these studies also found higher risk for repeat infection among men (5,13). Men who identified as homosexual or bisexual were at highest risk for repeat STDs (13). A separate study demonstrated that having one or more new sex partners was predictive of reinfection (63). Inconsistent or no condom use (58,62) and having a sex partner who is a sex worker (5) have also been identified as correlates of repeat infection.

Conversely, other studies have examined the relationship between repeat STDs and sexual behavior but have failed to find significant differences in the sexual behavior of repeaters and nonrepeaters (3,21,62). These studies examined a variety of sexual behaviors such as number of sex partners, a new sex partner in the last 30 to 60 days, commercial sex, and condom use. Only one of these studies identified a significant difference in a single sexual behavior. This study found that repeaters were more likely at their initial clinic visit to report failing to use condoms (62).

Male studies. In contrast, studies limited to men or that separately examine men have fairly consistently identified some sexual behaviors as correlates of repeat STDs. Probably the most consistent finding is that male repeaters are more likely to report multiple sex partners than male nonrepeaters (5,35,47,64,65). Additionally, a history of STDs (before study period) has been associated with acquiring STDs by men in multiple studies (9,15,29,47,66,67). Another finding that has been demonstrated in more than one study is an association between inconsistent or no condom use and repeat STDs in men (29,53). Finally, other sexual behaviors have been associated with repeat STDs in men in only one study. These behaviors include having a higher frequency of sex acts per month, having sex with a partner that was met the same day (35), fathering a greater number of children (53) and having sex with a commercial sex worker (5).

Female studies. Identifying behavioral correlates of repeat infection in women in the United States has been less successful. One study found that adolescent females with multiple sex partners had a higher risk of repeat infection (12); however, other studies have failed to replicate this finding about female adolescents and young adults (8,10,11,16,31,55,60). In fact, many of these studies failed to identify any behavioral predictors of acquiring repeat STDs (8,10,11,16,60). A study of adolescent women in Indianapolis found that inconsistent condom use and having gonorrhea rather than chlamydia or trichomonas vaginalis at the initial visit were significantly related to repeat infection in adolescent women (12). In univariate analysis, another study identified a failure to use condoms at the most recent sexual experience as a predictor of repeat STDs, but this association was not found in multivariate analyses (31). Some research indicates that women who are coinfected with both chlamydia and gonorrhea at their initial visit are more likely to acquire a subsequent infection (26,29,32). Given the lack of consistent behavioral predictors, it would appear as though for women that repeated STDs may be largely a function of their sex partners' risky behavior. For example, a sex partner who is high risk, a core group member, or is unaware of their infection and remains untreated can cause reinfection in women who are monogamous.

Given the mixed findings for behavioral risk of men and women, it may no longer make sense to compare the repeat infection status of women with that of men. Although the majority of studies show that men are more likely to be repeaters than women, women are also most vulnerable to the sequelae of STDs and should not be overlooked in terms of repeat infections. Finally, we argue that different behaviors of men and women can result in different levels of risk for repeat infections.

The Context of Behavioral Risk and Possible Interventions

To date, there has been little research on effective intervention strategies for STD repeaters. However, there has been a fair amount of research that has focused on the context of behavioral risk—psychosocial, network, and spatial factors that may contribute to a person's risky sexual behavior. In this section, we summarize the relevant research and discuss possible intervention strategies at various levels—individual, network, etc. Researchers have suggested that a sole focus on individual-level risk factors may not be sufficient to eliminate racial disparities in STD rates given the role of social context and networks (68). Given the complexities associated with repeat infection and racial disparities in general, we argue that multi-level strategies may be the most effective.

Individual Level

Contextual Factors and Individual Risk Behaviors
Given that the most consistent individual-level predictors of repeat infection are age and race or ethnicity, social context appears to be an important factor in the acquisition of repeat infections (45). Additionally, the mixed findings for male repeaters and the lack of consistent behavioral risk factors associated with female repeaters enhance the importance of examining the context in which the behavioral risk occurs in order to understand more fully the complexities associated with repeat infection with STDs. We discuss the possible effect of psychological and other factors on sexual risk and possible intervention strategies in the following sections.

Psychological factors. A few studies have examined the psychological characteristics and functioning of repeaters in an attempt to determine whether psychological problems are more prevalent in this group. Specifically, research has looked at the relationship between STD repeaters and psychological disorders such as depression and antisocial personality disorder, personality dimensions, and other psychological problems such as anger. Studies in the United States, Eastern Europe, and Africa have all demonstrated associations between psychological factors and repeat STDs. A U.S. study of 2061 adolescents most of whom were female (76%), African American (72%), and with a low income found that STD repeaters were more likely to have depression and conduct problems than adolescents who did not acquire multiple infections (69). Lack of hope for the future was a common theme identified in a qualitative study of STD repeaters age 18 and older in Baltimore (70). The situation was viewed as so hopeless that many repeaters made a conscious choice not to have goals for their future. A separate qualitative study of adolescent STD repeaters in Jacksonville, Florida, found mental health issues such as anger, conduct disorders, and depression; however, this study found that many of the adolescent repeaters still had hope for their future (71). These findings suggest that psychological distress and an inability to focus on the future may hinder interventions focused on changing individual behavior.

Findings from two international studies are supportive of those in the United States. A quantitative study of 283 men in Belgrade found that male repeaters were more likely to have antisocial personality than men who did not have repeat STDs (57). A qualitative study of repeaters in Zimbabwe found that men and women varied in their responses to repeated infections with STDs (59). The men tended to focus on physical symptoms and fear of AIDS, while the women tended to be more focused on their feelings of sadness and distrust of their husbands.

Other behaviors. Finally, acquisition of repeat STDs also has been examined in relation to other individual-level behavioral factors. In a study of almost 400 women, childhood sexual abuse and sexual coercion were not related to repeat infection (72). However, two studies of men did find that other behavioral factors were associated with repeat STDs. Men who had a lower income and education level were more likely to experience repeat infections with chlamydia (9). Additionally, men who consumed more alcohol and who had been prosecuted for criminal offenses were more likely to have repeat STDs (35).

Possible Intervention Strategies

Several things became evident in our review of the literature on STD repeaters. First, African Americans, adolescents, and young adults (<25 years) are at highest risk for repeat infection. Second, men and women largely have different risk factors for repeat infection. Finally, the phrase "once a repeater always a repeater" may be on the mark, as STD history was a strong predictor of repeat infections in different studies. These findings suggest intervention strategies that may be useful at the individual level; however, as we argue in the following sections, an individual-level intervention with STD repeaters is probably not sufficient to address the extent of the problem.

At a minimum, individual-level interventions should be aware of the gender differences in sexual risk and sequelae and the effect of these factors on interventions. For instance, a basic sexual risk-reduction intervention is probably not useful for female repeaters, given that they engage in very few sexual risk behaviors. Risk reduction may be more useful for male repeaters, especially an intervention that focuses on mutual monogamy and, if this is not achievable, the use of condoms with casual partners. For women, interventions that focus on empowerment and condom negotiation are possibilities. A thorough discussion of behavioral risk reduction strategies is available in Chapter 2 of this book. Also, biomedical interventions such as frequent screening, preventive antibiotic therapy post exposure, and symptom recognition education may lower the duration of infectiousness and prevent sequelae. A more detailed discussion of biomedical risk reduction strategies is available in Chapter 4 of this volume.

Two other possible individual-level interventions for STD repeaters include mental health services and STD education. Given findings that are suggestive of mental health issues among repeaters, interventions that focus on mental health may be important for this population. Mental health issues may interfere with the repeater's ability to successfully modify or change his or her sexual risky behaviors. At a minimum, local public health departments could link STD repeaters to available individual level counseling services as appropriate. Many communities offer free or low-cost counseling to impoverished citizens. Also, in some areas it may be useful to provide specific STD information to clients of public STD clinics. For instance, it may be important to stress the relationship between chlamydia and gonorrhea and complications such as PID, ectopic pregnancy, and infertility. This type of intervention would be most appropriate for clients who are concerned about reproductive health (i.e., want children). Also, two studies have demonstrated that repeaters are concerned about acquiring HIV (59,70). STD education about the STD-HIV transmission link may be useful in these situations. However, it is worth noting that education-only is typically not a sufficient intervention strategy, and repeaters in Baltimore were keenly aware of their HIV/STD risks (27).

Finally, some repeat infections are reinfections due to an untreated sex partner. Many repeaters viewed partner notification as important and indicated that they would notify their sex partner (70); however, patient referral is at most 50% effective at getting partners treated (73–79). Consequently, other partner services strategies should be considered for this high-risk population and their partners. Expedited partner therapy (EPT), or patient-delivered partner treatment (PDPT), is more effective than patient referral in treating sex partners of persons infected with gonorrhea and chlamydia (75,76). Enhanced patient referral through a booklet containing tear-out partner cards may also be useful (76), especially in situations where PDPT is not feasible. Another option is for the health department to offer provider referral for sex partners of repeaters. Chapter 7 of this volume provides more information on effective strategies for partner services. Finally, rescreening repeaters may also help to identify asymptomatic reinfections that are due to an untreated partner.

The major drawback to individual-level risk reduction interventions for repeaters is that there are limited sexual behaviors that are predictive of repeat infections. However, we have discussed individual-level interventions such as EPT that may effectively reduce some repeat infections. In the following sections, we shall discuss alternative intervention strategies.

Social Level

Gonorrhea has been characterized as a "social disease" (80), and racial disparities in STD prevalence have been well established (18). One study found that African Americans have a much higher rate of mixing between the core and periphery (81), meaning that an African American who is not a member of the STD core (or is a member of the "periphery") has a much higher chance of selecting a sex partner who is a core group member than persons of other racial and ethnic groups. Research also has shown that the overwhelming majority of African American women have African American male partners but only half of the partners of African American men are African American women (82). Differences in sexual mixing patterns in these subpopulations can result in different levels of STD risk (82). Lauman and Youm (81) noted that these network characteristics may explain the racial and ethnic disparities in STD prevalence. These general findings demonstrate that social relationships may be important to examine in relationship to repeat infection. The few studies that have done so as well as possible intervention strategies are discussed in the next two sections.

Social Factors

Social networks. Subgroups in the population that have high prevalence rates of gonorrhea, defined as 20% or higher, have been referred to as the STD "core" (49). It has been argued that most gonorrhea cases are a result of this core group and that the core sustains endemic gonorrhea (49). McEvoy and Le Furgy (4). were among the first to classify STD repeaters as members of the core group. In a longitudinal examination of clinic attendance and repeat infection with gonorrhea, data suggested that a core group of clinic clients existed (4) Clinic clients with repeat gonorrhea spent a median of 130 days in this core group. Further analysis of the data revealed that blacks spent significantly more time in the core group (median = 197 days) than did whites (median = 98.5 days).

One study has specifically examined male STD repeaters in relation to their social networks. Findings from the study indicate that acquiring a new sex partner was not related to an increased risk for a subsequent STD (83). In fact, participants who acquired a new sex partner that was outside of their social network were at less risk of a subsequent infection (83).

Partner factors. The bulk of research on STD repeaters has focused on individual-level factors as related to the index patient (i.e., demographics, sexual behavior). Less research has examined the risk behaviors of sex partners. Again, this research is limited to qualitative data collection methods. One study of adolescents in Jacksonville found that the issue of trust and eventual betrayal was a recurring theme for STD repeaters (30). In some instances, repeaters who were monogamous acquired an STD due to their partners' risky sexual behavior. Similarly, a study of adult repeaters in Baltimore also identified repeaters who reported only one sex partner, yet acquired repeat infections (27). In Zimbabwe, one-third of the women who acquired repeat infections from their husbands reported that condoms would protect them from STDs but that their husbands refused to use them (59).

Qualitative studies also have demonstrated an imbalance in the main relationship dynamics for STD repeaters. The notion of trust in a relationship as a barrier to condom use was a common theme of female adult repeaters (70). Women reported that their main partner accused them of having another sex partner when they asked the main partner to use condoms. STD repeaters also reported a lack of financial resources and in some instances relied on their main partner for financial support (70). A power imbalance in a main relationship as well as partner violence was reported by female adolescent repeaters (30).

These findings, coupled with the lack of sexual behaviors associated with repeat infections in females, suggest that partners' risky sexual behaviors are an important, if neglected, area for future study.

Spatial factors (geographic clustering). Another promising area of research is the focus on environmental factors such as neighborhood or geography. A study of adolescent and adult repeaters in San Francisco examined sociodemographics and included a neighborhood variable that combined city planning region and STD prevalence (23). The study found that African Americans had the highest rates of repeat gonorrhea and repeat chlamydia, and that for males and females, city planning region was related only to repeat gonorrhea. The authors suggested that these findings indicated that core groups may play a role in the transmission of gonorrhea but not of chlamydia (23). A study of gonorrhea repeaters in Baltimore found that gonorrhea repeaters clustered together spatially more than nonrepeaters even though gonorrhea prevalence was not significantly correlated geographically with repeat infections (84). Similarly, a study of gonorrhea repeaters in San Diego found that the strongest predictor of repeat gonorrhea was residence in the high morbidity region of the county (6).

Social and family support. Qualitative studies in both the United States and Africa have explored the social support systems of STD repeaters. Two of these studies focused on adult repeaters (27,59) while one focused on adolescent repeaters (30). Studies of adult repeaters suggest that they lack sufficient social support. One common theme among both male and female repeaters was that their relationships often began as a response to crisis (27). Participants who discussed a lack of social support and then experienced a crisis often turned to their sex partner for support (70). In contrast, an African study of married men and women found that men talked to their friends about their infections with STDs but many women indicated that they were too embarrassed to discuss personal issues such as these with their friends (59).

Similar to what we found for social support and partner risk behaviors, little attention has been paid to the role of family factors in acquisition of repeat STDs. The studies that have examined these factors have been limited to qualitative methods. A common theme identified among female adolescents who experienced repeat infections of gonorrhea or chlamydia in Jacksonville was the presence of inadequate parenting (30). Two parental issues that recurred in the girls' lives were absent fathers and parents who failed to appropriately supervise or to be involved with their daughters (30). Similarly, a recurring theme among adult repeaters in Baltimore was that the lack of parental involvement as children and the lack of parental support in adulthood left the men and women feeling as though they had to deal alone with personal health issues, such as STDs (70).

Possible Intervention Strategies
Network interventions. As noted previously, not all repeaters are at risk for STDs solely as a result of their own risky sexual behavior. Female repeaters often have no clearly identified risky sexual behaviors; yet, repeat STD rates remain high in this population. Additionally, national data show that there is little difference in the sexual behaviors of White and African American

women age 15 to 44 years in the United States. The median number of lifetime sex partners for white women is 3.6 compared with 4.1 for African American women (85). Of white women, 7.8% have never had sex, and 10.2% have had 15 or more sex partners in their lifetime. The corresponding numbers for African American women are 7.7% and 8.8%, respectively.

One study of African Americans found that network factors were important in transmission of STDs (86). Respondents were more likely to have a sex partner with chlamydia or gonorrhea when the partner had a concurrent sex partner who was outside of the local network. Additionally, the study found that participants were more likely to have a sex partner outside of their local network when there was a mean age difference of two or more years between partners (86). The limited research that is available on the sexual and social networks of repeaters indicates that characteristics of sexual networks are associated with repeat infection (83).

As a result, the social and sexual networks of STD repeaters are an extremely important, yet understudied, issue. Research that demonstrates the amount of overlap between core groups or those with multiple partners and STD repeaters would be valuable. A better understanding of repeaters' sexual and social networks may yield a useful network intervention that interrupts the chain of transmission. In clinic settings or through surveillance systems, repeaters can be easily identified and targeted for network-level interventions.

Place-based interventions. Research on geographic and spatial factors indicates that an intervention that is geographic or place-based may be appropriate. Additionally, it is often difficult to identify and locate repeaters or core group members, and research suggests that people may migrate in and out of the core group (87). Consequently, place-based interventions may be more feasible in some settings. Although there is a lack of place-based research with STD repeaters, place-based interventions have been successful when used for a syphilis outbreak (88). Additionally, a study of townships in South Africa that had complex sexual networks in which new partners were often acquired used key informants to identify places where interventions can be delivered to those at highest risk (89). We think that it would be beneficial to develop research focusing on place-based interventions for STD repeaters.

Provider Level

Possible Intervention Strategies
Provider education. Primary care, adolescent, and emergency care providers need to be aware of the effect of repeat STD infections on both individual and community health. It is essential for clinical care providers to assess the risks of their sexually active adolescent and young adult patients to determine the sex of their sex partners, the number of partners, condom use, and their history of prior STDs, particularly bacterial STDs. This information is needed to plan screening and other services. STD programs should take the lead and provide this information for providers. They should develop and evaluate brief risk assessment forms for their use, and, if possible, provide prevention case management services (see Programmatic Level "Possible Intervention Strategies," later in this chapter) through the STD clinic or assist major providers in the development and delivery of prevention case management services to

their patients with repeat infections. Prevention case management services for STD repeaters are discussed more fully below under "Prevention Case Management."

Programmatic Level

Possible Intervention Strategies

Considering the importance of repeat infection on individual health (e.g., sequelae) and community health (e.g., core groups and community transmission), it is essential for public STD programs to take the lead in addressing repeat infections from both a behavioral risk-reduction and biomedical perspective. An initial step is to assess the magnitude of repeat infections by developing routine surveillance for repeat gonorrhea, chlamydia, and syphilis infection. Given existing reportable disease surveillance systems, it should be easy to determine the overall community rates of repeat STDs and the associated demographic risk factors. A recent evaluation (6) described the various definitions and procedures that could be applied in a repeat gonorrhea surveillance system by using routine gonorrhea morbidity reports. These procedures could also be used for chlamydia as well as primary and secondary syphilis. The evaluation used a widely accepted definition of repeat gonorrhea–two or more infections more than 30 days and less than 365 days apart. Using such an approach, a nationwide epidemiologic description of persons with repeat infections can be developed.

The next step is to offer persons with repeat infection individual-level behavioral risk reduction and biomedical services to reduce the occurrence of repeat infection or to identify asymptomatic repeat infections in need of treatment that will decrease the duration of infectiousness. "Prevention case management" services can be offered to STD clinic clients, as well as to other community members with repeat infections. Private providers, clinics, managed care organizations, and university HIV treatment services can be encouraged to provide such services to their patients following STD program guidance and assistance.

Programs also should be encouraged to develop pathogen-specific repeat case interview data collection forms to further identify risky behaviors and to elicit information about partners and social/sexual networks. Programs could work in collaboration with researchers to develop the techniques for collecting network information and to evaluate network and other intervention services.

Finally, for infections that often are asymptomatic (e.g., chlamydia and some gonorrhea) rescreening programs are needed to identify persons with repeat infection and determine needed services. CDC has suggested that rescreening women several months after an initial infection may be an effective method of identifying additional morbidity (90). Additionally, Richert and colleagues (48) have proposed screening all persons with STDs within 6 months of their initial diagnosis.

Prevention case management. Since 1996, STD clinic clients in San Diego County with repeat STDs have been offered "prevention case management" services that include behavioral risk reduction counseling and a biomedical component (91). Clients with two bacterial STDs within 24 months or HIV infection and any bacterial STD are offered this service, which includes quarterly STD screening, HIV counseling and testing, STD symptom recognition education, risk-based hepatitis screening and vaccination, risk-based preventive treatment, behavioral risk-reduction counseling, and a "fast track" card for head-of-the-line privileges for subsequent STD clinic visits. Clients with concerns about what might be STD symptoms or a high-risk sexual exposure are encouraged to seek evaluation as soon as possible (using "fast track" privileges) so that diagnosis and treatment can be provided. From 1998 through 2004, approximately 210 clients were enrolled each year and 53% participated in the program to some extent (i.e., one or more visits) (91). In 2002, 150 prevention case management clients made 453 visits to the clinic. Of those who participated, 69 (46%) acquired an STD, and 13 of them were identified through screening asymptomatic clients. For those clients who reported STD symptoms, 59% sought health care within two days of symptom onset. Unfortunately, as a result of a lack of evaluation personnel, a more rigorous evaluation has not yet been performed on this service.

Conclusions: Recommendations for Practice and Future Research

Recommended Practices for Reaching This Population

STD repeaters are an important population for STD prevention and control purposes, and public health practitioners should be aware of the extent to which interventions for this population are needed. Given inconsistent research findings on behavioral risk factors for repeat infection and the importance of contextual factors, we have argued that individual-level interventions may be necessary, but such interventions are probably not sufficient to deal with this problem. It is critical that health care providers and other public health professionals receive education about the importance of repeat infection, both from an individual patient health perspective (i.e., the prevention of sequelae such as PID and tubal infertility) and from a public health perspective (i.e., repeaters may be core transmitters who play a substantial role in STD spread).

There are several steps that public health practitioners can take to start dealing with STD repeaters:

- Educate health care providers who provide services to a number of STD cases about the enormity and importance of repeat infections. These providers could be identified through notifiable disease reporting.
- Include STD repeaters in routine surveillance systems to make it easier to identify and intervene with this high-risk population. Information on methods of incorporating repeaters into surveillance systems is available (6).
- Establish prevention programs or prevention case management services for repeaters in pubic STD programs.
- Consider making STD repeaters a priority population for partner services (e.g., for gonorrhea and possibly chlamydia). If repeaters are interviewed by disease investigation specialists or other health department personnel, vital network information could be collected and used to develop appropriate interventions.

Implementation Issues: Challenges and Possible Solutions

As we have discussed, although there has been much research on STD repeaters, this research has resulted in inconsistent findings and a dearth of behavioral risk factors for repeat infection. The social context in which sexual risk behavior occurs and potential co-morbidity with psychological disorders appear to be important contributors to repeat infection. It is often very difficult to alter social environments, and psychological disorders may interfere with the success of risk reduction interventions that focus exclusively on individual behavior. Given that repeaters' needs may go beyond traditional STD care, it could be beneficial for public health practitioners to develop partnerships or collaborations with other organizations whether at the national (e.g., National Institute of Mental Health—NIMH, Substance Abuse and Mental Health Services Administration—SAMHSA) or local level (e.g., public mental health services, drug treatment programs). Although it may be difficult to forge such relationships, once established they can be extremely beneficial.

Future Research

Additional research is needed to help public health practitioners better understand the complexities associated with repeat infections and intervene with this high-risk group. We have argued that there really may be two different types of repeaters:

1. those who do *not* exhibit such typical risk behaviors as multiple sex partners but are at risk for repeat infection as a result of their sex partners' behavior, and
2. those who are likely members of core groups as a result of their own risky sexual behavior and who contribute to STD transmission.

Research is needed to confirm this hypothesis and better describe these types of repeaters. Additionally, research should focus on the characteristics and behavior of the repeaters who are likely members of an STD core group (e.g., have multiple sex partners). It would be helpful to understand more about the role that STD repeaters play in core groups and disease transmission. Information about the social and sexual networks of STD repeaters is crucial.

Finally, we desperately need to develop effective interventions at multiple levels: individual, partner, network, provider, and community (through targeted places). As stated by Brooks and colleagues (1) back in 1978, "intensive follow-up of the small number of high-risk repeaters and their contacts could result in a major reduction in the number of reported cases of gonorrhea." More recently, Rothenberg (92) has stated that "rediscovering the importance of the repeat infection is manifest." While it may not always be feasible to develop and sustain multi-level interventions, a focus on interventions beyond the individual level is essential. To date, STD repeaters have often been overlooked in terms of prevention activities; however, this population likely plays an important role in STD transmission in many communities. Although it is often difficult to determine how to allocate limited resources, intervening with this population may prove to be cost-effective.

References

1. Brooks GF, Darrow WW, Day JA. Repeated gonorrhea: an analysis of importance and risk factors. *Journal of Infectious Diseases.* 1978;137:161–169.
2. Kinghorn G, Pryce D, Morton RS. Repeated gonorrhea in Sheffield: the size of the problem, epidemiologic significance, and personal characteristics of repeaters. *Sexually Transmitted Diseases.* 1982;9:165–169.

3. Klausner JD, Barrett DC, Dithmer D, Boyer CB, Brooks GF, Bolan G. Risk factors for repeated gonococcal infections: San Francisco, 1990-1992. *Journal of Infectious Diseases*. 1998;177:1766–1769.

4. McEvoy BF, Le Furgy WG. A 13-year longitudinal analysis of risk factors and clinic visitation patterns of patients with repeated gonorrhea. *Sexually Transmitted Diseases*. 1988;15:40–44.

5. Mehta SD, Erbelding EJ, Zenilman JM, Rompalo AM. Gonorrhoea reinfection in heterosexual STD clinic attendees: longitudinal analysis of risks for first reinfection. *Sexually Transmitted Infections*. 2003;79:124–128.

6. Gunn RA, Maroufi A, Fox KK, Berman SM. Surveillance for repeat gonorrhea infection, San Diego, California, 1995-2001. *Sexually Transmitted Diseases*. 2004;31:373–379.

7. Barnett SD, Brundage JF. Incidence of recurrent diagnoses of *Chlamydia trachomatis* genital infections among male and female soldiers of the US army. *Sexually Transmitted Infections*. 2001;77:33–36.

8. Burstein GR, Zenilman JM, Gaydos CA, et al. Predictors of repeat *Chlamydia trachomatis* infections diagnosed by DNA amplification testing among inner city females. *Sexually Transmitted Infections*. 2001;77:26–32.

9. Dunne EF, Chapin JB, Reitmeijer C, et al. Repeat *Chlamydia trachomatis*: rate and predictors among males. *National STD Prevention Conference;* 2004.

10. Hillis SD, Nakashima A, Marchbanks PA, Addiss DG, Davis JP. Risk-factors for recurrent *Chlamydia-trachomatis* infections in women. *American Journal of Obstetrics and Gynecology*. 1994;170:801–806.

11. Kissinger P, Clayton JL, O'Brien ME, et al. Older partners not associated with recurrence among female teenagers infected with *Chlamydia trachomatis*. *Sexually Transmitted Diseases*. 2002;29:144–149.

12. Fortenberry JD, Brizendine EJ, Katz BP, Wools KK, Blythe MJ, Orr DP. Subsequent sexually transmitted infections among adolescent women with genital infection due to *Chlamydia trachomatis, Neisseria gonorrhoeae*, or *Trichomonas vaginalis*. *Sexually Transmitted Diseases*. 1999;26:26–32.

13. Hughes G, Brady AR, Catchpole MA, et al. Characteristics of those who repeatedly acquire sexually transmitted infections. *Sexually Transmitted Diseases*. 2001;28:379–386.

14. Lundin RS, Wright MW, Scatliff JN. Behavioral and social characteristics of the patient with repeated venereal disease and his effect on statistics on venereal diseases. *British Journal of Venereal Diseases*. 1977;53:140–144.

15. Gunn RA, Fitzgerald S, Aral SO. Sexually transmitted disease clinic clients at risk for subsequent gonorrhea and chlamydia infections: possible 'core' transmitters. *Sexually Transmitted Diseases*. 2000;27:343–349.

16. Blythe MJ, Katz BP, Batteiger BE, Ganser JA, Jones RB. Recurrent Genitourinary chlamydial infections in sexually active female adolescents. *Journal of Pediatrics*. 1992;121:487–493.

17. Chacko MR, Smith PB, McGill L. Recurrent chlamydial cervicitis in young women at a family planning clinic. *Adolescent and Pediatric Gynecology*. 1989;2:149–152.

18. Centers for Disease Control and Prevention. Sexually transmitted disease surveillance, 2003. Atlanta, GA: U.S. Department of Health and Human Services; 2004.

19. Hillis SD, Coles RB, Litchfield B, et al. Doxycycline and azithromycin for prevention of chlamydial persistence or recurrence one month after treatment in women: a use-effectiveness study in public health settings. *Sexually Transmitted Diseases*. 1998;25:5–11.

20. Thorpe EM, Stamm WE, Hook EW, et al. Chlamydial cervicitis and urethritis: single-dose treatment compared with doxycycline for seven days in community based practices. *Genitourinary Medicine*. 1996;72:93–97.

21. Richey CM, Macaluso M, Hook EW. Determinants of reinfection with *Chlamydia trachomatis. Sexually Transmitted Diseases*. 1999;26:4–11.

22. McKee KT, Jenkins PR, Garner R, et al. Features of urethritis in a cohort of male soldiers. *Clinical Infectious Diseases*. 2000;30:736–741.

23. Ellen JM, Hessol N, Kohn R, Bolan GA. An investigation of geographic clustering of repeat cases on gonorrhea and chlamydial infection in San Francisco, 1989-1993: evidence for core groups. *Journal of Infectious Diseases*. 1997;175:1519–1522.

24. Bernstein KT. Repeat sexually transmitted diseases and core transmitters. *National STD Prevention Conference;* 2004.

25. Broussard D, Leichliter JS, Evans A, Kee R, Vallury V, McFarlane M. Screening adolescents in a juvenile detention center for gonorrhea and chlamydia: prevalence and reinfection rates. *The Prison Journal*. 2002;82:8–19.

26. Eberhart M, Liddon N, Goldberg M, Leichliter JS, Asbel L. The relationship between repeat infections and behavioral risk factors and clinician counseling: findings from a Philadelphia STD clinic. *National STD Prevention Conference;* 2002.

27. Erbelding EJ. Repeat STDs: why are STD clinic patients refractory to clinic-based interventions. *National STD Prevention Conference;* 2004.

28. LaMontagne DS, Baster K, Emmett L. Determinants of chlamydia re-infection: the role of partner change and treatment. *ISSTDR;* 2005.

29. Liddon N, Eberhart M, Leichliter JS, Goldberg M, Asbel L. Repeat infections among previously undiagnosed adolescents: findings from Philadelphia STD clinic records. *National STD Prevention Conference;* 2004.

30. McGhan C. Repeated acquisition of sexually transmitted infections: Feelings, perceptions, and explanations of adolescent girls. Dissertation. University of Florida; 2005.

31. Oh MK, Cloud GA, Fleenor M, Sturdevant MS, Nesmith JD, Feinstein RA. Risk for gonococcal and chlamydial cervicitis in adolescent females: Incidence and recurrence in a prospective cohort study. *Journal of Adolescent Health*. 1996;18:270–275.

32. Xu FJ, Schillinger JA, Markowitz LE, Sternberg MR, Aubin MR, Louis MES. Repeat *Chlamydia trachomatis* infection in women: analysis through a surveillance case registry in Washington State, 1993-1998. *American Journal of Epidemiology*. 2000;152:1164–1170.

33. Hillis SD, Owens LM, Marchbanks PA, Amsterdam LE, Kenzie M. Recurrent chlamydial infections increase the risks of hospitalization for ectopic pregnancy and pelvic inflammatory disease. *American Journal of Obstetrics and Gynecology*. 1997;176:103–107.

34. Kerani R, Whittington WLH, Holmes KK. Gonococcal reinfection in an urban population. *ISSTDR;* 2005.

35. Bjekic M, Vlajinac H, Marinkovic J. Behavioural and social characteristics of subjects with repeated sexually transmitted diseases. *Acta Derma Venereol*. 2000;80:44–47.

36. Westrom L, Eschenbach D. Pelvic inflammatory disease. In: Holmes KK, Sparling PF, Mardh P., Lemon SM, Stamm WE, Piot P, et al., eds. *Sexually Transmitted Diseases* 3rd ed. New York: McGraw-Hill; 1999;783–809.

37. Brunham RC, Binns B, McDowell J, Paraskevas M. *Chlamydia trachomatis* infection in women with ectopic pregnancy. *Obstetrics and Gynecology*. 1986;67:722–726.

38. Brunham RC, Peeling R, Maclean I, Kosseim ML, Paraskevas M. *Chlamydia trachomatis*-associated ectopic pregnancy: serologic and histologic correlates. *Journal of Infectious Diseases*. 1992;165:1076–1081.

39. Svensson L, Mardh P, Ahlgren M, Nordenskjold F. Ectopic pregnancy and antibodies to *Chlamydia trachomatis. Fertility and Sterility*. 1985;44:313–317.

40. Stamm WE. *Chlamydia trachomatis* infections: progress and problems. *Journal of Infectious Diseases.* 1999;179(Suppl 2):S380–S383.

41. Rein DB, Kassler WJ, Irwin KL, Rabiee L. Direct medical cost of pelvic inflammatory disease and its sequelae: decreasing, but still substantial. *Obstetrics and Gynecology.* 2000;95:397–402.

42. Washington AE, Katz P. Cost of and payment source for pelvic inflammatory disease: trends and projections, 1983 through 2000. *JAMA.* 1991;266:2565–2569.

43. Rein DB, Gift TL. A refined estimate of the lifetime cost of pelvic inflammatory disease (letter). *Sexually Transmitted Diseases.* 2004;(5):325.

44. Yeh JM, Hook EW, Goldie SJ. A refined estimate of the average lifetime cost of pelvic inflammatory disease. *Sexually Transmitted Diseases.* 2003;30:369–378.

45. Aral SO, Wasserheit JN. Social and behavioral correlates of pelvic inflammatory disease. *Sexually Transmitted Diseases.* 1998;25:378–385.

46. Beller M, Middaugh J, Gellin B, Ingle D. The contribution of reinfection to gonorrhea incidence in Alaska, 1983 to 1987. *Sexually Transmitted Diseases.* 1992;(1):41–46.

47. Sherrard J, Barlow D. Men with repeated episodes of gonorrhoea 1990-1992. *International Journal of STD & AIDS.* 1996;7:281–283.

48. Richert CA, Peterman TA, Zaidi AA, Ransom RL, Wroten JE, Witte JJ. A method for identifying persons at high risk for sexually transmitted infections: opportunity for targeting intervention. *American Journal of Public Health.* 1993;83:520–524.

49. Yorke JA, Hethcote HW, Nold A. Dynamics and control of the transmission of gonorrhea. *Sexually Transmitted Diseases.* 1978;5:51–56.

50. Thomas JC, Tucker MJ. The development and use of the concept of a sexually transmitted disease core. *Journal of Infectious Diseases.* 1996;174(Suppl 2):S134–S143.

51. Brunham RC, Plummer FA. A general model of sexually transmitted disease epidemiology and its implications for control. *Medical Clinics of North America* 1990;74:1339–1352.

52. Thomas JC, Weiner DH, Schoenbach VJ, Earp JA. Frequent re-infection in a community with hyperendemic gonorrhoea and chlamydia: appropriate clinical actions. *International Journal of STD & AIDS.* 2000;11:461–467.

53. Wagstaff DA, Delamater JD, Havens KK. Subsequent infection among adolescent African-American males attending a sexually transmitted disease clinic. *Journal of Adolescent Health* 1999;25:217–226.

54. Peterman TA, Lin LS, Newman DR, et al. Does measured behavior reflect STD risk? An analysis of data from a randomized controlled behavioral intervention study. *Sexually Transmitted Diseases.* 2000;27:446–451.

55. Whittington WLH, Kent C, Kissinger P, et al. Determinants of persistent and recurrent *Chlamydia trachomatis* infection in young women—Results of a multi-center cohort study. *Sexually Transmitted Diseases.* 2001;28:117–123.

56. McKee KT, Jenkins PR, Garner R, et al. Features of urethritis in a cohort of male soldiers. *Clinical Infectious Diseases.* 2000;30:736–741.

57. Bjekic M, Lecic-Tosevski D, Vlajinac H, Marinkovic J. Personality dimensions of sexually transmitted disease repeaters assessed with the Millon Clinical Multiaxial Inventory. *Journal of the European Academy of Dermatology and Venereology.* 2002;16:63–65.

58. Nuwaha F. Risk factors for recurrent sexually transmitted infections in Uganda. *East African Medical Journal.* 2000;77:138–142.

59. Pitts M, Bowman M, McMaster J. Reactions to repeated STD infections: psychosocial aspects and gender issues in Zimbabwe. *Social Science & Medicine.* 1995;40:1299–1304.

60. Burstein GR, Gaydos CA, Diener-West M, Howell MR, Zenilman JM, Quinn TC. Incident *Chlamydia trachomatis* infections among inner-city adolescent females. *JAMA.* 1998;280:521–526.

61. Batteiger BE, Fraiz J, Newhall WJ, Katz BP, Jones RB. Association of recurrent chlamydial infection with gonorrhea. *Journal of Infectious Diseases.* 1989;159:661–669.

62. Rietmeijer CA, Van Bemmelen R, Judson FN, Douglas JM. Incidence and repeat infection rates of *Chlamydia trachomatis* among male and female patients in an STD clinic—implications for screening and rescreening. *Sexually Transmitted Diseases.* 2002;29:65–72.

63. Orr DP, Johnston K, Brizendine E, Katz B, Fortenberry JD. Subsequent sexually transmitted infection in urban adolescents and young adults. *Archives of Pediatrics & Adolescent Medicine.* 2001;155:947–953.

64. Bjekic M, Vlajinac H, Sipetic S, Marinkovic J. Risk factors for gonorrhea: case-control study. *Genitourinary Medicine.* 1997;73:518–521.

65. Rubertone MV, Krauss MR. Behavioral risk factors and other predictors of repeated urethritis in a sexually transmitted disease clinic. *International Conference on AIDS;* 1993.

66. Crosby R, Leichliter JS, Brackbill R. Longitudinal prediction of sexually transmitted diseases among adolescents: Results from a national survey. *American Journal of Preventive Medicine.* 2000;18:312–316.

67. McKee KT, Jenkins PR, Garner R, et al. Features of urethritis in a cohort of male soldiers. *Clinical Infectious Diseases.* 2000;30:736–741.

68. Adimora AA, Schoenbach VJ. Social context, sexual networks, and racial disparities in rates of sexually transmitted. *Journal of Infectious Diseases.* 2005;191(Suppl 1):S115–S122.

69. Jackson-Walker S, Nitz K. Depression and behavior problems in urban adolescents: risk factors for recurrent sexually transmitted diseases? *Journal of Adolescent Health.* 1996;18:117.

70. Leichliter JS, Esterberg ML, Leonard L, Erbelding EJ. Repeat bacterial STDs among adults in Baltimore: a qualitative exploration of the context of sexual risk behaviors. 2005. (Unpublished manuscript).

71. McGhan C. Repeated acquisition of sexually transmitted infections: Feelings, perceptions, and explanations of adolescent girls. Dissertation, University of Florida, 2005.

72. Blythe MJ, Fortenberry JD, Orr DP. Child sexual abuse does not increase risk for recurrent sexually transmitted infections among high risk adolescent females. *Journal of Adolescent Health.* 1996;18:147.

73. Chacko MR, Smith PB, Kozinetz CA. Understanding partner notification (patient self-referral method) by young women. *Journal of Pediatric Adolescent Gynecology.* 2000;13:27–32.

74. Fortenberry JD, Brizendine EJ, Katz BP, Orr DP. The role of self-efficacy and relationship quality in partner notification by adolescents with sexually transmitted infections. *Archives of Pediatrics & Adolescent Medicine.* 2002;156: 1133–1137.

75. Golden MR, Whittington WLH, Handsfield HH, et al. Partner management for gonococcal and chlamydial infection: expansion of public health services to the private sector and expedited sex partner treatment through a partnership with commercial pharmacies. *New England Journal of Medicine.* 2005;352:676–685.

76. Kissinger P, Mohammed H, Richardson-Alston G, et al. Patient-delivered partner treatment for male urethritis: a randomized, controlled trial. *Clinical Infectious Diseases.* 2005;41:623–629.

77. Potterat JJ, Rothenberg RB. The case-finding effectiveness of self-referral system for gonorrhea: a preliminary report. *American Journal of Public Health.* 1977;67:174–176.

78. van de Laar MJ, Termorshuizen F, van den Hoek A. Partner referral by patients with gonorrhea and chlamydial infections. Case-finding observations. *Sexually Transmitted Diseases.* 1997;24:334–342.

79. Woodhouse DE, Potterat JJ, Muth JB, Pratts CI, Rothenberg RB, Fogle JS. A civilian-military partnership to reduce the incidence of gonorrhea. *Public Health Reports.* 1985;100:61–65.
80. Potterat JJ, Rothenberg RB, Woodhouse DE, Muth JB, Pratts CI, Fogle JS. Gonorrhea as a social disease. *Sexually Transmitted Diseases.* 1985;12:25–32.
81. Laumann EO, Youm Y. Racial/ethnic group differences in the prevalence of sexually transmitted diseases in the United States: a network explanation. *Sexually Transmitted Diseases.* 1999;26:250–261.
82. Aral SO, Hughes JP, Stoner B, et al. Sexual mixing patterns in the spread of gonococcal and chlamydial infections. *American Journal of Public Health.* 1999;89:825–833.
83. Ellen JM, Gaydos CA, Chung M, Willard N, Reitmeijer CA. Changes in sex networks and repeat STDS among male adolescents and young adults. Oral Presentation at 2004, National STD Prevention Conference. March 8–11, 2004, Philadelphia, PA.
84. Bernstein KT, Curriero FC, Jennings JM, Olthoff G, Erbelding EJ, Zenilman JM. Defining core gonorrhea transmission utilizing spatial data. *American Journal of Epidemiology.* 2004;160:5158.
85. Mosher WD, Chandra A, Jones J. Sexual behavior and selected health measures: Men and women 15-44 years of age, United States, 2002. Hyattsville, MD: National Center for Health Statistics; 2005. Advance data from vital and health statistics; Report No 362.
86. Ellen JM, Brown BA, Chung S, et al. Impact of sexual networks on risk for gonorrhea and chlamydia among low-income urban African American adolescents. *Journal of Pediatrics.* 2005;146:518–522.
87. Fichtenberg CM, Ellen JM. Moving from core groups to risk spaces. *Sexually Transmitted Diseases.* 2003;30:825–826.
88. Michaud JM, Ellen JM, Johnson SM, Rompalo AM. Responding to a community outbreak of syphilis by targeting sex partner meeting location: an example of a risk-space intervention. *Sexually Transmitted Diseases.* 2003;30:533–538.
89. Weir SS, Pailman C, Mahlalela X, Coetzee N, Meidany F, Boerma JT. From people to places: focusing AIDS prevention efforts where it matters most. *AIDS.* 2003;17:895–903.
90. Centers for Disease Control and Prevention. 1998 Guidelines for treatment of sexually transmitted diseases. 1998. Report No.: 47.
91. Gunn RA. Prevention case management for STD repeaters. 2005. Unpublished data.
92. Rothenberg RB. Recidivism redux. *Sexually Transmitted Diseases.* 2000;27:350–352.

16

Looking Inside and Affecting the Outside: Corrections-Based Interventions for STD Prevention

Samantha P. Williams, Ph.D., and Richard H. Kahn, M.S.

Injustice anywhere is a threat to justice everywhere. We are caught in an inescapable network of mutuality, tied in a single garment of destiny. Whatever affects one directly, affects all indirectly.

—Rev. Dr. Martin Luther King, Jr.

Liberty is to the collective body, what health is to every individual body. Without health no pleasure can be tasted by man; without liberty, no happiness can be enjoyed by society.

—Thomas Jefferson

In the United States, there are approximately 2.2 million adults housed in correctional facilities (1). Approximately 6.9 million, or 3.2% of the U.S. population, are under some form of correctional supervision (i.e., prison[1], jail[2], on probation[3] or parole[4]) (2,3). The number of U.S. citizens incarcerated has continued to increase since 1980. The number of U.S. inmates in prisons, jails, and on parole has more than tripled (2–4). The number of U.S. persons on probation has more than quadrupled from 1,118,097 in 1980 to over 4.1 million in 2004 (4). Many states are now spending almost as much money on building correctional institutions as is spent on building and maintaining institutions of learning (5–7), which has had its most profound effect on educational achievement among ethnic minorities and those with lower socioeconomic backgrounds (8).

---

[1] Confinement in a state or federal correctional facility to serve a sentence of more than one year. In some jurisdictions, the length of sentence which results in prison confinement is usually longer than one year.

[2] Confinement in a local correctional facility while pending trial, awaiting sentencing, serving a sentence that is usually less than one year, or awaiting transfer to another facility after conviction.

[3] Court-ordered community supervision of convicted offenders by a probation agency. In many instances, the supervision requires adherence to specific rules of conduct while in the community.

[4] Community supervision after a period of incarceration. Community supervision includes active or inactive supervision, or some other form of conditional release, such a mandatory release, following a term of incarceration.

Behavioral Interventions for Prevention and Control of Sexually Transmitted Diseases. Aral SO, Douglas JM Jr, eds. Lipshutz JA, assoc ed. New York: Springer Science+ Business Media, LLC; 2007.

Increased populations are disproportionately undereducated and minority. Over two-thirds (68%) of state prison inmates did not receive a high school diploma (9). Black and Hispanic males have a 1 in 4 and 1 in 6, respectively, lifetime chance of being incarcerated, which is considerably higher than white males, who have a 1 in 23 chance (10). Incarcerated individuals and those with incarceration histories are disproportionately affected by substance use and abuse, have higher rates of behavioral risk, and high prevalence of health challenges (11). The considerable prevalence of STDs/HIV in communities co-affected by high rates of incarceration (and the associated factors) is indicative of a failed societal effort to devise healthy communities and inhibit criminogenic motivations, as well as a failed public health effort to facilitate health care access and acquisition of optimal health.

In the United States, there is considerable mobility of individuals between corrections facilities and communities. Prisons hold the largest proportion of inmates at any given time, but jails have the highest rate of recidivism. Long-term prison incarceration may increase an inmate's risk of HIV exposure. However, with an estimated 15 million cases STDs (12), the almost 10-fold national prevalence of STDs in the general population, as compared with HIV, combined with the overlapping associative factors between incarceration and sexual risk, translates into an increase risk of STDs—simply because a person was arrested. In essence, incarceration and STD infection, for many, are kindred consequences resulting from challenged experiences and/or environments. Finding a history of one is strongly tied to having a history of the other; and a review of STD-focused behavioral interventions would be inadequate without a discussion on how STD prevention can be accomplished, via behavioral change, in correctional settings.

In this chapter, we will focus on the behavioral interventions directed at the prevention of STDs among correctional populations[5]. We will include a discussion of the contextual and criminogenic factors associated with incarceration, the consequential effects of such imprisonment on the individual, as well as an overview of the burden of STDs in the corrections populations. In the latter portion of the chapter, examples of behavioral interventions implemented in diverse venues, with diverse correctional populations will be described and the implications discussed.

STD Epidemiology and Burden in Corrections

In 1997, the Institute of Medicine called for expanded STD services for disadvantaged populations (13). The Institute recommended that detention facilities[6] provide comprehensive STD-related services, including counseling and education, screening, diagnosis and treatment, partner notification and treatment, as well as methods for reducing unprotected sex and drug use. This recommendation was reinforced by earlier (14) and subsequent publications (15), which illustrated the importance of early detection and treatment of

---

[5] A term used to refer to multiple populations within and released from confinement. The term is inclusive of those incarcerated in jail, prisons, and detention centers, as well as those released from the aforementioned facilities that are still under correctional supervision (i.e., parolees and probationers).

[6] Confinement in a minimum to moderate security setting, most often for juveniles; such facilities can also house adult offenders who have first and or minor offences.

STDs to HIV prevention efforts. Correctional settings have an opportunity to provide such services because they serve large populations of high-risk persons who have higher rates of substance abuse and risk behaviors, such as intravenous drug use and involvement in the commercial sex trade. These behaviors and high-risk lifestyles increase the prevalence of infectious diseases such as HIV/AIDS, tuberculosis, STDs, and hepatitis among inmates and those formerly detained (16–18).

STD Screening Guidelines

Standards for medical care in corrections facilities include laboratory or diagnostic tests to detect communicable diseases, including STDs, as part of the health assessment within 14 days of admission in jails (19) and within seven days in prisons and juvenile facilities (20,21). Not all facilities, however, routinely screen for STDs. In many facilities, the majority of inmates are released before getting a complete medical evaluation, and therefore, are not tested for STDs (22), or inmates are tested, but are released before they can be adequately treated according to CDC STD Treatment Guidelines (23).

Most facilities performing STD tests use results to diagnose and treat infections but do not routinely assess the burden of disease in their population. However, the prevalence of STDs in this population has been described in a variety of studies (24–27). These studies have shown a high prevalence of various bacterial STDs in people entering selected corrections facilities. However, limited data exist on the extent of viral STDs, with the exception of HIV and hepatitis B, which are common in many incarcerated populations (28).

Chlamydia and Gonorrhea

Although multiple studies and surveillance projects have found a high prevalence of STDs in persons entering jails and juvenile corrections facilities, the burden of disease for chlamydia and gonorrhea in the United States is highest for women aged 15 to 19 (29). Incarcerated adolescents are more likely than nonincarcerated adolescents to engage in substance abuse, come from racial or ethnic minority backgrounds and engage in risky behaviors such as unprotected sex and are therefore at high risk of chlamydial and gonococcal infection (30).

Gonococcal and chlamydial infections are fairly common in youth, particularly adolescents admitted to juvenile facilities (31). The reported prevalence of chlamydia ranges from 14% to 20% in female adolescent detainees (32–34) and 7% to 12% in male adolescent detainees (34–36). Among adolescent females entering 56 juvenile corrections facilities, the median facility positivity for chlamydia was 14.0% (range, 2.4% to 26.5%). In contrast, the median facility positivity for chlamydia was 7.2% (range, 1.2% to 22.7%) in adult females entering 32 corrections facilities. The median chlamydia positivity in adolescent males entering 81 juvenile corrections facilities was 5.8% (range, 1.0% to 27.5%). In contrast, the median Chlamydia positivity for adult males entering 35 corrections facilities positivity was 10.2% (range, 0.7% to 30.0%) (29). Two published studies assessed behavioral factors related to chlamydial infection in incarcerated adolescents. One study found that family structure (i.e., living with stepfamily) was associated with increased risk of infection (37). The other study found a weak association between chlamydia infection and exchanging sex for money and witnessing violence (38).

The median positivity for gonorrhea in adolescent females entering 34 juvenile corrections facilities was 4.5% (range, 0% to 16.6%), which is slightly higher than the median positivity for gonorrhea in adult females entering 26 corrections facilities (3.0%; range, 0% to 8.4%) (29). In contrast, the median positivity for gonorrhea in adolescent males entering 49 juvenile corrections facilities was 0.8% (range, 0% to 18.2%), and 2.6% (range, 0% to 33.8%) for adult males entering 27 facilities (29).

Syphilis

High rates of syphilis are not unexpected in corrections facilities, particularly adult facilities. In general, syphilis is more prevalent among incarcerated women (5.3%; range, 0% to 19%) than men (2.7%; range, 0.2% to 5.9%), and more prevalent in persons admitted to jails than juvenile facilities (29). In the United States, from 1999 to 2002, there were 7725 early syphilis cases reported from corrections facilities; this represents 12.5% of all such cases reported nationally (39). Some of the highest syphilis prevalence has been reported from New York City among men who have sex with men (40), and among women where 26% of female inmates tested upon admission had indications for syphilis treatment (41). Syphilis prevalence rates are often associated with drug use and prostitution (42). Lower rates of 2% to 10% have been reported for men entering jails (24,25). Studies in juvenile facilities show syphilis prevalence of less than 1% in boys and 0% to 2.5% in girls (43,32,35).

Hepatitis

Incarcerated persons have a high prevalence of infection with hepatitis viruses (18,28). It is estimated that 12% to 39% of all Americans with chronic hepatitis B virus (HBV) or hepatitis C virus (HCV) infections were releasees from a corrections facility during the previous year (18). One study found a HCV prevalence rate of 29.7% and a HBV prevalence rate of 25.2% among those entering the Maryland Division of Correction and the Baltimore City Detention Center (44). Interestingly, more jail detainees were infected with HCV than were prison inmates (31.1% vs. 26.4%, respectively), and the number of jail detainees ever infected with HBV was almost double that of prison inmates (29.9% vs. 16.4%). Behavioral and sexual risk factors and neighborhood socioeconomic characteristics (e.g., high poverty, unemployment) contribute to significantly higher rates of HBV in the incarcerated. However, the cycling of jail inmates between corrections facilities, their communities and sexual networks, combined with the possibility of high community prevalence of hepatitis infection, may explain the significant difference between the rates of HBV and HCV in jail detainees and prison inmates.

In response to the growing HBV burden on the health of correctional populations, the CDC publishes specific guidelines on the prevention and control of hepatitis infections in corrections settings (18). The CDC recommends that all juveniles and adults receiving a medical evaluation in a correctional facility be administered the HBV vaccine, unless they have proof of completion of the vaccine series or serologic evidence of immunity to infection. Although routine testing of juveniles for markers of HBV infection is not recommended nor is routine testing for HCV antibodies (anti-HCV), juveniles and adults with signs or symptoms indicative of viral hepatitis should have appropriate diagnostic testing. Given the higher prevalence of hepatitis infection within adult corrections facilities, routine testing of long-term inmates for chronic HBV infection is recommended to facilitate vaccination of contacts, implement risk-reduction counseling, and ensure medical evaluation of infected persons (18). In addition, adult inmates should be asked questions regarding risk factors for HCV infection at the time of their medical evaluation, and inmates reporting risk factors for HCV infection should be tested for anti-HCV. Adults and juveniles with signs or symptoms indicative of viral hepatitis should have appropriate diagnostic testing (18).

STDs and Arrest Charge

Very little information exists about the relationship between arrest code and disease. In Fulton County, Georgia, a study found a very high prevalence of gonorrhea in women (20%) and men (15%) arrested for sexual offences (45). In Connecticut, women arrested for drug possession and prostitution had a high prevalence of syphilis, 7% and 14%, respectively (42). In both of these settings, however, the prevalence in women arrested for other crimes was not reported. In Baton Rouge, Louisiana, women arrested for prostitution were seven times more likely (odds ratio [OR], 7.0; 95% confidence interval [CI], 1.5, 39.3) to have syphilis infection than women arrested for other reasons and men arrested for felony theft were over four times more likely (OR, 4.8; 95% CI, 1.8, 13.8) to have syphilis than men arrested for other reasons (27). In Los Angeles, there was no significant association between booking charge and syphilis infection in men (46).

STD Incidence in Correction Facilities

The incidence of STDs acquired within corrections facilities is unknown. However, syphilis outbreaks in corrections populations have occurred (47–49) and there is evidence of the association between risk behaviors and prevalence of chlamydia in juvenile detention facilities (48). Transmission of gonorrhea in detention centers has also been reported (50). The high prevalence of specific STDs such as chlamydia and gonorrhea contributes to the question of the cost-benefits of universal screening in U.S. jails (51). Although sexual activity is prohibited in corrections facilities in the United States, it does take place, and transmission of STDs and subsequent outbreaks are possible and likely to repeatedly occur.

STD Screening in Corrections Facilities

Considering the high prevalence of STDs in persons admitted to corrections facilities, testing and treatment is important for protecting the inmates, their babies, their sex partners, and the rest of the community. Detection and treatment of infection can prevent long-term sequelae, which are harmful for the patient and costly to society. Given the asymptomatic nature of many infections, especially in women, many persons will not seek care for STDs. In addition, many incarcerated persons do not have a regular source of medical care in the community, so the corrections facility may be the only point at which they can be tested and treated.

Inmates who are infected at the time of admission may transmit disease to others in the community upon release if not treated. Identification and treatment of cases in detention facilities should prevent future transmission of STDs. In a recent study (52), the effect of male jail screening on female chlamydia rates was examined. The investigators found that a high proportion of males screened in the jails were from neighborhoods that had high female chlamydia rates. Female chlamydia rates at a health center that served the neighborhood showed a 50% decrease from 8.2% to 4.4% since the inception of the jail screening program (1997 to 2002). An analysis of syphilis case detection methods in two cities with high rates of heterosexual syphilis found that while private physicians identified the largest number of cases in females, jail screening was the most productive case detection strategy for identifying high-risk females that were likely to transmit disease (53). Identifying inmates with STDs should also help to identify cases in the community if infected inmates are interviewed about their recent sex partners and the partners are evaluated. Women entering corrections facilities often have high rates of pregnancy, and they could transmit STD infection to their newborn.

Public Health and Public Safety: Competing Priorities

The corrections environment present many obstacles to screening for STDs. Obviously, the primary purpose of corrections facilities is incarceration; and the first obstacle to screening is the viewpoint that screening for STDs is unnecessary. The responsibility of the corrections authority to screen for certain communicable diseases such as tuberculosis is more easily understood than the necessity of screening for STDs. Some local laws require screening for STDs, especially syphilis, as part of intake screening. Successful STD screening is best accomplished when it is integrated into the intake process, thus interrupting the cycle of disease transmission. In local jurisdictions where the law does not require screening, corrections officials may be reluctant to participate in such a program. In areas of high incidence and prevalence of STDs, however, corrections officials have the responsibility and opportunity to contribute to reducing the spread of STDs. When an STD is identified, treatment protocols and reporting to the appropriate local public health departments should ensue.

It is important to note, however, that screening for STDs is different in jails and prisons; therefore, health care administrators and public health officials must strategically adapt STD screening programs to the specific corrections environment. In prisons, the rate of admission is generally low compared with that in jails. Prison intake areas are often housing units where inmates reside for days to weeks until all intake screening is accomplished. This permits most medical evaluations to be conducted and allows sufficient time to provide treatment and contact tracing for those inmates with STDs. The situation is different in jails where large numbers of inmates are admitted. Several hundred inmates may be admitted each day to large urban jails. Because of the large number of daily intakes and the short length of stay, there is usually not a single designated housing area for new inmates. In addition, it is often necessary to recall patients for treatment after the initial intake screening. In short, the abbreviated nature of the jail intake process and the number of daily jail discharges (which is significantly higher than that of prisons) makes complete assessment and treatment more difficult.

Screening for STDs involves multiple activities, including performing a screening test, and interpretation of test results. Collaborative relationships with local health departments accomplish follow-up of positive test results, treatment, contact tracing, and post-treatment testing.

Behavioral Risk and STDs in Corrections Populations

The greatest challenges to quelling the prevalence and incidence of STDs among incarcerated persons are the behaviors and social contexts that contribute to both incarceration and STD risk. Many people under correctional supervision were arrested in, and return to, urban low-income neighborhoods with significant social and educational challenges such as high rates of drug commerce, commercial sex work, and under-funded and/or over-crowded schools (54). Sexual risk factors most often associated with STD risk and incarceration include episodes of non-use of condoms while incarcerated (55), as well as prior to and after incarceration (56–58); exchange of sex for drugs, money, or both (59,60); multiple, concurrent, and new partners (59,60); sex with men who have sex with men (61–63); and sex with a partner who has one of the aforementioned risk factors (64). Other risk factors for both STDs and incarceration include drug use (18,65,66); STD history and co-infections (58,67), and an incarceration history (22,68, 69).

Risk Factors and Detained Youth

Most of the aforementioned risk factors also affect adolescent detainees who have considerable physical and emotional morbidity (70). Approximately 5.5% of youth 10 years and older are referred to juvenile court; most are male and ethnic minority. Findings from a study that used the Child Health Illness Profile, Adolescent Edition (CHIP-AE), a self-administered tool for assessing the health and well-being of the young, found that when compared with a group of males in school, detained young males report a poorer health status, and were more likely to live at or below the poverty level. The detained youth also reported more sexual activity, drug and alcohol use, and problem behaviors in school, as well as poorer academic performance, interpersonal skills, and less family involvement (71). In a similar study that examined the health status of both male and female ($n = 350$) offenders and their families, the author found that over 90% of the sample reported levels of physical and emotional discomfort. Over half of the young people (53%) had been abused, been physically injured (20%), or sustained a gunshot or stab wound (16%). It was further noted that family members, including the siblings of incarcerated young people, experienced similar health problems and criminogenic behaviors (72).

Risk, STDs, and Detained Youth

STDs such as, chlamydia and gonorrhea have long-term health consequences for adolescent girls including: pelvic inflammatory disease, infertility, ectopic pregnancy and chronic pelvic pain (73). Detained young people, however, have a higher risk of STDs. One study found a median chlamydia prevalence rate of 15.6% in girls and 7.6% in boys upon entry into corrections facilities (24). In a recently published STD prevalence report of youth in corrections facilities, 15.6% and 5.1% of more than 33,000 young females, and 5.9% and 1.3% of 98,296 young males tested positive for chlamydia and gonorrhea, respectively. Half of both the young females and males with gonorrhea were co-infected with chlamydia (34).

The prevalence of HCV is also higher for detained juveniles than those in the general population (74). A recent study that examined the prevalence of

HCV and risk factors of detained juveniles found that the mean age of sexual debut was less than 13 years for both males and females, more than 45% of the youth had a history of five or more partners, and 18% had a previous STD diagnosis (74).

STD Prevention Behavioral Interventions for Corrections Populations

Evidence regarding increased risk of STD acquisition prior to and following incarceration is considerable, but behavioral intervention efforts that focus on correctional populations, particularly those that are supervised outside correctional facilities, but not detained are limited (68). In one qualitative study that examined the sexual behaviors of women with incarcerated partners, the authors described how institutional constraints that limit couples' contact and intimacy during the incarceration period, as well as the conditions of parole, promoted unprotected sexual intercourse and other risky behavior following release from prison (75).

The remainder of this chapter examines interventions tailored for correctional populations. First, we review the challenges to intervening with correctional populations. A discussion of different types of interventions that have been utilized with correctional populations and within corrections facilities will follow. Finally, alternative approaches and strategies for behavioral STD interventions for correctional populations will be proposed.

Intervening Within Corrections Settings: Prerelease

Inmates do not routinely receive STD information before they are released from prison, jail, or as parolees or probationers (76). Yet, corrections facilities provide an excellent opportunity to intervene in the STD acquisition and transmission cycle. For some, arrest—though an unintended event—is the only time they may encounter a system of health care. Incarceration stays can be "teaching opportunities" whereby the inmate can learn about his or her health status, including STDs/HIV infection, and possibly how to modify their own risky behavior. More importantly, intervening in the "revolving door" process between corrections institutions and communities directly affects societal health and well-being (76).

Challenges to Prerelease Interventions

Considerable challenges to implementing STD/HIV prevention interventions within corrections settings include inmate turnout (particularly in jails), perceived interference with security, staffing, and the under-acknowledgement of sexual and drug use behaviors in corrections facilities. Most states do not employ harm-reduction strategies (e.g., condom availability) in corrections facilities, nor permit condoms to be brought into or bought within corrections facilities. Condoms as well as drugs are considered contraband, yet drug use persists in jails as does consensual and nonconsensual sex.

May and Williams (77) surveyed both corrections officers and inmates who participated in a weekly health information class, in a jail where free condoms were dispensed by the facility's health educators and distributed by a local

AIDS service organization. The survey did not directly inquire about inmates' sexual behavior inside the facility, but the survey did include questions about the inmates' and officers' *perceptions* of inmates' sexual behavior. The authors found that a little over half (55%) of the inmates and about two thirds (64%) of the officers supported the availability of condoms in the jails. Over half (58%) of the inmates did not believe that the condom availability in the jail led to increased sexual activity, but the majority (89%) of the inmates did not try to gain access to the condoms. Although both inmates and officers agreed that sexual activity took place in the facility, twice as many officers believed sex occurred in the facility as compared with the inmates (53% and 26%, respectively). There were inmates and officers who did not endorse the availability of condoms in the jail, and this opinion was generalized to all corrections facilities. Specifically, they believed a policy on condom availability in the jail endorsed same sex relationships and compromised institutional and personal safety by increasing the risk of fights, bartering, contraband trafficking and rape. Given the success of condom distribution programs such as the program initiated in Canada (78), the expressed belief of both guards and inmates may appear alarmist. However, there was a documented incident in Jamaica that occurred in 1997 when a government announcement to provide condoms to inmates led to an officer strike and prison riot that resulted in six deaths (79). For this and other reasons mentioned previously, many interventions that are implemented while inmates are detained are done for the purpose of effecting post-release behavior, and are typically implemented a short time prior to release.

Interventions for Men

Men are disproportionately represented within corrections facilities, yet behavioral interventions that focus on males are limited. Grinstead and colleagues (80) tested the effectiveness of a peer-led prerelease HIV-prevention intervention designed to reduce post-release HIV risky behavior. Male prison inmates within two weeks of release were recruited to evaluate a prerelease HIV-prevention intervention. A total of 414 participants were randomly assigned to the intervention group or to a comparison group. The intervention consisted of an individual session with an inmate peer educator. Participants completed a face-to-face survey at baseline, while they were incarcerated. High rates of preincarceration risky behavior were reported. Risky behavior during incarceration was omitted. Men were followed up post-release via phone contact. Although the study had a 43% follow-up rate, results from the follow-up telephone surveys supported the effectiveness of the prerelease intervention. Participants in the intervention group were significantly more likely to use a condom the first time they had sex after release from prison and also were less likely to have used drugs, injected drugs, or shared needles in the first two weeks after release from prison.

Grinstead and colleagues (81) also designed an eight-session prerelease intervention for HIV seropositive inmates to decrease sexual and drug-related risky behavior and to increase use of community resources after release. The intervention sessions were delivered at the prison by community service providers. The researchers found that a prerelease risk-reduction intervention for HIV seropositive inmates was feasible. Results supported the effectiveness of the program in reducing sexual and drug-related behaviors and in increasing use of community resources after release. Men who received the intervention reported more use of community resources and less sexual and drug-related risky behavior in the months following release.

Another project that was implemented with men in prisons is Project START, a multi-site intervention study that targeted 18- to 29-year-old men who were being released from prison (80,82,83). The intervention was based on a prevention case management model that focused on preventing sexual and drug-related risk that could lead to HIV, STD, or hepatitis infection. The intervention strategies included harm reduction, motivational interviewing, and problem solving. A secondary goal of the intervention was to prevent re-incarceration. In addition to assessing HIV, STD, and hepatitis risk (individualized risk assessment) and developing an individualized risk-reduction plan, the intervention focused on other life issues for men leaving prison such as finding employment, successfully completing parole, and re-establishing familial and other relationships. The intervention continued for three months following release from prison. The main finding of this study was that the enhanced intervention was successful in reducing risk. Specifically, participants who received the intervention had lower rates of sexual risk 24 weeks after release and re-incarceration compared to men in the single-session intervention.

Interventions for Women

Over the past 15 years, the number of women detained has increased by more than 130%, a larger increase than that of men (84). This notable increase, combined with evidence that most female detainees have histories or incarceration, drug use, sex exchange or some combination thereof, highlights the increasing need for behavioral intervention strategies that are female focused.

An intervention (85) that focused on reduction of risk and recidivism of incarcerated women was a pre-release program called the Women's HIV/Prison Prevention Program (WHPPP). Prior to release from a state prison, women categorized as being at the highest behavioral risk for recidivism, resumed drug use, and HIV infection were assigned to the WHPPP intervention group. The intervention consisted of rapport building between the participant, a physician, and a social worker, as well as a detailed discharge plan. Although the intervention was initiated prerelease, the intervention effects were measured post-release via implementation of the discharge plan. Seventy-eight women were included in the study during a three-year data collocation period; most of the women were ethnic minorities (55%); 25–35 years of age (55%); unmarried (90%); had children (72%); and displayed a variety of HIV risk behaviors. The control group were mostly white (65%), similarly aged women incarcerated in Rhode Island. Although the study did not find a significant effect on reported risky behavior, women in the intervention group had significantly lower recidivism rates than the control group at three months (5% vs. 18.5%, $p = 0.0036$) and at 12 months (33% vs. 45%, $p = 0.06$). Given the shared criminogenic factors, the authors extend the implications of the findings by presenting recidivism as a possible marker for high-risk behavior.

One other demonstration project that is worth mentioning compared two interventions, one based on social cognitive theory and the other based on a gender and power theory (86). Ninety incarcerated women who were exposed to either intervention and given psychosocial and skill-based assessment at three time points. Both interventions produced increased self-efficacy, self-esteem, AIDS knowledge, communication and condom application skills, as well as more positive attitudes towards prevention at both post-intervention and six-month time periods among participants. An interesting difference to highlight is that women in the social cognitive theory-based intervention showed greater improvement in condom application skills, while the women in the gender and power theory-based intervention showed greater commitment to change their risky behavior. The results of the study demonstrated that brief interventions in prison settings are feasible and beneficial, but more importantly, that interventions based on different theories or approaches can yield different results while still having an effect on risky behaviors.

Interventions for Youth

Those who encounter the corrections system in their youth are significantly more likely to become inmates in adulthood. In response, more intervention efforts have targeted detained young people. One intervention program based in Indiana implemented a knowledge-based informational intervention for incarcerated youth (87). The intervention consisted of four peer-based, interactive sessions that were developed from the National Network of Runaway and Youth Services. The objectives and questionnaire were based on the AIDS Risk Reduction Model (ARRM). Analyses were based on a sample of 196 detainees who were enrolled during the first year of the program, and on comparisons between pre- and post-intervention program questionnaires. The authors found that detainees demonstrated an increase in their ability to appropriately recognize and label risky behaviors, but they shoed no evidence of significant commitment to change their risky behaviors.

One class of interventions that have had varying outcomes for incarcerated youth are parenting and family interventions. The goal of such interventions is to prevent youth risky behavior through parental and family engagement. Woolfenden and colleagues (88) conducted a review of empirical studies that utilized family and parenting interventions in the management of conduct disorder and delinquency in incarcerated youth between 10 and 17 years. The intent of the review was to determine whether the interventions were effective. Randomized controlled trials were eligible for inclusion, and needed to include at least one objective outcome measure (e.g., arrest rates) or have used a measure that had been published and validated. Two reviewers independently reviewed all eligible studies for inclusion, for an end data set of eight trials. Between the studies, 749 children and their families were randomized to receive a family and parenting intervention or to be in a control group. Juvenile participants from seven of the studies had an incarceration history. Young people in the remaining study had conduct disorders, but had not had contact with the juvenile corrections system. The reviewers found that at follow-up, family and parenting interventions significantly reduced the time spent by detained youth in institutions, a significant reduction in re-arrest risk and in the rate of subsequent arrests at 1–3 years. However, no significant difference was found for psychosocial outcomes such as family functioning and youth risk behavior. The reviewers concluded that, although the interventions may reduce recidivism among youth with conduct disorder, the results need to be interpreted with caution owing to their heterogeneity.

Family interventions are a valued means of affecting risk behavior, even when family characteristics possibly contribute to risky behaviors. One recent study sought to examine the intergenerational prevalence and effect of criminal justice involvement, substance use, and HIV/AIDS on families (89). The authors determined lifetime prevalence of criminal justice involvement (CJI), substance use (SU), and HIV/AIDS in 62 families with a member (the index case) on parole or probation for a drug offense who also was enrolled in a community support program in New York City's Lower East Side. The family maps, or "genograms," were analyzed and coded (by age, sex, and relationship to the index) to identify all significant members with histories of SU, CJI, and HIV/AIDS. Of the 62 families (592 individuals total), most had at least one other member besides the index case with a history of SU (82%) and CJI (72%). Almost half of the families have at least one member with HIV/AIDS, 16% had two or more, and 10% had three or more. Most (88%) of the family members other than the index case ($n = 105$) who reported a history of CJI had a history of substance use as well. The findings demonstrated the extent to which many families with members who are also part of the correctional population, are struggling with the burdens associated with having multiple relatives who have substance use histories, are involved in the criminal justice system, or who are living with HIV/AIDS, or some combination of these. However, the findings also illustrate the important role family-focused interventions can play in reducing the high rates of familial drug use, incarceration, and other forms of CJI and HIV/AIDS.

Intervening Postrelease

Intervening with inmates post-release is an opportunity to affect risky behavior and community health. As stated earlier, inmates do not routinely receive information regarding STD before they are released from prison, jail, or as parolees or probationers (76). Prerelease intervention efforts typically target inmates exiting prison, specifically those with chronic health illnesses such as HIV (ideally as part of a post-release aftercare program). Those exiting prison, as distinct from jail, are more likely to have been exposed to health care services such as TB and STD screening. Postrelease intervention programs do not have the same structural or legal constraints as interventions conducted within corrections facilities, but they also may not have the same attendance by or commitment from the inmates. Unless mandated as part of probation or parole, the formerly "captive audience" is free to attend or not. Also, former inmates have other "life stabilizing" or "life restructuring" concerns that they must address post-release, such as finding a job, a place to stay, and family members with whom to reconnect. It is this aforementioned drive—the drive to reestablish one's life—that may influence participation, retention, and the effectiveness of an intervention.

Interventions for Probationers and Parolees

Probationers and parolees account for the largest segment of the criminal justice population in the United States (91). Of the almost 7 million people under correctional supervision, over 70% are released and living in the community. Many, once released from correctional institutions, yet under correctional supervision, continue to have the same challenges and engage in the same behaviors that may have contributed to their prior arrest(s). One study conducted in New York City examined the HIV risk behaviors, knowledge, and prevention education experiences of probationers and parolees. The authors found that probationers and parolees have high rates of unprotected sex, and limited exposure to effective HIV education and prevention interventions (68). Given the opportunity to engage in drug use, or sexual and other risky behaviors, the importance of risk-reduction interventions designed to meet the needs of probationers and parolees is more than apparent. However, such interventions have had mixed results, and earlier studies with probationers have found little intervention effect (91).

Recent studies have reported more, though modest, success. One study examined effects of a risk-reduction intervention with a sample of probationers in Delaware. Participants were randomly assigned to either an enhanced version of National Institute on Drug Abuse (NIDA) standard HIV Intervention or a Focused Intervention based on a cognitive thought-mapping model. Participants were given questionnaires at baseline and at two follow-up periods: three and six months post-intervention. Participants were also exposed to booster sessions. At baseline, participants reported injection and other drug use, and risky sexual behaviors. Comparisons of the six-month follow-up data found significant changes in attitudes and behaviors and supported the conclusion that brief interventions can significantly affect both drug use and risky sexual behaviors. However, there were no apparent differences between the different interventions, and the authors concluded that further work was needed to determine the appropriate program components for probationers.

Coordinated Services: Discharge Planning and Case Management

Most interventions for probationers and parolees that are implemented and more consistently successful fall under the category of coordinated services. Services are either offered during incarceration for post-release service access (discharge planning), or coordinated and monitored pre- and post-release as part of health care continuity for the chronically at-risk or ill (case management), or both. The term *discharge planning* is more often applied to inmates who are released without a chronic illnesses. If the inmate is scheduled to leave the corrections facility with an illness, then the inmate is more likely to get case management. Prevalence of HIV infection and AIDS cases in inmates of corrections facilities, especially for female inmates, has driven corrections-based case management.

One such program is Maryland's Prevention Case Management (PCM) program, which provided individual or group counseling to inmates nearing release to promote changes in risk behavior. Pretest and post test surveys were used to assess perceived risk, condom attitudes and condom use self-efficacy, self-efficacy to reduce injection drug and other substance use risk, and behavioral intentions. Over a four-year period, counselors attempted to maintain client contact logs, and documented session participation by participants. Both pre- and post-intervention data were available for 745 participants; client contact logs were available for 71% of the 745. Significant, positive changes were found in participant-reported condom attitudes, self-efficacy for condom use, self-efficacy for injection drug use risk, self-efficacy for other substance use risk, and intentions to practice safer sex post-release. However, data on reported sexual risk behaviors were not available (92).

Health Link is a self-described "model" program that was designed to assist drug-using jailed women in New York City to return to their communities, reduce drug use and HIV risk behavior, and avoid re-arrest. For one year after release, the program combined discharge planning and case management and offered women who participated ($n < 700$) direct services. Community service providers that served the participants were given training, technical assistance, and financial support. Program activities for the women included empowerment groups, referrals, crisis intervention counseling, and information. Despite the extensive follow-up services offered by the Health Link programs, retention rates were below 50% at 6 months and at 35% at one-year post-release. Comparisons of women enrolled in the Health Link programs and those who were not eligible for the program were conducted to determine preliminary program efficacy. The authors found that the two groups of women did not differ in age or criminal charges, but that the women enrolled in the program had an arrest rate that was lower than the comparison group (38% vs. 59%; $p = 0.02$). Through described lessons learned, the authors concluded that empowerment approaches and community organizing strategies can play an important role in reducing recidivism and the potential for health risk (93).

A more recent examination of the Health Link program's effectiveness was conducted by Needels and colleagues (94). By the time the research examined the program, both formerly incarcerated women and young males ($n = 1400$) had been enrolled in the New York City based program. The authors investigated the program's effect on rates of drug use, HIV risk, and re-arrest. Using data from interviews and hair analysis for drug testing (hair analysis is effective at detecting drug use in the previous year versus urine screening, which tests more recent drug use), the authors measured effects during a 1-year follow-up period after clients' release from jail. Intervention participants reported increased participation in drug treatment programs and weak evidence for reduced drug use. However, reductions in re-arrest rates and sexual or other risk behaviors were not found. The authors concluded that despite the hope of finding evidence of greater success in community reintegration or improved health for the enrolled participants, a well-executed case management program may make modest differences in select outcomes of former inmates.

Housing as an Intervention

Housing is a significant concern for exiting inmates. The longer an inmate is incarcerated, the more likely they are to lose "life stabilizers" such as housing (60,95). In one study that examined the characteristics of individuals receiving cash assistance, the authors explored the link between cash subsidies and risky behavior in a sample ($n = 1156$) of homeless and marginally housed (HMH) adults living in San Francisco (96). The participants were recruited and interviewed about subsidies, shelter, jail, and drug use. The authors found that most (87%) of the sample were previously homeless; one-fifth used injectable drugs; and 14% were HIV positive. For much (60%) of the sample, their income came from subsidies. Those who received subsidies were more likely not to be living on the streets, and were less likely to report injection drug use, exchange of money for sex or drugs, or recent incarceration. The authors concluded that the subsidized assistance was associated with less risky behavior. The benefits of subsidies (entitlements), in the context of interconnected strategies such as discharge planning and case management was previous found (97), and continues to be a viable option to consider when attempting to improve the quality and efficiency of pre- and post-corrections care.

Substance Treatment Services

Substance use treatment services are another type of intervention that utilizes behavioral change models and seeks to reduce risky (including sexual risk) behaviors of the formerly incarcerated with substance use histories. An early program with behavioral intervention elements was the Multistage Therapeutic Community Treatment Program (MTCT) that was instituted in the Delaware correctional system (98). The program consisted of an in-corrections facility substance use treatment, discharge planning and post-release treatment follow-up and maintenance services. For the analysis, prerelease baseline and six-month post-release outcome data were analyzed for 457 respondents. Comparisons were made between inmates who participated in the MTCT program: 1) only while in prison; 2) only once released (aftercare); or 3) during both times (transitional). Results showed that groups 2 and 3 had significantly lower rates of drug relapse and recidivism than group 1. Differences were also found for HIV risk, but these were not as robust as those previously mentioned.

The same team of authors conducted subsequent analyses on data from the Multistage Therapeutic Community Treatment Program (MCTC) program (99). The previous evaluation demonstrated efficacy for up to three years post intervention, though strongest for inmates who participated either in the post-release program, or both the pre- and post-release segments. The focus of the subsequent analysis was on the relative effect of the within-prison, transitional, and aftercare treatment components upon criminal recidivism and relapse to illicit drug use (99). The authors concluded that the participation in each component of the MCTC program is beneficial in reducing recidivism and drug use. However, the residential transitional program that combined prerelease substance treatment and post-release services such as discharge planning (transitional group) had a more enduring effect.

A five-year follow up of inmates who participated in the MCTC program phases was conducted to examine the program's effects on drug use and employment rates (100). Men who participated in transitional treatment (TT) that combined pre- and post-release treatment and services were compared to inmates who received standard post-release correctional supervision. The transitional treatment group had higher drug abstinence rates (32.2% vs. 9.9%); longer time period between relapse (28.8 months vs. 13.2 months); and a higher rate of employment after work release ended (54.6% vs. 45.4%).

Collectively, each of the described studies and many others not presented in this brief chapter, demonstrated that sexual, drug use, and recidivism risk intervention prior to release and continuing post-release, which covers the transitional period between prison and community, has substantial and persistent benefits even for inmates with extensive criminal histories.

Conclusions

The intent of this chapter has been to examine behavioral STD/HIV prevention interventions tailored for correctional populations, and to describe a selections of those that worked. A broader question for consideration is *how* STD prevention professionals can intervene with correctional populations who may have been disadvantaged upon entry into the corrections system, and who will likely be even more disadvantaged upon release. It is not unreasonable to understand how the correctional environment, in and of itself, can change the psychology and humanity that is necessary for a released inmate to fulfill societal, judicial, and familial expectations of redemption, restitution, and reconciliation. STD risk reduction and prevention becomes two more things that the formerly detained persons are expected to accomplish, in addition to re-establishing their lives.

Suggestions for enhancing the adoption of risk-reduction behaviors of correctional populations can be numerous and would look similar to those tailored for substance users, commercial sex workers, those who simply didn't know better, or those who knew better, but chose risk and the potential consequences. Harm reduction approaches that acknowledge how repeat offenses and STD infection can be part of the process of change would be welcomed additions to the body of intervention literature that focuses on correctional populations (101). What has become clear throughout this endeavor is that interventions that address sexual risk and also speak to criminogenic factors associated with incarceration can have a longer term effect. This can be accomplished by integrating STD prevention skills training and messages into recidivism-reduction efforts, as well as by integrating "life stabilizing" issues and strategies into STD prevention interventions which target correctional populations.

What is also needed are enhanced collaborations between corrections institutions, public health institutions, and community based organizations (102—105). Such collaboration, in the form of case management and discharge planning, is more likely to occur when HIV-infected inmates are to be released. Inmates with STDs, particularly those with repeat STD histories and viral STDs, would benefit from similar collaborative efforts given the risk of reinfection (i.e., STDs, in general) and the chronic nature of viral infections (i.e., HBV, HCV, HPV, and HSV). Adequate case management requires considerable resources, which may not be cost-effective or feasible for all STD-infected inmates; therefore, the suggestion of targeting inmates with repeat infection histories and viral STDs. Collaboration between the aforementioned institutions and those that assist with social services, as well as HUD (Housing and Urban Development) would also enhance STD prevention efforts for inmates and the communities to which they return.

More facility-specific suggestions include: 1) offering STD/HIV screening at intake and prior to release from extended stays; 2) tailoring and offering brief STD prevention interventions (106) in jail settings; 3) providing, at least, a list of STD/HIV screening and treatment community resources to released inmates (this is particularly important for inmates released within 72 hours because they may not have had the opportunity to be screened or to have received their results and treatment prior to release); 4) offering STD/HIV screening and STD prevention interventions with multiple sessions to long-term jail and prison inmates during incarceration and/or immediately prior to release; 5) mandating parolees and probationers to be screened for STDs during each year of their obligation, and if available, participate in at least one STD/HIV prevention education session or intervention program; and 6) encouraging released inmates who will not be supervised, to be screened within six months to one year after release and to participate in an STD/HIV prevention education session or intervention program.

In closing, the correctional population is rapidly growing and there are segments of the population about which we know very little. Populations such as incarcerated transgenders, exiting adults who were convicted as youth, youth convicted as adults, and weekend/evening program inmates have special needs, circumstances, and mobility patterns which play an underexplored role in the STD risk landscape. Specifically, we know little about how to affect their risk of STD acquisition and transmission, while incarcerated or once released. STD prevention professionals' contribution to correctional health does not have to be limited to screening and treatment. The field of STD prevention is multidisciplinary, and the traditional track-and-treat model can be enhanced through the use of behavioral interventions and the continued integration of STD professionals' expertise. It is through this integration that we will have the greatest public health impact; in general, and in correctional health care, specifically. It is through reflection and behavior change that the STD and HIV risk of correctional populations and communities can truly be augmented.

References

1. Bureau of Justice Statistics. *Prison and Jail Inmates at Midyear 2005.* Washington, DC: U.S. Department of Justice, NCJ 213133; 2006.
2. Bureau of Justice Statistics. *Prisoners in 2004.* Washington, DC: U.S. Department of Justice, NCJ 210677; 2005.
3. Bureau of Justice Statistics. *Correctional Populations in the United States, 1997.* Washington, DC: U.S. Department of Justice, NCJ 177613; 2000.
4. Bureau of Justice Statistics. *Probation and Parole in the United States, 2004.* Washington, DC: U.S. Department of Justice, NCJ 210676; 2005.
5. Ambrosio TJ, Schiraldi V. *From Classrooms to Cell Blocks: A National Perspective.* Washington, DC: Justice Policy Institute; February 1997.
6. Ambrosio TJ, Schiraldi V. *Trading Classrooms for Cell Blocks: Destructive Policies Eroding D.C. Communities.* Washington, DC: Justice Policy Institute, February 1997.
7. Connolly K, McDermid L, Schiraldi V, Macallair D. *From Classroom to Cell Blocks: How Prison Building Affects Higher Education and African American Enrollment in California.* Washington, DC: Center on Juvenile and Criminal Justice, Justice Policy Institute. 1996. Available at: http://eric.ed.gov/ERICDocs/data/ericdocs2/content_storage_01/0000000b/80/23/58/af.pdf
8. McDermid L, Schiraldi V, Macallair D. *From Classrooms to Cell Blacks: How Prison Building Affects Higher Education and African American Enrollment.* San Francisco, CA: Center on Juvenile and Criminal Justice; 1996.
9. Bureau of Justice Statistics. *Education and Correctional Populations.* Washington, DC: U.S. Department of Justice, NCJ 195670; 2003.

10. Bureau of Justice Statistics. *Lifetime Likelihood of Going to State or Federal Prison*. Washington, DC: U.S. Department of Justice, NCJ 160092; 1997.
11. Prison health: a threat or an opportunity. *Lancet*. 2005;366:1.
12. Cates W. Estimates of the incidence and prevalence of STDs in the United States: American Social Health Association Panel. *Sexually Transmitted Disease*. 1999;26(4 suppl):S2–S7.
13. Institute of Medicine. *The Hidden Epidemic: Confronting Sexually Transmitted Diseases*. Washington, DC: National Academy Press; 1997.
14. Wasserheit JN. Epidemiological synergy: Interrelationships between human immunodeficiency virus infection and other sexually transmitted diseases. *Sexually Transmitted Diseases*. 1992;19:61–77.
15. Centers for Disease Control and Prevention. HIV prevention through early detection and treatment of other sexually transmitted diseases–United States recommendations of the advisory committee for HIV and STD prevention. *MMWR*. 1998;47(RR-12):1–24.
16. Centers for Disease Control and Prevention. Syphilis screening among women arrestees at the Cook County Jail–Chicago, 1996. *MMWR*. 1998;47:432–433.
17. National Commission on Correctional Health Care. *The Health Status of Soon-To-Be-Released Inmates: A Report to Congress, Vol. 1*. Chicago: National Commission on Correctional Health Care; March 2002. Available at: http://www.ncchc.org/pubs/pubs_stbr.vol1.html
18. Centers for Disease Control and Prevention. Prevention and control of infections with hepatitis viruses in correctional settings. *MMWR*. 2003; 52(RR-1):1–27.
19. National Commission on Correctional Health Care. *Standards for Health Services in Jails*. Chicago: National Commission on Correctional Health Care; 2003.
20. National Commission on Correctional Health Care. *Standards for Health Services in Prisons*. Chicago: National Commission on Correctional Health Care; 2003.
21. National Commission on Correctional Health Care. *Standards for Health Services in Juvenile Detention and Confinement Facilities*. Chicago: National Commission on Correctional Health Care; 2004.
22. Parece MS, Herrera GA, Voigt RF, Middlekauff SL, Irwin KL. STD testing policies and practices in U.S. city and county jails. *Sexually Transmitted Diseases*. 1999;26:431–437.
23. Centers for Disease Control and Prevention. Guidelines for treatment of sexually transmitted diseases. *MMWR*. 2006;55(RR-11):1–94.
24. Mertz KJ, Voigt RA, Hutchins K, Levine WC; Jail STD Prevalence Monitoring Group. Findings from STD screening of adolescents and adults entering corrections facilities. Implications for STD control strategies. *Sexually Transmitted Diseases*. 2002;29:834–839.
25. Heimberger TS, Chang HG, Birkhead GS, et al. High prevalence of syphilis detected through a jail screening program. A potential public health measure to address the syphilis epidemic. *Archives of Internal Medicine*. 1993;153: 1799–1804.
26. Mertz KJ, Schwebke JR, Gaydos CA, Beideinger HA, Tulloch SD, Levine WC. Screening women in jails for chlamydial and gonococcal infection using urine tests: feasibility, acceptability, prevalence and treatment rates. *Sexually Transmitted Diseases*. 2002;29:271–276.
27. Kahn RH, Scholl DT, Shane SM, Lemoine AL, Farley TA. Screening for syphilis in arrestees: usefulness for community-wide syphilis surveillance and control. *Sexually Transmitted Diseases*. 2002;29:150–156.
28. Decker MD, Vaughn WK, Brodie JS, Hutcheson RH Jr, Schaffner W. Seroepidemiology of hepatitis B in Tennessee prisoners. *Journal of Infectious Diseases*. 1984;150:450–459.
29. Centers for Disease Control and Prevention. Sexually Transmitted Disease Survei-llance, 2004. Atlanta, GA: U.S. Department of Health and Human Services; 2004.

30. Harwell TS, Trino R, Rudy B, Yorkman S, Gollub EL. Sexual activity, substance use, and HIV/STD knowledge among detained male adolescents with multiple versus first admissions. *Sexually Transmitted Diseases*. 1999;26:265–271.

31. Weinstock H, Berman S, Cates W. Sexually transmitted diseases among American youth: incidence and prevalence estimates. *Perspectives on Sexual and Reproductive Health*. 2000;36:6–10.

32. Bell TA, Farrow JA, Stamm WE, Critchlow CW, Holmes KK. Sexually transmitted diseases in females in a juvenile detention center. *Sexually Transmitted Diseases*. 1985;12:140–144.

33. Morris RE, Legault J, Baker C. Prevalence of isolated urethral asymptomatic *chlamydia trachomatis* infection in the absence of cervical infection in incarcerated adolescent girls. *Sexually Transmitted Diseases*. 1993;20:198–200.

34. Kahn RH, Mosure DM, Blank S, et al. *Chlamydia trachomatis* and *Neisseria gonorrhoeae* prevalence and co-infection in adolescents entering U.S. juvenile detention centers, 1997-2002. *Sexually Transmitted Diseases*. 2005;32:255–259.

35. Oh KM, Cloud GA, Wallace LS, Reynolds J, Sturdevant M, Feinstein RA. Sexual behavior and sexually transmitted diseases among male adolescents in detention. *Sexually Transmitted Diseases*. 1994;21:127–131.

36. O'Brien SF, Bell TA, Farrow JA. Use of a leukocyte esterase dipstick to detect *Chlamydia trachomatis* and *Neisseria gonorrhoeae* urethritis in asymptomatic adolescent male detainees. *American Journal of Public Health*. 1988;78:1583–1584.

37. Robertson AA, Thomas CB, St. Lawrence JS, Pack R. Predictors of infection with chlamydia or gonorrhea in incarcerated adolescents. *Sexually Transmitted Diseases*. 2005;32:115-122.

38. Crosby R, Salazar LF, Diclemente RJ, Yarber WL, Caliendo AM, Staples-Horne M. Health risk factors among detained adolescent females. *American Journal of Preventive Medicine*. 2004;27:404–410.

39. Kahn RH, Voigt RF, Swint E, Weinstock H. Early syphilis in the United States identified in corrections facilities, 1999-2002. *Sexually Transmitted Diseases*. 2004;31:360–364.

40. Centers for Disease Control and Prevention. Primary and secondary syphilis among men who have sex–New York City, 2001. *MMWR*. 2002;51:853–856.

41. Blank S, McDonnell DD, Rubin SR, et al. New approaches to syphilis control: finding opportunities for syphilis treatment and congenital syphilis prevention in a women's correctional setting. *Sexually Transmitted Diseases*. 1997;24:218–226.

42. Farley TA, Hadler JL, Gunn RA. The syphilis epidemic in Connecticut: relationship to drug use and prostitution. *Sexually Transmitted Diseases*. 1990;17:163–168.

43. Alexander-Rodriguez T, Vermund SH. Gonorrhea and syphilis in incarcerated urban adolescents: prevalence and physical signs. *Pediatrics*. 1987;80:561–564.

44. Solomon L, Flynn C, Muck K, Vertefeuille J. Prevalence of HIV, syphilis, hepatitis B, and hepatitis C among entrants to Maryland correctional facilities. *Journal of Urban Health*. 2004;81:25–37.

45. Conrad GL, Kleris GS, Rush B, Darrow WW. Sexually transmitted diseases among prostitutes and other sexual offenders. *Sexually Transmitted Diseases*. 1981;8:241–244.

46. Cohen D, Scribner R, Clark J, Cory D. The potential role of custody facilities in controlling sexually transmitted diseases. *American Journal of Public Health*. 1992;82:552–556.

47. Wolfe MI, Xu F, Patel P, et al. An outbreak of syphilis in Alabama prisons: correctional health policy and communicable disease control. *American Journal of Public Health*. 2001;91:1220–1225.

48. Smith WH. Syphilis epidemic in a southern prison. *Journal of the Medical Association of the State of Alabama.* 1965;35:392–394.
49. Kelly P, Bair R, Baillargeon J, German V. Risk behaviors and the prevalence of chlamydia in a juvenile detention facility. *Clinical Pediatrics.* 2000;39:521–527.
50. Alcabes P, Braslow C. A cluster of cases of penicillinase-producing neisseria gonorrhoeae in an adolescent detention center. *NYS Journal of Medicine.* 1988;88:495–496.
51. Kraut-Becher JR, Gift TL, Haddix AC, Irwin KL, Greifinger RB. Cost-effectiveness of universal screening for chlamydia and gonorrhea in US jails. *Journal of Urban Health: Bulletin of the New York Academy of Medicine.* 2004;81:453–471.
52. Steiner K, Kent C, Goldenson J, Snell A, Klausner J. Screening in jails is associated with a decrease in community prevalence of Chlamydia: San Francisco, 1997-2002. Presentation at the International Society for Sexually Transmitted Research (ISSTDR) in Amsterdam, July 10-13, 2005. Abstract #0146.
53. Kahn RK, Peterman TA, Pierce G., Arno J, Coursey EJ, Berman S. Which control strategies identify likely transmitters. Presentation at the International Society for Sexually Transmitted Research (ISSTDR) in Amsterdam, July 10-13, 2005. Abstract TO-502.
54. Hammett TM, Gaiter JL, Crawford C. Reaching seriously at-risk populations: health interventions in criminal justice settings. *Health Education and Behavior.* 1998;25:99–120.
55. Saum CA, Surratt H, Inciardim JA, Bennett RE. Sex in prison: exploring the myths and realities. *The Prison Journal.* 1995;75,413–430.
56. Braithwaite R, Arriola K. Male prisoners and HIV prevention: a call for action ignored. *Men's Health Forum.* 2003;93:759–763.
57. MacGowan R., Margolis, A., Gaiter J., Morrow, K., Zack, B., Askew, J., McAuliffe, T., Sosman, J.M., Eldridge, G.D; Project START Study Group. Predictors of risky sex of young men after release from prison. *International Journal of STD and AIDS.* 2003;14:519–523.
58. Hammett TM, Harmon MP, Rhodes W. The burden of infectious disease among inmates of and releases from US correctional facilities, 1997. *American Journal of Public Health.* 2002;92:789–1194.
59. Wohl AR, Johnson D, Jordan W, et al. High risk behaviors during incarceration in African-American men treated for HIV at three Los Angeles public medical centers. *Journal of Acquired Immune Deficiency Syndrome.* 2000;24:386–392.
60. Williams SP, Sperling C. The Development of an STD Prevention Intervention for Substance-Using Men Newly Released from Jail. Oral presentation at the Centerforce Summit on Correctional Health in San Francisco, Sept. 5-7, 2005.
61. Centers for Disease Control and Prevention. Internet use and early syphilis infection among men who have sex with men: San Francisco, California, 1999-2003. *MMWR.* 2003;52:1229–1232.
62. Centers for Disease Control and Prevention. Increases in fluoroquinolone-resistant *Neisseria gonorrhoeae* among men who have sex with men—United States, 2003, and revised recommendations for gonorrhea treatment. *MMWR,* 2004;53:335–338.
63. Wong W, Kent CK, Kahn RP, Klausner JD. Incidence of primary and secondary syphilis among HIV-infected men in San Francisco, 2001. In: Program and abstracts of the 40th meeting of the Infectious Disease Society of America. Chicago, IL: IDSA; October 2002.
64. Centers for Disease Control and Prevention. High-risk sexual behavior by HIV-positive men who have sex with men: 16 sites, United States, 2000-2002. *MMWR.* 2004;53:891–894.
65. Bureau of Justice Statistics. *Prisoners in 2002.* Washington, DC: U.S. Department of Justice, NCJ 200248; 2003.

66. Bureau of Justice Statistics. *Substance Abuse and Treatment of State and Federal Prisoners, 1997.* Washington, DC: U.S. Department of Justice, NCJ 172871; 1999.

67. Fleming DT, Wasserheit JN. From epidemiological synergy to public health policy and practice: the contribution of other sexually transmitted diseases to sexual transmission of HIV infection. *Sexually Transmitted Infections.* 1999;75,3–17.

68. Belenko S, Langley S, Crimmins S, Chaple M. HIV risk behaviors, knowledge, and prevention education among offenders under community supervision: a hidden risk group. *AIDS Education and Prevention.* 2004;16:367–385.

69. Beltrami JF, Cohen DA, Hamrick JT, Farley TA. Rapid screening and treatment for sexually transmitted diseases in arrestees: a feasible control measure. *American Journal of Public Health.* 1997;87:1423–1426.

70. American Academy of Pediatrics, Committee on Adolescents. Health care for children and adolescents in the juvenile correctional care system. *Pediatrics.* 2001;107:799–803.

71. Forrest CB, Tambor E, Riley AW, Ensmiger ME, Starfield B. The health profile of incarcerated male youths. *Pediatrics.* 2000;105:286–291.

72. Shelton D. Health status of young offenders and their families. *Journal of Nursing Scholarship.* 2000;32:173–178.

73. Aral S, Holmes KK. Sexually Transmitted Diseases in the AIDS Era. *Scientific American.* 1991;264:62–69.

74. Murray K, Richardson L, Morishima C, Owens J, Gretch D. Prevalence of hepatitis C virus infection and risk factors in an incarcerated juvenile population: a pilot study. *Pediatrics.* 2003;111:153–157.

75. Comfort M, Grinstead O, McCartney K, Bourgois P, Knight K. "You cannot do nothing in this damn place": Sex and intimacy among couples with an incarcerated male partner. *Journal of Sex Research.* 2005;42:3–12.

76. Rapposelli KK, Kennedy MG, Miles JR, et al. HIV/AIDS in correctional setting: A salient priority for the CDC and HRSA. *AIDS Education and Prevention.* 2002;14(5 Supp B):103–113.

77. May JP, Williams EL. Acceptability of condom availability in a U.S. jail. *AIDS Education and Prevention.* 2002;14 (5 Supp B):85–91.

78. Jurgens R. HIV/AIDS in Prisons: Final Report. Canadian AIDS Society & Canadian HIV/AIDS Legal Network. 1996. Available at: http://epe.lac-bac.gc.ca/100/200/300/reseau_jur_cdn_vih_sida/vih-sida_prison e/html/www.aidslaw.ca/Maincontent/issues/prisons/complete.pdf

79. Becker M. Six dead in Jamaica condom riots. Reuters Newservice; August 22, 1997.

80. Grinstead O, Zack B, Faigeles B. Collaborative research to prevent HIV among male prison inmates and their female partners. *Health Education and Behavior.* 1999;26:225–238.

81. Grinstead O, Zack B, Faigeles B. Reducing post-release risk behavior among HIV seropositive prison inmates: the Health Promotion Program. *AIDS Education and Prevention.* 2001;13:109–119.

82. Grinstead O, Zack B, Faigeles B, Grossman N, Blea L. Reducing post-release HIV risk among male prison inmates: a peer-led intervention. *Criminal Justice and Behavior.* 2001;26:453–465.

83. Wolitski RJ. *Project START reduces HIV risk among prisoners after release.* Presented at the XV International Conference on AIDS, Bangkok, Thailand.; July 2004.

84. Haywood TW, Kravitz HM, Goldman LB, Freeman A. Characteristics of women in jail and treatment orientations: a review. *Behavioral Modification.* 2000;24:307–324.

85. Vigilante KC, Flynn MM, Affleck PC, et al. Reduction in recidivism of incarcerated women through primary care, peer counseling, and discharge planning. *Journal of Womens' Health.* 1999;8:409–415.

86. St. Lawrence JS, Eldridge GD, Shelby MC, Little CE, Brasfield TL, O'Bannon RE. HIV risk reduction for incarcerated women: a comparison of brief interventions based on two theoretical models. *Journal of Consult and Clinical Psychology*. 1997;65:504–509.

87. Schlapman N, Cass PS. Project: HIV prevention for incarcerated youth in Indiana. *Journal of Community Health Nursing*. 2000;17:151–158.

88. Woolfenden SR, Williams K, Peat J. Family and parenting interventions in children and adolescents with conduct disorder and delinquency aged 10-17. *Cochrane Database System Review*. 2001;(2):CD003015.

89. Barreras RE, Drucker EM, Rosenthal D. The concentration of substance use and criminal justice involvement in the families of drug offenders. *Journal of Urban Health*. 2005;82:162–170.

90. Martin SS, O'Connell DJ, Inciardi JA, Surratt H, Beard RA. HIV/AIDS among probationers: an assessment of risk and results from a brief intervention. *Journal of Psychoactive Drugs*. 2003;35:435–443.

91. Lurigio AJ, Petraitis J, Johnson BR. Joining the front line against HIV: an education program for adult probationers. *AIDS Education and Prevention*. 1992;4:205–218.

92. Bauserman R, Richardson D, Ward M, et al. HIV Prevention with jail and prison inmates: Maryland's Prevention Case Management Program. *AIDS Education and Prevention*. 2003;15:465–480.

93. Richie BE, Freudenberg N, Page J. Reintegrating women leaving jail into urban communities: a description of a model program. *Journal of Urban Health*. 2001;78:290–303.

94. Needels K, James-Burdumy S, Burghardt J. Community case management for former jail inmates: its impacts on rearrest, drug use, and HIV risk. *Journal of Urban Health*. 2005;82:420–433.

95. Williams SP, Sperling C, MISTERS Project Team. STD prevalence and risk factors of men newly released from jail. Oral Presentation as part of symposium, *The Bugs They Bring In and Take Out: Recent Epidemiological Information from CDC*. American Corrections Association (ACA) Winter Conference, Nashville, TN; January 28, 2006.

96. Riley ED, Moss A., Clark RA, Monk SL, Bangsberg DR. Cash benefits are associated with lower risk behavior among the homeless and marginally housed in San Francisco. *Journal of Urban Health*. 2005;82:142–150.

97. Pollack H, Khoshnood K, Altice F. Health care delivery strategies for criminal offenders. *Journal of Health Care Finance*. 1999;26:63–77.

98. Martin SS, Butzin, CA, Inciardi JA. Assessment of a multistage therapeutic community for drug-involved offenders. *Journal of Psychoactive Drugs*. 1995;27:109–116.

99. Butzin CA, Martin SS, Inciardi JA. Evaluating component effects of a prison-based treatment continuum. *Journal of Substance Abuse Treatment*. 2002;22: 63–69.

100. Butzin CA, Martin SS, Inciardi JA. Treatment during transition from prison to community and subsequent illicit drug use. *Journal of Substance Abuse Treatment*. 2005;28:351–358.

101. Prochaska JO, Velicer WF, Rossi JS, et al. Stages of change and decisional balance for twelve problem behaviors. *Health Psychology*. 1994;13:39–46.

102. Ehrmann T. Community based organizations and HIV prevention for incarcerated populations: three HIV prevention program models. *AIDS Education and Prevention*. 2002;14:75–84.

103. Dubik-Unruh S. Peer Education Programs in Corrections: curriculum, implementation and nursing interventions. *Journal of the Association of Nurses in AIDS Care*. 1999;10:53–62.

104. Hogben M, St. Lawrence JS. HIV/STD risk reduction interventions in prison settings. *Journal of Women's Health and Gender-Based Medicine*. 2000;9: 587–592.

105. Skolnick A. Correctional and community health care collaboration. *Journal of the American Medical Association.* 1998;279:98–99.
106. Metcalf CA, Douglas JM Jr, Malotte CK, et al. Relative efficacy of prevention counseling with rapid and standard HIV testing: a randomized, controlled trial (RESPECT-2). *Sexually Transmitted Diseases.* 2005;32:130–138.

STDs Among Illicit Drug Users in the United States: The Need for Interventions

Salaam Semaan, Dr.P.H., Don C. Des Jarlais, Ph.D., and Robert M. Malow, Ph.D.

The magnitude of STDs other than HIV in drug users who engage in heterosexual behaviors has not been well assessed in the scientific literature. Similarly, the profile of effective STD risk-reduction interventions for drug users is limited because few interventions have been developed beyond HIV prevention to reduce the risk for the sexual transmission of bacterial and viral STDs in this population. The lack of data on STDs in drug users and on relevant interventions is in marked contrast to the extensive literature on hepatitis B and C(1–4) and HIV (5–8) in drug users.

We aim in this chapter to review and summarize the literature on STDs (excluding HIV) in drug users who engage in heterosexual behaviors and to describe the existing profile of STD-related prevention and control activities specific to drug users. We review three bacterial STDs—syphilis, gonorrhea, and chlamydia—and two viral STDs—hepatitis B and genital herpes. We focus primarily on the scientific studies conducted with heterosexual drug users in the United States, that were published between 1995 and early 2005. Although control of infection with human papilloma virus (HPV) is important for control of cervical cancer, it is worthwhile noting that only two studies were found that mentioned HPV among drug users (9,10), despite the imminent and recent availability of a vaccine for HPV.

Definition of the Population and Scope of the Studies Reviewed

We define drug users in this chapter as those who are addicted to the use of opiates (e.g., heroin), cocaine (e.g., freebase and crack), and methamphetamine (meth), and who are at risk for infection with STDs, other than HIV, through heterosexual behaviors. We use the term *injection drug users* (IDUs) to refer to those who primarily inject heroin, cocaine, or speedball (a combination of heroin and cocaine) and who may or may not also have smoked crack or snorted heroin. Recent trends of heroin use include snorting heroin because of its purity and the perceived perception of reduced risk for getting infected with HIV. By definition, crack smokers smoke primarily crack cocaine and may or may not also have injected drugs in the past. We use the term *meth users* to refer to those who abuse methamphetamine (other

Behavioral Interventions for Prevention and Control of Sexually Transmitted Diseases. Aral SO, Douglas JM Jr, eds. Lipshutz JA, assoc ed. New York: Springer Science+ Business Media, LLC; 2007.

terminology has been used in the literature for meth, such as "speed" and "crystal").

Over the past decade, three major groups of studies were conducted with drug users. One group of studies recruited only IDUs; another recruited only crack cocaine smokers; and a third recruited both IDUs and crack cocaine smokers, often analyzing the data for both groups combined. More recently, several studies with heterosexual meth users have been published. Our chapter and terminology reflect this literature. We use the term *IDUs* when the studies reflect injectors of heroin. We use the term *crack cocaine smokers* when the studies reflect this population only. We use the combined term *IDUs and crack cocaine smokers* for studies or results that included both IDUs and crack cocaine smokers. We use the term *meth users* when the studies reflect this population.

In this chapter, we report rates of STDs in drug users recruited from drug-treatment settings and from other settings including "streets" and other community-based settings. This population of drug users is at high risk for infection with HIV and with STDs. There are limited analyses and published data on STDs in the drug-using population as assessed in general household population surveys. While these surveys collect data on the rates of STDs in the general population and on the extent of drug use by this population, limited analysis has been conducted on the extent of STD rates in the drug-using population. Some studies, using national general population data, include drug use as a control variable in multivariate analyses (11–13). In spite of the availability of the general population use data, we did not find published studies that present national estimates of the rates of STDs in drug-using members of the general population. While the sample size may be small, it seems valuable to analyze the publicly available national data to assess the prevalence of STDs in drug-using members of the general population. Due to space limitation, we do not review in this chapter the association between use of alcohol and other club drugs (e.g., ecstasy, GHB, ketamine, and Rohypnol) and sexual risk behaviors (14–20). It remains important to reach these users with effective prevention and treatment efforts.

Drug Addiction

The use of illicit drugs produces profound degrees of physical tolerance and dependence, compulsive use and abuse, and addiction (21). Drug users develop a tolerance to the euphoria commonly produced with stimulant drugs. This euphoria is often referred to as a "high" or as a "rush." Drug users often increase their drug use to intensify and prolong the euphoric effects, and they gradually spend more time and energy obtaining and using drugs. Once addicted, the primary purpose of the drug user is to seek and use drugs. The drugs literally change the brains and behaviors of the users. Accordingly, addiction is defined as a chronic, relapsing disease, characterized by compulsive drug seeking and use, and by molecular changes in the brain.

Drug users adopt different routes to administer the drugs. The principal routes of administration are intranasal, intravenous, and inhalation. Snorting is the process of inhaling the drug through the nostrils, where it is absorbed into the blood stream through the nasal tissues. Injecting releases the drug directly into the blood stream and heightens the intensity of its effects. Smoking involves inhaling the smoke or the vapor into the lungs, where its absorption into the blood stream is as rapid as by injection. Although addiction is associated with risky sexual behaviors and infection with STDs, there are differences in the risk involved, depending on the drug of abuse and on the route of administration.

Drug Use and STDs

The addictive and intoxicating effects of illicit drugs alter judgment and inhibition, often causing impulsive and unsafe sexual behaviors. Impulsivity and depression have also been associated with drug use (22). Although different drugs affect sexual behaviors differently, drug use is usually associated with increased sexual activity, high-risk sex, and with infection with HIV and other STDs (23). High-risk sexual behavior includes engaging in unprotected sex (sex without the use of a condom), exchanging sex for drugs or money, having multiple sex partners, and having anonymous partners.

Heroin is a highly addictive drug. It is both the most abused and the most rapidly acting of the opiates. Heroin is processed from morphine, a naturally occurring substance extracted from the seed pod of certain varieties of poppy plants. It is typically sold as a white or brownish powder or as the black sticky substance known on the streets as "black tar heroin."

The short-term effects of heroin abuse appear soon after a single dose and disappear in a few hours. After an injection of heroin, the user reports feeling a surge of euphoria, accompanied by a warm flushing of the skin, a dry mouth, and heavy extremities. Following this initial euphoria, the user goes "on the nod," with alternately wakeful and drowsy states. Mental functioning becomes clouded owing to the depression of the central nervous system.

Heroin is believed to reduce sexual activity and to impair sexual arousal (24). However, when heroin users are not under the influence of heroin, they seem to engage in sexual activity at a rate that does not seem to be very different from the average person who does not use drugs, in terms of number of sex partners and frequency of vaginal intercourse (25,26).

Cocaine is a powerfully addictive drug and a strong nervous central system stimulant that interferes with the reabsorption process of the neurotransmitter dopamine. The buildup of dopamine is associated with the euphoria commonly reported by cocaine abusers. Coca leaves are the source of cocaine. There are basically two forms of cocaine: the hydrochloride salt and the "freebase." The hydrochloride salt, or powdered form of cocaine, dissolves in water and, when abused, can be taken intravenously or through the nose. Freebase refers to a compound that has not been neutralized by an acid to make the hydrochloride salt. Crack is the street name given to the freebase form of cocaine and is smokable. This form of cocaine, crack, comes in a rock crystal that can be heated and its vapors smoked. The term "crack" refers to the crackling sound heard when the crystal is heated.

In some people, the effects of cocaine use include hyperstimulation, reduced fatigue, mental clarity, and increased sexual activity. Cocaine's effects appear almost immediately after a single dose and disappear within a few minutes or hours. The duration of these immediate effects depends on the route of administration. The faster the absorption of cocaine, the more intense is the high and the shorter is the duration of its effect. The "high" from snorting is relatively slow in onset and it may last 15 to 30 minutes in some people. The "high" from smoking may last 5 to 10 minutes and can be experienced in less than 10 seconds.

In some people, the use of cocaine and crack is associated with an increase in sexual activity because of the perceived increases in libido and the binge pattern of consuming the drugs. Users of cocaine and crack might engage in high-risk sex behaviors, including unprotected sex, anonymous sex, a high number of sex partners, and trading sex for money or drugs (25,27–31).

Methamphetamine is a powerfully addictive stimulant that drastically affects the central nervous system (32). Methamphetamine is being used by different populations throughout the United States (33–36). The drug is made easily in clandestine laboratories with relatively inexpensive over-the-counter ingredients (33). The availability and production of methamphetamine are being reported in diverse areas of the country, particularly rural and suburban areas, prompting concern about more widespread use. Methamphetamine is a white, odorless, bitter-tasting crystalline powder that easily dissolves in water or alcohol. It causes increased activity, decreased appetite, and a general sense of well-being. It also prolongs stamina and increases sexual pleasure (37–39).

Methamphetamine is classified as a psychostimulant, as is cocaine, and, like cocaine, it results in an accumulation of the neurotransmitter dopamine, which produces the feelings of euphoria experienced by the user. In contrast to cocaine, which is quickly removed and almost completely metabolized in the body, methamphetamine has a much longer duration of action, and a larger percentage of the drug remains unchanged in the body. This results in methamphetamine being present in the brain longer, which ultimately leads to prolonged stimulant effects that can last 6 to 8 hours. After the initial "rush" associated with methamphetamine use, there is typically a state of high agitation that in some individuals can lead to violent behavior.

Methamphetamine comes in many forms and can be smoked, injected, snorted, or ingested. Immediately after smoking the drug or injecting it intravenously, the user experiences an intense rush that lasts only a few minutes and is described as extremely pleasurable. Snorting or oral ingestion produces euphoria—a "high" but not an intense "rush." Snorting produces effects within 3 to 5 minutes, and oral ingestion produces effects within 15 to 20 minutes. As with other stimulants, methamphetamine is most often used in a "binge and crash" pattern. Because tolerance for methamphetamine occurs within minutes—meaning that the pleasurable effects disappear even before the drug concentration in the blood falls significantly—users try to maintain the high by binging on the drug.

While research indicates that methamphetamine can increase the libido in users, long-term methamphetamine use may be associated with decreased sexual functioning, at least in men. Additionally, methamphetamine seems to be associated with rougher sex, which may lead to bleeding and abrasions. Among people who engage in heterosexual behaviors, methamphetamine use has been associated with risky sexual behavior (34,39–45), with infection with HIV (35,46) and with infection with STDs (40). The literature on the association between methamphetamine use and STDs in men who have sex with men is well documented and is covered elsewhere (47,48).

Importance of STD Control for Drug Users

Assessment of STDs in drug users is important for several reasons. First, the association between drug use and STDs in drug users has considerable public health importance not only for drug users (49,50) but also for populations who do not use drugs and who may have sex with persons who use drugs. Second, sexual transmission of HIV in IDUs may be becoming as prevalent as injection-related transmission of the disease (51,52). Third, the rates of STDs, mostly prevalence rates, are higher in subgroups of drug users (53), including those who exchange sex for crack (54–56), and those who use noninjection drugs (49,57–59). Fourth, the synergy between HIV and other STDs, especially syphilis and genital herpes, facilitates HIV transmission (60–64). Fifth, a modest proportion of HIV-positive IDUs (65,66) and a small proportion of male IDUs who have sex with men (67) engage in high-risk same-sex behaviors. Finally, the general health problems or consequences of infection with STDs are also important for drug users (17,68–70). These six reasons justify the need to boost efforts aimed at assessing and controlling STDs in drug users.

Assessment of STDs in Drug Users

Data Sources
Existing national STD databases and results from research studies on STDs in high–risk populations, such as sex workers and incarcerated people, do not provide estimates of the rates of STDs in drug users. For example, the national STD surveillance system does not usually collect or report data on the number of STD cases in drug users and does not provide information on STD rates by drug-use behaviors (71). Although many sex workers use illicit drugs, data on STDs in this population are not usually provided for those who do or who do not use drugs (72–76). Similar restrictions apply to data from incarcerated populations. Although many persons in jails and prisons are incarcerated because of drug use, data on STDs in incarcerated populations are not usually provided according to drug use (77–79). As a result, there are few data sources that provide estimates on the prevalence and incidence rates of STDs in drug users.

A limited number of research studies that often were part of HIV research projects form the primary source of information on the rates of STDs in drug users. In this chapter, we focus primarily on the studies conducted with drug users since the mid-1990s, allowing for a review of a decade of research studies on STD rates in drug users.

Approach to and Highlights of Data Review
Since the mid-1990s, most studies of drug users relied on biologic markers, such as serologic tests of blood samples or assays of urine samples, to test for STDs in drug users. Because estimates of STD rates depend on the laboratory tests used, we mention in this chapter the types of the tests used to assess STDs in drug users and also the clinical significance of the positive test results. Most of the studies reported that their staff members informed the study participants of the positive test results and reported the relevant information to state health departments. Data based on biologic markers have limitations if used with populations who have low STD prevalence and incidence rates, especially in short-term longitudinal studies or in intervention studies. However, data based

on biologic markers provide a different perspective from that provided by self-reported data on the lifetime history of diagnoses with STDs. The life time data show the propensity of drug users to get infected with bacterial STDs repeatedly (80). Additionally, data based on biologic markers allow, to a certain extent, comparison of the STD rates between drug users and other populations.

Most of the published studies on STDs in drug users used cross-sectional data and conducted bivariate analysis for subgroups of drug users. Few studies conducted regression analysis to examine the independent variables associated with STD infection rates. Still fewer studies provided incidence data. We provide in this chapter estimates of the STD rates in several subgroups of drug users, including information on the age distribution of the study participants, because STD rates are age-dependent. The age distribution is important, when available data allows for comparing STD rates between populations.

Based on the information reported in the literature, we structure our summaries on the rates of STDs among drug users by enumerating the subgroups of drug users who have higher rates for each STD. This information is based on bivariate data and on results of regression analysis. Due to the low number of STD cases in drug users, few studies conducted multivariate analyses of variables associated with STD rates.

In terms of reporting data on rates of STDs in drug users, we present first incidence data, followed by overall prevalence data, and then by prevalence data for different subgroups of drug users. We describe these subgroups of drug users according to certain variables that include sociodemographic variables, sex-risk variables, drug use variables, and venue of recruitment of drug users (e.g, from drug-treatment centers or from other venues, referred to in this chapter as in-treatment and out-of-treatment drug users). We then present the results of the regression analysis, enumerating the variables that were controlled for in the regression analysis. Based on the available data, we present results of the regression analysis for variables associated with prevalent infection and with incident infection, and, as data allow, separately for males and for females.

Syphilis

The association between syphilis and crack use was identified in the 1990s (81–83), and continues to be important, especially in those who exchange sex for money or drugs (84,85).

Several recent studies assessed syphilis seropositivity rates in drug users (49,85–90). These studies used a nontreponemal test such as the rapid plasma reagin test followed by the use of a confirmatory treponemal test such as the microhemagglutination test. Positive tests indicate past or current infection, which would require a clinical examination and taking a history to determine the stage of infection with syphilis and the course required for treating the infected person and the infected sex partners (91,92).

Overall, the data on syphilis seropositivity, on incidence rates, and on correlates of infection with syphilis suggest that syphilis continues to be a problem for drug users. Based on the available bivariate data and results of regression analysis, it seems that syphilis is especially problematic for certain subgroups of drug users, including crack cocaine users, female IDUs, those with multiple partners, those infected with HIV, those who reported having had a previous infection with syphilis, those who have had a history of STDs, and those who reported recent initiation of injection drug use.

In terms of incidence data, one study assessed incidence rates in IDUs. High incidence rates (26/1000 person-years) were reported for IDUs, with a very high incidence rate (187/1000 person-years) reported in the subgroup that included male IDUs who had sex with men, bisexuals, and women IDUs who had sex with women (90).

In terms of prevalence data, review of the studies of syphilis in drug users showed seropositivity rates ranging from 2% to 6% for drug users who were in drug treatment (85–88), and from 1% to 6% in recent studies of out-of-treatment drug users (49,89,90). Three of the four in-treatment studies reported data on the age of the participants, with a median age in the high 30s. In the out-of-treatment studies, two studies had an eligibility age range for the participants between 18 and 30 years. The third study reported a median age of 43 years.

With respect to rates in subgroups of drug users, higher rates of syphilis were reported in African-American drug users. For example, rates ranging from 6% to 8% were reported among African-American drug users (87,89,93). Mixed results were obtained with respect to age, with higher rates (12% in 18–25-year-old IDUs) reported in younger IDUs in-treatment (88), and in older (2% in 20–29 years vs. 7% ≥40 years) drug users in-treatment (94). Higher rates were reported in crack users (9%) (85), female IDUs (13%) (49), drug users with multiple partners (14% among those with >5 partners during the 4 weeks prior to data collection) (94), female drug users who reported having had a previous syphilis infection (33%) (89), and in HIV-positive drug users (42%) (95).

Two recent studies conducted regression analysis and controlled for confounding variables. Results of regression analysis from one study (87), showed that participants who reported ever having had an STD had higher syphilis seropositivity rates. This study controlled for the following confounding variables: age, sex, race, use of injection drugs, needle sharing, history of treatment for drug abuse, use of crack cocaine, history of selling sex, and having had more than five partners in the past four weeks. Controlling for age and race, regression results of another study (89) showed that, among women, those who reported a previous infection with syphilis had higher syphilis seropositivity rates.

In terms of variables associated with seroconversion rates, results of a recent study that conducted regression analysis and controlled for confounding variables showed that recent initiation of injection drug use and having had multiple sex partners were associated with syphilis seroconversion (90). This study controlled for age, sex, race, and exchanging of sex for money.

Maternal drug use, especially crack cocaine, was found to be associated with congenital syphilis in a few studies conducted in the 1990s (96,97). Data from the national surveillance system show that cases of congenital syphilis have continued to decline; from 432 cases reported in 2003 to 353 in 2004 (98). However, the national surveillance system does not provide the number of cases of congenital syphilis attributed to drug-using pregnant women. Nevertheless, most cases of congenital syphilis are easily preventable if women are screened for syphilis and are treated early during prenatal care.

Gonorrhea

The overall prevalence rates reported for gonorrhea seem to be slightly lower than the rates reported for syphilis, as determined by several studies that tested for gonorrhea in drug users. These studies used nucleic acid amplification tests. Overall, the data showed that gonorrhea is a problem particularly in younger drug users, male crack users, female IDUs, female IDUs infected with HIV, those who exchange sex for money, and those with multiple partners.

In terms of incidence data, one study reported incidence rates of gonorrhea, with 0% and 1% reported in male and female IDUs respectively at the six-month follow-up period (99). In terms of prevalence data, several studies provided an overall prevalence rate for gonorrhea, ranging from 1% to 3%, with similar rates reported for drug users recruited from drug treatment facilities (85–87,94,100,101) and from other venues (49,99,102). In these studies, the age range of drug users recruited from drug treatment facilities was in the mid-to-high 30s. Those recruited from out-of-treatment facilities were in the age group of 18 to 30.

With respect to prevalence rates in subgroups of drug users, bivariate data show that higher rates were reported in female drug users than in male drug users. For example, in one study, 4% of females and 1% of males had gonorrhea (87). Other studies found a zero prevalence rate (94,101,102) or close to a 0% prevalence rate (99) in male drug users. Rates in white drug users appear to be lower than those in drug users of other racial or ethnic groups. One study, showed that 1% of white drug users and 3% of African-American drug users had gonorrhea, respectively (87). Data on age show higher prevalence rates in younger drug users. For example, one study reported a prevalence of 4% among those who were younger than 20 years (87). Higher rates were reported in male crack users (11%) (49), female IDUs (13%) (49), those who exchanged sex for money (5%) (99), and in female IDUs who were HIV positive (4%) (99).

One study examined multivariate correlates of prevalent gonorrhea among female IDUs (99). Controlling for race, this study found that younger age at the time of penetrative sexual debut and having received money for sex were significant correlates of higher gonorrhea rates.

Chlamydia

Most of the studies that assessed gonorrhea rates in drug users also assessed chlamydia rates. The overall prevalence rates reported for chlamydia seem to be higher than the rates reported for gonorrhea and somewhat similar to or slightly lower than the rates reported for syphilis. The studies assessed the magnitude of chlamydial infections in drug users by using nucleic acid amplification tests, mainly the ligase chain reaction test. The data show higher rates of chlamydia in female crack users, female IDUs, those who trade sex, those with multiple partners, those who reported having had other STDs, and those who had a previous chlamydial infection.

Using the ligase chain reaction test, one study reported incidence rates for chlamydia, with 2% reported in male IDUs, and 4% reported in female IDUs at the six-month follow-up period (99). In terms of prevalence data, the results of studies with drug users showed overall rates ranging from 1% to 5% (49,85–87,94,99–102). In these studies, drug users recruited from out-of-treatment facilities were younger (18–30 years) than those recruited from treatment facilities, who had a median age in the late 30s.

With respect to prevalence rates in subgroups of drug users, bivariate data showed that rates were lower in white drug users. For example, data in one study showed that 4% and 6% of white male and white female drug users had chlamydia compared with 9% and 5% of African American males and African American females, respectively (99). As with gonorrhea, the rates of chlamydia appear to be lower in older drug users. For example, 2% of those who were older than 25 years had chlamydia, and 6% of those who were 25 years old or younger had chlamydia (102). Higher rates were reported in female crack users (14%) (49), female IDUs (13%) (49), those who engaged in the sex trade (8%) (99), those who had multiple partners (9% in those with >5 partners in the 4 weeks prior to data collection) (87), those who reported previous infection with chlamydia (14% in male IDUs who reported having had chlamydia in the year prior to data collection) (99), and in those who reported having had other STDs (33% in male and female IDUs who reported having had genital herpes in the year prior to data collection) (99). Similar rates were reported in drug users recruited from treatment facilities (85–87,94,100,101) and in those who were not (3,49,102).

One study examined independent correlates of prevalent chlamydial infection by conducting regression analysis separately for males and females (99). In male IDUs, and controlling for history of forced sex, the regression results showed that being younger, African American, and being younger at time of penetrative sexual debut were associated with higher rates of chlamydial infection (99). In female IDUs, the regression results showed that being younger at time of penetrative sexual debut and having received money for sex were associated with higher rates of chlamydial infection (99).

Summary information on the pattern of these three bacterial STDs in drug users is presented in Table 1.

Hepatitis B

While the hepatitis B virus (HBV) is transmitted to drug users primarily through the parenteral route (103), sexual transmission of HBV in drug users is also common (104–106) via semen and vaginal fluids. Several studies assessed prevalence of HBV among drug users. Most of the studies assessed prevalence of HBV by testing for the presence of antibodies. A positive result for HBcAb indicates past or current infection with HBV.

Several studies show that most (50–70%) IDUs become infected with HBV within 5 years of beginning to inject (107). Incidence rates of 3.5 cases per 100 person-years were reported in HIV-positive recent users of injection drugs and 1.9 cases per 100 person-years in HIV-positive recent users of non-injection drugs (108). In HIV-negative IDUs, incidence rates of 10.0 cases per 100 person-years were reported (109).

For in-treatment drug users, prevalence rates ranged from as low as 11% (101) to as high as 67% (110,111). Rates as high as 80% were reported in female IDUs (112). In one study with drug users in the age group 15–30 years, prevalence rates of HBV were much higher in IDUs than in noninjection drug users (37% vs. 19%), with noninjection drug use defined as sniffing, smoking, or ingestion of cocaine, crack, or heroin (113).

A low (10–25%) proportion of IDUs and those who live in high-risk neighborhoods perceive themselves to be at risk for HBV infection (105,114,115). Although a recommendation was first made in 1982 to vaccinate IDUs (116), a high proportion of IDUs and their sex and injection partners are not vaccinated

Table 1 Summary information on the rates of bacterial STDs in drug users[a].

	Syphilis	Gonorrhea	Chlamydia
Incidence rate	26/1000 person years (93)	0% among male IDUs at 6 months follow-up (99) 1% among female IDUs at 6 months follow-up (99)	2% among male IDUs at 6 months follow-up (99) 4% among female IDUs at 6 months follow-up (49,85–90)
Prevalence rate	Seropositivity rate: 1–6% (85,86)	Prevalence rate: 1–3% (49,85–87,94,99-102)	Prevalence rate: 1–5% (88)
Demographic variables[b]	Higher among African Americans (6–8%) (87,89,93) Mixed results with respect to age 12% among 18–25 IDUs (94) 2% among 20–29 years and 7% among >40 years (85)	Higher (4%) among females (87) Lower (1%) among whites (87) Higher among younger drug users (4% among <20 years old) (87)	Lower among whites (4% among white males and 6% among white females) (99) Lower among older drug users (2% among <25 years old) (102)
Drug-related variables[b]	Higher (9%) among crack users (49) Higher (13%) among female IDUs (49)	Higher (11%) among male crack users (49) Higher (13%) among female IDUs (49)	Higher (14%) among female crack users (49) Higher (13%) among female IDUs (94)
Sex-related variables[b]	Higher (14%) among those with >5 partners past 4 weeks (99)	Higher (5%) among those who exchange sex for money (99)	Higher (8%) among those who trade sex (87) Higher (9%) among those with >5 partners past 4 weeks (89)
Health-related variables[b]	Higher (33%) among females with previous syphilis infection (95) Higher (42%) among HIV-positive drug users (99)	Higher (4%) among HIV-positive female IDUs (99)	Higher (33%) among those with other STDs (99) Higher (14%) among those with previous chlamydial infection (87)
Multivariate correlates of prevalent infection[c]	History of an STD (OR[d] = 11.7) (89) Self-report of previous infection with syphilis (OR = 10.3) (99)	Among female IDUs: younger age of penetrative sexual debut (OR= 1.27) (99), and having received money for sex past six months (OR = 5.17) (99)	Among male IDUs: younger age (OR= 0.89) (99), younger age of penetrative sexual debut (OR = 0.91) (99), and being African-American (OR = 2.92) (99) Among female IDUs: younger age of penetrative sexual debut (OR = 1.16) (99) and having received money for sex past six months (OR = 1.96) (90)

Multivariate correlates of incident infection[c]	Recent initiation into drug use (HR[e] = 4.6) (90) Multiple sex partners (HR = 7.8) (71)	Not reported in the literature reviewed for this chapter	Not reported in the literature reviewed for this chapter
Comparison data[f]	Median seropositivity rate: 7.5% (range, 2.4–10.7%) for women entering adult corrections facilities (71) Median seropositivity rate: 2.3% (range, 0.2–8.3%) in men in adult corrections facilities (127,128)	4.2% median positivity rate among women <20 years old from juvenile detention centers, substance abuse treatment programs, school-based clinics and organizations serving street or homeless youth (126) 1%: prevalence rate in prisons and jails (71) Median positivity: 5.7% (range, 0.5–15.9%) in women entering juvenile corrections facilities (127,128)	13.8% median prevalence rate among women <20 years old from juvenile detention centers, substance abuse treatment programs, school-based clinics, and organizations serving street or homeless youth (126) 2.4%: prevalence rate in prisons and jails (71) Median positivity: 15.9% (range, 2.7–33.5%) in adolescent women entering juvenile corrections facilities

[a] The numbers in parenthesis refer to the citation numbers in the reference list.
[b] Based on bivariate results reported in the referenced studies.
[c] Based on regression results reported in the referenced studies. The variables are statistically significant at $p = 0.05$.
[d] OR, odds ratio.
[e] HR, hazard ratio.
[f] Selected sources.

for hepatitis B. However, a higher (reaching 86% vs. 10%) proportion of drug users recruited from drug treatment settings have been vaccinated for HBV compared to drug users recruited in primary health care clinics (117–119) Given that IDUs become infected with HBV very early in their injection years, IDUs need to be vaccinated with the hepatitis B vaccine at least as soon as they start injection. A high proportion of IDUs with HBV are also infected with HIV and with HCV (3).

Genital Herpes

Review of the data on biologic markers of genital herpes (herpes simplex virus–2, HSV-2) reported in four studies conducted with drug users shows that IDUs and crack cocaine smokers have high rates of HSV-2. Variation in prevalence rates by sociodemographic factors mirrors the variation in rates seen in other populations, with lower rates reported in younger, white, and male drug users. Higher prevalence rates have been found in subgroups of drug users, especially in male drug users who have sex with men, those who trade sex, those with multiple partners, those with a history of incarceration, and those who were HIV-positive.

The studies assessed HSV-2 serologically by using a blood test that detected HSV-2 antibodies. A positive test indicates life-long infection. The studies showed high prevalence rates, ranging from 38% to 61% (85,87,89,120). Two studies with IDUs in drug-treatment (85,87) reported identical rates (44%), and similar (38%) (89) or higher (61%) (120) rates were reported in out-of-treatment drug users. Rates were two or three times higher in females than in males, and were as high as 75% in female drug users who were in drug-treatment (87), and as high as 81% in out-of-treatment female drug users (120). Rates were higher in African-American drug users than in those of other racial or ethnic backgrounds and were as high as 57% in a study with out-of-treatment drug users (89) and as high as 64% in a study with in-treatment drug users (87). Higher rates were reported with older age (<20 years: 15% vs. ≥40 years: 57%).

In terms of sex-related behaviors, high rates were found in those with a history of selling sex versus those without such a history (74% vs. 41%) (87), male drug users who had sex with men (50%) (89), and women who traded sex (81%) (89). Drug users who had a history of incarceration had higher rates than those who did not report an incarceration history (65% vs. 50%) (89). Higher rates were found in HIV-positive drug users (93% in females and 78% in males) than in those who were HIV-negative (89).

In terms of significant independent correlates obtained in regression analysis, higher prevalence rates of HSV-2 were associated with an age over 30 years, being female, and with African-American ethnicity (87). This study controlled for the following confounding variables: use of injection drugs, needle sharing, having a history of treatment for drug abuse, history of STDs, use of crack cocaine, and history of selling sex. In another study (89), regression analysis was conducted separately for females and males. In males, and controlling for age, the regression results showed that being African American, having had more than 30 lifetime opposite sex partners, being HIV positive, and ever been incarcerated were significantly associated with higher rates of HSV-2 (89). In females, and controlling for age and for lifetime number of opposite sex partners, the regression results showed that higher rates of HSV-2 were associated with being African American, having engaged in sex trade in the previous six months, and having used heroin daily in the past 6 months (89).

Overall Summary of the STD Rates Among Drug Users

The paucity of national data on STDs in drug users makes it hard to determine the co-infection rate with HIV. This paucity of data also makes it hard to compare STD rates in drug users with those reported in populations at high risk for STDs. The data on STDs in drug users are available from research studies, while the data on STDs in other populations are available from large household surveys or from the STD national surveillance system.

Despite the paucity of the data on STDs in drug users and the limitations of the data, results of research studies conducted with drug users in different settings and cities indicate that STDs are common in drug users. The socio-demographic pattern of STDs in drug users appears to be consistent with the pattern observed in other populations. Additionally, several subgroups of drug users have higher rates of STDs than other drug users.

In general, the data show that STDs are common in drug users, with higher rates for viral STDs than for bacterial STDs. The results also show that, if we adjust for age, rates of bacterial STDs in drug users will probably fall somewhere between the low STD rates reported in surveys of the general population (11–13,121) and the high STD rates reported for minority adolescents (71,122,123). However, rates of viral STDs in drug users are most probably higher than those reported for any other population (11–13). Data on STD rates were similar for drug users recruited from drug treatment facilities and those recruited from other venues. This similarity is attributed to the fact that tests for STDs were done at the time of entry of drug users to drug treatment facilities.

The variation in the rates of bacterial STDs in drug users according to sociodemographic characteristics (e.g., race, ethnicity, sex) appears to be consistent with the variation observed in other populations. Higher rates of bacterial STDs are reported in drug users who are younger, of a racial or ethnic background other than white, and in females. The same pattern is seen for genital herpes, with the only exception of age, where both for drug users and for other populations higher rates are seen in those who are older. The higher rates of bacterial STDs seen in female drug users, for example, are likely to be explained by the sex differences that contribute to the variation in infection rates in women, including the increased likelihood of asymptomatic infection, the different types of drugs used by women, especially crack cocaine, and the practice of exchanging sex for money or drugs. Transmission of genital herpes to drug users is influenced by sex-related factors. Transmission of other viral STDs to drug users, especially HIV and hepatitis B, is influenced more by drug-related factors than by sex-related factors, although the role of sexual transmission should not be neglected (26,124).

As noted, higher STD rates are seen in subgroups of drug users. These subgroups include crack users, drug users who are incarcerated, those with multiple partners, those who trade sex for money or drugs, those who previously have had STDs, and those who are infected with HIV. Though data on STD rates among drug users who use methamphetamine are limited, the association of methamphetamine use with high-risk sexual behaviors (38–44,125) makes it important to reach drug users who use methamphetamine with prevention and treatment messages.

In summary, the review of the literature on STDs in drug users suggests that the observed rates, although lower than those seen in the general young population aged 15–24 (122), still require the attention of health care providers and public health practitioners to reduce these rates. It may be possible to focus prevention efforts on subgroups of drug users. Table 1 presents a brief summary comparison of the STD rates reported among drug users with those reported in other populations. The table provides summary information from a few selected sources (71,126–128).

Sexual Interactions and Mixing Patterns

Sexual mixing patterns associated with STD transmission include sexual interactions between injectors and noninjectors, between injectors and other high-risk populations such as sex workers, and between drug users and low-risk populations such as people who do not use drugs (59,129–134). These sexual mixing patterns form important bridges in STD transmission (135–137).

Many investigators have argued that social and sexual network characteristics of populations are the primary determinants of risky sexual behaviors and are associated with important determinants of infection with STDs (138–142). Sexual network and sexual mixing variables have explained differences in HIV prevalence in IDUs, as well as differences in STD prevalence and incidence rates in populations who are not drug users (143–150). However, several research questions remain about the association between sexual mixing and STDs in drug users. For example, it is important to know whether sexual network characteristics of noninjection drug users and of new injectors are predictors of infection with STDs. Some researchers have also argued that communication about sexual risk behaviors between IDUs may vary by race and ethnicity (143,151–153). To test this hypothesis, it is important to collect and analyze data by race and ethnicity on the kinds of risk-relevant communication with sex partners and to assess how such communication is related to risky sexual behaviors and to infection with STDs.

Several HIV prevention activities have been implemented with drug users, based on the network theory (152–155). These interventions were effective in reducing HIV risk behaviors of study participants and of their sex and drug-injection partners. It is also important to conduct similar network-based interventions to evaluate their effectiveness in reducing STD rates among drug users.

Working with Drug Users

The Context for Prevention and Treatment

In developing appropriate prevention and treatment interventions for STDs, it is important to consider the contextual factors that influence drug addiction and the relationship between drug use and risky sexual behaviors. The drug-sex relationships can be, in part, affected by the powerful forces of addiction and the context in which drugs are obtained and used. Addiction is associated with a compulsive urgency to use a drug and a willingness to take a greater sex risk to obtain the drug. Reasons for risky sexual behaviors associated with STD transmission can be both direct (e.g., unprotected sexual encounters) and indirect (e.g., impaired judgment, such as in partner selection; having multiple or anonymous partners; or trading sex for money to buy drugs).

An example of the effects and context of addiction is the association between crack and infection with HIV (81,156,157), and with syphilis (84). Crack-addicted women are often poor and have low education (84). They often exchange sex for crack or money to support their drug habits. Their addiction needs to be understood in the context of poverty, racism, and unequal sexual power relationships (156,157).

Substance abuse treatment has been shown to be associated with reduction in HIV transmission risk behaviors and with increased protection from HIV infection (158–161). Many studies show that drug abusers in treatment stop or reduce their drug use and related risky behaviors including risky injection practices and unsafe sex (161). Other studies emphasize the need for integrating effective sex-risk reduction programs into drug treatment facilities, especially for drug-using women (162). Drug abuse treatment has been considered an important component in a comprehensive strategy for HIV prevention (163). Drug treatment programs provide drug users with current information on HIV/AIDS and other diseases, counseling and testing services, and with referrals for medical and social services (86). However, the effect of drug treatment on infection with STDs has not been explored, and it remains an important area worthy of research and program efforts. Delivery of STD treatment in substance abuse treatment facilities can serve as an effective means to control STDs among drug users in-treatment (163,164).

Drug treatment is based on the premise that drug abuse is preventable and that drug addiction is treatable (165). In addition to pharmacologic interventions, behavioral interventions can also decrease drug use in patients who are in treatment for drug addiction (166). Providing the optimal combination of treatment and social services is critical to successful outcomes. Treatment tends to be more effective when drug abuse is identified early (158–161). For optimal effect, substance abuse treatment must be readily available and accessible to drug users (156,157).

Behavioral treatment options usually include residential and outpatient approaches. These treatment options include cognitive-behavioral interventions and contingency management therapy (168). Cognitive-behavioral interventions are designed to help modify the patient's thinking, expectations, and behaviors, and to increase skills in coping with various life stressors. Contingency management therapy uses a voucher-based system by which patients earn "points" based on negative drug tests, which they can exchange for items that encourage healthful living. For example, drug treatment has been shown to decrease cocaine use from an average of 10 days per month at baseline to 1 day per month at six-month followup by noninjection cocaine abusers (169). Reduction in cocaine use was associated with an average 40% decrease in HIV risk, mainly as a result of fewer sex partners and less unprotected sex (169,170). Therapeutic communities or residential programs with planned lengths of stay of 6 to 12 months, offer another alternative to those in need of treatment for cocaine addiction. These communities focus on resocialization of the addict, and they can include on-site vocational rehabilitation and other support.

In terms of pharmacological treatment, there is a broad range of treatment options. Methadone, a synthetic opiate medication that blocks the effects of heroin for about 24 hours and eliminates withdrawal symptoms, has a proven record of success when prescribed at a high enough dosage for people addicted to heroin (171). Buprenorphine is a recent medication and is different from methadone in that it offers less risk for addiction and can be dispensed in the privacy of a doctor's office (171). Buprenorphine/naloxone (Suboxone) is a combination drug product formulated to minimize abuse (172,173).

No medications are currently available to treat cocaine addiction. Several medications, though, are currently being investigated for their safety and efficacy in treating cocaine addiction (170). Current research activities involve evaluating medications to alleviate the severe craving that people-in-treatment for cocaine addiction often experience. Topiramate and modafinil, two marketed medications, have shown promise as potential cocaine treatment agents (169,170). Additionally, baclofen, a GABA-B agonist, has produced encouraging results in a subgroup of cocaine addicts with heavy use patterns.

There are currently no particular pharmacological treatments for dependence on methamphetamine (174,175). Cognitive behavioral interventions are currently the most effective treatments for methamphetamine addiction. Methamphetamine recovery support groups also appear to be effective adjuncts to behavioral interventions that can lead to long-term drug-free recovery.

Combined pharmacological and behavioral treatments for drug abuse have a demonstrated effect on HIV risk behaviors and incidence of HIV infection (168). For example, recent research demonstrates that when behavioral therapies are combined with methadone treatment, approximately one half of the study participants who report injection drug use at intake report no such use at study exit (168). While these findings suggest strategies for achieving reductions in sexual and drug-related risk behaviors, studies are still needed to determine the long-term effectiveness of such interventions.

Drug abuse and addiction are complex problems involving biologic changes in the brain as well as behavioral changes and a myriad of social, familial, and environmental factors. Therefore, treatment of addiction must address a variety of problems. Treatment strategies need to assess the psychobiological, social, and pharmacological aspects of the patient's drug abuse. Integration of both behavioral and pharmacological treatments may be the most effective approach for treating addiction. Equally important is providing drug users with social services to help them adhere to medical regimens. One approach is the model adopted and evaluated in the CDC multi-site, randomized trial Antiretroviral Treatment Access Studies (ARTAS) (176). This model links and promotes the utilization of social and health services for low-income minorities, including those in drug abuse treatment. The innovation is to manage people according to their strengths in negotiating service support and in enlisting the support of significant others.

Challenges in Addressing Risky Behaviors

It is critical to address two major barriers when working with drug users. The first barrier relates to the question of who is responsible for the problem of drug addiction. The second barrier relates to the societal prejudices toward drug users.

There is a strong tension between two notions when it comes to the question of who is responsible for the problem of drug addiction. The first notion is the personal responsibility for one's health and for being free from drug addiction. The second notion is the role of society and its infrastructure in disease prevention and in adoption of healthful behaviors (177,178). While the ideologies of personal responsibility and of societal responsibility are overlapping, they are often posed against each other in explaining the propensity of people for addiction to drugs. Historically, these two notions have influenced public health efforts and resource allocation and have had ethical and legal ramifications (179–182).

An emphasis on individual culpability or on "blaming the victim" has held people rather than the social environment responsible for the causes of drug addiction (181). However, placing a premium on individual responsibility rather than on the social values of equity and distributive justice and on the role of structural factors (183) can do more damage than good, both to individuals and to society (184). According to a "blaming the victim" mentality, those who do not adopt a healthful life style are labeled as weak or are considered at fault. People may then react to messages about personal responsibility for health with feelings of guilt, shame, or frustration especially when they cannot adopt the style considered to be healthful by others. Risk-taking is then considered to have a moral dimension (185,186), leading some people to stigmatize others and to discriminate against them. Consequently, some people may delay treatment for drug addiction or for disease when these consequences are seen by others as the result of one's personal behavior.

Harm Reduction Strategies

While some prefer absolute messages about health protection and prefer to promote health as a virtue rather than as a value, others believe in harm reduction strategies (187). By definition, the harm reduction approach aims to provide messages and interventions to protect people from greater harm when they are engaging in potentially harmful practices, such as drug use (188,189). When people do not want to or when they cannot refrain from risky sexual practices or from drug use, the ethical principle of beneficence justifies providing risk-reduction messages and interventions to protect these people from debilitating consequences. The harm reduction approach justifies offering information and services to help people avoid certain risks, but it does not imply acceptance of practices judged by others as antisocial, immoral, or as an attempt at legalizing illicit drugs. Those who believe in harm reduction as one strategy in a comprehensive approach in the control of HIV and STDs argue that the mere provision of information about safer sex practices or about safer drug injection practices does not mean that such behaviors are sanctioned or are normative. There is evidence that harm reduction approaches, such as needle-exchange programs and pharmacy sales of sterile syringes, may be effective in controlling HIV infection in drug users (190–193). Needle exchange programs are services dedicated to providing needles and syringes, including exchange of used needles and syringes for sterile needles and syringes clean replacements. Pharmacy-based distribution allows for sale of sterile syringes. These programs are important given the parenteral risk for infection with HIV and the fact that some drug users are not able or are not willing to stop use of injection drugs.

Needle exchange programs have been associated with reductions in needle reuse, sharing of syringes, and other injection equipment, as well as with reductions in HIV seroconversion rates (193,194). The incidence of HIV in IDUs who use needle exchange programs has been shown to be less than one third of the HIV incidence in IDUs who do not use these programs (192–194). Restricted syringe access has been shown to be associated with injection-related risk behaviors (195,196). Participation in needle exchange programs has been associated with improved access to health care and drug treatment (192). The available evidence indicates that needle exchange programs do not result in either increased use of illicit drugs or in first-time drug use (192). Access to sterile injection equipment through pharmacies has been associated with reduced rates of needle sharing and of HIV transmission (189,197).

Although effects of needle exchange programs, access to clean needles, and drug treatment programs have been associated with reductions in transmission of HIV and of hepatitis C, their effect on reducing STDs in drug users has yet to be evaluated. However, it is expected that while these programs present a blood-borne transmission prevention approach, they can contribute to reducing STD rates among drug users. These programs are especially important, given that a small proportion of drug users who need drug treatment have access to drug treatment programs. Moreover, syringe exchange programs help gain the trust of an under-served population (181,198). Despite the evidence on their effectiveness, harm reduction interventions still raise strong emotional responses and political controversy.

Delivery of Health Services to Drug Users

Working with drug users requires compassion and patience. Health care providers and public health practitioners need to work with drug users in a supportive climate that does not stigmatize them and that keeps their information confidential. In working to control the HIV epidemic in drug users, many HIV-interdisciplinary teams have worked respectfully with IDUs (199–203). These teams demonstrated an understanding of how personal and structural determinants influence risk for addiction and for HIV infection (205). This understanding was demonstrated in training recovering drug addicts to work as agents for delivering risk-reduction messages to other drug users in community-based outreach programs, in peer-driven interventions, and in needle exchange programs (204,205). Similar positive attitudes are needed while working with drug users to reduce their risk for infection with STDs. Many investigators and health care providers with experience or willingness to work with drug users have established good rapport with drug users and have been successful in improving prevention and control outcomes (202,203). Several principles have been advocated as critical for improving the prevention and treatment outcomes among drug users (202,203). These principles include informing drug users about the importance of seeking health care and of adhering to medical regimens; encouraging health care providers and public health practitioners to learn about referral services available for drug users; showing drug users respect; and avoiding common pitfalls such as unrealistic expectations, moralizing, and withholding therapy.

Prevention and Treatment Efforts for STD Control

The Profile of Prevention and Treatment Activities

Similar to efforts aimed at controlling STDs in other populations, efforts to control STDs in drug users should aim to interrupt and to reduce transmission of infection and to prevent the development of disease, complications, and sequelae. Primary prevention at the individual level includes behavioral interventions that focus on information, education, and communication skills between partners, and on the use of barrier methods. Individual-level secondary and tertiary prevention strategies include promoting appropriate health care-seeking, including vaccination, screening, testing, case finding, syndromic management, partner notification and management, and a supportive health care sector. Targeted interventions include working with drug users who are sex workers, those who have high rates of sexual partnerships, and those known to be HIV-positive. Equally important is the need to reach drug users in their early years of drug use and to reach those who do not self-identify as drug users. This is important to interrupt the development of greater drug problems and also to avoid adverse health consequences such as infectious diseases. Treatment of drug addiction, prevention of drug use, and preventing the transition from use of non-injection drugs to injection drugs are also important.

Behavioral Interventions and Programs with Drug Users

Reviews of the scientific literature and of the best practices show that very few research interventions or systematic programmatic efforts have been implemented specifically to prevent and control STDs in drug users (6,206–208). For example, a review of studies published between 1988 and 1996 for 48 behavioral interventions implemented with drug users showed that none of these studies evaluated the effect of the interventions on the prevalence or incidence of STDs (209). There are many reasons for this lack of STD intervention research and programs with drug users. The reasons include the myths about difficulties of working with drug users, funding opportunities, limitations in advocacy on behalf of the drug users, and the belief that getting infected with STDs is not as important as getting infected with HIV or with hepatitis C.

However, HIV risk-reduction interventions and programs which aim to reduce risky sexual behaviors that might cause HIV focus on the same behaviors that put people at risk for infection with STDs. These efforts might well have had a small effect, though not well-quantified, on controlling STDs in drug users. It is important to add explicit information about how each of the bacterial and viral STDs is transmitted sexually to any HIV-specific intervention (210). Such specificity about infections is important because it might be associated with the adoption of relevant preventive and curative measures, and also because drug users are capable of responding to health education messages (5–7). It remains important, though, to develop messages that contain sufficient specificity about different STDs without becoming so complex that they are not understood by many members of the target population. Because results of many HIV-intervention studies (205) and the data from the national surveillance system for HIV and AIDS show that drug users can reduce their risk for HIV infection (211), it follows that drug users may be capable of reducing their risk for infection with STDs. It is important though to make note of the differences in factors that influence motivation for risk reduction for HIV and not necessarily for STDs so as to ensure that interventions to reduce STDs are likely to be effective (210,212). For example, it has been noted that HCV may not raise as much concern and generate as much behavior change in IDUs as does HIV (213). However, it has been only recently that HIV prevention programs have begun to address HCV transmission explicitly, particularly transmission through sharing of drug preparation equipment.

From a behavioral perspective, drug users need to be informed about safer practices for the prevention of bacterial and viral STDs. They need to learn how correct and consistent condom use can reduce the risk for transmission of many of the bacterial and viral STDs. Drug users need to know that condoms offer some protection from the skin-to-skin and skin-to-sore transmission of STDs such as HPV, genital herpes, and syphilis and offer better protection against discharge-related STDs such as chlamydia and gonorrhea (214,215). While abstinence prevents the transmission of STDs, drug users also need to know that reducing the number of sex partners, knowing the infectious and treatment status of partners, and communication with partners about safer sex practices are important strategies in reducing the risk for infection with STDs. Equally important is telling drug users how to inform their partners about positive STD test results, about the need for testing and treatment of STDs, and about how to reduce the risk for violence or any other unintended negative consequences associated with partner notification (216). Providing information and counseling to drug users, along with providing opportunities for role playing and demonstration of learned skills, could be important for ensuring that drug users adopt safer behaviors. These suggestions for STD risk-reduction interventions are based on the work conducted with drug users for the prevention of HIV. It is our assumption that such interventions can be extended and modified to include STDs. Involving drug users as role models and as agents for change is also critical. Similar to the efforts and pay-offs realized in involving drug users in HIV prevention efforts (205), participation of drug users in STD prevention efforts might also be important to control STDs (70,217,218). Although treatment of STDs is not unique to drug users in the same way that HIV treatment is, getting their "buy-in" might be equally important in STD prevention and control efforts.

From a clinical perspective, informing drug users about symptom recognition and about the fact that many STDs are asymptomatic is also an important step in controlling STDs in drug users. Informing drug users about the importance of seeking medical care and follow-up is critical. While these needs are not unique to drug users, they become more important with drug users, given the instability in their social lives (70,202). Effective treatment often includes providing a consistent support and a simplified medical regimen to counter the irregular life style influenced by drug abuse and addiction (219–221). Drug users need to learn about the importance of taking medications and completing the medication regimen because inconsistent adherence to medications results in development of bacterial and viral resistance. Drug users need to learn about the synergy between HIV and other STDs and that treatment for STDs decrease the risk for infection with and transmission of HIV. Another key learning objective and public health strategy for this population is the importance of getting vaccinated for hepatitis B.

Efforts aimed at controlling STDs in drug users also include those that intend to reduce drug-related risky behaviors. Drug-related risk reduction includes abstaining from drugs, enrolling in drug treatment, switching to non-injection drugs, and using needle exchange programs.

Targeted Interventions

Targeting prevention and treatment efforts to particular subgroups of drug users and particular STDs is important. For example, crack cocaine users can benefit from targeted interventions because they have higher rates of particular bacterial STDs, especially syphilis. Sex workers form another special group that can benefit from targeted interventions (221). Although the proportion of sex workers who use drugs is estimated to be high, such data are not collected regularly. Interventions to prevent initiation of drug use by female sex workers as well as harm reduction efforts with female sex workers who use drugs are urgently needed.

Incarcerated populations are also at high risk for STDs, given their drug use history, yet a high proportion of them get little or no treatment for drug addiction or for infection with STDs (223). Many incarcerated women have been arrested for sex work. A recent study found that jails with a high prevalence of chlamydia and gonorrhea represent a feasible and cost-effective setting to test and treat women at high risk for STDs (224).

Integration of services is an important component in preventing STDs. A recent study found large increases between 1997 and 2001 in the proportion of STD clinics that offered to its patients hepatitis B vaccine (from 61% to 82%), provided information (49% to 84%), and gained access to federal vaccine programs (48% to 84%) (225). A coordinated and well-funded approach at facilities frequented by drug users, such as STD clinics, HIV counseling and testing sites, needle exchange programs, drug treatment facilities, corrections facilities, and emergency rooms is needed to improve STD prevention and treatment efforts with drug users (100,101,226–230). Integration of services for drug users has been successful in many settings, but such integration needs to be adopted on a wider scale and needs sufficient funds and trained personnel.

Conclusion

The popularity of different and emerging illicit drugs and their strong addictive power contribute to the risk for infection with STDs through unsafe sexual behaviors. This chapter is intended to review the rates of STDs in drug users and to suggest relevant public health activities for prevention and control of STDs in drug users. The results reviewed in this chapter demonstrate a need for more data on STD rates in drug users including data on the prevalence and incidence rates of different STDs in different subgroups of drug users. Even more important is the need to develop tailored and targeted interventions for different subgroups of drug users and for different STDs. Because few interventions specifically focus on reducing STDs in drug users, there is a need for STD-specific interventions and for identifying whether and how these interventions, especially in the use of behavioral theoretical models (231), should differ from HIV interventions.

Programmatic challenges include integration of services and training of personnel to cover different STDs and to overcome the myths of working with drug users. Funding mechanisms for conducting research and programmatic activities related to STD control in drug users should be more extensive and integrated. Identifying and implementing on a wider scale effective strategies and interventions is critical in the process of using scarce resources to prevent and control STD infections in drug users.

While preventing initiation of drug use is the best means to prevent the negative consequences associated with drug abuse, working with those who use illicit drugs remains a critical strategy in preventing and reducing health consequences associated with drug use. Specialists from different disciplines, including behavioral and social scientists, health care providers, and public health practitioners, need to work together to improve the profile of evidence-based interventions for drug users and to put in place a rapid mechanism for transfer of interventions from research to practice. Delivery of preventive and curative STD services to drug users must be provided in a humane and professional fashion, assuring delivery of the full spectrum of care.

Acknowledgments: The authors thank Ms. Cecile Punzalan for participating in the literature review on the rates of STDs among drug users. The findings and conclusions in this chapter are those of the authors and do not necessarily represent the views of the Centers for Disease Control and Prevention.

References

1. Backmund M, Reimer J, Meyer K, Gerlach JT, Zachoval R. Hepatitis C virus infection and injection drug users: prevention, risk factors, and treatment. *Clinical Infectious Diseases.* 2005;40:S330–S335.
2. Eotlin ER, Edlin BR, Kresina TF, Raymond DB, et al. Overcoming barriers to prevention, care, and treatment of hepatitis C in illicit drug users. *Clinical Infectious Diseases.* 2005;40:S276–S285.
3. Des Jarlais DC, Diaz T, Perlis T, et al. Variability in the incidence of human immunodeficiency virus, hepatitis B virus, and hepatitis C virus infection among young injecting drug users in New York City. *American Journal of Epidemiology.* 2003;157:467–471.
4. Murrill C, Weeks H, Castrucci B, et al. Age-specific seroprevalence of HIV, hepatitis B virus, and hepatitis C virus infection among injection drug users admitted to drug treatment in 6 U.S. cities. *American Journal of Public Health.* 2002;92: 385–387.
5. Des Jarlais DC, Friedman SR. Fifteen years of research on preventing HIV infection among injecting drug users: what we have learned, what we have done, what we have not done. *Public Health Reports.* 1998;13:19–30.
6. Semaan S, Des Jarlais DC, Sogolow E, et al. A meta-analysis of the effect of HIV prevention interventions on the sex behaviors of drug users in the United States. *Journal of Acquired Immune Deficiency Syndrome.* 2002;30:S73–S93.
7. van Empelen P, Kok G, van Kesteren NMC, ven den Borne B, Bos AER, Schaalma HP. effective methods to change sex-risk among drug users: a review of psychosocial interventions. *Social Science and Medicine.* 2003;57:1593–1608.
8. Ksobiech K. A meta-analysis of needle sharing, lending, and borrowing behaviors of needle exchange program attenders. *AIDS Education and Prevention.* 2003;15: 257–268.
9. Shah KV, Solomon L, Daniel R, Cohn S, Vlahov D. Comparison of PCR and hybrid capture methods for detection of human papillomavirus in injection drug-using women at high risk of human immunodeficiency virus infection. *Journal of Clinical Microbiology.* 1997;35:517.
10. Stover CT, Smith DK, Schmid DS et al. Prevalence and risk factors for viral infections among human immunodeficiency virus (HIV)-infected and high-risk HIV uninfected women. *Journal of Infectious Diseases.* 2003;187:1388–1396.

11. McQuillan GM, Kruszon-Moran D, Kottiri BJ, Curtin L, Lucas JW, Kington RS. Racial and ethnic differences in the seroprevalence of 6 infectious diseases in the United States: Data from NHANES III, 1988-1994. *American Journal of Public Health*. 2004;94:1952–1958.

12. Kruszon-Moran D, McQuillan GM. Seroprevalence of six infectious diseases among adults in the United States by race/ethnicity: Data from the third national health and nutrition examination survey, 1988-1994. Hyattsville, MD: National Center for Health Statistics; 2005. Report No.: Advance data from vital and health statistics: no.352.

13. Tien PC, Kovacs A, Bacchetti P et al. Association between syphilis, antibodies to herpes simplex virus type 2, and recreational drug use and hepatitis B virus infection in the women's interagency HIV study. *Clinical Infectious Diseases*. 2004;39: 1363–1370.

14. Cook RL, Clark DB. Is there an association between alcohol consumption and sexually transmitted diseases? A systematic review. *Sexually Transmitted Diseases*. 2005;32:156–164.

15. Cohen DA, Ghosh-Dastidar B, Scribner R et al. Alcohol outlets, gonorrhea, and the Los Angeles civil unrest: a longitudinal analysis. *Social Science & Medicine*. 2006.

16. Markos AR. Alcohol and sexual behavior. *International Journal of STD and AIDS*. 2005;16:123–127.

17. Zenilman JM, Hook EW, Shepherd M, Smith P, Rompalo AM, Celentano DD. Alcohol and other substance use in STD clinic patients: relationships with STDs and prevalent HIV infection. *Sexually Transmitted Diseases*. 1994;21:220–225.

18. Palepu A, Raj A, Horton NJ, Tibbetts N, Meli S, Samet JH. Substance abuse treatment and risk behaviors among HIV-infected persons with alcohol problems. *Journal of Substance Abuse Treatment*. 2005;28:3–9.

19. Maxwell JC, Spence RT. Profiles of drug users in treatment. *Substance Use & Misuse*. 2005;40:1409–1426.

20. Maxwell JC. Party drugs: Properties, prevalence, patterns, and problems. *Substance Use & Misuse*. 2005;40:1203–1240.

21. Uddo M, Malow RM, Sucker PB. Opioid and cocaine abuse and dependence disorders. In: Sutker P, Adams H, eds. *Comprehensive Handbook of Psychopathology*. New York: Plenum; 1993;477–503.

22. Semple SJ, Zians J, Grant I, Patterson TL. Impulsivity and methamphetamine use. *Journal of Substance Abuse Treatment*. 2005;29:85–93.

23. Rawson RA, Washton A, Domier CP, Rieber C. Drugs and sexual effects: Role of drug type and gender. *Journal of Susbtance Abuse Treatment*. 2002;22:103–108.

24. Smith DE, Moser C, Wesson DR, et al. A clinical guide to the diagnosis and treatment of heroin-related sexual dysfunction. *Journal of Psychoactive Drugs*. 1982;14:91–99.

25. Semaan S, Kotranski L, Collier K, Lauby J, Halbert J, Feighan K. Temporal trends in HIV risk behaviors of out-of-treatment drug injectors and injectors who also smoke crack. *JAIDS*. 1998;19:274–281.

26. Des Jarlais DC, Semaan S. Interventions to reduce the sexual risk behavior of injecting drug users. *International Journal of Drug Policy*. 2005;16S:S58–S66.

27. Logan TK, Leukeld C. Sexual and drug use behaviors among female crack users: a multi-site sample. *Drug and Alcohol Dependence*. 2000;58:237–245.

28. Hoffman JA, Klein H, Eber M, Crosby H. Frequency and intensity of crack use as predictors of women's involvement in HIV-related sexual risk behaviors. *Drug and Alcohol Dependence*. 2000;58:227–236.

29. Baseman J, Ross M, Williams M. Sale of sex for drugs and drugs for sex: An economic context of sexual risk behavior for STDs. *Sexually Transmitted Diseases*. 1999;26:444–449.

30. Semaan S, Kotranski L, Collier K, Lauby J, Halbert J, Feighan F. Temporal trends in HIV risk behaviors among out-of-treatment women crack users: the need for drug treatment. *Drugs and Society*. 1998;13:13–33.

31. Santibanez SS, Garfein RS, Swartzendruber A, et al. Prevalence and correlates of crack-cocaine injection among young injection drug users in the United States, 1997–1999. *Drug and Alcohol Dependence*. 2005;77:227–233.

32. Anglin MD, Burke C, Perrochet B, Stamper E, Dawud-Noursi D. History of the methamphetamine problem. *Journal of Psychoactive Drugs*. 2000;32: 137–141.

33. Lineberry TW, Bostwick M. Methamphetamine abuse: a perfect storm of complications. *Mayo Clinic Proceedings*. 2006;81:77–84.

34. Farabee D, Prendergast M, Cartier J. Methamphetamine use and HIV risk among substance-abusing offenders in California. *Journal of Psychoactive Drugs*. 2002;34:295–300.

35. Gibson DR, Leamon MH, Flynn N. Epidemiology and public health consequences of methamphetamine use in California's Central Valley. *Journal of Psychoactive Drugs*. 2002;34:313–319.

36. Kral AH, Lorvick J, Edlin BR. Sex- and drug-related risk among populations of younger and older injection drug users in adjacent neighborhoods in San Francisco. *JAIDS*. 2000;24:162–167.

37. von M.C., Brecht ML, Anglin MD. Use ecology and drug use motivations of methamphetamine users admitted to substance use treatment facilities in Los Angeles: an emerging profile. *Journal of Addictive Diseases*. 2002;21:45–60.

38. Semple SJ, Patterson TL, Grant I. The context of sexual risk behavior among heterosexual methamphetamine users. *Addictive Behaviors*. 2004;29:807–810.

39. Semple SJ, Grant I, Patterson TL. Negative self-perceptions and sexual risk behavior among heterosexual methamphetamine users. *Substance Use & Misuse*. 2005;40:1797–1810.

40. Semple SJ, Patterson TL, Grant I. Determinants of condom use stage of change among heterosexually-identified methamphetamine users. *AIDS and Behavior*. 2004;8:391–400.

41. Semple SJ, Grant I, Patterson TL. Female methamphetamine users: social characteristics and sexual risk behavior. *Women and Health*. 2004;40(3):35–49.

42. Yen CF. Relationship between methamphetamine use and risky sexual behaviors in adolescents. *Kaohsiung Journal of Medical Science*. 2004;20:160–165.

43. Molitor F, Ruiz JD, Flynn N, Mikanda JN, Sun RK, Anderson R. Methamphetamine use and sexual and injection risk behaviors among out-of-treatment injection drug users. *American Journal of Drug & Alcohol Abuse*. 1999;25:475–493.

44. Semple SJ, Patterson TL, Grant I. The context of sexual risk behavior among heterosexual methamphetamine users. *Addictive Behaviors*. 2004;29:807–810.

45. Centers for Disease Control and Prevention. Methamphetamine use and HIV risk behaviors among heterosexual men—preliminary results from five northern California counties, December 2001–November 2003. *Morbidity and Mortality Weekly Report*. 2006;55:273–277.

46. Wohl AR, Johnson DF, Lu S, et al. HIV risk behaviors among African American men in Los Angeles County who self identify as heterosexual. *Journal of Acquired Immune Deficiency Syndrome*. 2002;31:354–360.

47. Fenton KA, Bloom F. STD prevention for men who have sex with men in the United States. In: Aral SO, Douglas JM, eds, Lipshutz JA, Assoc. ed. *Behavioral Interventions for Prevention and Control of sexually Transmitted Diseases,*. New York, NY: Springer-SBM; 2007.

48. Mansergh G, Purcell DW, Stall R, et al. CDC consultation on methamphetamine use and sexual risk behavior for HIV/STD infection: summary and suggestions. *Public Health Reports*. 2006;121:127–132.

49. Friedman SR, Flom PL, Kottiri BJ, et al. Drug use patterns and infection with sexually transmissible agents among young adults in a high-risk neighborhood in New York. *Addiction*. 2003;98:159–169.
50. Tyndall M, Patrick D, Spittal P, Li K, O'Shaughnessy M, Schechter M. Risky sexual behavior among injection drug users with high HIV prevalence. *Sexually Transmitted Diseases*. 2002;78 :S170–S175.
51. Strathdee S, Galai N, Safaeian M, et al. Sex differences in risk factors for HIV seroconversion among injection drug users: a 10-year perspective. *Archives of Internal Medicine*. 2001;161:1281–1288.
52. Kral AH, Bluthenthal RN, Lorvick J, Gee L, Bacchetti P, Edlin BR. Sexual transmission of HIV-1 among injection drug users in San Francisco, USA: Risk-factor analysis. *Lancet*. 2001;357:1397–1401.
53. Weber MP, Schoenbaum EE. Heterosexual transmission of HIV infection in intravenous and non-intravenous drug-using populations. *Archives of AIDS Research*. 1991;5:45–47.
54. Des Jarlais D.C., Wenston J, Sotheran JL, Maslansky R, Marmor M. Crack cocaine use in a cohort of methadone maintenance patients. *Journal of Substance Abuse Treatment*. 1992;9:319–325.
55. Chaisson R, Baccheti P, Osmond D, Brodie B, Sande M, Moss A. Cocaine use and HIV infection in intravenous drug users in San Francisco. *Journal of the Medical Association*. 1989;261:561–565.
56. Edlin BR, Irwin KL, Faruque S. Intersecting epidemics: crack cocaine use and HIV infection among inner-city young adults. *New England Journal of Medicine*. 1994;331:1422–1427.
57. Friedman SR, Flom PL, Kottiri BJ, et al. Prevalence and correlates of anal sex with men among young adult women in an inner city minority neighborhood. *AIDS*. 2001;15:2057–2060.
58. Friedman SR, Flom PL, Kottiri BJ, et al. Consistent condom use in the heterosexual relationships of young adults who live in a high-HIV-risk neighborhood and do not use "hard drugs". *AIDS Care*. 2001;2001:3–285.
59. Flom PL, Friedman SR, Kottiri BJ, et al. Stigmatized drug use, sexual partner concurrency, and other sex risk network and behavior characteristics of 10-24 year old youth in a high-risk neighborhood. *Sexually Transmitted Diseases*. 2001;28: 598–607.
60. White RG, Orroth KK, Kornromp EL, et al. Can population differences explain the contrasting results of the Mwanza, Rakai, and Masaka HIV/sexually transmitted disease intervention trials? A modeling study. *Journal of Acquired Immune Deficiency Syndrome*. 2004;37:1500–1513.
61. Gray R, Wawer M, Sewankambo N, et al. Relative risks and population attributable fraction of incident HIV associated with symptoms of sexually transmitted diseases and treatable symptomatic sexually transmitted diseases in Rakai District, Uganda. Rakai Project Team. *AIDS*. 1999;13:2113–2123.
62. Grosskurth HMF, Todd J, Mwijarubi E, et al. Impact of improved treatment of sexually transmitted diseases on HIV infection in rural Tanzania: randomized controlled trial. *Lancet*. 1995;346:530–536.
63. Hitchcock P, Fransen L. Preventing HIV infection: lessons from Mwanza and Rakai. *Lancet*. 1999;353:513–515.
64. Freeman EE, Weiss HA, Glynn JR, Cross PL, Whitworth JA, Hayes RJ. Herpes simplex virus 2 infection increases HIV acquisition in men and women: Systematic review and meta-analysis of longitudinal studies. *AIDS*. 2006;20:73–83.
65. Knight KR, Purcell D, Dawson-Rose C, Halkitis PN, Gomez CA, and the seropositive urban injectors study team. Sexual risk taking among HIV-positive injection drug users: contexts, characteristics, and implications for prevention. *AIDS Education and Prevention*. 2005;17:76–88.

66. Purcell DW, Metsch LR, Latka M, et al. Interventions for seropositive injectors - research and evaluation: an integrated behavioral intervention with HIV-positive injection drug users to address medical care, adherence, and risk reduction. *Journal of Acquired Immune Deficiency Syndrome*. 2004;37:S110–S118.

67. Maslow CB, Friedman SR, Perlis TE, Rockwell R, Des Jarlais DC. Changes in HIV seroprevalence and related behaviors among male injection drug users who do and do not have sex with men: New York City, 1990-1999. *American Journal of Public Health*. 2002;92:382–384.

68. Knowlton AR, Hoover DR, Chung SE, Celentano DD, Vlahov D, Latkin CA. Access to medical care and service utilization among injection drug users with HIV/AIDS. *Drug and Alcohol Dependence*. 2001;64:55–62.

69. French MT, McGeary KA, Chitwood DD, McCoy CB. Chronic illicit druguse, health services utilization and the cost of medical care. *Social Science & Medicine*. 2000;50:1703–1713.

70. Kanno MB, Zenilman J. Sexually transmitted diseases in injection drug users. *Infectious Disease Clinics of North America*. 2002;16:771–780.

71. Centers for Disease Control and Prevention. Sexually Transmitted Disease Surveillance, 2003. Atlanta, GA: Department of Health and Human Services; 2004.

72. Harcourt C, Donovan B. The many faces of sex work. *Sexually Transmitted Infection*. 2005;81:206.

73. Jones DL, Irwin KL, Inciardi J, et al. The high-risk sexual practices of crack-smoking sex workers recruited from the streets of three American cities. The multi-center crack cocaine and HIV infection study team. *Sexually Transmitted Diseases*. 1998;25:187–193.

74. Paone D, Cooper H, Alperen J, Shi Q, Des Jarlais DC. HIV risk behaviors of current sex workers attending syringe exchange: The experiences of women in five U.S. cities. *AIDS Care*. 1999;11:269–280.

75. Parsons JT. Researching the world's oldest profession: introduction to the special issue on sex work research. *Journal of Psychology and Human Sexuality*. 2005;17:1–3.

76. Bellis DJ. Reduction of AIDS risk among 41 heroin addicted female street prostitutes: effects of free methadone maintenance. *Journal of Addictive Diseases*. 1993;12:7–23.

77. Peugh J, Belenko S. Substance-involved women inmates: challenges to providing effective treatment. *The Prison Journal*. 1999;79:23–44.

78. Niveau G. Prevention of infectious disease transmission in correctional settings: a review. *Public Health*. 2006;2005:1–9.

79. Altice FL, Springer SA. Management of HIV/AIDS in correctional settings. In: Mayer KH, Pizer HF, eds. *The AIDS Pandemic: Impact on Science and Society*. San Diego: Elsevier Academic Press; 2005;449–487.

80. Des Jarlais DC, Semaan S. HIV and other sexually transmitted infections in injection drug users and crack cocaine smokers. In: Holmes K, Sparling PF, Mardh PA, Lemon SM, Stamm WE, Wasserheit JN, eds. *Sexually Transmitted Diseases*, 4th Ed. New York: McGraw Hill; in press.

81. Gunn RA, Montes JM, Toomey KE, et al. Syphilis in San Diego County 1983-1992: Crack cocaine, prostitution, and the limitations of partner notification. *Sexually Transmitted Diseases*. 1995;22:60–66.

82. Fullilove RE, Fullilove MT, Bowser BP, Gross SA. Risk of sexually transmitted disease among black adolescent crack users in Oakland and San Francisco. *JAMA*. 1990;263:851–855.

83. DeHovitz JA, Kelly P, Feldman J, et al. Sexually transmitted diseases, sexual behavior, and cocaine use in inner-city women. *American Journal of Epidemiology*. 1994;140:1125–1134.

84. Sharpe TT. *Behind the Eight Ball: Sex for Crack Cocaine Exchange and Poor Black Women*. Binghamton, NY. The Haworth Press, Inc; 2005.

85. Ross MW, Hwang LY, Zack C, Bull L, Williams ML. Sexual risk behaviors and STIs in drug abuse treatment populations whose drug of choice is crack cocaine. *International Journal of STD & AIDS*. 2002;13:769–774.

86. Bachmann LH, Lewis I, Allen R, et al. Risk and prevalence of treatable sexually transmitted diseases at a Birmingham substance abuse treatment facility. *American Journal of Public Health*. 2000;90:1615–1618.

87. Hwang LY, Ross MW, Zack C, Bull L, Rickman K, Holleman M. Prevalence of sexually transmitted infections and associated risk factors among populations of drug users. *Clinical Infectious Diseases*. 2000;31:920–926.

88. Gourevitch MN, Hartel D, Schoenbaum EE, et al. A prospective study of syphilis and HIV infection among injection drug users receiving methadone in the Bronx, NY. *American Journal of Public Health*. 1996;86:1112–1115.

89. Plitt SS, Sherman SG, Strathdee SA, Taha TE. Herpes simplex virus 2 and syphilis among drug users in Baltimore, Maryland. *Sexually Transmitted Infections*. 2005;81:248–253.

90. Lopez-Zetina J, Ford W, Weber M, et al. Predictors of syphilis seroreactivity and prevalence of HIV among street recruited injection drug users in Los Angeles County, 1994-1996. *Sexually Transmitted Infections*. 2000;76:462–469.

91. Musher DM. Early syphilis. In: Holmes KK, Sparling PF, Mardh PA, Lemon SM, Stamm WE, Piot P, et al., eds. *Sexually Transmitted Diseases*, 3rd Ed. New York: McGraw-Hill; 1999;479–485.

92. Sparling PF. Natural history of syphilis. In: Holmes KK, Sparling PF, Mardh PA, Lemon SM, Stamm WE, Piot P, et al., eds. *Sexually Transmitted Diseases*, 3rd Ed. New York: McGraw-Hill; 1999;473–478.

93. Lopez-Zetina J, Ford W, Weber M, et al. Predictors of syphilis seroreactivity and prevalence of HIV among street recruited injection drug users in Los Angeles County, 1994-1996. *Sexually Transmitted Infections*. 2000;76:462–469.

94. Liebschutz JM, Finley EP, Braslins PG, Christiansen D, Horton NJ, Samet JH. Screening for sexually transmitted infections in substance abuse treatment programs. *Drug and Alcohol Dependence*. 2003;70:93–99.

95. Williams ML, Elwood WN, Weatherby NL et al. An assessment of the risks of syphilis and HIV infection among a sample of not-in-treatment drug users in Houston, Texas. *AIDS Care*. 1996;8:671–682.

96. Klass PE, Brown ER, Pelton SI. The incidence of prenatal syphilis at the Boston city hospital: a comparison across four decades. *Pediatrics*. 1994;94:24–28.

97. Webber MP, Lambert G, Bateman DA, Hauser WA. Maternal risk factors for congenital syphilis: a case-control study. *American Journal of Epidemiology*. 1993; 137:415–422.

98. Centers for Disease Control and Prevention. Sexually Transmitted Disease Surveillance, 2004. Atlanta, GA: U.S. Department of Health and Human Services; 2005.

99. Latka M, Ahern J, Garfien RS, et al. Prevalence, incidence, and correlates of chlamydia and gonorrhea among young adult injection drug users. *Journal of Substance Abuse*. 2001;13:73–88.

100. Lally MA, Alvarez S, Macnevin R, et al. Acceptability of sexually transmitted infection screening among women in short-term substance abuse treatment. *Sexually Transmitted Diseases*. 2002;29:752–755.

101. Gunn RA, Lee MA, Callahan DB, Gonzales P, Murray PJ, Margolis HS. Integrating hepatitis, STD, and HIV services into a drug rehabilitation program. *American Journal of Preventive Medicine*. 2005;29:27–33.

102. Plitt SS, Garfein RS, Gaydos CA, Strathdee SA, Sherman SG, Taha TE. Prevalence and correlates of *Chlamydia trachomatis, Neisseria gonorrhoeae, Trichomonas vaginalis* infections, and bacterial vaginosis among a cohort of young injection drug users in Baltimore, Maryland. *Sexually Transmitted Diseases*. 2005;32:446–453.

103. Levine OS, Vlahov DA, Koehler J, Cohn S, Spronk AM, Nelson KE. Seroepidemiology of hepatitis B virus in a population of injecting drug users: association with drug injection patterns. *American Journal of Epidemiology.* 1994;142:341.

104. Estrada AL. Epidemiology of HIV/AIDS, hepatitis B, hepatitis C, and tuberculosis among minority injection drug users. *Public Health Reports.* 2002;117: S126–S134.

105. Kottiri BJ, Friedman SR, Euler GL, et al. A community-based study of hepatitis B infection and immunization among young adults in a high-drug-use neighborhood in New York City. *Journal of Urban Health.* 2005;82:479–487.

106. Rich JD, Anderson BJ, Schwartzapfel B, Stein MD. Sexual risk for hepatitis B virus infection among hepatitis C virus-negative heroin and cocaine users. *Epidemiology and Infection.* 2005;30:1–7.

107. Rich JD, Ching CG, Lally MA, et al. A review of the case for hepatitis B vaccination of high-risk adults. *American Journal of Medicine.* 2003;114:318.

108. Kellerman SE, Hanson DL, McNaghten AD, Fleming PL. Prevalence of chronic hepatitis B and incidence of acute hepatitis B infection in human immunodeficiency virus-infected subjects. *Journal of Infectious Diseases.* 2003;188: 571–577.

109. Hagan H, McGough J, Thiede H, Weiss N, Hopkins S, Alexander E. Syringe exchange and risk for infection with hepatitis B and C viruses. *American Journal of Epidemiology.* 1999;49:203–212.

110. Thiede H, Hagan H, Murrill CS. Methadone treatment and HIV and hepatitis B and C risk reduction among injectors in the Seattle area. *Journal of Urban Health.* 2000;77:331–345.

111. Strathdee SA, Latka M, Campbell J, et al. Factors associated with interest in initiating treatment for hepatitis C virus (HCV) infection among young HCV-infected injection drug users. *Clinical Infectious Diseases.* 2005;40:S304–S312.

112. Tortu S, McMahon JM, Hamid R, Neaigus A. Women's drug injection practices in East Harlem: an event analysis in a high-risk community. *AIDS and Behavior.* 2003;7:317–328.

113. Kuo I, Sherman SG, Thomas DL, Strathdee SA. Hepatitis B virus infection and vaccination among young injection and non-injection drug users: Missed opportunities to prevent infection. *Drug and Alcohol Dependency.* 2004;73:69–78.

114. Seal KH, Ochoa KC, Hahn JA, Tulsky JP, Edlin BR, Moss AR. Risk of hepatitis B infection among young injection drug users in San Francisco: opportunities for intervention. *Western Journal of Medicine.* 2000;172:16–20.

115. Heimer R, Clair S, Gran LE, Bluthenthal RN. Hepatitis-associated knowledge is low and risks are high among HIV-aware injection drug users in three U.S. cities. *Addiction.* 2002;97:1277–1287.

116. Zimet GD, Mays RM, Fortenberry JD. Vaccines against sexually transmitted infections: Promise and problems of the magic bullets for prevention and control. *Sexually Transmitted Diseases.* 2000;27:49–52.

117. Mezzelani P, Venturini L, Turrina G, Lugoboni F, Des Jarlais DC. High compliance with a hepatitis B virus vaccination program among intravenous drug users. *Journal of Infectious Diseases.* 1991;163:923.

118. Rodrigo JM, Serra MA, Aparisi L, et al. Immune response to hepatitis B vaccine in parenteral drug abusers. *Vaccine.* 1992;10:801.

119. Borg L, Khuri E, Wells A, et al. Methadone maintained former heroin addicts, including those who are anti-HIV-1 seropositive, comply with and respond to hepatitis B vaccination. *Addiction.* 1999;94:493.

120. Ross MW, Hwang LY, Leonard L, Teng M, Duncan L. Sexual behavior, STDs and drug use in a crack house population. *International Journal of STD and AIDS.* 1999;10:224–230.

121. Miller WC, Ford CA, Morris M, et al. Prevalence of chlamydial and gonococcal infections among young adults in the United States. *Journal of American Medical Association*. 2004;291:2229–2236.
122. Weinstock H, Berman S, Cates W. Sexually transmitted diseases among American youth: Incidence and prevalence estimates, 2000. *Perspectives on Sexual and Reproductive Health*. 2004;36:6–10.
123. Dicker LW, Mosure DJ, Berman SM, Levine W, and the regional infertility prevention program. Gonorrhea prevalence and coinfection with chlamydia in women in the United States, 2000. *Sexually Transmitted Diseases*. 2003;30: 472–476.
124. Strathdee SA, Sherman SG. The role of sexual transmission of HIV in injection and non-injection drug users. *Journal of Urban Health*. 2003;80:iii7–iii14.
125. Semple SJ, Grant I, Patterson TL. Negative self-perceptions and sexual risk behavior among heterosexual methamphetamine users. *Substance Use & Misuse*. 2005;40:1797–1810.
126. National Commission on Correctional Health Care. A report to Congress. Prevalence of communicable disease, chronic disease, and mental illness among the inmate population. Available at: www.ncchc.org.
127. Wang SA, Matson SC. Implementing adolescent STD and reproductive health services in non-traditional settings. Presentation made at the annual meeting of the society of adolescent medicine, Boston, MA; 2002.
128. Wang SA, Rietmeijer CA, Matson SC, et al. Monitoring STD prevalence and reproductive health care among adolescent women in special settings in the United States, 1999-2001. Presentation made at the National STD Prevention Conference, San Diego, CA; 2002.
129. Stevens SJ, Erickson JR, Estrada AL. Characteristics of female sexual partners of injection drug users in southern Arizona: implications for effective HIV risk reduction interventions. *Drugs and Society*. 1993;7:129–142.
130. Montgomery SB, Hyde J, De Rosa CJ, et al. Gender differences in HIV risk behaviors among young injectors and their social network members. *American Journal of Drug & Alcohol Abuse*. 2002;28:453–475.
131. Evans JL, Hahn JA, Page-Shafer K, et al. Gender differences in sexual and injection risk behavior among active young injection drug users in San Francisco (the UFO Study). *Journal of Urban Health*. 2003;80:137–146.
132. Miller M, Neaigus A. Networks, resources and risk among women who use drugs. *Social Science & Medicine*. 2001;52:967–978.
133. Neaigus A, Miller M, Friedman S, et al. Potential risk factors for the transition to injecting among non-injecting heroin users: a comparison of former injectors and never injectors. *Addiction*. 2001;96:847–860.
134. Miller M, Neaigus A. Sex partner support, drug use and sex risk among HIV-negative non-injecting heroin users. *AIDS Care*. 2002;14:801–813.
135. Friedman SR, Curtis R, Neaigus A, Jose B, Des Jarlais D. *Social Networks, Drug Injectors' Lives, and HIV/AIDS*. New York: Kluwer Academic/Plenum Publishers; 1999.
136. Friedman SR, Neaigus A, Jose B, et al. Sociometric risk networks and risk for HIV infection. *American Journal of Public Health*. 1997;87:1289–1296.
137. Williams ML, Atkinson J, Klovdahl A, Ross MW, Timpson S. Spatial bridging in a network of drug-using male sex workers. *Journal of Urban Health*. 2005;1: i35–i42.
138. Aral SO. Patrons of sex partner recruitment and types of mixing as determinants of STD transmission: limits to the spread of sexually transmitted infections. *Venereology*. 1995;8:240–242.
139. Aral SO. Patterns of sexual mixing: mechanisms for or limits to the spread of STIs? *Sexually Transmitted Infections*. 2000;76:415–416.

140. Potterat JJ, Phillips-Plummer L, Muth SQ, et al. Risk network structure in the early epidemic phase of HIV transmission in Colorado Springs. *Sexually Transmitted Infections.* 2002;78 (Suppl 1):i159–i163.

141. Potterat JJ, Muth SQ, Rothenberg RB et al. Sexual network structure as an indicator of epidemic phase. *Sexually Transmitted Infections.* 2002;78 (Suppl 1):i52–i58.

142. Jolly AM, Muth SQ, Wylie JL, Potterat JJ. Sexual networks and sexually transmitted infections: a tale of two cities. *Journal of Urban Health.* 2002;78:433–445.

143. Kottiri B, Friedman S, Neaigus A, Curtis R, Des Jarlais DC. Risk networks and racial/ethnic differences in the prevalence of HIV infection among injection drug users. *JAIDS.* 2002;30:95–104.

144. Friedman S, Curtis R, Neaigus A, Jose B, Des Jarlais D. *Social Networks, Drug Injectors' Lives and HIV/AIDS.* New York: Plenum; 1999.

145. Friedman SR, Aral S. Social networks, risk-potential networks, health, and disease. *Journal of Urban Health.* 2001;78:411–417.

146. Neaigus A, Miller M, Friedman SR, Des Jarlais DC. Sexual transmission risk among non-injecting heroin users infected with HIV or hepatitis C. *Journal (sp.) of Infectious Diseases.* 2006;84:359–363.

147. Neaigus A, Friedman S, Jose B, et al. High-risk personal networks and syringe sharing as risk factors for HIV infection among new drug injectors. *Journal of Acquired Immune Deficiency Syndrome and Human Retrovirology.* 1996;11:499–509.

148. Friedman SR, Jose B, Neaigus A, et al. Multiple racial/ethnic subordination and HIV among drug injectors. In: Singer M, ed. *The Political Economy of AIDS.* Amityville: Baywood Press; 1998:105–127.

149. Friedman SR, Sufian M, Des Jarlais DC. The AIDS epidemic among Latino intravenous drug users. In: Glick R, Moore J, eds. *Drugs in Hispanic Communities.* New Brunswick: Rutgers University Press; 1990;45–54.

150. Friedman SR, Sotheran JL, Abdul-Quader A, et al. The AIDS epidemic among Blacks and Hispanics. *Milbank Quarterly.* 1987;65:455–499.

151. Latkin CA, Knowlton RA. Micro-social structural approaches to HIV prevention: a social ecological perspective. *AIDS Care.* 2005;17:S102–S113.

152. Latkin CA, Sherman S, Knowlton A. HIV prevention among drug users: outcome of a network-oriented peer outreach intervention. *Health Psychology.* 2003;22:332–339.

153. Latkin CA, Hua W, Forman VL. The relationship between social network characteristics and exchanging sex for drugs or money among drug users in Baltimore, MD. *Internat J STD AIDS.* 2003;14:770–775.

154. Latkin CA, Mandell W, Oziemkowska M, et al. Using social network analysis to study patterns of drug use among urban drug users at high risk for HIV/AIDS. *Drug and Alcohol Dependency.* 1995;38:1–9.

155. Latkin CA, Mandell W, Vlahov D, Oziemkowska M, Celantano DD. The long-term outcome of a personal network-oriented HIV prevention intervention for injection drug users: the Safe study. *American Journal of Community Psychology.* 1996;24:341–364.

156. DeHovitz JA, Kelly P, Feldman J, et al. Sexually transmitted diseases, sexual behavior, and cocaine use in inner-city women. *American Journal of Epidemiology.* 1994;140:1125–1134.

157. Williams PB, Ekundayo O. Study of distributions and factors affecting syphilis epidemic among inner-city minorities of Baltimore. *Public Health.* 2001;115:387–393.

158. Farrell M, Gowing L, Marsden J, Ling W, Ali R. Effectiveness of drug dependence treatment in HIV prevention. *International Journal of Drug Policy.* 2005;16:67–75.

159. Metzger DS, Navaline H, Woody GE. Drug abuse treatment as HIV prevention. *Public Health Reports.* 1998;113:97–106.

160. Metzger DS, Navaline H. Human immunodeficiency virus prevention and the potential for drug abuse treatment. *Clinical Infectious Diseases*. 2003;37:S451–S456.
161. Prendergast ML, Urada D, Podus D. Meta-analysis of HIV risk-reduction interventions within drug abuse treatment programs. *Journal of Consulting and Clinical Psychology*. 2001;69:389–405.
162. Latka MH, Wilson TE, Cook JA et al. Impact of drug treatment on subsequent sexual risk behavior in a multisite cohort of drug-using women: a report from the Women's Interagency HIV study. *Journal of Substance Abuse Treatment*. 2005;29:329–337.
163. Sorensen J, Copeland A. Drug abuse treatment as an HIV prevention strategy: a review. *Drug and Alcohol Dependence*. 2000;59:17–31.
164. Pollack HA, D'Aunno T, Lamar B. Outpatient substance abuse treatment and HIV prevention: an update. *Journal of Substance Abuse Treatment*. 2006;30:39–47.
165. Cami J, Farre M. Drug addiction. *New England Journal of Medicine*. 2003;349:975–986.
166. Rowe CL, Liddle HA. Treating adolescent substance abuse: State of the science. In: Liddle HA, Rowe CL, eds. *Adolescent Substance Abuse: Research and Clinical Advances*. Cambridge: Cambridge University Press; 2006.
167. Iguchi MY, Stitzer ML, Bigelow GE, Liebson IA. Contingency management in methadone maintenance: effects of reinforcing and aversive consequences on illicit poly drug use. *Drug and Alcohol Dependence*. 1998;22:7.
168. Shroeder JR, Epstein DH, Umbricht A, Preston KL. Changes in HIV risk behaviors among patients receiving combined pharmacological and behavioral interventions for heroin and cocaine dependence. *Addictive Behaviors*. 2005.
169. Woody GE, Gallop R, Lubrosky L, et al. HIV risk reduction in the National Institute on Drug Abuse Cocaine Collaborative treatment Study. *Journal of Acquired Immune Deficiency Syndrome*. 2003;33:82–87.
170. Dackis CA, Kampman KM, Lynch KG, Pettinati HM, O'Brien CP. A double-blind, placebo-controlled trial of modafinil for cocaine dependence. *Neuropsychopharmacology*. 2005;30:205–211.
171. Coffin PO, Blaney S, Fuller C, Vadnai L, Miller S, Vlahov D. Support for buprenorphine and methadone prescription to heroin-dependent patients among New York city physicians. *American Journal of Drug & Alcohol Abuse*. 2006;32:1–6.
172. Caldiero RM, Parran TV, Adelman CL, Piche B. Inpatient initiation of buprenorphine maintenance vs. detoxification: can retention of opioid-dependent patients in outpatient counseling be improved? *The American Journal on Addictions*. 2006;15:1–7.
173. Fischer G, Ortner R, Rohrmeister K, et al. Methadone versus buprenorphine in pregnant addicts: a double-blind, double-dummy comparison study. *Addiction*. 2006;101:275–281.
174. Cretzmeyer M, Sarrazin MV, Huber DL, Block RI, Hall JA. Treatment of methamphetamine abuse: Research findings and clinical directions. *Journal of Substance Abuse Treatment*. 2003;24:267–277.
175. Rawson RA, Gonzales R, Brethen P. Treatment of methamphetamine use disorders: An update. *Journal of Substance Abuse Treatment*. 2002;23:145–150.
176. Gardner LI, Metsch LR, Anderson-Mahoney P, et al. Efficacy of a brief case management intervention to link recently diagnosed HIV-infected persons to care. *AIDS*. 2005;19:423–431.
177. Tesh SN. *Political Ideology and Disease Prevention Policy*. New Brunswick, NJ: Rutgers University Press; 1988.
178. Minkler M. Personal responsibility for health? A review of the arguments and the evidence at century's end. *Health Education and Behavior*. 1999;26:140.
179. Roy DJ. Injection drug use and HIV/AIDS: an ethics commentary on priority issues. *Health Canada*. 2000.

180. Marantz PR. Blaming the victim: the negative consequences of preventive medicine. *American Journal of Public Health.* 1990;80:1186–1187.
181. Rhodes T, Singer M, Bourgois P, Friedman SR, Strathdee SA. The social structural production of HIV risk among injection drug users. *Social Science and Medicine.* 2005;61:1026–1044.
182. Friedman SR, Cooper HLF, Tempalski B, et al. Relationships of deterrence and law enforcement to drug-related harms among drug injectors in U.S. metropolitan areas. *AIDS.* 2006;20:93–99.
183. Becker MH. A medical sociologist looks at health promotion. *Journal of Health and Social Behavior.* 1993;34:1–6.
184. Guttman N, Salmon CT. Guilt, fear, stigma and knowledge gaps: ethical issues in public health communication interventions. *Bioethics.* 2004;18(6):531–552.
185. Elliott R. Drug control, human rights, and harm reduction in the age of AIDS. *HIV AIDS Policy Law Review.* 2004;9:86–90.
186. Wynia MK. Science, faith and AIDS: the battle over harm reduction. *American Journal of Bioethics.* 2005;5:3–4.
187. Marlatt, GA, ed. *Harm Reduction: Pragmatic Strategies for Managing High-Risk Behaviors.* New York: Guilford; 1988.
188. Wodak A, Cooney A. Effectiveness of sterile needle and syringe programs. *International Journal of Drug Policy.* 2005;16:S31–S44.
189. Cotton-Oldenburg NU, Carr P, DeBoer JM, Colison EK, Novotny G. Impact of pharmacy-based syringe access on injection practices among injecting drug users in Minnesota. 1998-1999. *Journal of Acquired Immune Deficiency Syndrome.* 2001;27:183–192.
190. Hagan J, Thiede H. Changes in injection risk behavior associated with participation in the Seattle needle exchange program. *Journal of Urban Health.* 2000;77:369–382.
191. Vlahov D, Junge B, Brookmeyer R, et al. Reductions in high risk drug use behaviors among participants in the Baltimore needle exchange program. *Journal of Acquired Immune Deficiency Syndrome and Human Retrovirology.* 1997;16:400–406.
192. Vlahov D, Junge B. The role of needle exchange programs in HIV prevention. *Public Health Reports.* 1998;113:75–80.
193. Des Jarlais DC, Marmor M, Paone D, et al. HIV incidence among injecting drug users in New York City syringe exchange programs. *Lancet.* 1996;348:987–991.
194. Des Jarlais DC. Research, politics and needle exchange. *American Journal of Public Health.* 2000;90:1392–1394.
195. Broadhead RS, van Julst Y, Heckathorn DD. The impact of a needle exchange's closure. *Public Health Reports.* 1999;114:439–447.
196. Rich JD, Dickinson B, Liu K. Strict syringe laws in Rhode Island are associated with high rates of reusing syringes and HIV risks among drug users. *Journal of Acquired Immune Deficiency Syndrome and Human Retrovirology.* 1998;18:S140.
197. Gostin LA. Legal and public policy interventions to advance the population's health. In: Gostin LA, ed. *Promoting Health: Intervention Strategies from Social and Behavioral Research.* Washington, D.C.: National Academy Press; 2000:390–416.
198. Strathdee SA, Celentano DD, Shah N, et al. Needle exchange attendance and health care utilization promote entry into detoxification. *Journal of Urban Health.* 1999;76:448–460.
199. McKnight C, Des Jarlais DC, Perlis T, et al. Update: Syringe exchange programs—United States, 2002. *Morbidity and Mortality Weekly Report.* 2005;54:673–676.
200. Hahn J, Page-Shafer K, Lum P, Ochoa K, Moss A. Hepatitis C virus infection and needle exchange use among injection drug users in San Francisco. *Hepatology.* 2001;34.

201. Kresina TF, Khalsa J, Cesari H, Francis H. Hepatitis C virus infection and substance abuse: medical management and developing models of integrated care. *Clinical Infectious Diseases*. 2005;40:S259–S262.
202. Edlin BR, Kresina TF, Raymond DB, et al. Overcoming barriers to prevention, care, and treatment of hepatitis C in illicit drug users. *Clinical Infectious Diseases*. 2005;40:S276–S285.
203. Edlin BR. Hepatitis C prevention and treatment for substance users in the United States: acknowledging the elephant in the living room. *International Journal of Drug Policy*. 2004;15:81–91.
204. Needle RH, Trotter RT, Singer M, et al. Rapid assessment of the HIV/AIDS crisis in racial and ethnic minority communities: an approach for timely community interventions. *American Journal of Public Health*. 2003;93:970–979.
205. Needle RH, Burrows D, Friedman SR, et al. Effectiveness of community-based outreach in preventing HIV/AIDS among injecting drug users. *International Journal of Drug Policy*. 2005;16S:S45–S57.
206. Manhart LE, Holmes KK. Randomized controlled trials of individual-level, population-level, and multilevel interventions for preventing sexually transmitted infections: what has worked? *The Journal of Infectious Diseases*. 2005;191: S7–S24.
207. Exner TM, Gardos S, Seal DW, Ehrhardt AA. HIV sexual risk reduction interventions with heterosexual men: the forgotten group. *AIDS and Behavior*. 1999;3:347–358.
208. Ward DJ, Rowe B, Pattison H, Taylor RS, Radcliff KW. Reducing the risk of sexually transmitted infections in genitourinary medicine clinic patients: A systematic review and meta-analysis of behavioral interventions. *Sexually Transmitted Infection*. 2005;81:386–393.
209. Semaan S, Kay L, Strouse D, et al. A profile of U.S.-based trials of behavioral and social interventions for HIV risk reduction. *Journal of Acquired Immune Deficiency Syndromes*. 2002;30 (Suppl 1):S30–S50.
210. Pinkerton SD, Layde PMDW CHW, et al. All STDs are not created equal: An analysis of the differential effects of sexual behavior changes on different STDs. *Internat J STD AIDS*. 2003;14:320–328.
211. Quan VM, Steketee RW, Valleroy L, Weinstock H, Karon J, Janssen R. HIV incidence in the United States, 1978–1999. *JAIDS*. 2002;31:188–201.
212. Kotranski L, Semaan S, Collier K, Lauby J, Halbert J, Feighan K. Effectiveness of an HIV risk reduction counseling intervention for out-of-treatment drug users. *AIDS Education and Prevention*. 1998;10:19–33.
213. Ompad D, Fuller C, Vlahov D, Thomas D, Strathdee S. Lack of behavior change after disclosure of hepatitis C virus infection among young injection drug users in Baltimore, Maryland. *Clinical Infectious Diseases*. 2002;35:783–788.
214. Holmes KK, Levine R, Weaver M. Effectiveness of condoms in preventing sexually transmitted infections. *Bulletin of the World Health Organization*. 2004;82:454–461.
215. Warner L, Newman DR, Austin HD, et al. Condom effectiveness for reducing transmission of gonorrhea and chlamydia: the importance of assessing partner infection status. *American Journal of Epidemiology*. 2004;159:242–251.
216. Semaan S, Klovdahl A, Aral SO. Protecting the privacy, confidentiality, relationships, and medical safety of sex partners in partner notification and management studies. *The Journal of Research Administration*. 2004;35:39–53.
217. Friedman SR, Des Jarlais DC, Sotheran JL, Garber J, Cohen H, Smith D. AIDS and self-organization among intravenous drug users. *International Journal of Addiction*. 1987;24:97–100.
218. Sufian M, Friedman SR, Curtis R, Neaigus A, Stepherson B. Organizing as a new approach to AIDS risk reduction for intravenous drug users. *Journal of Addictive Diseases*. 1991;10:89–98.

219. Dawson-Rose C, Shade SB, Lum PJ, Knight KR, Parsons JT, Purcell DW. Health care experiences of HIV positive injection drug users. *Journal of Multicultural Nursing & Health*. 2005;11:23–30.

220. Seal KH, Kral AH, Lorvick J, McNees A, Gee L, Edlin BR. A randomized controlled trial of monetary incentives vs. outreach to enhance adherence to the hepatitis B vaccine series among injection drug users. *Drug and Alcohol Dependence*. 2003;71:127–131.

221. Harcourt C, Donovan B. The many faces of sex work. *Sexually Transmitted Infection*. 2005;81:206.

222. Oliva G, Rienks J, Udoh I, Smith CD. A university and community-based organization collaboration to build capacity to develop, implement, and evaluate an innovative HIV prevention intervention for an urban African American population. *AIDS Education and Prevention*. 2005;17:300–316.

223. Conklin TJ, Lincoln T, Tuthill RW. Self-reported health and prior health behaviors of newly admitted correctional inmates. *American Journal of Public Health*. 2000;90:1939–1941.

224. Kraut-Becher JR, Gift TL, Haddix AC, Irwin KL, Greifinger RB. Cost-effectiveness of universal screening for chlamydia and gonorrhea in US jails. *Journal of Urban Health*. 2004;81:453–471.

225. Lally MA, Macnevin R, Sergie Z et al. A model to provide comprehensive testing for HIV, viral hepatitis, and sexually transmitted infections at a short-term drug treatment center. *AIDS Patient Care & STDs*. 2005;19:298–305.

226. Strauss SM, Astone JM, Des Jarlais DC, Hagan H. Integrating hepatitis C services into existing HIV services: The experiences of a sample of U.S. drug treatment units. *AIDS Patient Care & STDs*. 2005;19:78–88.

227. Litwin AH, Soloway I, Gourevitch MN. Integrating services for injection drug users infected with hepatitis C virus with methadone maintenance treatment: challenges and opportunities. *Clinical Infectious Diseases*. 2005;40:S339–S345.

228. Clanon KA, Mueller J, Harank M. Integrating treatment for hepatitis C virus infection into an HIV clinic. *Clinical Infectious Diseases*. 2005;15:S362–S366.

229. Pugatch DL, Levesque BG, Lally MA et al. HIV testing among young adults and older adolescents in the setting of acute substance abuse treatment. *JAIDS*. 2001;27:135–142.

230. Lally MA, Macnevin R, Sergie Z, et al. A model to provide comprehensive testing for HIV, viral hepatitis, and sexually transmitted infections at a short-term drug treatment center. *AIDS Patient care and STDs*. 2005;19:298–305.

231. Albarracin D, Gillette JC, Earl AN, Glasman LR, Durantini MR, Ho MH. A test of major assumptions about behavior change: a comprehensive look at the effects of passive and active HIV prevention interventions since the beginning of the epidemic. *Psychology Bulletin*. 2005;131:856–897.

Part 4

Understanding Methods

18

Quantitative Measurement

Mary McFarlane, Ph.D., and Janet S. St. Lawrence, Ph.D.

In order to ascertain whether any behavior needs intervention, the form that intervention should take, or whether an intervention is effective, careful attention must be paid to measurement. Measurement exists in many forms throughout public health, ranging from clinical applications to monitoring, surveillance, and intervention efforts. We count the number of infected individuals, measure the effective dose of medications, and measure a variety of physical characteristics of our patients. Measuring behavior, however, is a complicated business, requiring careful forethought regarding the exact information we want to gather. In most cases, we will be unable to directly observe the behaviors that put people at risk—or reduce their risk—for STDs. Thus, we must rely on questionnaires, interviews, role-play scenarios, biological outcomes, and other forms of measurement to assess a person's risk for STD. Each type of measurement can provide important contributions to the knowledge of behavioral risk for STD. Ideally, the information obtained from the various measurement methods will converge to provide a coherent picture of the behaviors that lead to disease transmission, and how to intervene upon them.

In this chapter, we will address several different forms of measurement that can provide useful information in the context of a behavioral intervention. In addition, we will discuss the methods by which researchers can determine whether their measurements, whatever their type, are "accurate." That is, we will discuss the extent to which different measurements can adequately represent the true nature of the behaviors we measure. In the literature related to self-reported behaviors, the term *accuracy* is rarely used, but instead we focus on evaluating the *reliability* and *validity* of instruments. These terms are used to refer to the quality of a number of different kinds of measurement in public health.

Types of Measurement

Directly Observed Behaviors

We have already referred to measurement that incorporates the direct observation of behaviors, which is exactly that: a researcher observes an individual for a specific time period or while the individual is engaged in a particular

Behavioral Interventions for Prevention and Control of Sexually Transmitted Diseases.
Aral SO, Douglas JM Jr, eds. Lipshutz JA, assoc ed. New York: Springer Science+
Business Media, LLC; 2007.

activity. The researcher carefully records the behaviors that he or she observes during the specified time period. This method of measurement is particularly difficult when the topic is sexual behavior. Masters and Johnson (1966, 1979) performed research on the physiology of the human sexual response cycle by directly observing participants engaging in sex in laboratory settings. In these studies, it was clear that a researcher was conducting a study, and the participants were well-informed as to what was expected of them. In contrast, Humphreys (1970) conducted *participant-observation research*, in which he served as the "lookout" for gay men engaging in sex in public places, such as restrooms. His role as a lookout (i.e., a participant not in the actual sexual act, but in the hiding of it) enabled him to directly observe the sexual behavior as it occurred. Humphreys then used the license-plate numbers of the men's cars to trace them, and interviewed them in their homes afterward. Naturally, this particular study yielded a wealth of data about behavior, but it also violated a long list of scientific and ethical principles. Most critically, the participants in this study were not given the opportunity to refuse to participate, did not provide informed consent, and were in fact unaware that they were participating in a research study. The Humphreys study illustrates just a few of the problems with participant-observation research in sexual behavior, and it is difficult to imagine a situation in which such direct observation would be possible today.

While it may not be possible to directly observe sexual behavior per se, it is possible to observe a number of behaviors that may be related to it. For example, a researcher can sit in a busy nightclub and observe single individuals, couples, and individuals who pair off by the end of the night. The researcher may be interested in the amount of time a person spends talking to a potential sex partner before leaving the club, what social rituals are observed, and so on (1–3). Similarly, a researcher may log in to a chat room or bulletin board to watch the interactions that facilitate sexual contact between two other internet users (4).

While studies of directly observed behavior can yield rich information about the nature of sexual behavior, it is imperative that researchers pay close attention to the scientific and ethical issues involved in such efforts. For example, in most situations, it is ethically unacceptable for a researcher to deceive the people he or she is observing. If approached, it is usually appropriate for the researcher to acknowledge his or her role and to be honest about the research efforts. Finally, it is critical for researchers to remain as objective and uninvolved in the behavior as possible, lest the recorded observations be biased by the researcher's experiences. It is usually a good idea to have more than one researcher observing behavior, so that individual *observer biases* can be illuminated and reduced by comparing observations.

Directly Observed Proxy Behaviors

As we have discussed, it is rarely possible to obtain data on sexual behavior by direct observation. In some cases, however, it is possible to gather data on a different behavior that is closely related to the behavior in question; that is, we observe a *proxy* for the behavior that we cannot feasibly observe directly. For example, we may want to measure the consistent and correct condom use of our respondents. As a part of this query, we want to determine how skilled the participants are at removing a condom from its packet and correctly putting it on the penis. It is clearly impossible for us to (directly) observe the participant engaging in this behavior; however, we can bring the respondent to a research setting and ask him or her to place a condom on a model of a penis. By determining whether the respondent engaged in the proper steps required for this process, we can gauge his or her skill level with respect to correct condom use. Obviously this is an imperfect solution, because applying a condom in a research setting is different than applying a condom during the sexual act itself; however, the former may represent the best *proxy behavior* for correct condom use that we can feasibly observe. Other proxies for prevalence of condom use may include searching for discarded condom packets in party venues and monitoring sales of condoms from vending machines (5).

Condom use with a model of a penis has been used as a proxy measure in several studies of preventive behavior (6). Other proxy behaviors that have been observed include behaviors related to sexual negotiation skills. For example, if a health educator is trying to determine whether women can successfully convince their partners to use condoms, he or she might ask the women to engage in role-playing tasks to demonstrate their skills. In the role-playing scenarios, a research assistant will play the male role, refusing to use condoms and making a variety of arguments against condoms. The woman (study participant) will react to those arguments and refusals, and the researcher will observe her responses and negotiation skills. Again, this is clearly an imperfect measure of the woman's ability to negotiate in a true sexual situation. However, we are unlikely to be able to observe her reactions in a natural setting, so we measure the proxy behavior.

Self-Reported Behaviors

Another solution to our problem of measuring behaviors that we cannot observe is to ask questions regarding a person's sexual behavior. This is, of course, a highly personal, often taboo, topic for people to discuss, so strong attention to details such as respondent comfort, interviewer rapport (if applicable), and asking exactly the right questions in the culturally accepted manner is merited. In the arena of respondent comfort, it is imperative to ensure that the respondent is as comfortable as possible with the questions being asked and the method in which they are being asked. For example, a series of questions asked by a doctor during a medical exam may be perceived by the patient as a part of routine care. These same questions asked by a research assistant might be construed as offensive.

In public health programs and in behavioral research, the most common methods of acquiring answers to questions are individual interviews, in which a staff member asks questions of the participant and notes the responses on a form, and paper-and-pencil surveys, in which a respondent reads each question and writes the answer on the survey form. There are advantages and disadvantages to each method, and there are interesting alternatives to these common strategies.

Individual interviews are often preferable because staff members can ensure that respondents understand the questions, that the responses are appropriately noted, and that any comments from the respondents are properly considered. In addition, many skilled interviewers are able to establish a rapport with respondents, which is thought to increase the respondent's willingness to answer questions openly and honestly. It is possible, however, that respondents would prefer not to talk to an interviewer about sexual behavior, and would rather complete a paper-and-pencil questionnaire.

Paper-and-pencil instruments have the advantage of cost savings, ease of administration, privacy, and the lack of need for an interviewer presence. For purposes of privacy and nonjudgmental survey environment, a paper-and-pencil instrument may be ideal. However, limitations include the inability to determine whether respondents understood the questions and responded to each and every one appropriately. Asking respondents to follow "skip patterns" on paper-and-pencil questionnaires is often tedious, and the sheer length of questions written on paper may be intimidating to persons of low literacy.

In an effort to create an efficient, objective, impersonal questionnaire that avoids the problems of interpersonal discomfort, low literacy, and interviewer time, investigators have created surveys using a variety of technological advances. Some of these methods, such as audio computer-assisted self-interviews (A-CASI), have proven useful in encouraging the reporting of sensitive information in some settings. Indeed, the use of A-CASI has been shown to enhance data quality when compared to other survey methods; specifically, respondents were more likely to report sensitive behaviors using these automated systems (7–9). Using such systems, the respondent is able to hear the interview being read, select the response on the computer, automatically proceed through the survey and its component skip patterns, and avoid disclosure to a person asking questions. Still, it may be the case that some people prefer to interact with people rather than computers, and this should be determined prior to expending the resources required to program an A-CASI questionnaire. Similarly, telephone administration of questionnaires has some appeal for researchers who prefer to engage respondents outside of the clinic setting using personal contact that is not face-to-face. An excellent review of the various administration modes is included in an article by Schroder et al. (10).

Scholars have debated whether self-reported sexual behavior is accurate, believable information (11). One of the factors that may detract from the accuracy of such data is memory error, which can in turn be affected by several issues. For example, the frequency of the behavior being measured may affect the responses provided by the participant. If a young man has had sexual intercourse with only one woman, one time, then his response is fairly easy to remember accurately. However, if this same young man has had sex with more than eight partners, more than three times each, then he may not recall specific information with as much accuracy. In general, response accuracy decreases with the increasing frequency of a given behavior (12). In fact, as behavioral frequency increases, people tend to begin rounding their numbers (12). For example, someone who has had sex with 13 partners may round to 15, thus providing a less accurate estimate.

Another research issue that may influence the accuracy of self-reported data is the type of data gathered. For example, if we ask someone how frequently he has engaged in oral sex in the past three months, the answer may be less accurate than simply asking if he has engaged in this behavior at all. This makes sense; after all, if someone engaged in oral sex, he is likely to recall it and report that he has done so, but he may not accurately report the number of times this behavior has occurred. However, in this case we must ask ourselves which type of data we prefer—a rough estimate of frequency or a simple statement of incidence? The use of frequency data, which can easily be transformed into incidence data if necessary, is intuitively preferable; however, investigators often use simple yes/no questions in order to save time and respondent effort.

Finally, the length of the recall period and the methods used to motivate recall of sexual behaviors during that period are strongly related to the accuracy of self-reported data. Asking an adolescent to think back over the past month may be very different than asking an adult who is out of school to consider the same time period. The adolescent can be provided with school-related cues, such as school vacations or football games, but adults may not have such salient "landmarks" available in the past month. In contrast, adults may simply recall information over this time period more accurately than adolescents. Literacy skills play a role in recall as well as the degree to which behaviors fluctuated over the course of the recall period (13).

In order to enhance recall of sexual behavior, some researchers have used techniques such as a time line follow-back method, in which a calendar is used to review the recall period and note when sexual behaviors occurred (13). This technique has been shown to produce stable estimates of frequency of sexual behavior. In general, each population will have separate issues related to recall and accuracy of self-reported behavior, and these should be investigated prior to collecting this type of data.

In addition to the fluctuations in accuracy that are incurred as described above, self-reported behavioral data may be influenced by the desire to project a personal image of one sort or another. For example, in different situations a man may want to over-report his sexual behavior to appear virile, or may want to under-report it to appear responsible and safe. A person may not wish to admit to his or her sexual activities with members of the same sex, or may wish to de-emphasize sexual practices that are considered taboo in some cultures. The desire to report the data that participants think researchers want to hear is called social desirability bias (14,15).

Taken together, there are clearly threats to the accuracy of self-reported sexual behavior. However, these measures are usually the only representation of sexual behavior that we can feasibly obtain. Thus, researchers and program staff must use care to avoid as many of the aforementioned threats as possible.

Cognitive Measures

In addition to measuring actual behaviors, we often want to measure the respondents' knowledge, attitudes and perceptions (KAP) of sex, sexual risk, disease, or condom use. These constructs are measured in a variety of intervention settings. Because these constructs do not represent observable behaviors, but rather are "latent" and based in the respondents' thought processes, we refer to them as *cognitive measures*. The distinction between measuring an observed behavior and measuring a latent construct is critical. Suppose we want to measure an athlete's foot speed. This can be accomplished using straightforward methods, such as time trials of an observable behavior (running). On the other hand, suppose we want to measure the same person's intelligence, a characteristic that we cannot see or measure directly. This is a latent (unobservable) construct, and the best we can do is collecting several measures that assess various types of intelligence (verbal skills, spatial thinking, memory, and reasoning). These measures are all statistically related to each other, and we say that they are all interrelated because they all measure some piece of the latent construct we call "intelligence."

Along these lines, we cannot know a person's true, underlying tendency toward STD-related behavior because it is an unobservable concept. We can, however, measure KAP that are all related to risk for STD. Knowledge measures, obviously, are questions or groups of questions that assess a respondent's knowledge of a particular topic, such as human papillomavirus, or syphilis. Knowledge is most often assessed using true/false or multiple-choice questionnaires, in which there is a correct response and one or more "distractors" (incorrect alternatives). Attitudes are more subjective constructs, reflecting a person's thoughts, feelings, opinions, or positions on particular topics. These also are measured with surveys; however, a key difference between attitude scales and knowledge assessments is that there is no "correct" response to attitude questions. Perceptions are generally defined as an individual's impressions, insights, intuitions, or subjective assessment of a particular object or topic. For example, one patient may perceive a diagnosis of syphilis as immensely disturbing, while another may perceive it less negatively. A clinic's location may be a perceived barrier for some patients but not for others. Knowing the clinic staff can be perceived as humiliating for one patient but comforting for another.

Separate from KAP, but theoretically related, are cognitive measure can be called intentions, such as the intention to change sexual risk behavior or reduce substance use. Intentions have been measured in behavioral interventions because of the assumption that a change in intentions is necessary (but not always sufficient) for a change in behavior to occur. The use of intentions, and the many social-cognitive theories that encompass these constructs, are described in Chapter 2 (16,17).

Why should we measure these cognitive variables? There are several reasons, starting with the fact that many of the cognitive variables have been shown to be related to actual sexual behaviors, as well as transmission or acquisition of infections. In the usual circumstances of behavioral research, when we cannot afford to study enough people to allow us to detect differences in actual disease or behavior rates, it may be helpful to measure cognitive variables. In so doing, we rely on the assumption that there is an important relationship between these variables and biological outcomes, i.e., changes in the cognitive variables (i.e., attitudes, intentions) will often result in changes in disease rates. One example of this hypothesized relationship may be that STD-related knowledge will lead to increased health-care seeking, which in turn results in reduced complications associated with STDs (18).

In addition, cognitive variables often serve as a *moderator* of relationships between two observable events or behaviors. For example, let us suppose that health-care seeking is related to a reduced probability of future STD. A cognitive variable such as knowledge can moderate this relationship as follows: health-care seeking has a stronger relationship to reduced infection rates among people who know more about STD than among people who know less about STD. In this case, we say that knowledge of STD moderates the relationship between health-care seeking and future infections.

Measuring Cognitive Variables

The construction of survey questions and instruments is a difficult, exacting process. For guidance on creating questionnaires and surveys, several accessible books and monographs are available from the SAGE Applied Social Research Methods Series (19–21).

Measurement error. In any classical measurement scenario, there are several more assumptions that must be made. These assumptions involve measurement error, or imprecision in the way we capture latent variables. The first assumption related to measurement error is that it is assumed to vary randomly. That is, no characteristic about a person is likely to make his or her measurement more or less erroneous. If we sum up these errors over a large group of respondents, then the average error is zero. Thus, while we may have random error in an individual's measurement, these random errors should cancel each other out when a large group of people are combined.

The second assumption is that the errors associated with one item on a survey are not related to the errors associated with any other item. This is because the errors occur at random, or by chance, and are not associated with any other item or error. Finally, we assume that the errors in measurement are not related to the value of the underlying construct that we are trying to measure. For example, people with more negative attitudes should not have greater measurement error than people with more positive attitudes, or vice versa.

Reliability. Why should we worry about measurement error? Measurement error is the key to determining how well our scale, questionnaire, or survey performs. Inversely related to measurement error is reliability, or the consistency of responses to a questionnaire provided by the same respondent under different conditions or on different occasions—or even using different sets of equivalent questions. If some portion of an individual's score (the error) can fluctuate as a result of these irrelevant, or random situations, then the reliability of a questionnaire is the degree to which the score stays the same in the face of these changing situations. For example, suppose an archer is shooting arrows at a bulls-eye in the middle of a target, and being an imperfect shot, she misses with some arrows. If the arrows are scattered all over the target, then we may say that her shot is unreliable. However, if the arrows are tightly clustered around the center spot, but randomly distributed to the left, right, top and bottom, then the archer is a reliable shooter because she achieves nearly the same result every time (19). If the archer's arrows systematically fall to the right of the target, then the error in measurement is not random, and we say that a *bias* has been introduced. Just as the archer tries to hit her target, we are trying to measure underlying, latent variables with as much reliability and as little bias as possible.

There are many different ways to assess reliability of questionnaires, and different forms of reliability may be more or less appropriate in different research circumstances. For example, test-retest reliability is assessed by computing the closeness of relationship between people's responses to a questionnaire taken at two different points in time. The time points may be a day apart, or a year or more, depending on the topic and the research agenda. A reliable questionnaire, using this definition, is one that produces the same results the second time as it did the first. It is useful to study test-retest reliability for traits that do not change over time; however, this construct is inappropriate for studying such constructs as mood or sexual behavior, which can change significantly over time.

A similar type of reliability is called alternative-form reliability. It is similar to test-retest reliability in that it requires an individual to complete a questionnaire at two different points in time. However, in alternative-form reliability, the questionnaire at the second time point is not the exact same questionnaire as at the first time point; rather, the second questionnaire is an alternative form of the first. The two questionnaires measure the same latent construct, but may contain different questions, different wording, etc. The similarity of results across the two sets of responses is the measure of reliability. This form of reliability assessment seeks to circumvent the possibility (prevalent in test-retest situations) that individuals will remember their responses to the first questionnaire, and use the exact same answers the second time. However, it is often difficult or impractical to create two separate questionnaires that measure the same construct.

A third form of reliability, split-half reliability, does not require two separate sets of responses from the same person. Instead, it divides the questionnaire in half, and computes the similarity in responses to the first half and responses to the second half. Intuitively, it is clear that this form of reliability is related to the consistency of an individual's responses across the two halves of the questionnaire. The obvious flaw is that there are multiple ways of dividing a questionnaire in half (i.e., beginning and end, odd and even), and the different "splits" might result in different levels of reliability.

In order to circumvent the problems with reliability assessments as identified above, most researchers rely on a measure of *internal consistency* called Cronbach's alpha (22). Computing Cronbach's alpha requires only one administration of the questionnaire to the study participants, and does not require alternative forms or creative methods of splitting the questionnaire. Instead, Cronbach's alpha is a function of the average relationship of each item to every other item in the questionnaire, or the average inter-item correlation. Interestingly, the alpha coefficient may also be interpreted as the average of all the reliability estimates we would obtain if we were to compute split-half reliability estimates using every possible division of the questionnaire, and then average those estimates. Cronbach's alpha can take on values from 0.0 to 1.0, with numbers above 0.80 being considered strong evidence for reliability. The coefficient can be somewhat arbitrarily improved by adding items to the questionnaire, but only if those items are related to the construct being measured. Thus, if the average inter-item correlation remains the same, we can increase the reliability of our questionnaire by increasing the length from four items to eight. However, this approach will provide diminishing returns as more items are added, and longer questionnaires are often undesirable in public health settings.

Validity. It is possible for a questionnaire to be quite reliable, returning consistent results as defined above, but not *valid*. The most common, general definition of *validity* is the degree to which a questionnaire measures what it was designed to measure. Ideally, we would be able to examine a person's responses to a questionnaire about sexual history, and then we would somehow tap into their entire store of memories about sexual encounters, and determine whether the responses to the questions adequately captured the reality of the person's sexual history. If the responses to the questionnaire were strongly related to the reality we found in the person's memory bank, we would say that the questionnaire was a valid measure of past sexual behavior.

Unfortunately, when we ask questions of our respondents, we rarely or never have a "gold standard" against which to compare the responses. Thus, we must turn to less perfect measures of validity. We might examine criterion-related validity, in which the responses to the questionnaire are compared with some other measure of the construct we are trying to capture. For example, suppose we administer a questionnaire to substance users on the occasion of their entrance to a treatment facility. The purpose of the questionnaire is to determine whether the prospective patient is likely to succeed in the drug rehabilitation program. We would validate this questionnaire by comparing it to the degree of success enjoyed by the patient after treatment. This is a special case of criterion validity called predictive validity, because the questionnaire predicts the occurrence of a future event. In concurrent validity, we would measure the degree to which the questionnaire was related to a contemporaneous event.

Another form of validity, content validity, is the extent to which a questionnaire captures all aspects of the construct it is trying to measure. For example, a questionnaire about depression that contained only items related to fatigue and apathy would not be considered valid under this definition. For such a questionnaire to be valid, the researcher must conduct a thorough review of the topic, enumerate its components (e.g., fatigue, apathy, sadness, hopelessness, weight changes, sleep changes, and so on), and develop questions that adequately measure each of the components. Content validity is difficult to measure or assess objectively, but must be established by meticulous scholarship, collaboration and exploration.

A complicated but important measure of validity is construct validity. Construct validity refers to the way in which a questionnaire is related to other measures. However, these other measures are not measures of the same construct, but rather measures of different constructs that are theoretically related to the topic of our questionnaire. For example, say we are creating a survey of women's abilities to negotiate condom use with their male partners. Background research, behavioral theories, and common sense might tell us the hypothesized relationship of our survey to other measures we might study. Negotiation ability might be positively related to self-reported condom use, but negatively related to the degree to which women fear their partner's anger. The ability to negotiate with a partner may be positively related to self-esteem, but not at all related to the age at first sexual intercourse. To establish this type of validity, we must examine all of the constructs we are measuring, generate reasoned and informed hypotheses about how they relate to one another, and then test these hypotheses with the data we obtain. When our survey is related to other measures as we hypothesized, then we have strong evidence for convergent validity. If our survey is unrelated to measures that we hypothesized should have little or no relationship to it, then we have evidence for discriminant validity.

Biological Outcome Measures

In addition to the cognitive, behavioral self-report, and behavioral measures described above, biological outcome measures can provide an additional data source. Public health practitioners generally place greater confidence in biological measures, believing they offer more valid information about the effectiveness of an intervention (23). This belief reflects skepticism about the reliability and validity of cognitive and behavioral self report measures, as well as an underlying assumption that the behavioral changes produced by an intervention should reduce HIV and STD incidence. In truth, there is no gold standard for measurement and whether the evaluation of behavioral interventions should include biological measures is a complex issue. Just as cognitive, behavioral self-report, and behavioral measures each have their own strengths and limitations, so do biological measures. Thus, just as one evaluates the reliability, validity, and feasibility of other types of measures, it becomes equally as important to examine the advantages and disadvantages of biological measures, especially when one disease is being used as a measurement proxy for another.

As discussed earlier, reliability and validity require thoughtful consideration when selecting cognitive or behavioral self report measures. In the case of the biological measures, the parallel terminology is the *specificity* and *sensitivity* of the tests. Sensitivity refers to the tests' accuracy in identifying people who are actually infected, the "true positives." Specificity refers to a test's ability to correctly identify people who are not infected, the "true negatives." Schachter and Chow (24) noted that even biological measures can be fallible: "there are no perfect diagnostic tests . . . if isolation of the bacteria or virus is the test being performed, then sensitivity is the problem because no culture test is 100% sensitive. However specificity is not a problem with this kind of test. The modern no culture tests may cause problems because of both specificity and sensitivity."

If the primary goal of an intervention is to reduce an STD in a population, it makes sense to use incidence of that STD as one of the outcome measures. It is also reasonable to assess STD incidence to support that a behavioral intervention interrupted disease transmission (25). If an intervention is designed to lower the incidence of chlamydia (CT) for example, biological tests for CT would be a logical outcome measure for the study. CT is prevalent in the United States, particularly in young adults, thus it may have an adequately high incidence to be a feasible outcome measure. In addition, this STD is readily cured. As a result, a sequence of screening, treatment and later re-screening can assess the outcome from intervention. However, this straightforward relationship is not present for all diseases. When biological and self-report data are not congruent with one another, it cannot be concluded that the behavioral measures are faulty and the biological measures are meaningful (11). The reasons for this cautionary statement about the complexity of using behavioral measures or biological measures as a proxy for one another are described below.

First, if the primary goal of an intervention is to prevent HIV transmission, then incidence of HIV infection is unlikely to be a feasible measure, especially in the United States, where prevalence is very low (11). When an intervention is intended to reduce HIV transmission, the use of STD biomarkers as a surrogate for HIV introduces a flawed assumption that any change that reduces HIV incidence will be reflected in STD tests. For a number of reasons, this is not necessarily the case. There is no simple linear relationship between STDs and HIV, especially when STD data are being used as a surrogate for HIV data (26). Measurable changes in STD incidence may or may not reflect changes in HIV incidence. In reality, the relationship between a given STD and HIV incidence is equally as complex as the relationship between self-reported behavior and HIV incidence (11).

The prevalence or incidence of a disease will also need to be considered. If prevalence and incidence are low in the sample, then a very large sample will be needed to detect a small, but potentially meaningful, change in STD or HIV incidence (27). Aral and Peterman (27) illustrated the relationship between prevalence, incidence, and sample sizes. They noted that an intervention whose goal is to have an 80% likelihood of detecting a difference at an alpha of .05 will need to have 313 persons in each of the intervention and control arms to be able to detect an increase from 20% to 30% condom use. On the other hand, if the outcome of interest is a decrease from 10% to 8% in gonorrhea incidence in STD clinic patients, then 3312 subjects would be needed for each arm of the study. In a general population sample where disease prevalence is considerably lower than in STD clinic patients or with a different disease that has a lesser prevalence, these numbers would be even greater. In order to detect a decrease in HIV incidence from 0.5% to 0.4%, Aral and Peterman (27) reported that 72,307 subjects would be needed in each arm of the study. Thus, the introduction of biomarkers can have a substantial impact on both the implementation demands and the cost of the research, given the potential need to greatly increase sample size, pay for collection and processing the specimens, and provide treatment to those who are found to be infected.

In addition, all tests are not of equal cost or complexity. Some are more costly than others. Some may require specialized equipment that is not readily available and the researchers also must ensure the quality of their laboratory's performance. In field studies, stringency in the collecting, storage, transportation, and analysis of samples may be lacking and a reference laboratory to corroborate the findings may be required (11).

Some biological tests are invasive, requiring a blood sample or a vaginal or penile swab. When these tests are employed, participant refusals may increase. This, in turn, biases the study's results since the results from the biological tests may not accurately represent those who refused to undergo the test. Thus, qualities of a test may bias the obtained results if the test is perceived as being onerous and generates refusals from participants who are not willing to complete that aspect of the assessment.

Additionally, biological tests can only reflect relatively recent or current behaviors (25). If a behavior occurs only rarely, the test may not be useful. For adolescents, sexual behavior is often episodic and intermittent. This poses a complicating factor to any exclusive reliance on biological measures.

Even the meaning of a positive test result can be subject to some uncertainty. Many tests cannot reveal whether a positive result is detecting a new, or incident, infection. With a bacterial STD, the results cannot always indicate whether the person has acquired a new infection or whether they may previously have been infected but the pre-existing infection was not detected, not treated, or was unresponsive to the treatment that was provided. If the STD is viral then the test often cannot disentangle whether this is a new infection or is a recurrence of a pre-existing infection.

Another complication is that there is not a straightforward linear relationship between condom use and disease incidence. Both the condom measurement strategy and characteristics of the disease can complicate any interpretation of the results. Condom use is most often measured as a self-reported behavior. Zenilman and colleagues (28) concluded there was no relationship between self-reported condom use and STD incidence when disease prevalence was comparable in condom users and nonusers. The problem was that the self-reports in the Zenilman et al study assessed reported consistency of use, but did not provide any information about correct use. When investigators have assessed correct application of a condom onto a penile model, errors were observed in 25% to 58% of the samples' participants (25,29–32). St Lawrence and colleagues (31) found that only 51% of a community sample of 445 African American women could put a condom onto a penile model correctly. Warner et al. (32) asked college men who reported using condoms to quantify the number of times they experienced problems in the preceding month. They found that 31.9% of the men reported putting the condom on inside out and then flipping it over; 17% initiated intercourse without a condom and interrupted later to put on the condom; 12.8% reported breakage during intercourse; 8.5% began intercourse with a condom and removed it before ejaculation; and 6.4% reported that the condom fell off during intercourse or withdrawal. Note that these same participants could all validly report using a condom, yet they were still susceptible to transmitting or acquiring an STD or HIV because of incorrect use. Thus, the findings from the study of Zenilman et al. may have reflected measurement artifact because they ignored the issue of correct use (28).

Different STDs also have very different transmissibility, infectiousness, and exposure probabilities. This means for some diseases, condoms are more effective in preventing transmission than for others (33,34). As a result, the relationship between condom use and biological measures is not a simple linear correspondence, despite the evidence that correct and consistent condom use is more effective than not using a condom for all STDs. In addition, transmissibility can vary greatly by gender, age, and the probability of being exposed to a pathogen is determined by the prevalence of disease in the person's sexual network.

Taken together, these issues illustrate why using a biological measure to asses a behavioral intervention is complex. Biological measures can make an additive contribution to understanding an intervention's outcome, but cannot be used as the solitary standard for measuring a behavioral intervention. Mathematical modeling studies are being used in an effort to quantify the potential changes in incidence given specific behavioral changes, but until the relationships between behavioral and biomedical measures are more precisely quantified, one measure cannot be used as a surrogate for the other. The best results are probably to be obtained when sound measures from each of the four measurement domains can be employed and show consistent patterns of change.

Summary and Conclusions

Each domain of measurement, whether cognitive, self-report, behavioral, or biological, offers a partial contribution to the interpretation of outcome following a prevention program. Overall an aggregate approach to measurement using all available measurement domains is, under optimal conditions, the best approach. When all four measurement domains converge, showing parallel change, confidence in an intervention's effectiveness is strengthened. Thus, it is most useful to assess the outcome from a behavioral intervention using multiple measurement domains (cognitive, behavioral, self-reported behaviors, and biological measures) given that we are unable to directly measure the behaviors in an actual sexual episode and must necessarily rely on surrogate, analogue, self-report, and proxy measures. However, when cost or sample size precludes the use of biologic measures, there is substantial evidence to suggest that the other measurement domains can yield reliable and valid evidence of a behavioral intervention's impact.

References

1. Aral SO, St. Lawrence JS. The ecology of sex work and drug use in Saratov Oblast, Russia. *Sexually Transmitted Diseases*. 2002;29:789–805.
2. Aral SO, St Lawrence JS, Tikhonova L, Safarova E, Parker KA, Shakarishvili A, Ryan CA. The social organization of commercial sex work in Moscow, Russia. *Sexually Transmitted Diseases*. 2003;30:39–45.
3. Aral SO, St. Lawrence JS, Dyatlov R, Koslov A. Commercial sex work, drug use, and sexually transmitted infections in St. Petersburg, Russia. *Social Science in Medicine*. 2005;60:2181–2190.
4. Bull SS, McFarlane M. Soliciting sex on the Internet: what are the risks for sexually transmitted diseases and HIV? *Sexually Transmitted Diseases*. 2000;27:545–550.
5. Steinfirst JL, Cowell SA, Presley BA, Reifler CB. Vending machines and the self-care concept. *Journal of the American College of Health*. 1985;34:37–39.
6. Crosby R, DiClemente RJ, Wingood GM, Sionean C, Cobb BK, Harrington K, Davies S, Hook EW 3rd, Oh MK. Correct condom application among African-American adolescent females: the relationship to perceived self-efficacy and the association to confirmed STDs. *Journal of Adolescent Health*. 2001;29:194–199.
7. Turner CF, Villarroel MA, Rogers SM, Eggleston E, Ganapathi L, Roman AM, Al-Tayyib A. Reducing bias in telephone survey estimates of the prevalence of drug use: a randomized trial of telephone audio-CASI. *Addiction*. 2005;100:1432–1434.
8. Perlis, TE, Des Jarlais, DC, Friedman, SR, Arasteh, K, Turner, CF (2004). Audio-computerized self-interviewing versus face-to-face interviewing for research data collection at drug abuse treatment programs. *Addiction*. 2004;99:885–896.
9. Rogers SM, Willis G, Al-Tayyib A, Villarroel MA, Turner CF, Ganapathi L, Zenilman J, Jadack R. Audio computer assisted interviewing to measure HIV risk behaviours in a clinic population. *Sexually Transmitted Infections*. 2005;81:501–507.
10. Schroder KE, Carey MP, Vanable PA. Methodological challenges in research on sexual risk behavior: II. Accuracy of self-reports. *Annals of Behavioral Medicine*. 2003;26:104–123.
11. Pequegnat W, Fishbein M, Celentano D, Ehrhardt, A, Garnett G, Holtgrave D, Jaccard J, Schacter H, Zenilman J. NIMH/APPC workgroup on behavioral and biological outcomes in HIV/STD prevention studies: a position statement. *Sexually Transmitted Diseases*. 2000:27:127–132.
12. Kauth MR, St. Lawrence JS, Kelly JA. Reliability of retrospective assessments of sexual risk behavior: a comparison of biweekly, three-month, and twelve-month self-reports. *AIDS Education and Prevention*. 1991;3:207–215.
13. Catania JA, Gibson DR, Chitwood DD, et al. Methodological problems in AIDS behavioral research: influences on measurement error and participation bias in studies of sexual behavior. *Psychological Bulletin*. 1990;108:339–362.
14. Rosenthal R, Persinger GW, Fode KL. Experimenter bias, anxiety, and social desirability. *Perception and Motor Skills*. 1962;15:73–74.
15. King M, Bruner G. Social desirability bias: a neglected aspect of validity testing. *Psychology and Marketing*, 2003;17:79–103.
16. Choi KH, Yep GA, Kumekawa E. HIV prevention among Asian and Pacific Islander American men who have sex with men: a critical review of theoretical models and directions for future research. *AIDS Education and Prevention*. 1998;10 (3 Supp):19–30.
17. Abraham C, Sheeran P. Modeling and modifying young heterosexuals' HIV-preventive behaviors; a review of theories, findings, and educational implications. *Patient Education and Counseling*. 1994;23:173–86.

18. Van Devanter N, Messeri P, Middlestadt SE, Bleakley A, Merzel CR, Hogben M, Ledsky R, Malotte CK, Cohall RM, Gift TL, St. Lawrence JS. A community-based intervention designed to increase preventive health care seeking among adolescents: the Gonorrhea Community Action Project. *American Journal of Public Health*, 2005;95:331–337.

19. Carmines EG, Zeller RA. *Reliability and Validity Assessment*. Thousand Oaks, CA: SAGE Publications; 1979. Applied Social Research Methods Series.

20. DeVellis RF. *Scale Development: Theory and Applications*. Thousand Oaks, CA: SAGE Publications; 1991. Applied Social Research Methods Series.

21. Fowler FJ. *Improving Survey Questions: Design and Evaluation*. Thousand Oaks, CA: SAGE Publications; 1995. Applied Social Research Methods Series.

22. Cronbach LJ. Coefficient alpha and the internal structure of tests. *Psychometrika*, 1951;16:297–334.

23. NIMH Collaborative STD/HIV Prevention Trial. Behavioral and biologic endpoints for international trials to prevent sexually transmitted infections and HIV. 2007; Manuscript in preparation.

24. Schachter J., Chow JM. The fallibility of diagnostic tests for sexually transmitted disease: the impact on behavioral and epidemiologic studies. *Sexually Transmitted Diseases*. 1995;22:191–196.

25. Fishbein M., Pequegnat W. Evaluating AIDS prevention interventions using behavioral and biological outcome measures. *Sexually Transmitted Diseases*. 2000;27:101–110.

26. Pinkerton SD, Layde PM, DiFranceisco W, Chesson HW; NIMH Multisite HIV Prevention Trial Group. All STDs are not created equal: An analysis of the differential effects of sexual behaviour changes on different STDs. *International Journal of STD & AIDS*. 2003;14:320–328.

27. Aral SO, Peterman TA. A stratified approach to untangling the behavioral/biomedical outcomes conundrum. (Editorial) *Sexually Transmitted Diseases*. 2002;29: 530–532.

28. Zenilman JM, Weissman CS, Rompalo ASM, et al. Condom use to prevent incident STDs: the validity of self-reported condom use. *Sexually Transmitted Diseases*. 1995;22:5–21.

29. Crosby R, Salazar LF, DiClemente RJ, Yarber WL, Galiendo,AM, Staples-Horne M. Accounting for failures many improve precision: Evidence supporting improved validity of self-reported condom use. *Sexually Transmitted Diseases*. 2005; 32: 513–515.

30. Kamb ML, Fishbein M, Douglas JM, et al.; Project RESPECT Study Group. HIV/STD prevention counseling for high risk behaviors: results from a multicenter, randomized controlled trial. *Journal of the American Medical Association*. 1998; 280:1161–1167.

31. St. Lawrence JS, Wilson TE, Eldridge GD, Brasfield TL,, O'Bannon RE. Community-based interventions to reduce low income, African American women's risk of sexually transmitted diseases: a randomized controlled trial of three theoretical models. *American Journal of Community Psychology*. 2001;29:937–964.

32. Warner L, Clay-Warner J, Boles J, Williamson J. Assessing condom use practices: implications for evaluating method and user effectiveness. *Sexually Transmitted Diseases*. 1998; 998:273–277.

33. Cates W., Holmes KK. Re: Condom efficacy against gonorrhea and nongonococcal urethritis. *American Journal of Epidemiology*. 1996;143:843–844.

34. Warner L., Stone K, Magalliuso M, Buehler JW, Austin HD. Condom use and risk of gonorrhea and chlamydia: a systematic review of design and measurement factors assessed in epidemiologic studies. *Sexually Transmitted Diseases*. 2006;3:36–51.

Qualitative Methods

Pamina M. Gorbach, M.H.S., Dr. P.H., and Jerome Galea, M.S.W.

Qualitative research is broadly defined as a set of interpretative, material practices that make the world visible by turning it into a series of representations (e.g., field notes, observations, interview recordings) through the study of things in their natural settings (1). In sexually transmitted infection (STI)/HIV research, qualitative research is the study of the words and the significance of certain behaviors and seeks to answer why people practice certain behaviors and to describe the social organization of sexual interactions. Qualitative data are words such as those collected verbatim in interviews or as transcribed in observation notes. This is to be contrasted with *quantitative* research, which is the study of numbers and often focuses on "how many" people practice "which different behaviors." The aim of quantitative research is to find numerical patterns in responses to survey questionnaires or observed behaviors, the results of which indicate the magnitude of people's decisions and behaviors and how these are distributed across a study population. Both quantitative and qualitative research are essential to study the complex factors that sustain and feed STI epidemics throughout the world and work together to design interventions that change the course of such epidemics by reducing transmission. This chapter will examine how qualitative methods are applied within STI/HIV research; outline the main types of qualitative research approaches used in STI/HIV research, including advantages and disadvantages of each application; and discuss different sampling approaches. Contemporary examples of each method are given throughout.

STI/HIV Qualitative Research

Qualitative research is used in a number of different ways by researchers working on STI/HIV (Figure 1), but the three most common applications are as follows:

1. *The formative stage*: qualitative research can serve as a tool to generate ideas or a preliminary step in developing a quantitative study or intervention. In this case, qualitative research is conducted before a survey or intervention is designed and the data are used to develop a second and usually larger study.

Behavioral Interventions for Prevention and Control of Sexually Transmitted Diseases. Aral SO, Douglas JM Jr, eds. Lipshutz JA, assoc ed. New York: Springer Science+ Business Media, LLC; 2007.

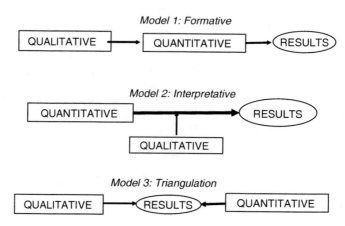

Figure 1 Uses of qualitative methods.

2. *Results interpretation*: qualitative research can help explain the result of a quantitative study (e.g., a subsample of a study population could be interviewed to assist in the understanding of quantitative patterns).
3. *Triangulation of data:* when qualitative and quantitative data are collected simultaneously, the results of both data collection efforts can be analyzed together, compared, and findings can be interpreted based on both sources of data. In this way, convergence patterns would be sought to develop or corroborate an interpretation (2).

When reading qualitative research, the method used and how it was applied must be understood for correct interpretation of findings. In a very practical sense, it is important to know how generalizable the results are (or are not) to gauge the level of relevance to local settings.

Review of Different Qualitative Methods: Advantages and Disadvantages for STI/HIV Research

Much of qualitative research may be considered "ethnographic research," which is the "work of describing a culture" with the purpose of seeking to understand another way of life from the native point of view (3). This involves the collection of data about behaviors, beliefs, knowledge, world view, attitudes, and a population's values and provides the background against which certain aspects of people's behavior can be meaningfully explained. The purpose of ethnographic research is to understand another way of life from the point of view of those who live it. The goal is to grasp another's point of view; to see the world as he or she sees it. Therefore, the core of ethnography is concerned with attaching *meaning* of actions and events to the people that understanding is sought of. Meaning is both *place* and *culture* specific. In every society people make constant use of complex meaning systems to organize their behavior, understand themselves and others, and to make sense of the world in which they live. Meaning can be expressed directly through words, but many meanings are assumed and communicated only indirectly through words and behavior. These systems of meaning constitute their culture; ethnography always implies a theory of culture. Culture can be defined as "acquired knowledge that people use to interpret experience and generate social behavior" (3). It is important to recognize that in a single country there can be many different cultures. Qualitative methods are especially useful in ethnographic research because they record the actual language and actions of respondents from their own perspective. Although qualitative methods can be applied in research that is not ethnographic, this is its most common application in the field of STI/HIV.

Qualitative data can be collected in various ways. The most commonly used methods in STI/HIV research are one-on-one interviews (or in-depth interviews), focus groups, and naturalistic observations; each are described in detail below. It is important to consider when to use such methods. While the data gathered through all these methods are rich and provide contextual depth, some are more appropriate given the study topics addressed or the design (Table 1). For example, in-depth interviews may be better suited than focus groups when the research questions are highly sensitive and respondents are being asked to report on their practice of potentially non-normative behaviors. Research shows that when responses from the same individuals are compared from focus groups and in-depth interviews, clear differences emerge between what individuals report one-on-one to what they report in a group setting (see reference below). In focus groups, social norms and normative group behaviors are emphasized. Thus, sensitive behaviors may not be reported as often as in one-on-one interviews, as shown in one study that compared results from focus groups and one-on-one interviews with the same adolescent females and found that risk behaviors in group settings were underreported (4). Therefore, to obtain accurate reports of sexual behavior, especially if the behaviors in question are considered "non-normative," in-depth interviews may be a more appropriate methodology. But there are exceptions, as in the case of individuals who are already accustomed to informal exchange about the topic themselves—such as commercial sex workers discussing condom use—for whom focus groups could work despite the sensitive nature of the topic (5).

One-on-One Interviews or In-Depth Interviews

The in-depth interview is one strategy used for getting people to talk about what they know and is an intensive and intimate opportunity to hear in detail from one individual (6). In-depth interviews help to understand the meanings behind the behavior by extracting the language of the respondent or study participant. Therefore, research questions arise out of the respondent's culture. The explicit objective of an in-depth interview is to understand the respondent's experience from his/her point of view. The respondent's language thus represents the data; "the words people use provide the structure and categorization of their experience" (7). This type of interview allows respondents the freedom to choose their own words, context, and manner to describe their experiences, thereby permitting the emergence of cognitive data. The content of such interviews is structured according to an interview guide that specifies the exact topics to be covered and specific questions for each respondent while maintaining an open-ended response format, which allows the interviewer to probe with follow-up questions when clarification is necessary.

Table 1 Comparison of three qualitative methods used for text analysis.

Method	Approach	Best for	Not recommended	Published example
One-on-one interviews	In-depth interviews about a person's personal perceptions regarding a specific experience. Interviewees may be selected at random. Interview guide outlines open-ended questions. Interviewer has flexibility to add follow-up questions/probes as appropriate.	Delicate subject matter, personal experiences. When time, money, and equipment are available, as well as private space.	Topics that are "too" sensitive (e.g., where anonymity cannot be assured), with very shy or untalkative subjects, when private space or sufficient time to analyze data are not available.	Don't ask, don't tell: patterns of HIV disclosure among HIV positive men who have sex with men with recent STI practising high risk behavior in Los Angeles and Seattle. Gorbach PM, Galea JT, Amani B, Shin A, Celum C, Kerndt P, Golden MR. *Sex Transm Infect.* 2004 Dec;80:512–517 (ref. 28).
Key informant interviews	In-depth interviews about a person's viewpoint, observations, and experiences, usually regarding an external issue. Interviewees are purposefully selected based on their background and experience with the issue; they are seen as "experts" on the given topic due to their knowledge or experiences. Interview guide is normally standardized so that all key informants are asked the same questions.	Rapid uptake of viewpoints from those "In the Know" regarding an issue, particularly useful in public policy issues. Good for identifying other key informants to interview.	When verbatim language or "slang" terms are sought. When actual behaviors and experiences are necessary—these provide only proxy reports. Since interviewees are chosen specifically for their background and experience (and not randomly), their viewpoints are inherently biased.	HIV risk and prevention in a post-vaccine context. Newman PA, Duan N, Rudy ET, Johnston-Roberts K. *Vaccine.* 2004;22:1954–1963 (ref. 29).
Focus groups	Group interviews that learn not only about individual opinions regarding the focus matter but the group's reactions, as a collective, as well.	Issues that will eventually affect people on a group level (rather than or in addition to only the individual level).	Sensitive topics where self-censorship occurs due to social desirability bias.	Environmental barriers to HIV prevention among incarcerated adolescents: a qualitative assessment. Freedman D, Salazar LF, Crosby RA, DiClemente RJ. *Adolescence.* 2005;40:333–343 (ref. 30).

In such interviews the interviewer is the "eyes and ears" of the study. The function of the interviewer is to serve as a link between those who seek the facts and the respondents who furnish the answers. The interviewer obtains information from the point of view of the respondents and supplies the researchers with information for analysis. The interviewer is involved in a very important act of communication and must be carefully trained and supervised in how to conduct such interviews. The information heard and recorded during an interview must be accurate and complete so as not to bias or distort the content. An in-depth interview is like a series of friendly conversations into which the interviewer slowly introduces new elements that assist the respondents to respond as informants. The interviewer guides the respondent into discussion on the topics of interest. An important component of such interviews is the establishment of rapport, or a harmonious relationship between the interviewer and the respondent characterized by a basic sense of trust between the respondent and the interviewer that allows for a free flow of information (3). Both the interviewer and respondent must have positive feelings about the interviews, perhaps even enjoy them. But rapport does not necessarily mean deep friendship or profound intimacy between two people. It is important that interviewers understand how an interview is different from a social conversation. In a social conversation, two people exchange information, ideas, opinions, and feelings. In an interview, however, one person—the interviewer—records the information, ideas, opinions and feelings of the other person—the respondent—and should not share his/her own feelings, opinions or attitudes on the topic area, instead remaining completely neutral. However, because the interviewer must encourage the respondent to share their feelings he or she must show interest in what the respondent is saying so that a thorough understanding is obtained.

Since the interviewers ask the respondents to speak about their personal thoughts, feelings, attitude, etc., it is essential to protect all respondent information gained during the study. This concerns the interview itself as well as extraneous observations of the respondent's family or activities. An interviewer must recognize the importance of maintaining confidentiality because very personal questions are often asked and situations observed. In order to get honest answers from respondents, privacy must be protected both during the interview (by using a private space free of distractions) as well as after (by using study ID numbers instead of names to identify participants; deleting references using names of people; changing identifying information to disguise a participant if those data are to be singled out in a report; etc.).

As the name implies, one-on-one interviews are generally conducted between two people—one interviewer and one respondent. The interviewer follows a "guide" of topics written by the study investigators and is instructed to ask probing and follow-up questions. A key characteristic of qualitative interviews is that not all interviews have to be the same; the point is to engage the respondent to use their own words to express their ideas, experiences, or opinions. Some interview guides are more structured and contain wording of a series of actual questions to be asked of all respondents. Such a format ensures that a minimum set of questions is asked of all study participants. But even when questions are supplied in a qualitative interview, the interviewers are still instructed to ask follow-up questions that are not prewritten. A final format is when individuals are asked to describe situations more loosely and "narratives" of their experiences are recorded that are less structured. One example of this approach was a study addressing reputed rising rates of unprotected anal intercourse (UAI) among men who have sex with men (MSM) in San Francisco, in which detailed narratives of a recent incident of UAI were collected from 150 MSM (8).

Advantages

Information from in-depth interviews is very detailed and can provide explanations of why behaviors are practiced, not just who practices them and how often. Data reflect how people think and talk about their experiences and provide conceptualizations of behavior, allowing researchers to see the exact words that respondents use amongst themselves. This method lends itself well to applications where the subject matter is complex and the respondents are knowledgeable, when there is highly sensitive subject matter, when respondents are geographically dispersed, or when peer pressure and social desirability are barriers to honesty.

Disadvantages

Since relatively few people are usually interviewed in one-on-one interviews and statistical sampling methods are rarely used, the results are limited in nature and not generalizable to a population in the same way as quantitative data. It is rarely possible to conclude that *many* people think a certain way, since respondents are often selected by convenience. Additionally, the interviews may be very long, produce an abundance of data, and are often difficult and time consuming to analyze. Social desirability can cause some respondents to say what they believe the interviewer wants to hear rather than stating what is true for them. Finally, unless explicit decision rules about coding of data and intercoder reliability rates are included, it may be difficult to determine how much the researcher's opinions influence what the data means.

When reviewing, reading, or analyzing data (published or unpublished), these key questions listed below will help make sense of—and critique—the data:

1. Who dominated the interview? Tape recordings/transcripts should be 80–90% from the respondent, not from the interviewer; otherwise the data are "diluted" by the researcher.
2. How were questions asked? Were there leading questions (e.g., "So, would you say you were scared to come to this clinic because of the stigma with STIs?")? Look for the actual interview questions asked to get a clear sense of how they were phrased to the respondent.
3. How were the data recorded? Qualitative data relies on the precise capture of the respondent's words. The gold standard would be to audio record the interview and, while simultaneously taking field notes, capture nonaudible data (e.g., frowning, smiling, other body gestures). Audio-recorded interviews can then be transcribed verbatim in order obtain direct quotations that illustrate qualitative themes and help increase the credibility of the findings. Be suspicious of qualitative data that provide no direct quotes.
4. What was the coding process used to develop the qualitative themes? Two different people can read an interview transcript and arrive at very different conclusions about the intent of the respondent. Qualitative interviews are best coded by two different people who later compare their codes with each other to measure a "coding concordance" rate; the higher the rate of intercoder reliability, the more likely it is that the data were objectively analyzed. Look in the article's methods and/or results section to see how the researchers processed and analyzed their data.

Structured In-Depth Interviews with Key Informants

Key informants are individuals who are "hand picked" to be interviewed specifically because of criteria such as their knowledge, age, experience, or reputation and who provide information about their culture from that very specific point of view. They may be seen as "experts" in their culture (or around a specific event or experience). These individuals are chosen often in the preliminary stages of research to help identify which subjects, and/or where and how they should be interviewed, to provide proxy information about the behaviors, attitudes, and beliefs of the target research population and, often, to assist in gaining access to them. The same methodology used for structured interviews can be used for key informant interviews. Key informant interviews should be open-ended, but a set of prewritten questions should be asked of *all* persons to be interviewed, with specific questions included to address each key informant's area of expertise. The questionnaire should include probes and encourage key informants to provide information beyond the questions drafted. An example of a research project that included key informant interviews addressed the recent change in California to a non-name system for HIV case reporting. To study the acceptability of this system, key informant in-depth interviews of health department surveillance staff, laboratory personnel, health care providers, and clinic staff along with focus groups of community members were analyzed (9). The findings from this study show how the experiences and opinions of key informants are essential data when considering the impact of health system changes.

Advantages

Key informants are hand picked to perform a specific role based on their position, knowledge, skill set, and connections. Thus, they can act as agents of observation in circumstances that would be difficult or impossible for the researcher to directly access.

Disadvantages

The same disadvantages for one-on-one interviews apply to key informant interviews, but there are some additional drawbacks to consider. Precisely *because* of the way in which they are selected (i.e., *for* their position, knowledge, skill set and connections rather than in an unbiased fashion), the information obtained cannot and should not be taken as anything more than their perceptions rather than direct observations (10). Key informants provide proxy reports of the behavior of study populations of interest but are not always members themselves of this population. Data are never generalizable to the experience of the population.

Focus Group Interviews

This method, born out of market research for consumer products in the 1950s, contrasts to the earlier methods described in that it relies on *group process* and dynamics to explore a common topic area. They are particularly useful in gauging how people react to new ideas (or product evaluation), pricing, or for idea generation, problem identification or marketing strategies such as slogan or logo design. It is important to keep in mind that a focus group interview is, by definition, an *interview* (not a discussion, support group, problem-solving group, etc.) that is *focused* (11). The group moderator presents specific questions to the group participants (usually 6–10) and guides the members in exploring the issue. A typical focus group interview lasts approximately 1.5–2 hours and includes welcoming remarks; explanation of group guidelines (e.g., confidentiality and respect for each other's opinions); introductions/ice breaker; interview questions; closing remarks (brief summary, thanking participants); and, usually, refreshments.

Since a key element of this methodology is the group process or interaction between members as the questions are considered and answered, it is best that participants are heterogeneous as a group (e.g., by sex, age, ethnicity, background, etc.) and unknown to each other so that friendship biases are limited. It is suggested that the research team be comprised of a moderator and a note-taker/process observer (5). The moderator's role is vital in the group process so that the session stays on topic/focused, all members have a chance to speak (and no one dominates the session), and group guidelines are adhered to. Thus, it is important that the moderator be experienced with how groups function, have strong leadership and listening skills, and be able to engender a sense of trust among the group participants. The note-taker handles the logistical components such as audio-tape recording the session, note-taking, and monitoring the group environment.

An example of the application of focus groups to a STI prevention research project is one that collected data to inform the development of a safer-sex intervention for women who have sex with women. The individuals involved in the focus groups were recruited from those with the same sexual orientation (lesbian and bisexual women) and among those from a narrow age group (aged 18–29). Topics included the acceptability of use of barrier methods (gloves or condoms) in sexual encounters between women as well as perceptions of STI risk for women who have sex with women (12).

Advantages

The main advantage of the focus group interview is its cost effectiveness and short data turnaround time, since in a few hours data from several people can be gathered simultaneously. Additionally, some people are more comfortable and talk more openly in group settings when they see that other group members may share their feelings and opinions. Also, the focus group interview collects information on social norms (4), which is lost during single-interviewee methods. The interaction in focus groups may also stimulate new ideas and allow participants to reflect differently than if only describing their own experiences (6). Focus groups are particularly useful for obtaining feedback on study design, language, and images and can be extremely helpful in the development of an intervention.

Disadvantages

The disadvantages with this method are directly related to the topic material and group composition, since some issues don't lend themselves to public discussion. For example, it can be difficult to access actual practice of very personal or sensitive behaviors due to embarrassment or shame. Also, the size of the group limits the number of questions that can be asked; in a usual session, only about 10 questions are attempted. Finally, focus groups that collect data about social norms from individuals within a group who either have behaved or have beliefs outside these norms may be inhibited from sharing them in a relatively public setting—limiting the researcher's access to non-normative behaviors (4). As with other qualitative methods, focus groups suffer from the same problem with generalizability. Given the way most of the sampling is done for focus groups, the results are not generalizable.

Naturalistic or Participant Observations

For some research questions, there are practices best accessed by direct observation, since interview-based techniques are considered merely "accounts" or reports of practices. The observations, however, allow the researcher learn how something factually works rather than relying on a personal account of an activity or event which may contain a mixture of how something is and how it should be (13); in other words, observation allows the study of a subject in real time and in a naturalistic setting (6). Observations may be differentiated as covert vs. overt; nonparticipant vs. participant observations; systematic vs. unsystematic, observation in natural vs. artificial situations; and self-observation vs. observing others.

Because of the highly personal nature of human sexuality, and the illegal status of drug use in most countries, it is difficult to apply the use of observations to STI research and therefore, they are rarely applied. However, this approach can still be useful. One example of "naturalistic observations" was conducted in studies on commercial sex in Russia (14,15). In these studies, naturalistic observations were defined as being in the situation where the action to be observed was taking place—without calling attention to oneself in any way. The observation might be formalized using frequency recordings (unobtrusively) or a more global impression formation but the observer does not directly participate in the events taking place (personal communication, Jan St. Lawrence). Researchers in the Russian studies observed sex worker recruitment and solicitation in multiple settings and were able to record the roles of different players in this business, including how the authorities interacted with commercial sex activities.

Advantages
The major advantage of naturalistic observations is that the researcher is able to witness the target event first hand rather than rely on a "filtered" account or story from a respondent.

Disadvantages
Particularly in STI/HIV research, since sexual behaviors are often of interest, naturalistic observations (both covert and overt) are often not feasible or present ethical challenges. Also, with overt observations, data collected may be due to social desirability.

Integrating Multiple Methods

While most research projects employing qualitative methods choose one of those listed above for their study, there are others that utilize more than one method. Studies designed to collect data for the purpose of program design often use such an approach that integrates findings collected from the different methods to collect data from users of a health program, practitioners who practice within it, and experts who evaluate its impact. An example is from a study conducted in Kenya as formative research for a STI control and HIV/AIDS home care project. Methods utilized included key informant interviews, focus group discussions, and in-depth interviews. Findings were used for development of educational materials about health seeking behavior and clinic design (16).

Now that the major qualitative approaches have been explored, it is important to understand the variety of sampling designs employed. Every (reputably) published journal article of a qualitative study should clearly describe in its methods section how the target population was selected. As with quantitative studies, understanding how subjects were selected for participation will assist in the understanding and use of the information learned from the research.

Sampling Designs: Moving Toward More Systematic (Representative) Samples

Most books and journal articles on qualitative research that detail sampling methods give general guidelines for "purposive" samples or "illustrative" samples. Purposive sampling is defined as selecting participants for their ability to provide rich information (5). The emphasis is on finding respondents who are informative and talkative, but not necessarily representative. It has been suggested that samples should be large enough to "adequately answer the research questions" until the information being collected becomes redundant (5). This is also described as reaching "saturation." The justification for this approach is that, since statistical analyses are not performed, the assumptions regarding nonvalidity without random sampling do not apply. This removes the random sampling contingency and frees investigators to adopt other sampling approaches. A side effect of this approach is that qualitative research has been subsequently plagued by claims that it is "illustrative" and with findings that are merely descriptive. This poses an inherent contradiction—a goal of qualitative research is to collect information "representative" of the range of experiences, perspectives, and behaviors relevant to the research question (5) but to achieve representativeness, systematic sampling is necessary and the steps necessary to do so are rarely employed in qualitative studies. Issues around lack of systematic sampling are compounded by the usually small sample sizes (recommended to be less than 40) in most qualitative studies (10). Certainly, qualitative studies should be relatively small because of the large amount of data produced by each respondent—often pages and pages of text. The emphasis is then on a lot of data collected from a few subjects. However, the basic principles of systematic sampling can be easily applied to qualitative research to enhance the representativeness of the samples, therefore strengthening the utility of the findings. Some examples are provided below.

Drawing Independent Samples Using Systematic Approaches

One approach that can be used is to systematically select individuals from within set locations that are also systematically selected. A good example of this is an approach called venue-based sampling, often used in survey research of hard-to-reach populations. In this approach, spaces or locations where subjects of interest congregate (called venues) are identified as are the specific days and time periods when subjects congregate. Next, the venues and the days are divided into time sampling units (composed of days and time-periods) called venue day time units (VDTs). These VDTs then are considered the primary sampling units for the study. The result is also a two-stage sampling process beginning with the random selection of VDTs from the sampling frame, followed by systematic sampling of the individuals within these VDTs. (17) A good example of this sampling method at the community level is the "PLACE Method" (Priorities for Local AIDS Control Efforts), which has been extensively used outside of the United States (18). In this case, venue-based sampling quickly identities those most at risk of acquiring and transmitting HIV to help determine where AIDS prevention programs should be focused.

Although designed for survey research, this method can be adapted for use in qualitative studies. The division of the number of subjects needed for each locale is merely smaller, so instead of sampling 50 individuals from each venue, 5 might be selected from 5 separate venues, yielding a sample of 25 total respondents. Given the systematic design that incorporates random selection, these 25 respondents would be representative of the larger population and the findings could be generalized.

Embedding a Sample in a Quantitative Survey: Utilizing Other Sampling Frames

Another approach to drawing a random sample is to embed a qualitative study within a large survey that is using a random sampling approach. Once the subjects are selected into the large quantitative survey, the qualitative component could randomly select 25 subjects from the list of survey respondents (using a random number for a random start, then a sampling interval based on dividing the number needed by the total sample size and adding that consecutively in the list from the first selected).

General Analytic Approaches

Applying Theory

One approach to analysis of qualitative data involves utilization of an existing theory or conceptual framework and application of it to empirical data. Categories and themes in an established theory are drawn on and tested with empirical data collected from interviews or focus groups. The theory may be adapted accordingly in the discussion of results. This process is also known as theory testing.

An example is the application of the Dual Process Model, an established theory of how individuals process and respond to an illness threat posed by onset of symptoms. This theory was tested for its cross-cultural applicability as well as the durability of its constructs when applied to symptoms of reproductive health tract infections (RTIs). First, the theory was modified for the particular health issue (RTIs) (Figure 2), then its constructs were incorporated into an open-ended ethnographic interview guide and 32 women in Vietnam were interviewed. The constructs were also used to guide the development of a codebook, and content analysis was performed on these codes. Findings were that this individually based model was not well suited in a cultural context where women preferred to manage problems collaboratively, relying on their peer network to form illness representations. While the model assumes a pattern of "self-regulation" in interpreting their symptoms, in Vietnam, decision making about illness and coping strategies was done through a group process. Finally, some of the components of the model were not suited to this cultural context and, as a consequence, duration, and cure were less salient than the immediacy of a health threat, and women tended to not take action on symptoms until they interfered with their daily responsibilities (19).

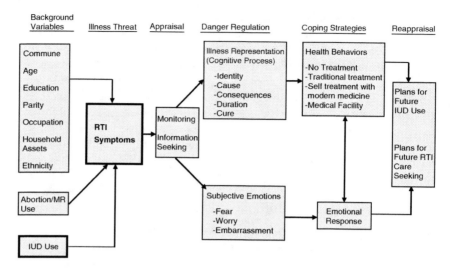

Figure 2 Conceptual model of women's risks and responses to RTI symptoms in Vietnam (applications of Leventhal's Dual Process Model) (19).

Behavioral theories and psychosocial theories that have utility for STI research abound. It is useful to apply them in research to see whether they help explain a specific study population's behavior or they can be used to develop an intervention. Some theories specific to STI that have been developed include the AIDS Risk Reduction Model as applied to microbicide research (20), the Theory of Gender and Power as applied to developing interventions for HIV-related exposures and risks for women (21), or the Stage of Change Theory for clinic-based risk reduction counseling interventions (22).

Developing Theory
Rather than utilizing an existing theory as described above, another approach is to develop a theory through qualitative research. The mainstay of theory development among qualitative research is an approach known as "grounded theory." This is defined as the building of theory firmly *"grounded"* in the empirical data of a cultural description (3). Concepts surface from the raw data and are examined and analyzed to form broad thematic headings or categories that are divided into explanatory and descriptive categories. These are often conceptual frameworks, rather than "theories." The difference is that theories begin as hypotheses and become formalized after undergoing scientific testing and being empirically substantiated, whereas conceptual frameworks are less formal. In either form, the purpose is to provide a fresh structure for how to conceptualize an issue in STI research.

An example of grounded theory is the formulation of different types of concurrent partnerships, defined as a sexual partnership in which one or more of the members has other sexual partners with repeated sexual activity with at least the original partner. Initially, concurrent partnerships were characterized as a single entity, with the emphasis on the overlap in timing rather than the dynamics within the partnerships that could lead to variations in risk behavior and the duration of these overlaps, especially among individuals with and at high risk for STIs. Therefore, semi-structured interviews with heterosexuals (108 with gonorrhea, chlamydial infection, or nongonococcal urethritis and 120 from high STI prevalence and randomly selected neighborhoods) were conducted to identify patterns of concurrency in STD clinics and community samples. This study identified six main forms of concurrency (Figure 3): experimental, separational, transitional, reciprocal, reactive, and compensatory. Experimental concurrency, overlapping short-term partnerships, was most common. Patterns were also identified by gender, with men practicing concurrency to avoid becoming partnerless during partnership disintegration. Yet more women, especially STI patients, reported reactive concurrency, recruiting new partners rather than leaving partners with other partners. The findings also revealed that concurrency clustered by age and during separation and transitioning between partners was socially acceptable. Because concurrent partnerships were found in all groups studied, it is suggested that it is a pattern linked to individuals' life stage and carries some social acceptability (23).

Using Theories in Analysis: Thematic Analysis

To either test or develop a theory, analytical categories must be formed to describe and explain the social phenomena studied (24). The categories may be derived inductively, that is, come from the data in development of grounded theory described above, or deductively by applying components of a formal theory (i.e., applied theory). This term refers to the identification of common themes and exploration of differences in how these themes are expressed and applied in a particular cultural context. This approach is conducted by a careful review of written transcripts noting specific words used by respondents to understand their systems of meaning (3). In a thematic analysis, the first step is to code the text. A code is defined as an abbreviation or symbol used to classify words in the text by categories. The process of coding is the process of identifying categories of meaning (25) and is accomplished by indexing the data by assigning these codes to discrete data units such as a group of sentences or paragraph. A set of decision rules should be elaborated clearly to assign codes to text, and these should be clearly described in a codebook that is shared by all members of the research team and developed following an iterative process (26).

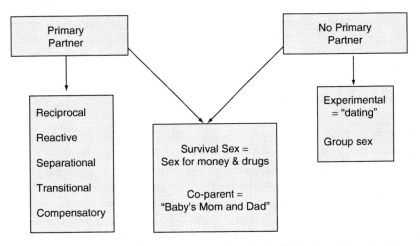

Figure 3 Patterns of concurrent partnerships for individuals with and without a primary partner (23).

It is advisable to have more than one person code the text as described above. Either all the text can be coded twice—once by each of two coders–or a subset can be randomly selected for double coding. Whichever method is selected, the numbers of shared codes and discrepant codes can be calculated to produce a level of intercoder agreement. Moreover, when discrepant coding is found, coders and investigators should discuss the differences in order to resolve disparities and further clarify definitions in the codebook. Using more than one coder may improve the consistency and reliability of analyses (24).

Following the guidelines laid out in an extremely comprehensive guide to qualitative data analysis, the next step after the data are coded is to conduct searches of the text by the coded categories. This brings up "chunks" or portions of verbatim text from the interviews or focus groups that were assigned the code of interest. In order to analyze these segments of text for each code, tables or matrices are a useful approach to organizing the data. The matrix should display identified categories by groups of respondents. Short quotes or summarizing remarks from coded text are entered into appropriate boxes in the matrix by category following a precise set of decision rules and criteria (25).

Once a matrix is created, the following steps are useful in identifying themes: look for patterns; build a logical chain of evidence; make contrasts and comparisons; look for clusters of issues around a topic; count *carefully*—not to communicate distributions of ideas but to capture whether or not this was a theme or issues expressed by most participants or by a few. There are also steps that may be followed to verify the themes identified: follow-up on surprises; triangulate by reviewing data from other interviews, or other sources of data such as from surveys; make some *if-then* tests to see whether the rationale works; check out rival explanations; obtain feedback from informants, experts, colleagues, and other members of the research team to see whether the identified themes have salience.

To summarize, the process of data analysis includes the following steps:

1. Data collection: conduct interviews/focus groups
2. Data management: interview/focus group recording transcription
3. Choice of theoretical approach: grounded or applied
4. Determination of analytic approach: case or cross-case
5. Coding of transcripts
6. Data reduction: create matrices, displays
7. Analysis and identification of themes
8. Conclusions: presentation of themes

Presentation of Findings in Reports and Manuscripts

There are two main formats in which qualitative data are presented in the STI/HIV literature. The choice of which to use should be based on the audience to which the information is being presented and the location where it is being presented. However, it should be noted that, even with broad categories of places for presentation and publication, there is variation. For example, if the qualitative data are being analyzed for publication in a journal, there are some formats more common to certain journals than to others. Restrictions by journals such as article length and number or size of tables and figures vary as well and affect data presentation choices. Different formats may be more common or acceptable at different conferences as well, and careful consideration about format should also be undertaken when presenting to community groups or community agencies. Following are two commonly used formats.

Quotations in Text
This is the most common format for presenting qualitative data. Actual words, phrases, sentences and even verbatim paragraphs from quotations of interview or focus group texts are placed directly into a report, manuscript, or presentation as data. An example of this is from a study in North Carolina where statements made by focus group participants are woven in the text to support the author's points (27).

Quotations in Tables
Another format for presenting qualitative data that is particularly suited to medical and public health journals is the use of tables with embedded quotations. Because journals restrict the article length, when quotations are embedded in text as described above, the words in the quotations are included in the word count of the manuscript. This has a twofold negative effect: authors are forced to write less substantively about the data and present less of their data in the pressure to meet the manuscript length restrictions. While there are journals from the social science disciplines (such as *Social Science and Medicine*) or specific to qualitative research (such as *Qualitative Research* or *Qualitative Health Research*), these journals may be read less often by those in the STI/HIV field than the journals specific to STIs (such as *Sexually Transmitted Diseases* and *Sexually Transmitted Infections*). Using tables to present quotations is a format that allows more of the actual study data to be presented, thereby allowing more of the participants' actual words to be heard. Since the quotations are in tables, their word count is not included in the text word count. An example of such a table is presented as Table 2, which is a table of quotations on reasons why HIV-positive men who have sex with men chose whether or not to disclose their HIV status to sexual partners (28). In this table, themes are presented in one column, the quotations that represent the theme are in the next column, and basic descriptor information about the respondent from whom each quotation comes is in the final column (examples of these include gender, age, ethnicity, sexual orientation, STI status, or recruitment site). The text of the manuscript or report should then refer to each quotation presented to interpret and explain what it captures and represents.

Themes: Tables and Models
Figures or tables of themes can also serve an important role in bringing together findings of a qualitative research study. Qualitative researchers should remember to take a step back from their data during the analysis phase and consider how the themes are interwoven and what overall story they tell about the research subject of interest. The theory tested or developed through the study may serve this purpose, or the themes identified may work together in a larger pattern that merits explanation. Therefore, presentation of themes or patterns identified around the research question can be useful ways to provide a summary of findings.

Table 2 Representative quotes by theme.

Theme	Representative quote	Age	Ethnicity
It's nobody's business	(1) "This is a medical condition that I've got and why should I tell everybody?" (Seattle)	43	W
	(2) "… it was nobody's business but mine." (Los Angeles)	27	AA
In denial	(3) "Me in denial about the status, me not want nobody to know. Ruin me image." (Los Angeles)	44	AA
Low viral load	(4) "I get regular blood work done, monitor my viral loads, and things of that sort…I know it isn't entirely true, but I tend to think that if your viral load is low, and your immune system is strong, that you probably have less of the virus forcing through your body." (Seattle)	40	W
	(5) "There was no conversation and I ended up fucking him—again, the false sense of security that my viral load is zero. I don't feel too bad about it." (Seattle)	49	AS
Fear of rejection	(6) "Some guys I talk to, they're like, this guy was so hot I wasn't going to talk about anything because I didn't want to blow my chance to have sex with him." (Seattle)	41	W
	(7) "I just … sometimes it don't always pay to be—to tell people—because a lot of times it just runs them off, you know …?" (Los Angeles)	42	W
	(8) "I feel like you've treated me like I should be wrapped in saran warp from head to foe." (Los Angeles)	39	W
Just sex	(9) "I feel like it wasn't even important because I don't really know him and he doesn't really me. And all it's about … is just a sexual thing." (Los Angeles)	41	AA
	(10) "… if I'm never going to see them again and it's a casual experience, I'm not necessarily interested in going down that road [disclosure]" (Seattle)	35	W
Drug use	(11) "I guess the effect of the crystal was just so exhilarating, I guess, it didn't even enter my mind to even say anything." (Los Angeles)	34	W
	(12) "The crystal meth impaired my judgment, and all I could care about was just getting laid, you know." (Los Angeles)	40	H
	(13) "In the heat of the moment, the drugs, you know, wanting to have sex…that's it." […] I mean, you're—you're—you're up there, and you like, hey, I got to have me some sex. And I'm going to do anything to get it." (Los Angeles)	35	W
Public place	(14) "Total anonymity in a bathhouse or the park, you're not going, 'oh, before you put your mouth there you should know [that I'm positive]." (Seattle)	40	W
	(15) "… there were of other people standing around [at the park]…the environment…it just didn't seem appropriate, I guess." (Los Angeles)	22	H
	(16) "… a bar, it's more like a social place, and it, they're here, they're to have, supposed to have fun, dance drink whatever, and to bring that up, it would, it would probably kindo, awfully, turn off the other person." (Los Angeles)	47	AA
Type of sex Partner wants to use a condom	(17) "No, I didn't tell him my status, because he wanted to use a condom, so I figured why tell him, if he always want, if he wants to use a condom so why tell him?" (Los Angeles)	40	AA

Theme	Quote	Age	Ethnicity
No anal sex	(18) "I mean I knew I wasn't going to take off all my clothes and, and have...anal sex with him, so, I was just like you know I kept my mouth shut and, and then do what I have to do, and that was that." (Los Angeles)	27	AA
Only receptive anal sex	(19) "Being the receptive anal partner, probably less infective, less of a concern." (Seattle)	49	AI
Gave oral sex	(20) "... it was just um one of those things where, you know, I gave somebody oral sex, and, and...I just didn't feel it was necessary because of the low risk, or whatever, of HIV." (Los Angeles)	39	H
	(21) "If I'm only giving him head and we're kissing, there's no need to tell him." (Seattle)	38	W
Partner asks or discloses first	(22) "If they were to ask me straight out, I would tell them straight out." (Seattle)	41	W
	(23) "[I disclosed] because he asked." (Seattle)	52	W
	(24) "If they would've told me they were HIV then I would've felt more comfortable, and told them I was."	39	W
	(25) Yes, [I told him I was HIV positive] because he told me that he was positive too."	27	AA
Feelings for partner	(26) "He was a really sweet guy. It was like, OK, this could lead somewhere. Who knows? This could be a lot of fun. Who knows? This could lead somewhere. I am going to let him know." (Seattle)	51	W
	(27) "... If you make a bond on an emotional level, I certainly feel more obligated to divulge my status because I might want to continue a relationship with them." (Seattle)	35	W
	(28) "Well the reason because I wanted him to be in my life and I felt that he had a right to know." (Los Angeles)	45	AA
Responsibility	(29) "I don't think it's fair and I think they should have an option to have sex or not to have sex...don't want to ruin his life and, you know . . ." (Los Angeles)	45	AA
	(30) It's not like something you want to spread around...it's like killing people." (Los Angeles)	33	W
Fear of arrest	(31) "There is a legal issue. You have to." (Seattle)	44	W
	(32) "I heard stories about you can go to jail for like attempted murder and I don't want to have to go through that. I'm 46 years old and what little time I have left on this earth. I would like to enjoy it outside of a jail." (Los Angeles)	47	AA
	(33) "Like I said, it is considered murder if you slept with somebody then that person had one time thing with you and he goes and gets and he knows who you are, it is a risk, it's a felony rap, it's a murder rap on you, you know?" (Los Angeles)	44	H
	(34) "For one thing, you know that I found out, there are cases of murder or manslaughter..." (Los Angeles)	39	W

Ethnicity: AA, African-American; W, white; H, Hispanic; AS, Asian.

Conclusions

STI/HIV providers and those creating programs and policies often look to study reports and journal articles to provide a "big picture" concept of the factors influencing the behavioral choices of individuals at risk, or how multiple socioeconomic forces work together to perpetuate STI epidemics. Qualitative research serves an important role in elucidating how and why individuals acquire and transmit STIs by allowing their perspectives and voices to be heard by the professionals who work with them. By allowing the direct expression and words of real people to become part of our research and interpretation of what is human behavior, qualitative research provides unique insights into STI/HIV research problems. It is important to remember that qualitative research is essential but not sufficient for effective programs to be designed to reduce STI/HIV epidemics. Numerical (quantitative) data about the distribution and frequency of behaviors are also necessary, and it is only through both listening to people's voices and analyzing the impact of these voices that programs that work can be designed.

References

1. Denzin NK, Lincoln YS. *The Landscape of Qualitative Research: Theories and Issues*, 2nd Ed. Thousand Oaks, CA: Sage Publications, 2003.
2. Mays N, Pope C. Qualitative research in health care. Assessing quality in qualitative research. *BMJ*. 2000;320:50–52.
3. Spradley JP. *The Ethnographic Interview*. New York: Holt, Rinehart, and Winston, 1979.
4. Helitzer-Allen D, Makhambera M, Wangel A. Obtaining sensitive information: the need for more than focus groups. *Reproductive Health Matters*. 1994;3:75–82.
5. Ulin PR, Robinson ET, Tolley E. *Qualitative Methods in Public Health: A Field Guide for Applied Research*. San Francisco, CA: Family Health International and Jossey-Bass, Inc., 2005.
6. Goering PN, Streiner DL. Reconcilable differences: the marriage of qualitative and quantitative methods. *Can J Psychiatry*. 1996;41:491–497.
7. Bauman LJ, Adair EG. The use of ethnographic interviewing to inform questionnaire construction. *Health Educ Q*. 1992;19:9–23.
8. Sheon N, Crosby MG. Ambivalent tales of HIV disclosure in San Francisco. *Soc Sci Med*. 2004;58:2105–2118.
9. Koester KA, Maiorana A, Vernon K, et al. HIV surveillance in theory and practice: assessing the acceptability of California's non-name HIV surveillance regulations. *Health Policy*. 2006;78(1):101–110.
10. Patton MQ. *Qualitative Evaluation and Research Methods*, 2nd Ed. Newbury Park, CA: Sage Publications, Inc., 1990.
11. Patton MQ. *Qualitative Evaluation and Research Methods*, 3rd Ed. Thousand Oaks, CA: Sage Publications, Inc., 2002.
12. Marrazzo JM, Coffey P, Elliott MN. Sexual practices, risk perception and knowledge of sexually transmitted disease risk among lesbian and bisexual women. *Perspect Sex Reprod Health*. 2005;37:6–12.
13. Flick U. *An Introduction to Qualitative Research*. Thousand Oaks, CA: Sage Publications, Inc., 1998.
14. Aral SO, St Lawrence JS. The ecology of sex work and drug use in Saratov Oblast, Russia. *Sex Transm Dis*. 2002;29:798–805.
15. Aral SO, St Lawrence JS, Tikhonova L, et al. The social organization of commercial sex work in Moscow, Russia. *Sex Transm Dis*. 2003;30:39–45.

16. Moss W, Bentley M, Maman S, et al. Foundations for effective strategies to control sexually transmitted infections: voices from rural Kenya. *AIDS Care*. 1999;11:95–113.

17. Muhib FB, Lin LS, Stueve A, et al. A venue-based method for sampling hard-to-reach populations. *Public Health Rep*. 2001;116(Suppl 1):216–222.

18. Weir SS, Pailman C, Mahlalela X, Coetzee N, Meidany F, Boerma JT. From people to places: focusing AIDS prevention efforts where it matters most. *AIDS*. 2003;17:895–903.

19. Gorbach PM, Hoa DT, Eng E, Tsui A. The meaning of RTI in Vietnam—a qualitative study of illness representation: collaboration or self-regulation? *Health Educ Behav*. 1997;24:773–785.

20. Severy LJ, Tolley E, Woodsong C, Guest G. A framework for examining the sustained acceptability of microbicides. *AIDS Behav*. 2005;9:121–131.

21. Wingood GM, Scd, DiClemente RJ. Application of the theory of gender and power to examine HIV-related exposures, risk factors, and effective interventions for women. *Health Educ Behav*. 2000;27:539–565.

22. Coury-Doniger P, Levenkron JC, Knox KL, Cowell S, Urban MA. Use of stage of change (SOC) to develop an STD/HIV behavioral intervention: phase 1. A system to classify SOC for STD/HIV sexual risk behaviors—development and reliability in an STD clinic. *AIDS Patient Care STDS*. 1999;13:493–502.

23. Gorbach PM, Stoner BP, Aral SO, WL HW, Holmes KK. "It takes a village": understanding concurrent sexual partnerships in Seattle, Washington. *Sex Transm Dis*. 2002;29:453–462.

24. Pope C, Ziebland S, Mays N. Qualitative research in health care. Analysing qualitative data. *BMJ*. 2000;320:114–116.

25. Miles MB, Huberman AM. *Qualitative Data Analysis: An Expanded Sourcebook*, 2nd Ed. Thousand Oaks, CA: Sage Publications, 1994.

26. MacQueen KM, McLellan E, Kay KA, Milstein B. Codebook development for team-based qualitative analysis. *Cultural Anthropology Methods*. 1998;10:31–36.

27. Adimora AA, Schoenbach VJ, Martinson FE, Donaldson KH, Fullilove RE, Aral SO. Social context of sexual relationships among rural African Americans. *Sex Transm Dis*. 2001;28:69–76.

28. Gorbach PM, Galea JT, Amani B, et al. Don't ask, don't tell: patterns of HIV disclosure among HIV positive men who have sex with men with recent STI practising high risk behaviour in Los Angeles and Seattle. *Sex Transm Infect*. 2004;80:512–517.

29. Newman PA, Duan N, Rudy ET, Johnston-Roberts K. HIV risk and prevention in a post-vaccine context. *Vaccine*. 2004;22:1954–1963.

30. Freedman D, Salazar LF, Crosby RA, DiClemente RJ: Environmental barriers to HIV prevention among incarcerated adolescents: a qualitative assessment. *Adolescence*. 2005;40:333–343.

20

From Data to Action: Integrating Program Evaluation and Program Improvement

Thomas J. Chapel, M.A., M.B.A., and Kim Seechuk, M.P.H.

While program evaluation is widely recognized as a core function of public health, differences in definition of "good evaluation practice" often lead to evaluations that are time consuming and expensive, and, most importantly, produce findings that are not employed for program improvement. This chapter offers simple, systematic guidelines to maximize the likelihood that the time and effort to evaluate will be translated into program improvement. The goal that findings be used for program improvement is fundamental to the discipline of program evaluation. An old adage says it best: "Research seeks to prove; evaluation seeks to improve." And evaluators have responded with a variety of approaches/frameworks whose central premise is "utilization-focused" evaluation—that no evaluation is good unless its results are used (1,2). This chapter emphasizes how early steps of a good evaluation process can build the conceptual clarity about the program that is needed to choose the right evaluation focus. It reinforces these points with case-specific advice for those doing STD interventions.

Programs can be "pushed" to do evaluation by external mandates from funders or authorizers or they can be "pulled" to do evaluation by an internally felt need to examine and improve the program. STD programs are likely no different. State and local STD programs are pushed to evaluate by a mix of evaluation mandates in cooperative agreements or foundation mandates—which in turn reflect demands on foundations by their boards or on funding agencies like the Centers for Disease Control and Prevention (CDC) by the Office of Management and Budget and the Government Performance and Results Act (GPRA) and Performance Assessment and Rating Tool (PART) processes.* Using the STD world as an example, CDC's Division of STD Prevention (DSTDP) now explicitly lists program evaluation as an essential activity within the Comprehensive STD Prevention Systems (CSPS) framework, and recent DSTDP *Performance Measures Guidance* (3) commits CDC's efforts to measuring performance and aligning with goals. This CDC emphasis is translated

---

* See the following for more discussion of the relationship of program evaluation to the Government Performance and Results Act (GPRA): http://www.gao.gov/new.items/gpra/gpra.htm, and to the Performance Assessment and Rating Tool (PART), http://www.whitehouse.gov/omb/part/

Behavioral Interventions for Prevention and Control of Sexually Transmitted Diseases. Aral SO, Douglas JM Jr, eds. Lipshutz JA, assoc ed. New York: Springer Science+ Business Media, LLC; 2007.

into pressure on states to evaluate; the *Program Operations Guidelines* require that programs monitor progress toward achievement of goals and objectives (4).

While external mandates such as these can be effective in motivating evaluation, it is preferable that programs be "pulled" by the internally felt need to evaluate, even when it is not required. And, indeed, more and more STD programs see the need for good evaluation as problems become more complex, efforts emphasize behavioral interventions with hard-to-reach audiences, and programs must deal with the complexities of communities and institutional structures. Community-wide surveillance measures tell only part of the story, and determining whether program efforts are effective—and why or why not—means delving into the innards of program efforts, understanding the sequence of milestones and markers for success, and unraveling the relationships between activities and outcomes. STD programs might be evaluated for the following reasons:

- to help prioritize activities and guide resource allocation;
- to inform funders of the program whether their contributions are being used effectively;
- to inform community members and stakeholders of the project's value;
- to provide information that can be useful in the design or improvement of similar projects.

Framework for Program Evaluation in Public Health: The CDC Example

CDC's Framework for Program Evaluation in Public Health (5) is a six-step approach to evaluation whose core assumption is that use of findings is most likely when the evaluation focus and design match the purpose and the potential use and user of the specific evaluation situation. CDC's framework intentionally employs broad definitions of both "evaluation"—"examination of merit, worth, significance of an object" (6)—and "program"—"any set of intentional, interrelated activities that aim for a common outcome"(5) so that practitioners at all levels would see program evaluation as something they needed and had the capacity to undertake.

The CDC framework includes six steps (Figure 1): 1) engage stakeholders; 2) describe the program; 3) focus the evaluation and its design; 4) gather credible evidence; 5) justify conclusions; and 6) use findings and share lessons learned.

The rationale underlying these steps is as follows: No evaluation is good just because the methods and analysis are valid and reliable, but because the results are used; getting use means paying attention to creating a "market" before you create the "product"—the evaluation itself. The evaluation focus is key to developing this market by ensuring the evaluation includes questions that are relevant, salient, and useful to those who will use the findings. Determining the right focus requires identifying key stakeholders (those besides the program who care about our efforts and their success) and understanding the program in all its complexity.

The steps are sequenced in a way that reinforces the idea that planning, performance measurement, and evaluation are integrated in a continuous cycle of continuous quality improvement loop:

- Planning—What *do* we do?

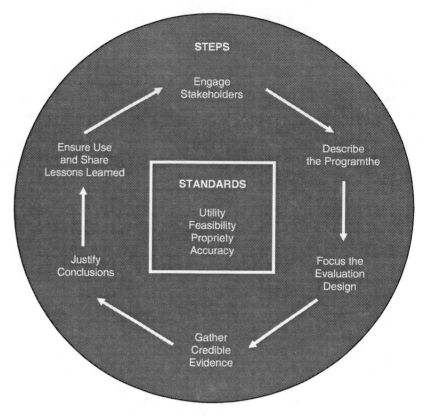

Figure 1 Evaluation framework.

- Performance measurement—*How* are we doing?
- Evaluation—*Why* are we doing well or poorly?
- Planning—What *should* we do?

A set of four evaluation standards (7) complement the six steps. They help broaden or constrain our thinking at any step by asking: 1) Who will use the information and how (utility)? 2) How many resources are available for evaluation (feasibility)? 3) What must be done to be proper and ethical (propriety)? 4) What approaches will produce the most accurate results, given the intended use (accuracy)?

The remainder of this chapter presents key insights at each step of the framework and illustrates them with some cross-cutting STD examples.

Applying Key Insights from the Framework

Engaging Stakeholders

Turning evaluation results into program improvement is often not under the control of evaluators or even of program staff members. Hence, programs that are committed to "use" of evaluation findings must pay attention to engaging "stakeholders," the array of people and organizations with vested interests in the program and its results.

Stakeholders for the typical public health program fall into three overlapping categories: 1) those involved in program operations; 2) those affected by the program; and 3) those who will use evaluation results (who may be part of the first two groups). For a state or local STD program, these categories might comprise the following stakeholders:

- STD program management
- STD program staff
- Other public health partners: family planning, laboratory, epidemiologists, etc.
- STD program clients
- Federal, state, and local funders of the program
- Private providers
- Community- or faith-based organizations that serve affected communities
- Schools
- Departments of corrections or jails
- Businesses that cater to the target community (e.g., gay baths or bars)
- Other public health partners (family planning, laboratory, epidemiologists, etc.)
- Community members at large
- Professional organizations (local chapter of AMA, NCSD)
- HIV care providers
- HIV community planning groups

These categories are broad; if the program desires use of evaluation findings, then within these three broad groups, the most important stakeholders are those who 1) will enhance the credibility of the evaluation or results, 2) will implement the evaluation's recommendations for program improvement, and 3) will help with or are responsible for the continued authorization or funding, or some combination of these.

Following are two STD case examples. Note who the key stakeholders are and the differences in the parts of the program of most interest to them:

- In a large metropolitan area, increases in infectious syphilis have been concentrated in the men who have sex with men (MSM) community. Most syphilis cases in MSMs are diagnosed by private providers rather than the STD clinic and most MSMs with syphilis have reported frequenting particular gay baths or bars in the metro area. As the STD program thinks about design and evaluation of prevention efforts, it might consider the following:

  - Physicians' concerns about patients' confidentiality and Health Insurance Portability and Accountability Act (HIPAA) may deter physicians from working with the health department or influence which types of data collection are acceptable or not, or both.
  - Business members may be concerned about prevention activities in their venues hurting business, but they may also desire to help protect their customers from STDs or from co-infection with HIV.

- A rural community is experiencing high chlamydia (CT) rates in adolescents. As the STD program thinks about design and evaluation of prevention efforts, it might consider the following:

  - Faith-based organizations may not participate unless prevention emphasizes safe-sex messages that include abstinence.

- Parents may fear that prevention activities will teach and induce their children to experiment with risky behaviors.
- Schools may fear the reaction of parents and the community to sex and drug education in the schools or schools may resist the disruption of the curriculum and the demands on teacher time.
- The community-at-large may fear that the evaluation will spread bad publicity about the community, thus hurting investment.

Knowing these needs, fears, and preferences of stakeholders early in the evaluation helps in a number of ways. If known early enough, this information can inform the design of the intervention and not just the evaluation. But even after the intervention is underway, the stakeholder information reminds us of outcomes that must be measured in the evaluation in order to keep these necessary stakeholders engaged in the process. For example, in the first case, business owners as citizens and potential members of the targeted community want to decrease STD rates in their community, but to keep them engaged in our interventions and evaluation as business owners, we must be attentive to the impact on their business, since cooperation or lack of cooperation from them will undermine prevention. Likewise, in the second case, since we must have schools, faith-based organizations, and parents engaged for CT prevention to be effective, then from the start we must be attentive to the outcomes that matter to them and we must include them in the evaluation. Note that including the stakeholders' needs and priorities in the evaluation does not ensure the answers they want, but only that the evaluation will include the questions that are most relevant and salient to them.

"Engaging stakeholders" sounds more complicated than it is. We may identify a host of stakeholders but conclude that only a few are essential for credibility, implementation, or continuation of the program. And most stakeholders may not want to be involved in every step of the evaluation. Determining the needs, opinions, and preferences of the few who must be engaged need not require extensive data collection; qualitative and simple methods are often enough.

Describing the Program

Before jumping into evaluation or planning, we want clarity on the following aspects of our program:

- *Need for the program:* The big public health problem on which the program hopes to make some impact.
- *Target groups:* Those people or organizations—other than the program and its staff—who need to change in some way to achieve the intended impact.
- *Outcomes:* The way(s) in which they need to change.
- *Activities:* The actions of the program and its staff that are intended to cause the target groups to change.
- *Inputs:* The necessary resources to mount the activities effectively, such as staff members, funds, and legal authority.

In the syphilis case, the public health need is to contain the sudden surge of syphilis cases in men; this appears from widening male-to-female case ratios as well as patient-identified risk to be in MSM. Target groups in this case include, among others, MSMs, the private providers who are diagnosing cases in the MSM community, and some of the businesses the targeted men frequent. We need interventions that will produce the following outcomes: MSMs will reduce risky behavior/adopt protective behavior; private providers will consistently report cases of syphilis to the HD to assure adequate treatment, and offer partner services, counseling, and follow-up; and businesses will participate in communication campaigns or screening events to encourage safe behaviors by their customers. Some key activities will include 1) conducting provider visits to inform providers about reporting regulations, services provided, etc.; 2) conducting grand rounds for targeted providers; and 3) conducting outreach to selected businesses and developing materials for distribution. Key inputs would include, among others, sufficiently trained staff and time to conduct visits and follow up on reports.

By contrast, in our rural community, the needs are identifying the best venues (e.g., high schools) for screening to detect early any increase in CT in adolescents and to prevent new cases that, if left untreated, might cause infertility. The target groups include the adolescents at risk, and, just as importantly, the schools who will host the screening and parents and those who can influence the school and the adolescents' behavior. The outcomes we need to cause in these groups are as follows: Adolescents need to agree to screening, adopt protective behaviors and avoid risky behaviors, and, if positive, complete treatment and partner counseling. Schools need to agree to sponsor screening on site and during school hours, and parents and community influencers need to endorse and encourage participation of adolescents in screening, or at least not publicly oppose these efforts. The activities to move these target group outcomes include outreach to schools and community organizations, campaigns with parents and adolescents, screening clinics that are set up in the schools, and referral and follow-up for counseling and treatment. Key inputs for this intervention include trained staff members and time, an inventory of appropriate materials, and existing relationships with the schools and community organizations. These components of any program are implemented against a backdrop that includes:

- *Stage of development:* How long the program has been underway.
- *Context:* The trends and forces in the larger environment that may affect the program's success or failure, such as history, demographics, competition, economics, and technology.

This backdrop will influence how or whether the intervention can be implemented, and, later on, which parts of it are suitable for evaluation. Both programs in our case examples are just getting underway; we would not yet expect significant progress in public health outcomes. Some important components of the context might include changing demographics of affected communities, which makes engaging and building trust with community organizations and neighborhoods more complicated; competition of STD programs for public health resources, especially with newly felt emergency preparedness needs; new technology—urine-based tests, self-administered risk assessments—that might make interventions simpler to implement; and the political or legislative climate of the community regarding such things as minor consent or condom distribution.

Logic models are a common way of depicting visually the relationship among some or all of these elements of the program description, focusing especially on showing the relationship between a program's activities and intended outcomes. There are many ways to construct logic models, but most start by generating of a list of activities—actions taken by the program and its staff—and outcomes—ways in which people or organizations other than the program need to change. The next step is to try to depict any logical sequencing with the list of activities and outcomes, i.e., the changes in knowledge, attitude, and belief (KAB) usually would precede behavior change, and formulation of materials would logically precede distribution of them. The resulting four-to-six column table may be all that is needed to lend clarity to discussions about the program and its evaluation. But, more often, final logic models will add columns for inputs and outputs. Or the content of the original four-to-six column table may be converted into a "flow chart" format that adds arrows that connect activities to their intended outcomes, or early outcomes to the later ones they are intended to influence.

Below, in Tables 1 and 2, the narrative program descriptions for our two case examples have been converted into simple logic models that depict the activities and outcomes. In listing the activities and outcomes, we have been sure to include outcomes that were identified as important to stakeholders in the discussions conducted earlier (these outcomes are marked with asterisks). When an evaluation focus is chosen in the next step, these serve as reminders of important outcomes that may need to be included in the evaluation.

These logic models are "snapshots" of the program and will change over time as evaluation, research, and daily experience show what is working and what is not. Also, these models could be made more detailed or less detailed, depending on the purpose for which they were drawn. In general, the dictum "less is more" is good advice. Keep the model simple; construct a macro-level

Table 1 Logic model: Preventing syphilis in MSMs in a large metro area.

Inputs	Activities	ST outcomes	MT outcomes	LT outcomes
If we have in place ...	And, if we do ...	Then ...	Then ...	Then ...
Trained staff for provider and business outreach and health communication	Outreach to and education for providers	Private providers will report all cases counsel at-risk patients promptly	Positive patients and partners will complete treatment	Disease transmission will be interrupted earlier to prevent further spread
Funds	Development of provider information and campaign materials	Patients will agree to HD treatment, and counseling and to partner services	Patients and partners will adopt protective behaviors and avoid risky behaviors	Prevalence and incidence of syphilis are reduced
Treatment and service capacity	Outreach to and information for business owners	Businesses will display campaign information	Customers of targeted businesses will adopt protective behaviors and avoid risky behaviors	
Relevant, supportive governmental regulation		Businesses will allow on-site screening as needed	Cooperating businesses and practices not adversely affected**	
			Patient confidentiality not compromised**	

Table 2 Logic model: Identifying and preventing CT in adolescents in a rural community.

Inputs	Activities	ST outcomes	MT outcomes	LT outcomes
If we have in place ...	And, if we do ...	Then ...	Then ...	Then ...
Staff Funds Inventory of prevention education materials	Outreach to schools and community organizations	Schools accept and sponsor clinics on site and during school hours	Students are screened	Prevalence and incidence of CT are reduced
Space, supplies, etc. to conduct testing	Information campaigns with parents and students	Parents and community influencers encourage screening campaign information	Early ID of CT is enhanced	Prevalence and incidence of infertility are reduced
Relationships with schools, parents, and community organizations	Screening clinics in the schools Referral and follow-up for treatment and counseling		Positive students seek and complete treatment Students adopt protective behaviors** and avoid risky behaviors** School day not adversely affected**	Reputation of town not adversely affected**

(i.e., "global") as the starting point, and use it as a template to "zoom in" for more detail on specific aspects of the program.

Focusing the Evaluation and Its Design

While the evaluation plan for a program may include indicators and data sources for every activity and outcome, the evaluation focus step identifies the specific parts of the whole program that need to be part of this evaluation this time. This focus will change over time as the purpose, use, and user of evaluation findings evolve. As noted, being attentive to changes in the purpose, use, and user of evaluation findings over time, ensures that the evaluation "product" has a ready "market."

Over the life of a program, all of the following types of questions are likely to be asked of a program:

- *Implementation/process:* Have the activities been implemented as intended?
- *Effectiveness/outcome:* Have the outcomes occurred as hoped?
- *Efficiency:* What level of resources was necessary to mount the activities and outputs?
- *Cost-effectiveness:* What level of resources was necessary to produce a change in any outcome or all outcomes?
- *Causal attribution:* Were any observed changes in outcomes due to our program and its efforts as distinguished from other factors?

Two of the four evaluation standards are used to determine which parts of the program need be part of the current evaluation focus. The "utility" standard asks:

- What is the purpose of the evaluation?
- Who will use the evaluation results?

- How will they use the evaluation results?
- Were key stakeholder needs identified in Step 1 that must be addressed to keep the stakeholders engaged?

The "feasibility" standard acts as a "reality check" to ensure that "useful" questions are realistic ones based on:

- *Stage of development of the program:* Is it too early in the program's life to expect the specific program component of interest to have occurred.
- *Program intensity:* The program is not intensive or strong enough to produce the program's outcome of interest.
- *Resources for measurement:* Easy-to-access data sources to collect information on the program component of interest do not exist nor do the resources to devise them.

By applying the utility and feasibility standards, the program can identify which components—i.e., what parts of the logic model—need to be part of the current evaluation. These components are converted into specific evaluation questions—i.e., implementation, efficiency, effectiveness, and causal attribution.

Because our two case examples are new programs, an early purpose and user of evaluation may be the program itself that wants to determine whether it could implement the many components of the program as intended. This evaluation would include mainly activities and inputs in the focus; indeed, at this early stage no outcomes may be included at all. Did the outreach to the various target audiences happen, and happen did they happen as extensively as was desired? Were campaign materials developed and screening clinics established? Were the necessary numbers and types of staff members available to mount this program as intended? Implementation questions such as these are called "process evaluation." Among other benefits, when outcomes are not achieved, good process evaluation helps determine whether the program was not the right intervention or whether it was a good intervention but poorly or inadequately implemented.

Both programs are addressing high rates of STD, either a sudden upsurge in incidence (MSM syphilis) or high-prevalence rates found in other venues with the same population (adolescents), and the interventions themselves are not without controversy. An early evaluation purpose may be to sustain the support of the community for the intervention; the department may still be the chief user of findings, but also may need to show somewhat reluctant partners that the effort is paying off. In this scenario, partners may care little about inputs or activities, but they need proof that early outcomes are occurring, such as providers' reporting, schools agreeing to host clinics, and parents and community organizations endorsing the prevention efforts. The partners may want to see such proof of some mid-term outcomes as positive patients being identified and referred to treatment, and patients reporting the adoption of protective behaviors. They also may want proof that their fears or special needs are being addressed: Was business adversely affected by the prevention activities on site? Was the curriculum or teacher workday significantly hurt by the clinics? Was the intervention not too intrusive to their practice, and was only appropriate information shared? Did the reputation of the town suffer?

Over time, certainly funders and authorizers will want some evidence that the program and these interventions are meeting accountability standards. In this scenario, the department is again the user of the evaluating findings, but the purpose is to prove to funders that their money has been spent well or is making progress on intended public health outcomes. Such an evaluation might include some measures of efficiency of activities: Is this a good use of limited resources, or are there other activities that are less resource-intensive that would achieve similar or acceptable results? This focus will almost certainly include long-term outcomes such as prevalence and incidence. It may include showing that reductions in prevalence and incidence are due to the efforts of the program, although demonstrating this conclusively is very hard in field settings and may require special research studies.

By understanding the needs and preferences of key stakeholders and the full complexity of the program before proceeding to evaluation, the early steps of the CDC evaluation framework ensure that the evaluation includes questions that are most important and relevant to those who can make program improvements.

Design choice, as with all elements of the evaluation focus step, will vary with purpose, use, and user, and with the time, resources, and expertise that can be brought to bear. In general, research and evaluation studies employ one or more of the following three designs:

- Experimental designs;
- Quasi-experimental design;
- Observational designs.

When the program is being asked not only whether outcomes have occurred but also whether those outcomes are attributable to the program and its efforts, and there is need to make this "causal attribution" case with a high degree of certainty, then research studies using experimental or quasi-experimental designs may be appropriate. Components and options for these studies are discussed elsewhere (8). But the emphasis of this chapter is on choosing the best design for more customary program evaluation studies where nonexperimental designs are either the only feasible choice or even a better choice than experimental designs. As the World Health Organization (WHO) has noted, "the use of randomized control trials to evaluate health promotion initiatives is, in most cases, inappropriate, misleading, and unnecessarily expensive" (9).

Some of the obstacles in implementing experimental or quasi-experimental designs are illustrated by our two cases. One can imagine choosing a comparison or control community for the syphilis intervention or assigning some but not all schools to in-school CT screening. However, even if the time, resources, and expertise were available to implement this design, it is fraught with potential problems. A comparison community would need to be one also experiencing an upsurge in syphilis in MSMs and it is unlikely that that community would do nothing to address the problem while it awaited the outcome of our intervention. Also, efforts in our community might spill over to the comparison community unless it were located far away, in which case cultural and geographic factors might make it a poor choice for comparison. If CT screening is implemented in some but not all schools, the adolescent grapevine is sure to spread word of the intervention, leading either to resistance in the schools with the intervention or ethical questions about withholding it from the other schools. While good design can address these problems, nonexperimental designs are more practical and may work adequately for the purpose at hand. If the community has good information on syphilis and CT rates, and, better yet, can disaggregate the data for demographic or geographic groups, then changes in rates after implementation of the intervention offer some initial "proof" that efforts are working. While circumstantial, this evidence can be supplemented by targeted surveys or other information to bolster the case. For example, do patients remember campaign messages? Do patients attribute their decision to be screened or to adopt protective behaviors to elements of the intervention? Do parents and organizations attribute their cooperation to outreach efforts of the health department?

The early steps of the framework are not the end of the story, but ensure that the remaining steps—selecting indicators and data sources, analyzing and reporting the data—are informed by clarity and consensus on what the program is and what is most important to evaluate. This ensures that the time and energy spent on data collection and analysis result in use of the findings.

Gathering Credible Evidence and Justifying Conclusions

Program components are often expressed in global or abstract terms. Indicators are specific, observable, and measurable statements that help define exactly what we mean. Indicators are needed for both the outcomes and the activities in the logic model. Outcome indicators provide clearer definitions of our global statement and help guide the selection of data collection methods and the content of data collection instruments. For example, "Positive students complete treatment" and "Parents and community organizations encourage screening campaign" are two outcomes in the CT logic model. The treatment indicator might specify the type of medical treatment, duration, or adherence to the regimen. Likewise, the parent and community indicator might include specific behaviors that indicate encouragement.

Indicators for program activities—usually called "process" indicators—provide specificity on what constitutes "good implementation" of the activities—not just "outreach," but "good outreach" or "enough outreach with the right organizations."

If the logic model listed "outputs," then some of the work has been done, since, as noted earlier, outputs are tangible, countable ways of documenting that the activities tool place. For outreach, outputs might include the number of visits made to a certain mix of community organizations, or the number of memoranda of agreement signed. These serve well as process indicators. Similarly, a program with a strategic plan may already have developed process or outcome objectives. If the objectives were written to be specific, measurable, action-oriented, realistic, and time-bound (so-called "SMART" objectives), then they may serve as indicators as well.

Programs can sometimes use indicators developed by others. Some large CDC programs have developed indicator inventories that are tied to major activities and outcomes for the program. An advantage of these indicator inventories is that they may have been pre-tested for "relevance" and accuracy, define the best data sources for collecting the indicator, and include many potential indicators for each activity or outcome, ensuring that at least one will be appropriate for your program, and, because many programs are using the same indicator(s), you can compare performance across programs or even construct a national summary of performance.† For example, the Division of STD Prevention has a performance indicator that measures the timely treatment of women with chlamydia at certain family planning sites. This indicator may be very useful to the Office of Population Affairs (OPA) that oversees Title X family planning clinics. Conversely, measures used by OPA may be of use to DSTDP as it looks at STD prevention and care in family planning clinics.

In selecting data collection methods and sources for indicators, the primary decision is whether existing data sources—secondary data collection—are available or whether new data must be collected—primary data collection. As was the case in choosing an evaluation focus, the program must balance "utility" (how useful the information is), against "feasibility" (how hard or expensive it will be to collect). Often, programs have limited funds for evaluation, and unless a particular outcome is of widespread interest and requires very accurate data, they will rely as much as possible on existing data sources. For STD programs, several secondary sources might exist such as laboratory or provider reports of reportable diseases, interview records for patients' syphilis, HIV or other STD, and laboratory reports of positive and negative tests completed by provider. However, these secondary data sources must be appropriate to the indicators. Some surveillance systems have the advantages of uniform definitions and ability to compare across jurisdictions, but do not allow for adding questions to the survey or disaggregation of data at the level of geography needed to examine the performance of the intervention.

Primary data collection methods fall into several broad categories:

- *Surveys*, including personal interviews, telephone, or instruments completed in person or received through the mail or e-mail;
- *Group discussions or focus groups*;
- *Observation*;
- *Document review*, such as medical records, but also diaries, logs, minutes of meetings, etc.

These methods may yield quantitative or qualitative data, or both, and, where evaluation questions are abstract or data quality is poor, programs are often advised to use multiple methods. The following checklist—based on the four evaluation standards—can reduce the data collection options to a manageable number:

- *Utility:*
  - Purpose and use of data collection—Do you seek a "point in time" determination of a behavior, or to examine the range and variety of experiences, or to tell an in-depth story?
  - Users of data collection—Will some methods make the data more credible with skeptics or with key users than with others?

- *Feasibility:*
  - Resources available—Which methods can you afford?
  - Time—How long until the results are needed?
  - Frequency—How often do you need the data?
  - Your background—Are you trained in the method, or will you need help from an outside consultant?

---

† While such an indicator inventory does not currently exist for DSTDP's grant program, the 12 new performance measures discussed earlier (CDC, NCHSTP, DSTDP, 2005) may play a similar role.

- *Propriety:*

  ○ Characteristics of the respondents—Will issues such as literacy or language make some methods preferable to others?
  ○ Degree of intrusion upon to program or participants—Will the data collection method disrupt the program or be seen as intrusive by participants?
  ○ Other ethical issues—Are there issues of confidentiality or safety of the respondent in seeking answers to questions on this issue?

- *Accuracy:*

  ○ Nature of the issue—Is it about a behavior that is observable?
  ○ Sensitivity of the issue—How open and honest will respondents be in responding to the questions on this issue?
  ○ Respondent knowledge—Is it something the respondent is likely to know?

In our two cases, surveillance data are a likely source to measure changes in long-term outcomes of incidence and prevalence, so long as those data can be disaggregated for just the communities with the interventions. By contrast, the short-term and mid-term outcomes will need to rely on primary data collection: surveys, interviews, or document reviews. The final methods chosen will depend on factors cited earlier, such as time, money, and credibility with stakeholders.

In our MSM syphilis scenario, data collection sources might include surveillance data to measure number and promptness of case reports; patient or partner interviews regarding self-reported, risky behaviors; reports of businesses that participate in outreach; numbers of condoms requested for distribution at these venues; number of clients accepting screening; or risk surveys with customers of the businesses. Physician outcomes might include physicians' surveys. But if there were doubts about the reliability of self-reported physician data or if heavy physician schedules would likely lead to low response rates, then direct observation or reports (logs) of the numbers of physicians who contact the HD or allow provider visits to be conducted might be a better choice.

With respect to CT screening of adolescents in schools, data sources would include logs or reports of the number of schools in a district that agree to participate; the number of students screened; number of parental consents received; and prevalence data from the site. For monitoring changes in students' risky behavior, risk questionnaires would be a good choice. But, if parents were hesitant about such risk questionnaires or were likely to demand to see the data, the threat to confidentiality would affect how honestly students would answer or would reduce the students' participation. Hence, some other source might be a better choice.

We talk of "justifying conclusions" and not "analyzing data" in order to emphasize that the evidence does not stand on its own, but is judged and interpreted through the prism of (potentially different) values that each stakeholder brings to the evaluation. Fortunately, the identification of any significant differences in values and standards was a core part of Step 1 and, as a result, the evaluation design should already reflect their priority outcomes and preferences for credible data collection. In this step, those values and priorities are used to interpret the evidence and judge the success of the program.

In our two cases, for example, while all parties might agree that a 50% reduction in syphilis rates is a significant achievement, if the bar or bath owners experienced a decrease in business or reputation, they may not see a 50% reduction as worth the loss to their livelihood. Others, such as advocacy organizations, may want to know which 50% experienced the reduction. Was the reduction across the board or was it confined to some income and ethnic groups but not to others? In the CT example, overall reduction in risky behavior is likely to be applauded by all stakeholders, but, as noted, faith-based organizations or parents may want to see increases in abstinence as distinguished from condom use as a safe-sex behavior or they might see increases in condom use as a bad thing.

Ensuring Use and Sharing Lessons Learned

Because the evaluation has been based on the six steps of the CDC evaluation framework, most of the seeds for ensuring use were sown earlier and are ready for harvest at this step. Key actions are obvious ones and include making recommendations and ensuring the recommendations are acted upon.

Making Recommendations

Remember, the underlying rationale of the framework is that using this approach is more likely to lead to use of findings. That is, if we choose questions of interest to stakeholders and measure activities and outcomes in a way that is both useful and feasible, then the findings will be used for program improvement. How might this play out in our two cases?

For the urban syphilis case, achieving our public health outcomes requires engagement of private providers, patients, and local businesses. And our evaluation focus included some outcomes of potential interest to them—"patient confidentiality is not compromised" and "businesses and practices are not adversely affected." Thus, our evaluation findings will not only determine whether we met outcomes on adoption of protective behaviors and reduction in disease transmission or not, it will determine, even if we did not, what factors we might address in the next cycle to achieve our outcomes. We might find that providers did their part, but that we did not convince businesses that there would be no adverse effect. As a result, we reached only those who presented for care. Bad as that sounds, these findings guide our action in the next round. Of all the elements of this intervention, we would put time and attention in the next round to reassuring business owners and gaining their support.

Findings would be used in a similar way in our rural CT case. By including in our focus a range of intermediate outcomes and not just the ultimate public health outcome we seek, the evaluation can direct strategic action in the next round. Our findings may show that positive students completed treatment, but that students as a whole did not adopt protective behaviors. Why? Other findings show that parents and community influencers opposed the content of the screening campaign. These findings tell us in the next cycle of program activity we may need to do some or all of the following: convince parents to accept our messages; change the messages even if they may be less powerful; or find some way to get information to students outside the school setting.

In both examples, the findings provide guidance because we have been careful to include an array of activities and outcomes from the logic model in the evaluation focus and because we made most of those selections based on the explicit purpose, user, and intended use of the findings. The result was relevant findings that could inform action.

Following are some examples from real STD projects where applying steps in the CDC evaluation framework led to findings that could guide program improvement:

- Because a state chlamydia screening program included partners in its evaluation focus and evidence-gathering decisions, all parties agreed in advance to the screening criteria, agreed on data to be collected, monitored data, and shared it periodically. When it appeared that several clinics were not adhering to the criteria, partners were able and willing to work with the clinics to help them adhere to the criteria, thus better using limited resources to screen populations most at risk.
- A syphilis elimination project employed a community partnership approach but wanted to ensure that the task force component was being implemented as intended. By including good process measures in their evaluation plan, they were able to identify several gaps between intention and reality. The findings were used to add activities such as an open house to recruit members from a target population, and helped the task force create an action plan with goals, objectives, and timelines to assure they stayed on track. Likewise, because they had a comprehensive logic model for their education and screening event component and had included stakeholders in choosing where to focus their education and screening evaluation, the findings were able to guide them in revising materials to include more information on STDs other than syphilis, increase the emphasis on risk-reduction messages, modify the content of the brochure so that the community found it less offensive, target locations of screening events based on prevalence and incidence data, and add HIV testing to the screening events.

Acting on Recommendations
Because the evaluation focus and data collection were decided on in conjunction with key stakeholders, the remaining steps to maximize use are as follows:

- *Preparation:* Giving early warning about themes and results to key evaluation audiences to prevent "blind-siding" them;
- *Feedback:* Allowing for review and response to early versions of results to encourage buy-in and utility and to get better sense of best format and emphasis;
- *Follow-up;*
- *Dissemination:* Sharing the results and the lessons learned from evaluation.

Of these, dissemination has been most enhanced by the work done in earlier steps. The market for the evaluation was created earlier; dissemination decisions are simple ones of working from audience to format. And much about this is known from the stakeholder engagement step where we should have asked what messages and delivery method would be of most value to them.

In the syphilis example, health care providers may likely be interested in receiving information in a relatively brief, nonintrusive way (routine faxes or mailings), or receiving the information in a format such as a "report card" that shows numbers of cases that they reported and timeliness of their reports compared to the mean of others. Likewise, we know that business owners want to know how their patrons react to the health communications campaign, and perhaps to understand the changing risky behaviors of their clients so that they may serve them better. But, as with providers, they probably want this in a simple, straightforward format.

In the second example, we may have determined in stakeholder engagement that students will be interested in disease rates and risky behaviors reported by their peers and will use these to establish social norms. Here, group venues such as a school assembly or student health fair might be best. School administrators will be interested in rates and risky behaviors reported so that they might begin to address the issues in the classroom regarding STD information, but are likely to prefer private channels so that the school reputation is not adversely affected.

Summary: The "Payoff"

The CDC framework and similar "utilization-focused" approaches arose from the observation that most evaluations did not lead to program improvement. By thinking about use and user from the start, these approaches aim to ensure that evaluation time and effort make a difference. Still, six steps are a lot, and a dogmatic approach to this or any framework can lead to wasted energy. The evaluation standards serve as a reminder that all evaluations are case-specific. Where the program is the only stakeholder and the intended outcome is clear and easy to measure, then we can zip through the early steps. But clear and easy evaluations are the exception, and paying at least cursory attention to engaging stakeholders and understanding the program will yield insights that ensure evaluation is focused on the parts of the program that matter most and result in findings that are used to improve the program.

References

1. Goodman RM. Principles and tools for evaluating community-based prevention and health promotion programs. *Journal of Public Health Management and Practice*. 1998;4:37–47.
2. Patton MQ. *Utilization-Focused Evaluation: The New Century Text*, 3rd Ed. Thousand Oaks, CA: Sage; 1997.
3. Centers for Disease Control and Prevention, National Center for HIV, STD, and TB Prevention, Division of STD Prevention. Measures Companion Guidance: Comprehensive STD Prevention Systems, Prevention of STD-Related Infertility, and Syphilis Elimination Program Announcement. June 2005.
4. Centers for Disease Control and Prevention, National Center for HIV, STD, and TB Prevention, Division of STD Prevention. Program Operations Guidelines for STD Prevention. Program Evaluation. January 2001.
5. Centers for Disease Control and Prevention. Framework for program evaluation in public health. *MMWR* 1999;48:1–40.
6. Scriven M. Minimalist theory of evaluation: the least theory that practice requires. *American Journal of Evaluation*. 1998;19:57–70.
7. Joint Committee on Standards for Educational Evaluation. *The Program Evaluation Standards: How to Assess Evaluations of Educational Programs*, 2nd Ed. Thousand Oaks, CA: Sage Publications; 1994.
8. Campbell DT, Stanley J. *Experimental and Quasi-experimental Designs for Research*. New York: Houghton Mifflin; 2005.
9. WHO European Working Group on Health Promotion Evaluation. Health promotion evaluation: Recommendations to policy-makers: Report of the WHO European working group on health promotion evaluation. Copenhagen, Denmark: World Health Organization, Regional Office for Europe, 1998.

21

Cost-Effectiveness Analysis

Thomas L. Gift, Ph.D., and Jeanne Marrazzo, M.D., M.P.H.

Cost-effectiveness analysis (CEA) is a commonly used tool to evaluate health care interventions. This chapter will introduce CEA, define it, and describe its limitations and its importance for analyzing behavioral interventions in HIV and STD prevention. The procedures used in conducting CEA and several examples follow.

Rationale for CEA of Behavioral Interventions

This section will define the reasons that CEAs are conducted for health care interventions generally; describe the limitations of CEAs; and briefly describe other economic analysis tools for health care interventions (cost analyses and cost-benefit analyses).

CEA Defined

CEA is a tool that has seen increasing use in recent decades as decision makers at all levels of health care provision seek to value alternative interventions (or programs, tests, or treatments). Although CEAs can be complex, and are often described using somewhat arcane terminology, the concept at the core of any CEA is fairly simple: to combine the net cost of a given intervention and its outcomes with its effectiveness, then use the resulting cost-effectiveness ratio to compare that intervention to alternative interventions that are aimed at accomplishing the same goal (be it changes in behavior, increases in good health outcomes, or decreases in bad ones). Cost-effectiveness ratios can be calculated differently depending on whether the given intervention must be chosen *instead of* the alternatives, or whether it can be combined *with* some of the alternatives. An example of the former approach is choosing an optimal interval for repeat testing of women diagnosed with *Chlamydia trachomatis* infection. An example of the latter approach is deciding whether to combine repeat testing for *C. trachomatis* with a behavioral intervention designed to reduce risk behavior subsequent to receipt of a positive test, in which case the behavioral intervention could be combined with any of the potential repeat testing intervals, or could even be done instead of repeat testing). Because CEA provides explicit quantitative ratios showing the tradeoffs made when

Behavioral Interventions for Prevention and Control of Sexually Transmitted Diseases. Aral SO, Douglas JM Jr, eds. Lipshutz JA, assoc ed. New York: Springer Science+ Business Media, LLC; 2007.

considering alternative interventions, it can aid in decision making about efficient allocation of resources.

CEA Limitations

There are some questions that CEA cannot answer, or that can be better answered by other forms of analysis. For example, CEA expresses intervention costs per unit of outcome. Typically, the outcomes chosen represent the final endpoints of the intervention under consideration, and are fairly straightforward. For STD-associated interventions, the outcomes of choice are usually the number of STD cases detected or prevented, or some other measure related to the sequelae of STDs (such as pelvic inflammatory disease [PID] in women following infection with *C. trachomatis* or *Neisseria gonorrhoeae*). Selecting appropriate outcomes for CEAs that incorporate behavioral interventions is more complex, as discussed in the next section. For any CEA in this area, an added complication is that programs with responsibilities for STD-related activities will often need to allocate resources among activities that address different STDs, including HIV. For example, assume that a program can choose between one of the following interventions: an HIV risk reduction intervention that has a net societal cost of $1.3 million per case of HIV averted (1996 U.S. dollars) (1), and a behavioral intervention based on motivational interviewing to encourage STD clinic attendees to return for repeat diagnostic testing, at a net societal cost of $345 per case of *C. trachomatis* or *N. gonorrhoeae* infection treated (2). Which activity represents a better use of resources? By themselves, these ratios do not provide the answer.

To address these questions, a variant of CEA, cost-utility analysis (CUA), has been developed. This approach uses derived outcome measures that are common across different interventions—usually quality-adjusted life years (QALYs) or disability-adjusted life years (DALYs) (3,4). QALY and DALY measures are generated using health-related quality of life weights that apply to health states with a referent of "perfect health" rather than to particular diseases. Therefore, two diseases that cause the same physical condition (and therefore the same reduction in perfect health) would have the same QALY or DALY impact when that condition occurs. For example, an ectopic pregnancy imposes the same level of disability, regardless of whether it results from a chlamydial or gonococcal infection. QALYs and DALYs have been estimated for outcomes related to STD and HIV infection and have been used in several studies (1,5–7).

All CEAs and CUAs, however, are subject to limitations. The analyses are often limited in scope and do not evaluate all potential options, even within a given program. For example, a behavioral intervention aimed at STD-related risk reduction that is not cost-effective if conducted with women aged 18–40 years might be cost-effective if restricted to women aged 18–24 years, if the latter group evidenced more frequent or serious risk behavior, or to such "high-risk" women within any given age group. Studies may not explore these options, either because of data limitations or other considerations, and thus fail to provide information on them. Other studies may not fully consider all of the potential alternative uses of resources used to conduct programs. For example, staff hired for the express purpose of delivering small-group behavioral sessions might alternatively also appropriately (within the limit of their roles)

support the adoption process. The model emphasized collaboration with prevention providers and community members. Experience with these projects demonstrated that the replication process is complex and that interventions need to be adapted to local circumstances (14). The notion of adaptation, while intuitive, leads to a number of critical questions. Foremost, to what extent must a program adhere to the principles of an original intervention, and to what extent can the intervention be adapted before it loses its effect? These principles fall into two categories: *core elements*, i.e., those elements that are generally considered to be those aspects of the intervention responsible for its effects, and *key characteristics*, i.e., elements that are thought to be more lenient and, while considered important for an intervention, can be changed within certain limits to better meet the needs of a community or agency (15). Therefore, in the example of the RESPECT brief counseling intervention, developing a personalized risk assessment and encouraging the client to take a first step towards risk reduction may be considered "core elements" of the intervention, whereas the HIV test may be considered a "key characteristic." This is an important distinction, since it implies that this counseling model could be expected to "work" outside the HIV testing environment as long as one adheres to the core elements.

Fidelity can thus be defined as the set of core elements that a program must adhere to and for which it must have quality assurance measures in place for the intervention to retain its effect (16). The problem is that most intervention studies have not included analyses to evaluate what intervention elements are critical to the outcome and which are less relevant. Therefore, while the lack of effect in certain replication attempts (17,18) may be due to lack of adherence to core elements (19), the identification of such elements and adherence to them (or the lack thereof) may lead to controversy (20,21). Furthermore, because these research interventions were found to be efficacious in the research setting before being recommended for dissemination, programs are not required (nor encouraged) to conduct outcome evaluation on the interventions they implement. While quality assurance protocols are always recommended, they are costly and not always completed. Clearly, this is an area for future research.

Dissemination (Roll-Out, Scale-Up)

The utility of an evidence-based intervention is ultimately determined by its dissemination, implementation, and continued use in program applications, a process often referred to as *technology transfer*. (22). Three general methods can be discerned by which academia and policy makers have usually attempted to influence this process. The first one consists of the publication of study results and recommendations based on scientific evidence and best practices. This is in essence a passive approach that relies on the assumption that the intended target of such publications, in this case the provider of prevention services, will a) be reached by them, b) be persuaded by them, and c) be willing and able to make the suggested program changes and adjustments. This approach may be effective for provider behaviors that are already largely driven by strict protocols that in turn are periodically revised based upon current guidelines. The CDC STD Treatment Guidelines (23) are a good example for this, but even here, the ultimate effectiveness, i.e., the adoption of and adherence to these guidelines, especially in primary care settings, is not known. In most circumstances, particularly for complex interventions, dissemination of research findings and recommendations is not sufficient, because such an approach does not take into consideration the various barriers to implementation and maintenance. (14).

A second, more proactive, strategy consists of a set of activities, including training, technical assistance, and capacity building, that seeks to reach out to service providers to educate them about new interventions, convince them to use them, and assist them with developing the necessary infrastructure and support for implementation and maintenance. In this context, the STD/HIV Prevention Training Centers (PTCs) have been among CDC's primary conduits for STI and HIV prevention training. (24). They are at the interface between academia and public health policy makers on the one hand and prevention and care providers on the other. Historically, this network of training centers was limited to the provision of STI clinical training. Over the past decade, though, training in behavioral and social interventions as well as training in partner services and program management has been added to their portfolio. Currently, CDC is relying on the PTCs as one of the main training sources for their Diffusion of Effective Behavioral Interventions (DEBI) program. This program has been designed as a national-level strategy to provide high-quality training and continuing technical assistance on selected evidence-based HIV/STD/viral hepatitis prevention interventions to state and community HIV/STD program staff. (25). This program can be considered the next step in the previously described REP project. As the PTCs are primarily charged with training, CDC is also supporting a network of Capacity Building Assistance Providers (CBAs) that are providing technical assistance and limited training for infrastructure development for community-based organizations involved in HIV prevention efforts (26).

Finally, a third mechanism to influence the adoption process is proscriptive: programs can be forced or strongly encouraged to adopt certain intervention protocols, contingent upon the funding they receive. For example, most states have contracts in place for the provision of HIV counseling and testing, and such contracts stipulate the qualification process of counselors, the types of training they must attend, and an array of other quality-assurance measures. In other areas of prevention, prevention programs have traditionally had significant freedom in how they conduct their programs. However, policy makers have grown increasingly frustrated by the "natural" adoption process through the passive and more proactive mechanisms described above or the lack of adoption altogether, and by the continuing concern that increasingly scarce resources may not be used optimally. As a result, funding agencies appear to be increasingly proscriptive in the way they provide support for prevention programs. Therefore, federal and state agencies increasingly require HIV prevention programs to select DEBI interventions as a condition for funding.

Thus, policy and/or funding priorities may override barriers to implementation, and can strongly influence intervention adoption, replication, and dissemination. Project RESPECT (now simply called RESPECT) is being targeted for national diffusion as an evidence-based intervention (EBI) for STI and HIV prevention programs, which will likely result in greater demand for its implementation. Still, while quality assurance protocols are one of several core elements of this DEBI that require adherence, adaptation of this intervention is likely, and it is unknown to what extent these requirements will be followed once roll-out and dissemination begins.

Adaptation

Thus far, we have described the dissemination of effective behavioral interventions as a more or less linear process from innovation to replication to dissemination into the program arena. A less kind observer might describe this process not so much as linear but as vertical: "from the top down." Inherent in this process is the notion that there is something inferior happening in the program area that must be replaced by something that will be far more efficacious. While there may be a general agreement that improvements can be made at the program level, such a condescending approach will obviously be detrimental to the adoption process. It seems to discount the value of the services that are currently provided and to dismiss the presented obstacles as excuses not to change the status quo. So, even as we have effective interventions and replication packages in hand; have decided what critical elements in an intervention must be adhered to in order to maintain effectiveness; and have created a dissemination taskforce that is capable of training and technical assistance, the critical interface with prevention programs must be examined. There are numerous variables operating at the program level that may interfere with the successful adoption of interventions. Therefore, this is an area of increasing interest and is worthy of its own research focus (27). Gandelman et al. (15) propose that effective behavioral interventions cannot be successfully implemented without thorough assessments of the community to which the intervention is targeted; the intervention considered for implementation; and the implementing agency. At the community level, the assessment addresses subpopulations at highest risk, specific risk behaviors, and determinants of risk behaviors, including cultural, religious, and familial patterns. On the basis of this assessment, a determination can be made as to what intervention should be selected and to what extent it should be adapted to best suit the prevention needs of the community. Finally, assessment of the agency includes the primary mission of the organization and how STI/HIV prevention fits within that mission; the perceived benefits of the intervention for the community served by the agency; its resources, strengths, and weakness; capacity of staff and management; and mechanisms for active synthesis, dissemination, and transfer (15).

Acknowledging the intricate interplay of these factors and the effects on the adoption process, the aforementioned STD/HIV Prevention Training Centers, have developed a separate curriculum for adapting evidence-based interventions, particularly for use with community-based organizations providing HIV prevention programs that is best utilized when it precedes intervention-specific training. One of the principles of this course is that the adoption process is a two-way street, "technology exchange," rather than "technology transfer" (15,22). It inherently acknowledges the expertise held by those working in the trenches of HIV and STI prevention and takes their experiences as the starting point for any changes that they desire to adopt and are capable of making. There is an interesting parallel with the principles of prevention counseling. Indeed, the adoption of prevention interventions by agencies can be viewed as a behavior change process at the program level, the principles of which are not necessarily different from behavior change processes at the individual level.

As an illustration, implications of these concepts for the two case studies will be described below.

Although Project RESPECT evaluated the brief counseling strategy recommended by CDC for use in HIV counseling and testing (28), it was very much an efficacy study in the sense that it was conducted in a research setting outside the clinic, using specially hired and trained counselors, and implementing a rigorous quality control protocol (13,29). Since the type of counseling evaluated in RESPECT had been the standard in CDC-supported HIV counseling and testing sites and resources for its implementation as well as training and quality assurance have historically been available for this purpose, we will not consider the adoption of the RESPECT findings in this setting. However, one of the reasons that this intervention has not been adopted in STI clinic settings to the extent hoped for is that it is perceived as a labor-intensive add-on service to an already very busy practice setting, requiring additional staff training members, and oversight, and thus monetary resources. To the degree that there might have been an interest in the implementation of the brief counseling intervention, the current policy that appears to value HIV testing over counseling (2) has not been encouraging. Interestingly, although the RESPECT study was primarily interpreted as demonstrating the efficacy of counseling as an HIV prevention intervention, the study findings should have provided ample reason to consider prevention counseling as a non-HIV STI prevention intervention in its own right. First, study subjects in RESPECT were recruited from STI clinics and were generally at higher risk for non-HIV STI than for HIV per se. In fact, men who have sex with men were excluded from the study. Second, the study results demonstrated significant reductions in non-HIV STI (used as proxy for HIV infection), particularly among adolescents and young adults, i.e., those at highest risk for non-HIV STI (30). Therefore, it could be argued that the significant utility of prevention counseling for the prevention of subsequent non-HIV STI should prompt a (re-)consideration of this intervention in STI clinic settings.

From an effectiveness perspective, there are two strengths generally present in STI clinics that could form a solid starting point for the adoption of prevention counseling in these settings. First, a sexual history is routinely taken, albeit usually in the form of closed-ended questions prompted by the clinic chart: number of sex partners, sex of partners, types of sex, condom use, etc. While this satisfies the data needs of programs and allows for the plotting of trend data, there is no compelling argument to suggest that this way of collecting information has prevention value. By contrast, the RESPECT intervention suggests that asking open-ended questions results in a more personalized and meaningful sexual history that forms the stepping-stone to the development of a prevention plan. Practical experience suggests that taking a sexual history using open-ended questions does not have to take more time than doing it the usual closed-ended way. Furthermore, switching to an open-ended format can be easily taught and would be acceptable if there would be less of a focus on "filling in the blanks." There also appears to be more logic in following an open-ended format with a limited number of closed-ended questions than the other way around.

Second, most clinicians in the STI clinic setting already spend a significant amount of time on counseling, not in the least because their patients expect them to. Given that many patients experience distress over the reason that brought them to the clinic, there is likely to be a "teachable moment" that may enhance the counseling effect. Unfortunately, the quality of counseling varies (greatly) by clinic and by clinician. Still, continual observation and training of clinicians, which is often already part of a clinical quality assurance or improvement protocol, could be used to identify individual counseling strengths and to suggest client-centered ways to enhance the clinician's counseling skills. Thus, rather than imposing an additional counseling intervention to the existing exam, the principles of prevention counseling can be incorporated into the way that clinicians interact with all clients as part of standard of care. Alternatively, utilizing trained non-clinicians, such as disease intervention specialists, counselors, or health educators, as STI clinic support staff may be acceptable in addition to or instead of clinician-delivered risk assessment or risk-reduction counseling.

Changing the standard of the clinician-patient interaction is also the focus of the model developed in the "Ask, Screen, Intervene" intervention, our second case study. Here, however, the development of the intervention was directly driven by the feasibility of implementation in the HIV care setting and the need to efficiently address this emerging issue. Rather than developing or awaiting academic efficacy research on intervention models, a collaboration was sought between HIV care providers and trainers, especially the AIDS Education and Training Centers and the STD/HIV Prevention Training Centers, as well as behavioral scientists at the CDC to develop an intervention based on the balance between proven effective behavioral interventions and the likelihood that such an intervention would be acceptable in clinical settings. The basic starting points of this intervention were that it be brief (an average of five minutes per interaction) and that it would maximize the continuing relationship between clinician and patient. Furthermore, the intervention was eclectic, in that it considered concepts from several individual interventions that appeared to enhance the counseling effect, such as RESPECT, stage-based counseling, motivational interviewing, and the use of loss- and gain-frame messages. Because of the importance of non-HIV STI in the continuing transmission of HIV, an STI screening component was incorporated into the intervention.

The synthesis of what are considered the essential components of different interventions into one prevention strategy is controversial, as it could be argued that the efficacy of such an eclectic intervention model has not been tested and that, in theory, each individual component could counteract one another rather than be synergistic. Still, the individual provider is more likely to adopt elements of interventions that appear to make sense to her/him and that he or she feels comfortable with than to selectively adopt one model over another. Selecting a single effective intervention is further impeded by the outward similarity of the different models, the difference between which are often subtle and likely to be lost in the translation process (22). Indeed, from a provider perspective, research needs may be greater in the area of the synthesis of effective interventions that take into account the strengths and weaknesses at the provider level than the development and evaluation of new intervention models.

Maintenance

The final stage in the adoption process is one where the new intervention has been effectively integrated into standard program operations and maintained over time. There are a number of factors that will help support this phase. First are changes in public health policy and priorities that promulgate the intervention as standard of care. Unfortunately, all too often, such new standards do not come with needed additional resources, and are thus negatively perceived as unfunded mandates. In such instances, changes toward new interventions cannot be made unless resources are shifted from other program areas. In the absence of additional funding, policy makers and funders must be aware of this dilemma and assist providers in prioritizing prevention services. Funders must also be aware of conflicting guidance and mandates. For example, the current CDC guidance on facilitating HIV testing in clinical settings (2) appears to be at odds with increasing the requirements for data collection related to HIV testing (31), resulting in confusion and creating an impediment for the implementation of a potentially important policy change.

A second factor supporting maintenance is composed of changes and support at the level of the institution or agency where the program is housed. A lack of buy-in and support from leadership and management does not stimulate program workers to change business as usual. Even if buy-in is achieved at the worker level, a (perceived) lack of support by the upper echelons in the organization will discourage workers from doing things differently. This challenge is often encountered in training situations where students are direct service providers and not their supervisors. Thus, innovations must often diffuse "upstream" before they are adopted as a standard in the agency. It must be recognized that successful adoption of new interventions requires change of the entire or a large part of the agency and not just front-line staff. Therefore, it is imperative that inclusion of agency leadership and managers should occur early in the adoption process.

A third factor is the recognition that "maintenance" is not a fixed but rather a dynamic process. Continual training and capacity building is needed to maintain the quality of the program. Furthermore, as the STI and HIV epidemics are changing, new prevention concepts are emerging, and old ones may be revisited. Consequently, prevention services must be regularly evaluated against this evolving backdrop and adapted to the new circumstances if recommended research-based interventions are to remain timely and relevant. This process will be achieved more easily if good connections exist between program workers, policy makers, and researchers.

From Efficacy to Effectiveness

Problems with the translation and dissemination of effective interventions from research into daily practice are not limited to HIV/STI prevention interventions. In fact, a body of research on this topic is emerging from the field of health promotion and chronic disease prevention that may provide a very useful guide in thinking about the transfer, translation, and dissemination process of STI/HIV interventions. A central theme in this discourse is the dichotomy between "efficacy" and "effectiveness." Glasgow et al. (8) propose that trials on intervention efficacy and "real world" effectiveness differ fundamentally along five dimensions using the RE-AIM evaluation framework. In this framework, R (reach) refers to the participation rate of those approached and to the representativeness of participants. These are likely to be very homogeneous and highly motivated in efficacy trials but much more heterogeneous in effectiveness settings. *E* (efficacy or effectiveness) relates to the type and effect of an intervention that is likely to be more standardized, intensive, and delivered in ways to maximize effect size in efficacy trials, while tending to be brief, feasible, adaptable and not requiring great expertise in effectiveness settings. *A* (adoption) concerns the setting/agency implementing the intervention. In efficacy research, involved settings have many resources and high-quality staff that are usually limited in number to reduce variability. At the effectiveness level, interventions must appeal to multiple and varied settings, and be adaptable so as to fit the setting's limitations. *I* (implementation) refers to quality and consistency with which the intervention is delivered, both of which are usually high and well-controlled by research staff in efficacy trials, but much more variable in program settings where staff members are scarce, have multiple competing demands, and often turn over quickly. Finally, *M* (maintenance) and costs are usually not issues at the efficacy level; resources are abundant and sustenance beyond the trial period is of no concern. By contrast, costs are a major concern for program effectiveness; many interventions are too costly as designed, to be implemented and maintained in real world (public health) settings (8).

Glasgow et al. point to the deficiencies of the traditional, linear model that begins with efficacy research and, through a "trickle down" process leads to changes in public health practice. Rather, they advocate for a greater focus on the end-users, i.e., the (public health) service providers and involve them in a participatory research process to focuses on effectiveness rather than efficacy (8).

The California HIV/AIDS Prevention Evaluation Initiative (started in 1995) may provide an example on how this may work in the real world of STI/HIV prevention. This initiative consists of four components: community collaborative research, community collaborative translation projects, training and technical assistance, and evaluation. The community collaborative research projects comprise 42 projects in a variety of communities at high risk for HIV infection, including minority MSM, HIV-infected inmates who were recently released, needle exchange users, sex workers, etc. Key features of these projects include a balanced collaboration between scientific and community investigators, direct grants to all collaborators, collaborative conceptualization, development, and implementation, and simultaneous support for research and prevention infrastructure. Factors associated with successful implementation of these projects included history of collaboration, higher proportion (>30%) of funds allocated to direct service provision, substantial and consistent collaboration during the development of the project, integration of the intervention with existing services, intervention delivered within community or with easy community access, the service organization being community-based versus large health care provider or health department, and the service organization having been in existence longer than 10 years (32). Questions still remain regarding the success of such projects when community-research collaborations are too costly or not feasible.

Evaluation

Evaluation as a general topic is discussed elsewhere in this volume (Chapter 20). For the purpose of this chapter, a few pertinent comments will be made. Unlike the evaluation in efficacy studies that focuses on behavioral and biomedical outcomes at the level of the individual, group, or community targeted by the intervention, evaluation of the adoption of behavioral interventions at the program level is often more process-oriented. In this context, a distinction is made in *process monitoring*, which is measured in terms of the quantity and quality of provider-delivered interventions, and in terms of process evaluation, which focuses on whether the intervention was implemented as it was originally intended. Thus, process monitoring may include the number of individual counseling sessions, the number of group meetings, or the frequency and length of outreach sessions and numbers of prevention materials distributed. *Process evaluation* would entail a more qualitative assessment of whether the program adheres to the principles of the intervention, i.e., core elements and key characteristics as mentioned above.

Though the focus of this chapter has been on the process of adopting behavioral interventions at the level of prevention programs, the ultimate goal is that these interventions will impact preventive behaviors by the at-risk populations they serve. These effects may be evaluated through *outcome monitoring*, i.e., measuring changes in the behavior of clients receiving the intervention (e.g., through pre- and post-intervention assessments) or a more rigorous *outcome evaluation* through comparisons with control groups not receiving the intervention. While the latter is akin to evaluation in efficacy research, the methods may be different, for example employing randomized time series and quasi-experimental designs (8). Finally, *impact evaluation* measures the overall impact of the intervention on behaviors and associated morbidity and mortality at the community level. In general, community surveys whether targeted at high-risk populations or of a more general nature can be used to evaluate trends in risk behavior in association to exposure to certain interventions. This is currently being done in the CDC-supported National HIV Behavioral Surveillance (NHBS) project that aims to systematically survey three high risk populations for HIV/STI-related risk behaviors: MSM, IDU and high-risk heterosexuals (33). In addition, available data sources may yield biological, behavioral, service and socio-political information that can be used as "prevention indicators" and be ecologically linked to the availability and density of prevention interventions (34,35).

Conclusion

Many important lessons have been learned from behavioral prevention research that, if applied generally, could have a significant impact on the effectiveness of STI/HIV prevention programs. However, numerous factors appear to influence an effective adoption process. Studying these factors and their interactions can provide tools to improve the linkages between academia, policy, program, and community. Such collaborations may facilitate the transition of interventions from research to practice, and, importantly, provide a framework in which the collaborating parties can inform one another to develop a more effectiveness-oriented research paradigm.

References

1. Centers for Disease Control and Prevention HIV/AIDS Prevention Research Synthesis Project. Compendium of HIV Prevention Interventions with Evidence of Effectiveness. Available at: http://www.cdc.gov/hiv/pubs/hivCompendium/ hivcompendium.htm. Accessed August 31, 2005.

2. CDC. Advancing HIV prevention: new strategies for a changing epidemic -United States, 2003. *MMWR -Morbidity & Mortality Weekly Report*. 2003;52:329–332.
3. CDC. HIV/AIDS Surveillance Report 2003. 2004;15.
4. CDC. Sexually Transmitted Disease Surveillance, 2003. Atlanta, GA: U.S. Department of Health and Human Services, September 2004.
5. CDC. Resurgent bacterial sexually transmitted diseases among men who have sex with men -King County, Washington 1997-1999. *MMWR*. 1999;48:773–777.
6. CDC. Increases in unsafe sex and rectal gonorrhea among men who have sex with men—San Francisco, California, 1994-1997. *MMWR Morb Mortal Wkly Rep*. 1999;48:45–48.
7. Wolitski RJ, Valdiserri RO, Denning PH, Levine WC. Are we headed for a resurgence of the HIV epidemic among men who have sex with men? *Am J Public Health*. Jun 2001;91:883–888.
8. Glasgow RE, Lichtenstein E, Marcus AC. Why don't we see more translation of health promotion research to practice? Rethinking the efficacy-to-effectiveness transition. *Am J Public Health*. Aug 2003;93:1261–1267.
9. CDC Advisory Committee on the Prevention of HIV Infection. *External Review of CDC's HIV Prevention Activities*. Atlanta: Centers for Disease Control and Prevention; 1995.
10. Fishbein M, Guinan M. Behavioral science and public health: a necessary partnership for HIV prevention [editorial]. *Public Health Rep*. 1996;111(Suppl 1):5–10.
11. Fisher JD, Fisher WA. Theoretical approaches to individual-level change in HIV risk behavior. In: Peterson J, DiClemente R, eds. *HIV Prevention Handbook*. New York: Kluwer Academic; 2000.
12. Kalichman S. *Preventing AIDS: A Sourcebook for* behavioral interventions. Mahwah, NJ: Lawrence Earlbaum Associates; 1998.
13. Kamb ML, Dillon BA, Fishbein M, Willis KL. Quality assurance of HIV prevention counseling in a multi-center randomized controlled trial. Project RESPECT Study Group. *Public Health Rep*. 1996;111(Suppl 1):99–107.
14. Neumann MS, Sogolow ED. Replicating effective programs: HIV/AIDS prevention technology transfer. *AIDS Educ Prev*. 2000;12(5 Suppl):35–48.
15. Gandelman A, DeSantis L, Rietmeijer C. Assessing community needs and agency capacity—an integral part of implementing effective evidence-based interventions. *AIDS Educ Prev*. 2006;18(4 Suppl. A):32–43.
16. Kelly JA, Heckman TG, Stevenson LY, et al. Transfer of research-based HIV prevention interventions to community service providers: fidelity and adaptation. *AIDS Educ Prev*. 2000;12(5 Suppl):87–98.
17. Flowers P, Hart GJ, Williamson LM, Frankis JS, Der GJ. Does bar-based, peer-led sexual health promotion have a community-level effect amongst gay men in Scotland? *Int J STD AIDS*. 2002;13:102–108.
18. Elford J, Bolding G, Sherr L. Peer education has no significant impact on HIV risk behaviours among gay men in London. *AIDS*. 2001;15:535–538.
19. Kelly JA. Popular opinion leaders and HIV prevention peer education: resolving discrepant findings, and implications for the development of effective community programmes. *AIDS Care*. 2004;16:139–150.
20. Hart GJ, Williamson LM, Flowers P. Good in parts: the Gay Men's Task Force in Glasgow—a response to Kelly. *AIDS Care*. 2004;16:159–165.
21. Elford J, Bolding G, Sherr L. Popular opinion leaders in London: a response to Kelly. *AIDS Care*. 2004;16:151–158.
22. Gandelman A, Rietmeijer CA. Translation, adaptation, and synthesis of interventions for persons living with HIV: lessons from previous HIV prevention interventions. *J Acquir Immune Defic Syndr*. 2004;37:S126–S129.
23. CDC. Sexually Transmitted Diseases Treatment Guidelines, 2002. *MMWR -Morbidity & Mortality Weekly Report*. 2002;51(RR-6).

24. National Network of STD/HIV Prevention Training Centers. Available at: http://depts.washington.edu/nnptc/index.html. Accessed August 24, 2005.
25. Diffusion of Effective Behavioral Interventions (DEBI). Available at: http://www.effectiveinterventions.org/. Accessed August 24, 2005.
26. CDC. Capacity building. Available at: http://www.cdc.gov/hiv/cba/default.htm. Accessed August 31, 2005.
27. Elford J, Hart G. If HIV prevention works, why are rates of high-risk sexual behavior increasing among MSM? *AIDS Educ Prev.* 2003;15:294–308.
28. CDC. Technical guidance on HIV counseling. *MMWR -Morbidity & Mortality Weekly Report.* 1993;42(RR-2):5–9.
29. Kamb ML, Fishbein M, Douglas JM Jr, et al. Efficacy of risk-reduction counseling to prevent human immunodeficiency virus and sexually transmitted diseases: a randomized controlled trial. Project RESPECT Study Group. *JAMA.* 1998;280:1161–1167.
30. Bolu OO, Lindsey C, Kamb ML, et al. Is HIV/sexually transmitted disease prevention counseling effective among vulnerable populations?: a subset analysis of data collected for a randomized, controlled trial evaluating counseling efficacy (Project RESPECT). *Sex Transm Dis.* 2004;31:469–474.
31. CDC. The changing epidemic. Available at: http://www.cdc.gov/hiv/HIV_3rdDecade/PDF/section3.pdf. Accessed August 30, 2005.
32. Aoki B. What does it take to implement a scientifically sound intervention in a community setting? Paper presented at: 2005 National HIV Prevention Conference, 2005; Atlanta, GA.
33. CDC. HIV prevalence, unrecognized infection, and HIV testing among men who have sex with men—five U.S. cities, June 2004-April 2005. *MMWR Morb Mortal Wkly Rep.* 2005;52:597–601.
34. Rugg DL, Heitgerd JL, Cotton DA, et al. CDC HIV prevention indicators: monitoring and evaluating HIV prevention in the USA. *AIDS.* 2000;14:2003–2013.
35. Page-Shafer K, Kim A, Norton P, et al. Evaluating national HIV prevention indicators: a case study in San Francisco. *AIDS.* 2000;14:2015–2026.
36. CDC. Incorporating HIV prevention into the medical care of persons living with HIV. Recommendations of CDC, the Health Resources and Services Administration, the National Institutes of Health, and the HIV Medicine Association of the Infectious Diseases Society of America. *MMWR Recomm Rep.* 2003;52(RR-12):1–24.
37. Fisher JD, Cornman DH, Osborn CY, Amico KR, Fisher WA, Friedland GA. Clinician-initiated HIV risk reduction intervention for HIV-positive persons: formative research, acceptability, and fidelity of the Options Project. *J Acquir Immune Defic Syndr.* 2004;37:S78–S87.
38. Richardson JL, Milam J, McCutchan A, et al. Effect of brief safer-sex counseling by medical providers to HIV-1 seropositive patients: a multi-clinic assessment. *AIDS.* 2004;18:1179–1186.

Part 5

Ethical and Policy Issues

23

The Ethics of Public Health Practice for the Prevention and Control of STDs

Salaam Semaan, Dr.P.H., and Mary Leinhos, Ph.D.

The goal of public health is to promote the health of all persons for the good of the entire population. While this is a straightforward intention, in practice, public health regularly raises ethical dilemmas that result primarily from conflicts between individual interests and community interests. With respect to sexual health, ethical public health practice is made all the more challenging by the private nature of sexual behavior, and by the social stigma associated with many sexual practices and sexually transmitted diseases (STDs).

This chapter provides an overview of the ethical topics that arise in STD prevention and control, in order both to heighten awareness and understanding of these issues and to provide readers with some guidance for articulating and exploring these issues. We examine the ethics of STD prevention and control in both public health practice and in the delivery of health care. Here, we circumscribe public health practice as the set of activities intended to improve the health of a specific community or population by preventing or controlling disease (1–3). We define delivery of health care as the provision of preventive and treatment services to individuals, including the use of screening and diagnostic tests and the implementation of vaccination programs (4,5).

We highlight in this chapter key concepts in the ethics literature and discuss their implications for several strategies used in STD prevention and control. Our aim is to support the work of health care providers and public health practitioners and provide them with tools to help ensure the ethical delivery of strategies to prevent and control STDs. The overview presented in this chapter is not meant to be all-inclusive, but rather illustrative of key ethical issues stemming from or influencing the implementation of various STD management strategies. The first section of the chapter provides background information on research ethics, bioethics, public health ethics, and the regulatory context; highlights key ethical concepts in public health; summarizes how paradigms of disease transmission influence ethical thinking and delivery of care; and presents a decision-making framework for articulating and responding to ethical challenges in public health. The purpose of this section is to provide a context as well as a useful and consistent approach for the ethical analysis of STD prevention and control. The second section of the chapter examines the ethical considerations that arise from the pursuit of several STD management

Behavioral Interventions for Prevention and Control of Sexually Transmitted Diseases.
Aral SO, Douglas JM Jr, eds. Lipshutz JA, assoc ed. New York: Springer Science+
Business Media, LLC; 2007.

strategies, including behavioral interventions, biomedical interventions, health-care-seeking interventions, partner management, social marketing interventions, structural interventions, internet-based interventions, and work with special populations. We conclude with a summary of key points for the ethical practice of STD management.

The Ethical Context of STD Prevention and Control

A useful approach for analyzing the ethics of STD prevention and control includes the set of ethical approaches and regulations that guide and govern public health research and practice as well as medical practice. We discuss the ethics of STD prevention and control from the perspectives of our heritage from medical and research ethics, and from the particulars of public health practice.

Research Ethics and Bioethics

The three ethical principles of respect, beneficence, and justice (6,7) are generally recognized as relevant to public health practice, clinical care, and public health research. For more than 20 years, these three ethical principles, articulated in the landmark Belmont Report (7), have guided medical research and clinical practice. The Belmont Report calls for investigators, and by extension, health care providers and public health practitioners, to treat the autonomy of people with respect (respect for persons); to maximize potential benefits and to minimize possible harms (beneficence and nonmaleficence); and to be fair in delivery of patient care (justice). The principle of respect requires treating participants and patients as autonomous individuals and obtaining their informed consent before they receive health care. Informed consent means that the individual has voluntarily agreed, based on solid knowledge and understanding of all relevant health care information, to receive health care or to choose among alternative treatments. The principle of beneficence requires that the risk to participants and patients be reasonable in relation to the anticipated benefits gained. The principle of justice requires that the benefits and burdens of health care be distributed fairly so that no single group, especially if disadvantaged, vulnerable, or minority, bears a disproportionate share of the risk or burden of disease.

These three major ethical principles—respect for persons, beneficence and nonmaleficence, and justice—are important tools that can assist health care providers and public health practitioners with making decisions and clarifying the rationale and the justifications for the decisions that need to be made. Shortly, we will review five global ethics concepts in STD management and a decision-making framework for public health ethics, which are both informed by these foundational ethical principles. Accordingly, it is important for health care providers and public health care practitioners to understand the ethical principles. Equally important is their ability to appropriately translate and apply these principles in delivery of care. Throughout the rest of the chapter, we will revisit these fundamental principles, illustrating their application in the prevention and control of STDs.

The Ethics of Public Health

While the ethics of medicine (8) and research (7) have been thoroughly articulated in scholarly discourse, ethical analysis and principles specific to public health practice were developed more recently (9). While there is an overlap in the ethical principles of the different disciplines, the ethical principles for public health differ from the ethical principles for medicine and research (10,11). The main differences lie in the emphasis of public health practice on the role of the community in disease prevention and control (12,13), and in balancing the need for protecting individual liberties while also serving the communal good (2,14–17).

Specialized codes of ethics play a major role in the ethics of public health. The Public Health Code of Ethics (13) was adopted recently by various public health organizations including the American Public Health Association. The code lists 12 ethical principles of public health practice. These principles highlight several thematic values including community participation; protection of both communities and individuals; appropriate collection, use, and sharing of information; and a holistic approach to public heath. The enumeration of thematic values, principles, and skills needed for the ethical practice of public health establishes a firm foundation for the ethics of public health. Professional codes of ethics, which guide many of the day-to-day activities of various health professionals, have long existed for physicians (18), nurses (19), and psychologists (20), as well as for other professions (21). Training public health practitioners and health care providers in the application of the public health code of ethics to the realm of STD prevention and control will help them in articulating ethical arguments and justifications in the delivery of STD prevention and control, and in rendering the relevant ethical issues more transparent.

Regulatory Context

In addition to the ethical theories, principles, and codes, the delivery of health care and public health practice is governed by federal and state laws and regulations, codes of ethics of relevant professional organizations, and institutional policies and procedures (2). Laws specific to STD prevention and control have been in place for many years, both at federal and state levels (22). Several ethical principles are codified as laws, such as those governing the application of the legal documents of informed consent and authorization and the protection of confidential information.

In medical care, informed consent is defined as the communication process between a patient and his or her physician that results in the patient's agreement to undergo a particular medical procedure or treatment. The concept of informed consent is rooted in medical ethics, codified as legal principle, and is based on the assertion that a competent person has the right to determine what is done to him or her. The American Medical Association recommends that its members disclose and discuss the following with their patients (23): a description of procedure, risks, benefits, uncertainties, alternatives, and likely outcomes if no treatment is elected; assessment of patient understanding; and acceptance of the intervention by the patient. Specific elements include the patient's diagnosis, if known; the nature and purpose of a proposed treatment or procedure; the risks and benefits of a proposed treatment or procedure; alternatives (regardless of their cost or the extent to which the treatment options are covered by health insurance); the risks and benefits of the alternative treatment and procedure; and the risks and benefits of not receiving or undergoing a treatment or procedure. The requirement for informed consent in spelled out in statutes and case law in all 50 states. Most health care institutions, including STD clinics, have policies that state which health interventions require a signed consent form. For example, surgery, anesthesia, and other invasive procedures are usually in this category. These signed forms are really the culmination of a dialogue required to foster the patient's informed participation in the clinical process and decision. In some instances, the patient consent appears as a paragraph in forms titled as admission and registration agreement forms or as confidential registration information forms. For a wide range of clinical exams, written consent is not required, but some meaningful discussion is needed. For example, a patient contemplating a certain screening test, diagnostic test, or treatment for an STD should be cognizant of the relevant arguments for and against this test or treatment, discussed in layperson's terms.

Although regulation of public health is intended to ensure the safety and welfare of the public, there are inherent trade-offs between protecting the health of the public on one the hand and the professional and economic cost to the public health system on the other hand (24,25). Laws, as part of the existing infrastructure and environment, shape the effectiveness of the public health system in the prevention and control of STDs and the vulnerability or resilience of persons at risk for STDs (25,26).

The most recent federal law relevant to STD prevention and treatment is the Health Insurance Portability and Accountability Act, known as the HIPAA Privacy Rule, that aims to protect the privacy of individually identifiable health data (27). HIPAA limits disclosure of "individually identifiable health information" to certain individuals, including one's family and friends, regardless of one's state of health. Since its implementation in April 2003, few articles have been written about the advantages of the HIPAA Privacy Rule in protecting the health data and several articles have been written about its unintended effect on the structure and cost of health care (28,29), including articles that addressed its ethical ramifications (30,31).

State laws, regulations, and case law often impose additional requirements to those required by the federal government (32). State laws, which vary significantly among states, address a wide range of topics including age of consent, responsibilities of surrogate decision makers, confidentiality of medical records, reporting requirements for STDs, delivery of medical care, and delegation of authority to perform medical procedures (24,33,34). The model state public health act was developed in 2003 through a collaboration between a federal, state, and a nongovernment organization. This model covers various topics, including the power of authority of public health officials and the privacy of public health information, and offers states a tool for reform of public health law (35).

Health care providers and public health practitioners are responsible for knowing the laws that govern their work in STD prevention and control. A pertinent question is whether health care providers and public health practitioners need to be concerned about the ethics of STD prevention and care, when these issues are already covered by relevant statutes. While the law provides limits on what can and cannot be done, it does not determine ethical behaviors. Some may argue that regulations and laws are not necessarily always ethically correct, creating a situation where it may be possible to conduct activities that are legal and in conformity with the regulations, but that are ethically flawed. For example, laws influence the ability of health care providers and public health practitioners to notify third parties, such as spouses and sex partners of their exposure to an STD (36–40). Some of these statutes have been criticized for exacerbating the problem of reconciling patient privacy and relevant parties' right to know (36).

One example of a controversial regulation is name-based HIV case reporting. As of March 2006, name-based HIV case reporting was prohibited by law in the state of California. Name-based reporting has been strongly criticized in California by many HIV/AIDS advocates, who instead favor a code-based reporting system due to confidentiality concerns. However, later, in spring 2006, name-based HIV case reporting was authorized in California. Opponents of name-based reporting argue that those named may be subject to discrimination and stigma, and that consequently such a system may be a deterrent to testing. However, delays in implementing name-based reporting may result in reductions of federal Ryan White CARE Act (RWCA) funding, and in reduced services to clients (41). On the other hand, code-based reporting has its own limitations such as the increased risk that duplicate records will be created. It is important to collect as much empirical data as possible to best weigh the risks and benefits in ethical controversies such as name-based HIV case reporting.

Of importance, the moral grounds for laws may change with biomedical advances or with new evidence on the best approaches to effective prevention. Relevant examples include the evolution in the requirements for explicit informed consent and for pre-test HIV counseling. Early in the epidemic, consensus emerged that voluntary testing with explicit informed consent was essential to encourage willingness to be tested and to protect individuals from discrimination and psychological harm (42). As relatively effective AIDS treatments became available in the 1990s and early diagnosis became more beneficial, physicians began to support routine HIV testing, given with presumed consent, although initially, federal and state policy continued to call for voluntary testing with explicit informed consent (43). Furthermore, as HIV testing became more acceptable to patients, it was realized that low acceptance of testing was associated with explicit informed consent, and that higher acceptance of testing was associated with presenting counseling and testing as routine rather than as optional (44). Clearly, as the epidemic progressed, and along with it, medical progress and societal attitudes, the moral arguments shifted from favoring testing with explicit written consent to testing with consent obtained as part of general consent for care in health care settings (45).

In 1993, guidelines were published recommending a client-centered approach to counseling (46). By applying this approach, the counselor helps the client to identify and to commit to a single step he or she can take to reduce HIV risk and to develop strategies for overcoming personal barriers to behavior change. While it is time intensive, client-centered counseling has been associated with a 20% reduction in new STD infection rates compared with the informational counseling approach (47) recommended a few years earlier (48). New recommendations encourage counseling in settings where risk behavior is discussed such as STD clinics, but does not require it as a mandatory component of HIV testing in health care delivery settings (45). Justifications for this shift include the fact that with the maturing of the HIV epidemic and the availability of potent antiretroviral therapies, HIV prevention efforts now prioritize both case finding of those with undiagnosed infection and access and adherence to HIV care and treatment, as well as prevention activities focused on ensuring adequate and sustained sexual and drug risk reduction across diverse populations (49,50).

Selected Ethical Concepts

There are several concepts and applications that lie at the core of public health ethics, including the ethics of STD prevention and control. Here we review five fundamental and far reaching public health concepts: informed consent and authorization; privacy and confidentiality; risk-benefit analysis; community protections; and considerations for special populations. Discussion of how these selected ethical concepts apply to STD prevention and control appears in the second section of this chapter as we elaborate more specifically on how these concepts apply to different STD interventions.

Informed Consent and Authorization

The processes and legal documents of informed consent and patient authorization stem from the ethical principle of respect for people. This ethical concept and related regulations require health care providers and public health practitioners to treat people as autonomous individuals in the delivery of health care. Informed consent refers to the process in which a patient agrees to treatment at the beginning of the provider-patient relationship (51). With the advent of the HIPAA Privacy Rule, the term authorization now specifically refers to the process of obtaining permission from patients to use or disclose their personal health information to a third party, for the purposes of health care delivery and reimbursement (51). Authorization forms for health care, must contain elements required by HIPAA, and also elements required by state laws where applicable (27).

Treating patients as partners and collaborators can improve the overall outcome of medical care by improving trust, facilitating communication, and improving compliance rates (52,53). The process of consent and authorization is even more important than the signed documents. Accordingly, it is important for patients and health care providers to discuss and understand the meaning of those documents and to be able to apply their knowledge in delivery of health care.

Privacy and Confidentiality

Although the concepts of privacy and confidentiality are related, they address different concerns. Privacy refers to how individuals share information about themselves with others, and confidentiality refers to how shared information is handled. While privacy is influenced by relational, cultural, and social characteristics, confidentiality is influenced by security measures. All patients want to be assured that their personal data are protected and that threats to privacy or breaches of confidentiality are prevented. Sound procedures need to be carefully developed, in advance, for handling files and for storing and transmitting data, for creating or eliminating linkages between medical data and identifiers, and for recontacting patients. Training staff members in the concepts and procedures for ensuring privacy and confidentiality, and for choosing appropriate steps and places to inform patients, their partners, and related family members about sensitive information, are important strategies as well.

Risk-Benefit Analysis

The concept of risk-benefit analysis stems from the ethical principles of benef-icence and nonmaleficence, which call on health care providers and public health practitioners to ensure that the benefits of health care are proportionate to the risks assumed by patients, population groups, and communities. The principle of beneficence calls for minimization of harm through the use of pro-cedures that are consistent with sound health care. Harm is defined as unde-sirable outcomes or adverse events encompassing physical, social, or emotional detriment that may affect people as a result of receipt of health care. Before implementation of procedures, as in the case of partner notification, health care providers and public health practitioners need to engage relevant individuals and families in a careful review of the risks and benefits (54). They also need to highlight the harms that may result and ensure that safeguards are in place to minimize unintended consequences.

Community Protections

Because of its collective focus, public health practice often places limits on the autonomy of individuals, particularly on their privacy and liberty (55) in the name of protecting the health of the community or the population. However, there is always a concern that efforts to override individual liberties for the col-lective good may result in abuse (56).

It has been argued that a set of five conditions must be met in order to jus-tify public health restrictions on individual liberties (57). These conditions are 1) demonstrating the effectiveness of the infringing intervention in protecting public health; 2) showing that the probable benefits outweigh negative conse-quences; 3) confirming the necessity of the intervention for achieving public health; 4) minimizing to the extent possible any infringement; and 5) actively providing public justification and explanation of such infringement. Other important remedies against abuse of authority include open admission that policies and practices may need revision in light of new evidence, and enlist-ment of affected populations in the decision-making and implementation processes (55).

It is important to protect communities from stigma, as stigma makes it harder to reach and serve the populations and individuals who are subjected to it. Efforts aimed at STD prevention and control should not contribute to stigma, intentionally or unintentionally. Empowering communities to be involved in decision-making processes while also showing respect for diver-sity and cultural competency are important. An important benefit of working with communities in planning and implementing public health strategies includes building community trust in public health institutions, which is vital to the success of many public health initiatives. Communities, especially dis-enfranchised ones, must be empowered with access to health resources, and with articulation and implementation of culturally sensitive health interven-tions (13,43).

Considerations for Special Populations

The need to consider the vulnerabilities of special populations stems from the ethical principle of justice, which requires that the benefits and burdens of health care be distributed fairly among people. Accordingly, disadvantaged, vulnerable, or minority groups or communities should not be asked to bear a disproportionate share of infection or disease burden. Two questions are usually relevant when considering the ethical principle of justice. First, are we systematically delivering preventive or curative care to people simply because of their ease of availability as opposed to reasons related to infection or disease burden? Second, are we systematically excluding groups of people who may benefit from health care? Systematic exclusion of certain population groups or communities violates the principle of justice, especially when these population groups or communities could benefit from public health practice and health care. It is important that efforts aimed at STD prevention and control not end up further marginalizing or stigmatizing special populations when they are already vulnerable and disenfranchised.

The absence of universal access to health care and the high disparities in disease rates between population groups raise relevant ethical issues of justice. Some health care intervention strategies are expensive, are delivered at few places, or are not covered by insurance. Low hepatitis B vaccination rates among drug users, for example, raises ethical concerns about distributive justice (58,59).

Paradigms of Disease Transmission

Having reflected on the role of key ethical concepts, it is also important to understand how paradigms of disease transmission can influence the ethical delivery of preventive and curative health care services. The STD interventions discussed in this chapter constitute a spectrum of public health strategies, representing four major, complementary disease transmission paradigms. These four paradigms—the biomedical, behavioral, health promotion, and structural paradigms—differ in their emphasis on the role of the microorganism, host, and environment in disease prevention and control. While these four paradigms are not mutually exclusive, the primary paradigm informing a particular public health intervention is associated with a typical set of ethical issues, as described in the second section of this chapter. Awareness of these disease transmission paradigms and their attendant ethical concerns may help anticipate and deal with ethical challenges ahead of implementation.

First, the biomedical paradigm of disease dynamics emphasizes various biomedical approaches (e.g., diagnostic tests, treatment, vaccination) in control of STD (60,61). Hence, the relationship of patients to health care providers and public health practitioners in clinical settings and practice, as addressed by the ethical principles of respect and autonomy, is of paramount importance (8). Second, the behavioral paradigm emphasizes the role of individual behaviors and responsibilities in determining health outcomes (62–64). Accordingly, the moral and cultural perspectives on proper and improper behaviors and the judgment ramifications reflected in perceptions of blame, stigma, and discrimination are relevant (65,66). The behavioral model also focuses on interactions between dyads, which highlight, for example, the ethical obligations of both partners in a sexual relationship and the public health practice of partner notification (67,68). Third, whereas the biomedical paradigm relies on biomedical tools to diagnose, treat, and prevent infection, the health promotion paradigm emphasizes the psychological and social determinants that are important in acquisition, transmission, prevention, and control of infection and disease (69,70). The health promotion paradigm reflects concerns associated with respect for persons and for communities. Fourth, the structural paradigm emphasizes the role of the social, economic, and legal context in influencing risk-taking behaviors and in explaining the variations in prevalence and incidence rates of infections and diseases (71,72). This paradigm is influenced by the perceptions of the role of the social infrastructure in prevention and control of infection and reflects concerns associated with the ethical principles of beneficence and justice (73). In the context of the structural paradigm, the ethical principle of beneficence requires protecting group dignity and preventing community harm, and the ethical principle of justice calls for ensuring equitable access to care. Efforts that focus on improving community access to health resources and on reducing population disparities in disease burden acknowledge that social inequities are a major cause of disease (74,75). The health and human rights perspective, which emphasizes the causes of social inequities and promotes the right to health, has begun to influence the ethics of disease prevention and treatment (10,76,77), and typically invokes the ethical principles of justice and respect for rights of persons and of communities.

Awareness of both the underlying disease transmission paradigms that affect STD interventions and the ethical principles can help health care providers and public health practitioners anticipate and avoid potential ethical dilemmas associated with interventions they consider implementing. Such foresight can save time, effort, money, and frustration.

A Framework for Ethical Analysis

We now present an ethical framework that may serve as a valuable tool to guide selected aspects of public health decision making (78). The framework involves 1) assessing the public health problem; 2) identifying and evaluating ethically acceptable options for addressing the problem; and 3) making and implementing decisions ethically. We can use in this framework the ethical concepts that we just reviewed.

In the first step, *assessing the public health problem*, it is important to articulate the threats and harms to the public's health, the goals of potential public health action, the ethical concerns that are at stake in the situation and the alternative courses of action, as well as the relevant laws, regulations, and sources of authority. It is of particular importance to research precedent cases and the historical context, and to explore analogies to other historical public health challenges.

Second, having sized up the public health problem, decision makers need next to determine and weigh the options. In *identifying and evaluating ethically acceptable options*, it is important to ascertain the stakeholders who will be affected by each alternative, the ethical claims of critical stakeholders, the impact on relationships (e.g., building and maintaining trust) affected by each option, and the ethical considerations that provide justification for an option. These ethical considerations include several questions. For example, is there a balance of benefits over harms (utility)? Are the benefits and burdens distributed fairly (distributive justice)? Are those affected participating in the decision-making process (procedural justice)? Are individual choices and interests respected? Are relationships respected through honesty, transparency, trustworthiness, promise-keeping, and protection of confidentiality? What useful guidance does the public health code of ethics or other professional guidelines provide?

Third, having assessed the options, decision makers need next to choose from among them. In order to *make and implement decisions ethically*, it is important to discuss whether the chosen public health action is likely to effectively achieve public health goals, given practical, political and economic factors, and to determine how ethical tensions and conflicts can be resolved. Questions to consider include: Can the conflicting ethical principles be balanced? Is the selected action the least burdensome to particular moral interests or the least restrictive alternative? If the burdens are great, is the action necessary to achieve an important public health goal? What roles might public health professionals play (e.g., mediator, authority, advocate, teacher) in implementation? What are appropriate roles for other government officials? How should the public and specific stakeholders be involved? How should the process of public justification take place?

Ethical Considerations in Selected STD Prevention and Control Strategies

The preceding section of this chapter presented a review of global ethical concepts and of key factors influencing the ethical context of public health, as well as a framework for ethical analysis of public health topics. These overarching concepts and tools for public health practice are applicable to the specific strategies used in STD prevention and control. We turn now to examine these overall concepts in specific STD management strategies presented in the other chapters of this book, including behavioral interventions, biomedical interventions, health-care-seeking interventions, partner management, social marketing interventions, structural interventions, Internet-based interventions, and working with special populations.

The Ethics of Behavioral Interventions

Behavioral interventions aim to effect behavioral change through 1) sharing with the target population information on specific infections and diseases and on risk-reduction strategies; 2) emphasizing motivational factors and providing information on risk-reduction skills, including skills in partner communication, sexual negotiation, resistance skills, and condom application; and 3) influencing peer norms. Behavioral interventions are delivered to individuals, dyads, groups, or communities.

In terms of the ethical principle of respect for persons, development of nonjudgmental attitudes about patient behaviors is important in fostering respectful relationships with patients. Ensuring that there is no harm to secondary subjects, whose consent was not obtained and about whom information was provided by primary informants, is important.

In terms of the ethical principle of beneficence, protecting private and confidential information and minimizing the potential for physical and sexual abuse is essential. If identities of individuals participating in behavioral interventions are not protected, there could be the risk of embarrassment or even the risk for more serious harm. Addressing the psychosocial effect of having an STD is also important (79,80). Health care providers and public health practitioners may encounter reportable situations, when there is evidence of abuse or neglect or the likely prospect of harm to self or to others. In most states, health care providers and public health practitioners have a legal obligation to report such situations to appropriate authorities. Behavioral interventions can raise speculative concerns about adverse behavioral outcomes, including increase in risky sexual behaviors or earlier sexual debut. Evidence to date supports the assertion that risk-reduction approaches (e.g., condom promotion) are no more likely, and sometimes less likely, than risk-avoidance approaches (e.g., abstinence-only education) to be associated with an unintended increase in other risk behaviors (e.g., increased unprotected sex or earlier sexual debut) (81–84). In terms of the ethical principle of justice, relevant ethical considerations include showing respect for diversity and providing culturally appropriate interventions.

The Ethics of Biomedical Interventions and Health-Care-Seeking Interventions

We define biomedical and health-care-seeking interventions as encompassing a wide array of interventions, including the provision of screening, diagnostic, and testing procedures, the use of vaccines and microbicides, and the delivery of treatment strategies (5). Biomedical interventions and health-care-seeking interventions share ethical considerations.

In terms of the ethical principle of respect, the duty to respect the autonomy of others, as operationalized in the processes and legal documents of informed consent or authorization calls for discussing the purpose of the intervention, its potential benefits, risks, and limitations. An important component of informed consent is the discussion that takes place before implementing the intervention. Counseling and informing patients is especially critical when the intervention is based on incomplete scientific knowledge, such as when the efficacy of a vaccine or treatment is not fully known, or when the positive predictive value of a test is low and the balance of potential benefits and harms is unclear, as is arguably the case for HSV-2 testing (85). However, if benefits of routine, presumed-consent testing become clear, as was established for screening of pregnant women for HIV when the efficacy of antiretroviral therapy against vertical transmission was established (86), requirements for consent and pre-test counseling may do more harm than good (43). It is critical that health care providers and public health practitioners keep abreast of the current medical literature and most recent recommendations for treatment, for the purpose of delivering effective and ethical care to their patients, including those with STDs.

Autonomy also mandates that patients make their decisions on a voluntary basis free from coercion from parents, family members, health care providers, public health practitioners, and even society. Patients have the right to explore their values, feelings, and coping styles before accepting an intervention, despite the emotionally charged arguments that can be made by significant others or in the family decision-making process because of differences in values or in coping with risk and uncertainty. In addition, health care providers and public health care practitioners need also to balance their own clinical or personal judgment about the best path for prevention or treatment with respect for the patient's wishes.

In terms of beneficence, it is equally important to discuss with patients how to inform third-party members, including affected family members, partners, or others who may not be aware that they are at risk for infection or disease.

It may be hard to convince patients that other affected members should know about a certain health situation or about certain test results, or to convince them of the importance of naming their partners or of having their partners tested or treated. Feelings of guilt, shame, fear of abuse, and fear of breakdown in relationships may be of concern to patients. These concerns need to be discussed with patients, and, when relevant, family members or significant others need to be included in the information and counseling sessions.

Protection of private and confidential information is critical for avoiding devastating consequences for individuals, families, communities, and society and for preserving beneficence. Patients highly value having assurances related to their privacy and to the confidentiality of their data (87). Health care providers, public health practitioners, and patients need to be clear about safeguards used in protecting patient information; who owns, controls, and has access to the information; how the information will be interpreted and used; and how people can be protected from harm that might result from improper disclosure or use of the information. HIPAA privacy rules identify personal health information as protected health information. Accordingly, health care providers cannot disclose private information to third parties without the signed authorization of the patients.

Ethical public health requires attentiveness to the needs of patients who are multilingual and to those or who are from different cultures. Health care providers and public health practitioners have the responsibility to ensure that patients and affected members hear the medical and scientific information in a language and cultural context that they can understand. Such clarity and comfort are critical elements in the decision-making process about one's health care. Providing the information in a culturally sensitive and scientifically appropriate manner that includes a balanced discussion of the health care procedures and the potential benefits and harms is an important ethical responsibility of health care providers and public health practitioners (52).

The vaccination of adolescents for STDs raises ethical issues related to the consent of parents or legal guardians for the procedure. While an effective vaccine for hepatitis B is already available, an effective vaccine for HPV has become available in 2006 (88–92). Ethical tension about adolescent vaccination stems from the fact that respect for autonomy usually implies accepting the choices that parents make on behalf of their children. However, it is important to recognize the cases where parental refusal to allow their children to get vaccinated may cause the children harm. Parental autonomy requires adequate disclosure of the benefits and possible harms of the vaccine and setting limits on the persuasive techniques that might be used in providing the information. A relevant question is whether adolescents should be provided with the information despite the objections of their parents or legal guardians, on the basis of the rights of children and youth (15). The attitudes of not only parents or legal guardians towards vaccination, but also those of health care providers and public health practitioners pose ethical concerns (93–97). Recent studies suggest that that a reasonable proportion of parents and health care providers (more than 70%) have favorable attitudes towards vaccinating adolescents against STDs (95,97). These studies also indicate the importance of recommendations of professional associations in shaping attitudes of parents and providers towards vaccinating adolescents against STDs (95,97). Health care providers, public health practitioners, and parents need to reflect on how their personal biases or beliefs may unintentionally shape the care they provide or allow. Accordingly, vaccine recipients need to receive rigorous informed consent, including counseling, information, and accurate and unbiased information about the risks and benefits of vaccines without inappropriately pressuring them to receive or not to receive the vaccine (98).

In keeping with the ethical principle of beneficence, it is important to ascertain that the children will not suffer physical or psychological harm if they do not get the vaccine. Carefully developed vaccination counseling procedures that provide information on the benefits and harms of accepting or refusing a vaccine should also include information about the benefits and harms of alternative strategies, including risk-reduction strategies and use of safer sex practices. In addition, ethical deliberations need to address the potential for post-immunization, changes in risk behavior, fueled by perceptions of invulnerability by vaccine recipients. Vaccination could paradoxically increase the prevalence of other STDs for which vaccines or treatments are not available. If vaccine recipients were to reduce their commitment to engage in safe behaviors, they will put themselves and others at risk for other STDs. Thus, in addition to information on the adverse effects and negative unintended consequences of vaccines, consideration should be given to providing age-appropriate information about other preventive strategies such as abstinence, monogamy, condom use, limiting the number of sex partners, and undergoing Pap testing.

While data are lacking as to whether vaccination for any STD is associated with increased sexual disinhibition, administering a particular vaccine for one STD without providing education on the risk for getting infected with other STDs presents a missed prevention opportunity for the patient and for public health. It is important for both the patient and the public to understand that receiving a vaccine for one STD will not protect against infection with other STDs.

Speculative risks will be raised with any new intervention, and the busy health professional must decide how best to make use of time spent in consultation with patients. Rather than subjecting the patient to a lengthy list of caveats and explanations that may be moot, health professionals are advised to probe and listen carefully to patients for concerns or beliefs they may have about the vaccination. The time that providers have for care and prevention is limited, but it may be wasted if patients' potential misconceptions are not addressed. The decision whether to counsel parents, teens, or both about sexual health will depend on factors such as the ethnic or cultural viewpoint of the family, age of the adolescent, the parent's agenda in pursuing the vaccination, and whether opportunities are created to consult privately with the adolescent (96). Possible scenarios should be enumerated and planned for ahead of time, in the context of the local client population.

Although vaccines represent a promising public health opportunity, they also raise ethical concerns about balancing individual liberties and communal health (98). While, for example, some people may have concerns about the medical adverse events associated with vaccination, in many circumstances, individual and community benefits on their own outweigh the risk of adverse events. Suggestions have been made for considering a set of seven ethical principles in prioritizing and planning vaccination programs (98). These principles suggest that vaccination programs 1) should target serious diseases that are public health problems; 2) must be effective and safe; 3) should be associated with small burdens and inconveniences; 4) should have favorable burden/benefits ratio in comparison with alternative vaccination schemes or preventive options; 5) should involve a just distribution of benefits and burdens; 6) should be voluntary unless compulsory vaccination is essential to prevent a concrete and serious harm; and 7) should honor and protect the public trust. Public health practitioners are well advised to consider these issues now in anticipation of STD vaccines currently in the development pipeline. For example, as mentioned earlier, recipients of a vaccine against a specific STD should know that such a vaccine does not protect them from getting infected with other STDs, and be aware of the importance of other prevention strategies against other STDs.

The Ethics of Partner Management

For effective STD prevention and control, it is important not only to treat the patient (also referred to as the index case) with effective medications for treatable STDs, but also to provide risk-reduction information, medical evaluation, and treatment of sex partners, through the practice of partner notification and management (99). This strategy provides benefit to the exposed (and often unknowing) partner of the index patient by reducing the chance for infection and re-infection, and to the community, by reducing ongoing transmission. However, these benefits must be balanced with respect to privacy of the person diagnosed with an STD.

Partner notification and management must always be voluntary on the part of infected persons and their partners. Furthermore, to increase cooperation and to show respect for those involved, the information obtained should be treated as confidential. Health care providers and public health practitioners should endeavor to not only provide science-based partner notification services, but also to deliver these services with knowledgeable, skilled, and trained staff in a nonjudgmental, sensitive, and culturally appropriate manner (54).

The potential for unintended negative consequences is a major concern in the practice of partner management, consistent with the ethical principle of beneficence (100). Such consequences include threats to privacy and confidentiality and the potential for breakdown in relationships between sex partners. With patient-delivered therapy, there is the additional concern about missed prevention and treatment opportunities for partners of the index patients, who could be infected with STDs other than those diagnosed in the index patients and for which they did not receive patient-delivered therapy (101). Absence of trust between patients and health care providers and absence of trust toward the health care system can lead to problems (53).

Another concern in the practice of partner management is missing prevention and treatment opportunities for unnamed sex partners. Hence, it is important for patients to understand the importance of knowing and naming their sex partners to ensure their treatment, and for health care providers and practitioners to emphasize to their patients their regard for privacy of persons and confidentiality of information.

Procedures to protect patients and partners should include truly informed consent and authorization processes, stringent procedures for handling data, incorporation of patient privacy measures into the physical space and into the operating procedures of the clinic, training staff members in privacy of persons and confidentiality of data, and use of culturally appropriate wording and delivery modes to reach and inform partners. Other approaches include training index patients in partner communication strategies, testing sex partners for STDs other than those diagnosed in the index patients, and informing the general public and those at risk for STDs about the importance of knowing and naming their sex partners in order to provide them with appropriate prevention and treatment services. Health care providers and public health practitioners also need to counsel patients about how to prevent or minimize the potential for family abuse, family violence, or the initiation of risky sexual encounters, should current relationships break down when they disclose STD infection to affected partners (54). Additional concerns relate to the provision of prescriptions or medications for the treatment of sex partners in the absence of laboratory testing, taking of a medical history, or a clinical examination, especially for partners who may be pregnant, have antibiotic allergies, or have antibiotic-resistant infections. Health care providers and public health practitioners need to educate index patients accordingly.

The Ethics of Structural Interventions and Social Marketing Interventions

These interventions aim to address the social, medical, and economic factors impacting disease transmission risk at the individual and population levels, and thus to reduce geographic and racial and ethnic disparities in health conditions (71,102). Large-scale public health communication campaigns aim to increase the awareness of disease transmission and the adoption of recommended prevention and treatment strategies, while structural interventions seek to induce changes at the societal level to change health behaviors and health outcomes (103). Over the past several years, public health practitioners have developed a variety of social marketing campaigns aimed at prevention and control of several STDs (104,105). These include several media campaigns aimed at control of syphilis outbreaks (105–108). In developing these campaigns, public health practitioners working in state and local STD health departments partnered with a diverse group of health professionals to reach the target audience with effective scientific information aimed at disease control and prevention. In developing such campaigns, it is important to pay attention to a number of ethics-related matters, including balancing scientific information with social values to induce risk-reduction behavior change.

Public health practitioners also need to be involved in the design and implementation of structural interventions, and to assess and improve the efficacy of those interventions. Over the past few years, such interventions have included closing or regulating bathhouses (110) and imposing STD prevention regulations on Nevada brothels (112–114). Compelling arguments have been made that structural and environmental interventions are an effective tool for HIV prevention in bathhouses (109–111). Stringent health testing requirements for sex workers in Nevada brothels, in place since the mid-1980s, mandate that brothel workers get weekly tests for chlamydia and gonorrhea and monthly tests for HIV and syphilis (112). The Nevada brothel industry voluntarily adopted mandatory condom-use policies in 1987, that got legally mandated by the state health department the following year (112). The mandatory condom policy is supported by brothel workers (112,113), and has met with acceptance by the majority of brothel clients in one study (114). There have been no cases of licensed sex workers contracting HIV since the STD testing policies were implemented. STD rates amongst these brothel workers are significantly lower than that of the general population (112), and are associated with one of the lowest published rates of condom breakage and slippage (114). While Nevada's brothel health regulations are effective, there is still a need to provide health benefits and services to brothel workers, who as independent contractors receive no employment benefits (112). More recently, public health practitioners from local health departments were involved in control of an HIV outbreak and the establishment of regulations concerning condom use for the adult film industry (115).

Harm at the population level or at the community level as well as stigma are major concerns that health care providers and public health practitioners need to recognize when they are engaging with social marketing interventions and structural interventions. Sometimes, production of pamphlets to accompany health messages may raise ethical questions because the illustrations or pictures used may challenge or reinforce discriminatory cultural norms or stigmatizing attitudes. The illustrations may also be seen by some as challenging important community norms or addressing sensitive issues in improper ways. Thus, it is advisable to engage representative community advisory boards in developing message design and depiction.

In terms of the ethical principle of beneficence, while some may argue that illustrations with strong shock tactics or with strong emotional appeal may be helpful in inducing behavior change, others believe that such depictions can be intrusive, lingering in the minds of the viewers and leaving a negative psychological effect. Using messages through depictions and statistics to motivate change and to facilitate persuasion without having people ignore the messages or see them as offensive is an important balancing act.

It is also important to consider whether the depictions show the persons with a certain health behavior or disease as victims, and to consider the effect of such depictions on others. A relevant concern is whether such depictions lead others to blame the sick people, to avoid them, to stigmatize them, to discriminate against them, or to say their disease was a punishment. Such consequences can already be devastating to vulnerable populations associated with stigmatized behaviors or certain medical conditions because such judgment by others can result in the internalization of self-blame and in the destruction of self-esteem (116).

In addition to avoiding stigma and victimization, the design and implementation of structural interventions and social marketing should anticipate and avoid other likely negative social implications of efforts to change health behaviors. While some practices are unhealthy, it is important to recognize that they may have cultural value or emotional importance, facilitate socialization, or provide coping mechanisms, and thus have some beneficent qualities. For instance, while the use of condoms is an important strategy in the prevention of HIV and certain STDs, condom use is not as widespread as expected because condom use affects sexual intimacy. When people have fewer options or substitutions, it is important to ask whether interventions can provide alternatives when asking people to stop some practices. As alternatives to unhealthful practices, can interventions provide people with other options for social solidarity, friendship, and bonding? For example, in the case of condoms, some people have adopted the option of not using condoms with primary partners for the sake of intimacy, and of using condoms with casual partners for the sake of sexual health. Another option used to reduce risk for HIV infection is serosorting, where individuals, regardless of their HIV status, engage in sexual risks only with those partners who they believe to be seroconcordant (117). Vaginal douching, while associated with an increased risk for pelvic inflammatory disease, ectopic pregnancy, cervical cancer, and infection with STDs (118,119), still carries particular cultural importance for certain populations (120–123). Interventions are starting to show success in reducing vaginal douching practices among adolescent and young adult women (124).

Social marketing and structural interventions should be designed and implemented with care so that health promotion does not turn the pursuit of health into a crusade with moral overtones that may do more harm than good (125). When good health is seen as a virtue rather than a value, those who engage in what are labeled as unhealthful behaviors may be made to feel unworthy and stigmatized at a time when there is a strong need to promote equity and a sense of inclusion. Also, the ethical principle of beneficence supports the need to clarify the risks of certain preventive measures or health outcomes, and the need to avoid asserting certainty when degrees of probability are more accurate, while still providing information in a clear way. Yet, presenting arguments for and against a certain behavior may distract those who are averse to ambiguity and risk and may decrease the effectiveness of the message. Messages should therefore be constructed to clearly communicate recommended actions (arrived at through systematic reviews and cost-benefit and cost-effectiveness analyses) as the primary theme, and secondarily to convey issues of associated risks and uncertainty tailored in a manner that is acceptable to the intended audience.

The Ethics of Internet Interventions

The Internet presents new challenges and opportunities for prevention and control of STDs and HIV (126). In response to using the Internet to meet sex partners which can be a sexual risk-taking behavior (127–129), public health practitioners and health care providers have started using the internet for prevention and control of STDs (130,131). These services can include providing health education and prevention messages on web sites that are frequented by populations engaging in high-risk behaviors via pop-up ads and links to web sites offering information on STD testing sites, STDs, and partner referral; making health educators available in chat rooms to answer health-related questions; and offering online test-result reporting, which might increase testing for HIV and STDs by preserving anonymity and decreasing the lag period from test to result.

A positive use of the Internet for STD prevention and control, for example, relates to a case involving seven persons with syphilis who met through an Internet chat room. In response to this case, a local health department worked with a marketing firm to enter the Internet chat room and to send electronic messages to hundreds of users about the syphilis cluster (129). As a result, the local health department was able to notify and evaluate approximately 40% of named sex partners. In another example, involvement of the index patient in partner notification via e-mail improved partner response rates (126). In the case of instant messaging (i.e., messages sent to a person logged into a chat room), nearly 50% of all persons contacted via this method by the health department responded and were evaluated for syphilis (126). Personalized messages, messages sent from an e-mail-provider or within an Internet service provider (ISP), and message headers about STD matters (132) have been used by health departments for prevention and control of STDs.

Concurrent with the use of the Internet for STD prevention and control, questions and scenarios about potential negative ethical ramifications, appropriate use of the Internet, and requests for guidelines about the ethical use of the Internet have emerged (133,134). For example, suggested practices for online partner notification have been published (135). In general, it is assumed that the same confidentiality rules apply to messages sent online as to those sent via telephone or mail. Although online referral makes ensuring the confidentiality of the contact more difficult, it is an efficient method for establishing initial contact with an otherwise inaccessible person and allows subsequent communication to occur.

In keeping with the ethical principle of respect, health care providers and public health practitioners must describe themselves and their activities clearly and completely in network communications. Ethical responsibilities for protecting the privacy of people and confidentiality of data shared on the Internet need to be taken seriously by health care providers and public health practitioners. One reason is that the Internet gives people the illusion their information is being kept confidential or anonymous. Accordingly, people may be more open or less cautious in their network communications. Another reason is that the Internet may present unexpected threats to privacy or alter people's perceptions about privacy. Health care providers and public health practitioners need to pay attention to how they communicate with their patients and how they safeguard private information (136). Furthermore, because some people share their computers and e-mail accounts with other household members or access them at home, heath care providers and public health practitioners need to be aware of resulting privacy issues and exercise caution about how they share information with their clients and patients.

The confidentiality of data transmitted over the Internet is a major concern related to the ethical principle of beneficence. For example, who is the responsible party when one's sexual orientation is revealed without consent by an automated computer process or by cross-referenced computer databases? Many people do not realize that their Internet conversations can be traced to their computers and their conversations could be used for purposes other than the originally intended reasons. Some users access the Internet in public settings, such as libraries or schools or at work where communication is not necessarily private.

The Ethics of STD Prevention and Control with Special Populations

There is an ethical obligation to reach populations who are at risk for STDs due to high-risk behaviors and other factors, and to provide access to STD prevention and treatment services to underserved and disenfranchised populations. These populations include groups such as incarcerated persons, adolescents, disempowered women, men who have sex with men (MSM), lesbians, and drug users. While some of these populations need targeted or focused interventions to reduce elevated risk behaviors and infection rates, it is equally important to consider relevant ethical ramifications.

The Incarcerated

Incarcerated people have higher rates of STDs than the general population and are likely to engage in high-risk behaviors after they are released (137,138). Ensuring a truly informed consent process, gaining the trust of the incarcerated population, and avoiding unintended negative consequences are three important ethical challenges (139).

It is important to obtain genuine consent from prisoners when they seek medical care and to treat incarcerated persons with respect (140). In many instances, a signed consent form is not required for routine examinations or treatment because inmates are considered to have given implied consent through presenting themselves for medical services. Prisoners are legally and morally entitled to the same rights of authorization, consent, or refusal of medical care and treatment as are free citizens, and should accordingly be treated in the same way in terms of respecting their autonomy. As examples are the Kansas and the Tennessee Departments of Corrections policies and procedure on consent to or refusal of medical treatment (141,142). However, courts have in some cases authorized corrections officials to forcibly treat prisoners (e.g., force-feeding or kidney dialysis), on the grounds that the state's interests were superior to the inmate's constitutional right to refuse treatment (143). Health care providers in correctional settings are advised to properly document refusal of treatment, conduct appropriate follow-up assessments, and work with correctional staff to keep refusal from developing into a more serious situation (143).

In keeping with the ethical principle of beneficence, health care providers and public health practitioners need to clarify to inmates at the outset of their interactions what collected information will be kept in confidence, and what collected information may be shared with staff members of corrections facilities. For example, because the chief concerns of staff members of corrections facilities are security and safety, health care providers and public health practitioners need to report to staff members of corrections facilities security breaches that could endanger prison staff or inmates. Health care providers and public health care practitioners also need to share with staff information relevant to safety and security that is learned about in private conversations with inmates. Because of this concern, it can be a challenge for health care providers and public health practitioners to maintain the privacy and confidentiality of inmates, and to gain their trust, owing to inmates' fears about how collected information will be used (144). Health care providers and public health practitioners may need to request that prison staff members search them upon entering detention facilities, lest they be blamed for such incidents as staff of corrections facilities getting stabbed with a pencil that an inmate might have obtained from health care providers or public health practitioners. Health care providers and public health practitioners must work conscientiously to prevent any unintended harmful consequences of their presence, which inevitably poses logistical challenges for both correctional facility staff and health care staff members.

Adolescents

Sexually active adolescents have high rates of STDs and may be less likely to obtain health care than other persons. Relevant barriers to receiving adequate sexual health care include limited financial resources, limited access to convenient care, a sense of invulnerability, feelings of embarrassment, and the desire to keep parents from knowing they are seeking STD care (145–147).

It is often the case that heath care providers or public health practitioners cannot have easy or direct access to adolescents independent of their parents, legal guardians, caretakers, school representatives, or other third-party members, raising ethical concerns about respect for both parents and adolescents (148,149). In conducting interventions with adolescents, it is generally appropriate to consider four factors: 1) the circumstances when consent cannot be obtained from parents or legal guardians (e.g., runaways, drug users, those having no contact with parents or legal guardians) and whether permission can be sought from an alternate group such as a shelter or an advocate; 2) the importance of the public health activity with adolescents; 3) the potential for harm or risk to the adolescent; and 4) the capacity of the adolescent to understand the nature of the public health activity. Some states have parental notification laws for adolescents who request reproductive health services. These laws may have the negative effect of reducing use of needed sexual health care services by adolescents and increasing incident STD rates or unintended pregnancy rates (146). Further ethical issues stemming from the principle of beneficence concern parents who may deny that their children are sexually active, or blame them for lack of self-control and discipline. In such situations, adolescents may hide and deny their sexual activity, and they may be less likely to seek out information on sexual health or to engage in risk-reduction behaviors.

To advance the ethical principle of justice, health care providers and public health practitioners can consult with the local community and the intended audience in the development of STD interventions to help ensure that any related stigma is minimized and that interventions have lasting effects. STD-related stigma can be particularly problematic for adolescents, especially in communities with high disease prevalence. Yet, adolescents have fewer effective institutional bases for community participation and for social or political mobilization, and consequently have greater difficulty advocating to combat stigma and to promote the health of their peer group. Thus, the entire community, and the intended audience including STD programs, must mobilize to acknowledge and confront STD-related stigma and provide accessible STD preventive and curative services to adolescents. Because some local communities may have conservative views about provision of comprehensive education and STD and reproductive health services to adolescents, health care providers and public health practitioners need to work with their patients and communities both to maximize the benefits of health care and to show respect for values and choices of their patients and communities, including adolescents and their parents (150,151).

Women Disempowered to Take Protective Health Measures

Although women have made great strides in achieving equal social status, many women are socially and materially dependent upon men and consequently have limited power to insist on the use of risk-reduction measures with their male partners (152–154). Different motivations affect women's communication with their partners, including fear of personal violence, abandonment, stigma, economic repercussions, and harsh judgment for socially unacceptable sexual behavior. Cultural expectations for some women to be passive make it more difficult for them to take responsibility for their sexual health and to prepare for the possibility of sexual encounters (155–157). This is important because of concerns related to the ethical principle of beneficence, especially when women get infected with an STD by partners who are not monogamous and when the women fear leaving their partners because of economic concerns or fear of harm or abuse. Health care providers and public health practitioners need to be careful not to perpetuate sex-related stigma in the design of STD interventions, such as reinforcing expected gender roles in the hope of reducing high-risk behavior. This ethical consideration aims to reduce harm and unintended consequences, and aims to achieve justice by providing women with equitable access to the benefits of health interventions. Ultimately, perpetuating gender inequities undermines the capacity of women to effectively take charge of their sexual health.

Lesbians and Men Who Have Sex with Men

Lesbians and men who have sex with men often encounter pervasive discrimination and homophobia. A number of STD clinics and other community-based sexual health services have been purposely established by and for gay and lesbian communities, precisely because mainstream sexual health services did not meet their needs, such as health histories and physical examinations that are geared toward exclusively heterosexual patients (158,159). In terms of the ethical principle of respect, health care providers and public health practitioners need to maintain a nonhomophobic attitude, to make a clear distinction between sexual behavior and sexual identity, to use gender-neutral terms, to communicate clearly and sensitively with patients, and to be vigilant against allowing personal attitudes to affect clinical judgment (160).

Drug Users

Drug users are also at increased risk for getting infected with STDs (161). Addiction, the prejudices that substance users face, and the criminalization of drug use make it a challenge for public health practitioners to work effectively with drug users. The fact that HIV transmission has been greatly reduced in injection drug users compared with other populations (162) speaks volumes about the readiness of drug users to take steps to protect their health and those of their sex and drug-injection partners. Addiction is defined as a chronic, relapsing disease, characterized by compulsive drug seeking and use, and by molecular changes in the brain (163). Use of illicit drugs unmistakably alters the brains as well as the behaviors of the users, who gradually spend more time and energy obtaining and using drugs and taking increased risky behaviors. The addictive and intoxicating effects of illicit drugs alter judgment and inhibition of users, and often cause impulsive and unsafe sexual behaviors (59). In observance of the ethical principle of respect, it is important to remember that people addicted to drugs have the same rights as people with other health conditions (164,165). While drug addiction affects all aspects of one's being, the societal marginalization of drug users and attendant lack of life opportunities is also responsible for the epidemic of drug addiction (75,166). A set of 13 principles has been advocated to manage health care delivery relationships with drug users (167,168). Some of these principles include informing drug users about the importance of seeking health care and adhering to medical regimens; encouraging health professionals to learn about referral services available to drug users and to treat drug users with respect; and avoiding common pitfalls such as unrealistic expectations, frustration, moralizing, and withholding therapy. Consistent with the ethical principle of justice, it is important to make drug treatment available and accessible to drug users, to address the societal causes of addiction, and to reduce the use of incarceration as a means of curbing drug addiction (166,169). Concerns about potential harm, such as in the case of needle-exchange programs, slowed implementation of public health activities, and may accordingly exacerbate health disparities. Although infection with HIV is nowadays not as fatal as it was in the 1990s, there is still no promise of a preventive vaccine. Thus, a range of HIV prevention efforts continues to be essential to reduce HIV rates among injection drug users. Syringe-exchange programs have become a major component of HIV prevention in most developed countries under the philosophy of harm reduction or risk reduction (170). However, increasing access to sterile syringes has been met with considerable controversy (171,172). Opponents of syringe-exchange programs have generally argued that increasing access to sterile syringes would simultaneously increase the number of injecting drug users, raise the frequency of injection among already active injection drug users, and appear to condone an illegal behavior (173). To date, many research studies and several major reviews of needle- and syringe-exchange literature have been conducted. All these studies and reviews have shown not only no increase in illicit drug injection associated with needle and syringe exchange, programs but also significant decreases in drug risk behaviors, and in infection with HIV (174,175). The scientific evidence shows that needle- and syringe-exchange programs, in conjunction with other HIV prevention programs, can be effective in reducing risk behavior and HIV infection among injection drug users (176,177). The review and research studies include those by the U.S. National Commission on AIDS (178), a report from the Consensus Development Conference held by the National Institutes of Health (179), a review by the National Academy of Sciences (180), a review by the Cochrane Collaboration (181), and a number of investigator-initiated research studies (174,182–186). When dealing with controversial health interventions, it is important to collect data on the intended and unintended outcomes to guide policy and program development.

Conclusion

Health care providers and public health practitioners have a responsibility to protect the rights and welfare of individuals and communities receiving STD prevention and care services. In STD management efforts, ethical concerns are critical in part because these efforts often involve exchange of private and identifiable information regarding sensitive topics—sex and STDs. Open and effective dialogue between health care providers, public health practitioners, patient representatives, community members, and ethicists can enhance the delivery of ethically and scientifically sound preventive and curative services. When all parties work together and cultivate a meaningful dialogue to learn about each other's concerns, they foster the development of collegial and respectful relationships that can enhance the ethical integrity of health care delivery and public trust in prevention and treatment programs.

Professional awareness and application of ethical guidelines and regulations can enhance the ethics of prevention and care. Continuous training in ethical justification and decision making is to be encouraged. Delivering medical care in an ethical way that meets the regulatory requirements need not be perceived as a burden, but rather as contributing to an ethically responsible standard of care. Commitment to the delivery of ethically sound health care is part and parcel of the public health commitment to excellence in promoting the health of the population.

Even with collaboration, guidelines, and training, societal changes and scientific progress will ensure that new ethical predicaments arise. Public health practitioners will want to anticipate and recognize situations that are likely to present ethical challenges in public health research and practice. In addressing such challenges, the following set of questions is useful to bear in mind: Are we respecting the rights of autonomous individuals? What is the probability of risk? What is the severity of risk? What is the likelihood of benefit? How invasive is the intervention? Can the burdens be minimized? How do we weigh benefits and burdens? Are we treating affected individuals fairly? Are we respecting the human rights of individuals? Are we influencing human rights in an unfair way?

In addition to striving for ethical public health practice, it is critical to document the ethical concerns, abuses, and justifications of ethical decision making that arise during the implementation and operation of STD interventions. Such documentation and collection of both qualitative and quantitative data will serve to enhance the ethical delivery of STD prevention and care, as the lessons from them are communicated and internalized.

General public health guidelines, as well as STD-specific guidelines, convey goals for public health programs to reduce morbidity and mortality, to identify and minimize the burdens of infection and disease, to reduce health disparities, to implement programs fairly, to minimize relevant preexisting social injustices, and to ensure that fair procedures are used to determine the burdens that are acceptable to a community. The guidelines for ethical delivery of health care support these goals, and it is important to recognize that delivery of health care, public health practice, and ethics share the same purpose—to reduce the burden of disease, and to protect people from harm. Competency in ethics-related principles and practice demonstrates respect for all persons and a capacity to protect and to reduce unintentional harms. Conveying not only the scientific and medical competence of public health, but also the ethical competence of public health will foster public trust, confidence, and cooperation in relation to public health activities, ensuring that STD prevention and treatment efforts serve the population as they were intended.

Acknowledgment: The authors thank Dr. John Arras of the University of Virginia for his comments on an earlier version of this chapter and Dr. Lynda Doll of the Centers for Disease Control and Prevention for a thoughtful discussion on the ethics of HIV and STD prevention and control. The findings and conclusions in this chapter are those of the authors and do not necessarily represent the views of the Centers for Disease Control and Prevention.

References

1. Kass N. An ethics framework for public health. *American Journal of Public Health*. 2001;91:1776–1782.
2. Gostin LO. Public health law in a new century, part II: public health powers and limits. *JAMA*. 2000;283:2979–2984.

3. The Council of State and Territorial Epidemiologists. Assessment of the distinctions between public health practice and research. Available at: http://www.cste.org/pdffiles/newpdffiles/cstephreserpthodgefinal 5 24 04 pdf 2005. Accessed August 3, 3005.

4. Padian N, Aral SO, Holmes KK. Individual, group, and population approaches to STD/HIV prevention. In: Holmes KK, Mardh PA, Sparling PF, Lemon SM, Stamm WE, Piot P et al., eds. *Sexually Transmitted Diseases*. 3rd Ed.. New York: McGraw-Hill; 1999;1231–1238.

5. Holmes KK, Ryan CA. STD care management. In: Holmes KK, Sparling PF, Mardh PA, Lemon SM, Stamm WE, Piot P et al., eds. *Sexually Transmitted Diseases*. 3rd Ed. New York: McGraw-Hill; 1999;653–667.

6. Amdur RJ, Bankert EA. *Institutional Review Board Management and Function*. Sudbury, MA: Jones and Bartlett Publishers; 2002.

7. The national commission for the protection of human subjects of biomedical and behavioral research. The Belmont report: Ethical principles and guidelines for the protection of human subjects of research. Washington, DC: U.S. Government Printing Office; 1978. Report No.: DHEW Publication No. (OS 78-0012).

8. Jecker NS, Jonsen AR, Pearlman RA. *Bioethics: An Introduction to the History, Methods, and Practice*. Boston: Jones and Bartlett Publishers; 1997.

9. Roberts MJ, Reich MR. Ethical analysis in public health. *Lancet.* 2002;359:1055–1059.

10. Callahan D, Jennings B. Ethics and public health. *American Journal of Public Health.* 2002;92:169–176.

11. Beauchamp DE. *New Ethics for the Public's Health*. New York, NY: Oxford University Press. 1999;1–382.

12. Beauchamp D. Community: The neglected tradition of public health. In: Beauchamp D, Steinbock B, eds. *New Ethics for the Public's Health.* New York: Oxford University Press; 1999.

13. Thomas JC, Sage M, Dillenberg J, Guillory VJ. A code of ethics for public health. *American Journal of Public Health.* 2002;92:1057–1059.

14. Bayer R, Fairchild AL. The genesis of public health ethics. *Bioethics.* 2004;18:473–492.

15. Pywell S. Vaccination and other altruistic medical treatments: should autonomy or communitarianism prevail? *Medical Law International.* 2000;4:223–243.

16. O'Neill O. Public health or clinical ethics: Thinking beyond borders. *Ethics and International Affairs.* 2004;16:35–45.

17. Bayer R, Colgrave J. Public health vs. civil liberties. *Science.* 2002;297:1811.

18. American Medical Association. *Code of Medical Ethics: Current Opinions with Annotations, 2004-2005.* Chicago: American Medical Association Press; 2004.

19. International Council of Nurses. The International Council of Nurses Code of Ethics for Nurses. Geneva, Switzerland: International Council of Nurses; 2006.

20. American Psychological Association. Ethical principles of psychologists and code of conduct. *American Psychologist.* 1992;47:1597–1611.

21. The Society for the Scientific Study of Sexuality. The Statement of Ethical Guidelines. Available at: http:///www.ssc.wisc edu/sss/ethics htm 2005.

22. Burris S, Gostin LO. The impact of HIV/AIDS on the development of public health law. In: Valdiserri RO, ed. *Dawning Answers: How the HIV/AIDS Epidemic Has Helped to Strengthen Public Health.* London: Oxford University Press; 2005.

23. American Medical Association. Code of Medical Ethics: Current opinions with annotations. Chicago, IL: American Medical Association Press; 2004;1–283.

24. Burris S, Gable L, Stone L, Lazzarini Z. The role of state law in protecting human subjects of public health research and practice. *Journal of Law, Medicine, and Ethics.* 2003;31:654–662.

25. Burris S. Law as a structural factor in the spread of communicable disease. *Houston Law Review*. 1999;36:1755–1786.

26. Burris S, Strathdee SA. To serve and protect? Toward a better relationship between drug control policy and public health. *AIDS*. 2006;20:117–118.

27. Centers for Disease Control and Prevention. HIPAA privacy rule and public health: guidance from CDC and the U.S. department of Health and Human services. *Mortality and Morbidity Weekly Report*. 2003;52 (suppl):1–20.

28. Hodge JG. Health information privacy and public health. *Journal of Law Medicine and Ethics*. 2003;31:663–671.

29. Moran M, Holloman S, Kassler W, Dozier B. Living with the HIPAA Privacy Rule. *Journal of Law, Medicine, and Ethics*. 2004;(Suppl):73–76.

30. Hodge JG, Gostin KG. Challenging themes in American health information privacy and the public's health: Historical and modern assessments. *Journal of Law, Medicine, and Ethics*. 2004;670–679.

31. Magnusson RS. The changing legal and conceptual shape of health care privacy. *Journal of Law, Medicine, and Ethics*. 2004;680–691.

32. Kaltman SP, Isidor JM. State Law. In: Amdur R, Bankert E, eds. *Institutional Review Board: Management and Function*. Boston: Jones and Bartlett Publishers; 2002:338–341.

33. Cason C, Orrock N, Schmitt K, Tesoriero J, Lazzarini Z, Sumartojo E. The impact of laws on HIV and STD prevention. *Journal of Law, Medicine, and Ethics*. 2002;30(Suppl):139–145.

34. Richards EP, Bross DC. Legal and political aspects of STD prevention: Public duties and private rights. In: Holmes KK, Mardh PA, Sparling PF, Lemon SM, Stamm WE, Piot P, et al., eds. *Sexually Transmitted Diseases*, 3rd Ed. New York: McGraw-Hill; 1999;1441–1448.

35. Hodge JG. The Turning Point Model State Public Health Act. *Journal of Law, Medicine, and Ethics*. 2003;31:716–720.

36. Acosta EA. The Texas communicable disease prevention and control act: are we offering enough protection to those who need it most. *Houston Law Review*. 1999;36:1819–1864.

37. Bernstein B. Solving the physician's dilemma: an HIV partner-notification plan. *Law and Policy Review*. 1995;6:127–136.

38. Gabel JB. Liability for "knowing" transmission of HIV: the evolution of a duty to disclose. *Florida State University Law Review*. 1994;21:981–1029.

39. Stroud KM. An Indiana doctor's duty to warn non-patients at risk of HIV infection from an AIDS patient. *Indiana State Law Review*. 1989;22:587–617.

40. Hermann DH, Gagliano RD. AIDS, therapeutic confidentiality, and warning third parties. *Maryland Law Review*. 1989;48:55–76.

41. California Performance Review. HHS14 make California's HIV reporting system consistent with its AIDS reporting system, and improve AIDS reporting. Available at http://cpr.ca.gov/report/cprrpt/issrec/hhs/hhs14.htm.

42. Bayer R, Levine C, Wolf SM. HIV antibody screening: an ethical framework for evaluating proposed programs. *Journal of the American Medical Association*. 1986;256:1768–1774.

43. Bayer R. AIDS and the making of an ethics of public health. In: Valdiserri R, ed. *Dawning Answers: How the HIV/AIDS Epidemic Has Helped to Strengthen Public Health*. New York: Oxford; 2003;135–154.

44. Irwin KL, Valdiserri RO, Holmberg SD. The acceptability of voluntary HIV antibody testing in the United States: a decade of lessons learned. *AIDS*. 1996;10:1707–1717.

45. Centers for Disease Control and Prevention. Revised recommendations for HIV testing of adults, adolescents, and pregnant women in health care settings. *Mortality and Morbidity Weekly Report*. 2006:55 (RR14);1–17.

46. Centers for Disease Control and Prevention. Technical guidance on HIV counseling. *Morbidity and Mortality Weekly Report*. 1993;42:11–17.

47. Kamb ML, Fishbein M, Douglas, et al. Efficacy of risk-reduction counseling to prevent human immunodeficiency virus and sexually transmitted diseases: Randomized control trial. *JAMA*. 1998;280:1161–1167.

48. Centers for Disease Control and Prevention. HIV counseling, testing, and referral standards and guidelines. Atlanta, GA: Centers for Disease Control and Prevention; 1994.

49. Janssen RS, Holtgrave DR, Valdiserri RO, et al. The serostatus approach to fighting the HIV epidemic: prevention strategies for infected individuals. *American Journal of Public Health*. 2001;91:1019–1024.

50. Centers for Disease Control and Prevention. Revised recommendations for HIV screening of pregnant women. *Morbidity and Mortality Weekly Report*. 2001; 50:59–86.

51. Leslie RS. Consent vs. authorization. Avoiding Liability Bulletin. Available at: URL: http://www.cphins.com/LegalResources/tabid/65/cid/57/sid/0/Default.aspx. Accessed March 30, 2006.

52. Anderson LM, Scrimshaw SC, Fullilove MT, Fielding JE, Normand J, Task Force on Community Preventive Services. Culturally competent healthcare systems. A systematic review. *American Journal of Preventive Medicine*. 2003;24:68–79.

53. Leape LL, Berwick DM, Bates DW. What practices will most improve safety? Evidence-based medicine meets patient safety. *Journal of the American Medical Association*. 2002;288:501–507.

54. Semaan S, Klovdahl A, Aral SO. Protecting the privacy, confidentiality, relationships, and medical safety of sex partners in partner notification and management studies. *The Journal of Research Administration*. 2004;35:39–53.

55. Bayer R, Fairchild A. The genesis of public health ethics. *Bioethics*. 2004;18:473–492.

56. Fairchild AL, Bayer R. Uses and abuses of Tuskegee. *Science*. 2000;284:919–925.

57. Childress JF, Faden RR, Gaare RDGL, et al. Public health ethics: mapping the terrain. *Journal of Law, Medicine, and Ethics*. 2002;30:170–175.

58. Blumberg BS, Fox RC. The Daedalus effect: changes in ethical questions relating to hepatitis B. *Annals of Internal Medicine*. 1985;102:390–394.

59. Semaan S, Des Jarlais DC, Malow RM. STDs among illicit drug users in the United States: the need for interventions. In: Aral SO, Douglas JM Jr, eds. Lipshutz JA, assoc ed. *Behavioral Interventions for Prevention and Control of Sexually Transmitted Diseases*. New York: Springer-SBM; 2007:397–430.

60. Fox JP, Hall CE, Elveback LR. *Epidemiology: Man and Disease*. New York: Macmillan; 1970.

61. Hill AB. The environment and disease: association or causation? *Proceedings of the Royal Society of Medicine*. 1965;58:295–300.

62. Prochaska JO, Velicer WF. The transtheoretical model of health behavior change. *American Journal of Health Promotion*. 1997;12:38.

63. Aggleton P. Promoting whose health? Models of health promotion and education about HIV disease. In: Albrecht G, Zimmerman R, eds. *The Social and Behavioral Aspects of AIDS, Advances in Medical Sociology*, 3rd Ed. Greenwich, CT: JAI Press; 1993;185–200.

64. Bandura A. Self-efficacy: toward a unifying theory of behavioral change. *Psychological Review*. 1977;84:191–215.

65. Douglas M. *Risk and Blame: Essays in Cultural Theory*. London: Routledge; 2005.

66. Parker R, Aggleton P. HIV and AIDS-related stigma and discrimination: a conceptual framework and implications for action. *Social Science and Medicine*. 2003;57:13–24.

67. Potterat JJ. Partner notification for HIV: running out of excuses. *Sexually Transmitted Diseases*. 2003;30:89–90.

68. Rothenberg R. The transformation of partner notification. *Clinical Infectious Diseases*. 2002;35 (Suppl 2):S138–S145.

69. Delor F, Hubert M. Revisiting the concept of "vulnerability." *Social Science & Medicine*. 2000;50:1557–1570.

70. Friedman SR, O'Reilly K. Sociocultural interventions at the community level. *AIDS*. 1997;11:S201–S208.

71. Sumartojo E, Doll L, Holtgrave, D., Gayle H, Merson M. Enriching the mix: incorporating the structural factors into HIV prevention. *AIDS*. 2000;14:S1–S2.

72. Blankenship KM, Bray SI, Merson MH. Structural interventions in public health. *AIDS*. 2000;14:S11–S21.

73. Ruger PJ. Ethics of the social determinants of health. *Lancet*. 2004;364: 1092–1097.

74. Muntaner C, Smith LL. Social capital, disorganized communities, and the third way: understanding the retreat from structural inequalities in epidemiology and public health. *International Journal of Health Services*. 2001;31:213–237.

75. Rhodes T, Singer M, Bourgois P, Friedman SR, Strathdee SA. The social structural production of HIV risk among injection drug users. *Social Science and Medicine*. 2005;61:1026–1044.

76. Mann J, Tarantola D, O'Malley J. Toward a new health strategy to control the HIV/AIDS pandemic. Global AIDS Policy Coalition. *Journal of Law, Medicine, and Ethics*. 1994;22:52.

77. Mann J, Gostin L, Gruskin S, et al. Health and human rights. In: Mann J, Gostin L, Gruskin S, Annas G, eds. *A Health and Human Rights Reader*. New York: Routledge; 1999;7–20.

78. Bernheim G, Neiburg P, Bonnie R. Ethics and the practice of public health. In: Goodman et al, ed. *Law in Public Health Practice*, 2nd Ed. Oxford University Press; 2006;43–62.

79. Vezina C, Steben M. Genital herpes: psychosexual impacts and counselling. *Canadian Journal of Contemporary Medical Education*. 2001;13:125–137.

80. Vezina C, Steben M. Psychosexual impacts of human papillomavirus. *Canadian Journal of Contemporary Medical Education*. 2001;13:139–153.

81. Jemmot JB, Jemmott LS, Fong GT. Abstinence and safer sex HIV risk-reduction interventions for African American adolescents: a randomized controlled trial. *JAMA*. 1998;279:1529–1536.

82. Blake SM. Condom availability programs in Massachusetts high schools: relationships with condom use and sexual behavior. *American Journal of Public Health*. 2003;93:955–962.

83. Kirby D. Effective approaches to reducing adolescent unprotected sex, pregnancy, and childbearing. *Journal of Sex Research*. 2002;39:51–57.

84. Smoak ND, Scott-Sheldon LAJ, Johnson BT, Carey MP, and the SHARP research team. Sexual risk reduction interventions do not inadvertently increase the overall frequency of sexual behavior: a meta-analysis of 174 studies with 116,735 participants. *Journal of Acquired Immune Deficiency Syndrome*. 2006;41:374–384.

85. Krantz I, Lowhagen G, Ahlberg BM, Nilstun T. Ethics of screening for asymptomatic herpes virus type 2 infection. *British Medical Journal*. 2004;329:621.

86. Centers for Disease Control and Prevention. Zidovudine for the prevention of HIV transmission from mother to infant. *Morbidity and Mortality Weekly Report*. 1994;43:287.

87. Pyper C, Amery J, Watson M, Crook C. Access to electronic health records in primary care—a survey of patients' views. *Medical Science Monitor*. 2004;10:SR17–SR22.

88. Unger ER, Duarte-Franco E. Human papillomaviruses: into the new millennium. *Obstetrics & Gynecology Clinics of North America*. 2001;28:653–666.

89. Centers for Disease Control and Prevention. Incidence of acute hepatitis B—United States, 1990–2002. *Morbidity and Mortality Weekly Report.* 2004;52:1252–1254.

90. Rupp R, Stanberry LR, Rosenthal SL. New biomedical approaches for sexually transmitted infection prevention: vaccines and microbicides. *Adolescent Medicine Clinic* 2004;15:393–407.

91. Zimet GD, Kee R, Winston Y, Perkins SM, Maharry K. Acceptance of hepatitis B vaccination among adult patients with sexually transmitted diseases. *Sexually Transmitted Diseases.* 2001;28:678–680.

92. Zimmerman RK. Ethical Analysis of HPV vaccine policy options. *Vaccine.* 2006;24:4812–4820.

93. Zimet GD, Mays RM, Sturm LA, Ravert AA, Perkins SM, Juliar BE. Parental attitudes about sexually transmitted infection vaccination for their adolescent children. *Archives of Pediatric Adolescent Medicine.* 2005;159:190–192.

94. Mays RM, Sturm LA, Zimet GD. Parental perspectives on vaccinating children against sexually transmitted infections. *Social Science & Medicine* 2004;58: 1405–1413.

95. Raley JC, Followill KA, Zimet GD, Ault KA. Gynecologists' attitudes regarding human papillomavirus vaccination: a survey of fellows of the American College of Obstetricians and Gynecologists. *Infectious Disease Obstetrics and Gynecology* 2004;12:127–133.

96. Rosenthal SL, Stanberry LR. Parental acceptability of vaccines for sexually transmitted infections. *Archives of Pediatric Adolescent Medicine.* 2005;159:190–192.

97. Mays RM, Zimet GD. Recommending STI vaccination to parents of adolescents: the attitudes of nurse practitioners. *Sexually Transmitted Diseases.* 2004;31:428–432.

98. Verweij M, Dawson A. Ethical principles for collective immunization programmes. *Vaccine.* 2004;22:3122–3126.

99. Centers for Disease Control and Prevention. *Partner Services: Program Operations Guidelines for STD Prevention.* Atlanta, GA: Centers for Disease Control and Prevention; 2000. Available at: http://www.cdc.gov/std/program/partners.pdf.

100. Steckler J, Bachman L, Brotman RA. Concurrent sexually transmitted infections (STIs) in sex partners of patients with selected STIs: implications for patient-delivered therapy. *Clinical Infectious Diseases.* 2005;40:787–703.

101. Kissinger PJ, Niccolai LM, Mangus M, et al. Partner notification for HIV and syphilis: effects on sexual behaviors and relationship stability. *Sexually Transmitted Diseases.* 2003;30:75–82.

102. Sumartojo E. Structural factors in HIV prevention: concepts, examples, and implications for research. *AIDS.* 2000;14:S3–S10.

103. Guttman N, Salmon CT. Guilt, fear, stigma and knowledge gaps: ethical issues in public health communication interventions. *Bioethics.* 2004;18:1467–8519.

104. Klausner JD, kent CK, Wong W, McCright J, Katz MH. The public health response to epidemic syphilis, San Francisco, 1999–2004. *Sexually Transmitted Diseases.* 2005;32:S11–S18.

105. Schmitt K, Bulecza S, George D, Burns TE, Jordhal L. Florida's multifaceted response for increases in syphilis among MSM: The Miami-Ft. Lauderdale initiative. *Sexually Transmitted Diseases.* 2005;32:S19–S23.

106. Chen JL, Kodagoda D, Lawrence MA, Kerndt PR. Rapid public health interventions in response to an outbreak of syphilis in Los Angeles. *Sexually Transmitted Diseases.* 2002;29:277–284.

107. Montoya JA, Rotblatt H, Mall KL, Klausner J, Kerndt PR. Evaluating "Stop the Sores": a community-led social marketing campaign to prevent syphilis among men who have sex with men, Los Angeles County, 2002–2003. International Society for Sexually Transmitted Disease Research Congress, Ottawa, Canada. 2003. Available at: http://lapublichealth.org/std/msm%20campaign%20evaluation.pdf.

108. Vega MY, Roland EL. Social marketing techniques for public health communication: a review of syphilis awareness campaigns in 8 US cities. *Sexually Transmitted Diseases*. 2005;32:S30–S36.

109. Wohlfeiler D. Structural and environmental HIV prevention for gay and bisexual men. *AIDS*. 2000;14:S52–S56.

110. Woods WJ, Binson D, Pollack LM, Wohlfeiler D, Stall RD, Catania JA. Public policy regulating private and public space in gay bathhouses. *Journal of Acquired Immune Deficiency Syndrome*. 2003;32:417–423.

111. Wohlfeiler D, Potterat JJ. Using gay men's sexual networks to reduce sexually transmitted disease (STD)/Human immunodeficiency virus (HIV) transmission. *Sexually Transmitted Diseases*. 2005;32:S48–S52.

112. Brents BG, Hausbeck K. State-sanctioned sex: negotiating formal and informal regulatory practices in Nevada brothels. *Sociological Perspectives*. 2001;44:307–332.

113. Albert A, Warner DL, Hatcher RA. Facilitating condom use with clients during commercial sex in Nevada's legal brothels. *American Journal of Public Health*. 1998;88:643–646.

114. Albert A, Warner DL, Hatcher RA, Trussell J, Bennett C. Condom use among female commercial sex workers in Nevada's legal brothels. *American Journal of Public Health*. 1995;85:1514–1520.

115. Centers fo Disease Control and Prevention. HIV transmission in the adult film industry–Los Angeles, California, 2004. *Morbidity and Mortality Weekly Report*. 2005;54:923–926.

116. Becker MH. A medical sociologist looks at health promotion. *Journal of Health and Social Behavior*. 1993;34:1–6.

117. Parsons JT, Schrimshaw EW, Wolitski RJ, et al. Sexual harm reduction practices of HIV-seropositive gay and bisexual men: serosorting, strategic positioning, and withdrawal before ejaculation. *AIDS*. 2005;19:S13–S25.

118. Zhang J, Thomas G, Leybovich E. Vaginal douching and adverse health effects: a meta-analysis. *American Journal of Public Health*. 1997;87:1207–1211.

119. Foxman B, Aral SO, Holmes KK. Interrelationships among douching practices, risky sexual practices, and history of self-reported sexually transmitted diseases in an urban population. *Sexually Transmitted Diseases*. 1998;25:90–99.

120. Oh MK, Funkhouser E, Simpson T, Brown P, Merchant J. Early onset of vaginal douching is associated with false beliefs and high-risk behavior. *Sexually Transmitted Diseases*. 2003;30:689–693.

121. Vermund SH, Sarr M, Murphy DA, et al. Douching practices among HIV-infected and uninfected adolescents in the United States. *Journal of Adolescent Health*. 2001;1:80–86.

122. Funkhouser E, Pulley L, Lueschen G, et al. Douching beliefs and practices among black and white women. *Journal of Women's Health and Gender-based Medicine*. 2002;11:29–37.

123. Koblin BA, Mayer K, Mwatha A, et al. Douching practices among women at high risk of HIV infection in the United States: Implications for microbicide testing and use. *Sexually Transmitted Diseases*. 2002;29:406–410.

124. Grimley DM, Oh MK, Desmond RA, Hook EW, Vermund SH. An intervention to reduce vaginal douching among adolescent and young adult women: a randomized, controlled trial. *Sexually Transmitted Diseases*. 2005;32:752–758.

125. Fitzgerald FT. The tyranny of health. *New England Journal of Medicine*. 1994;331:196–198.

126. Centers for Disease Control and Prevention. Using the internet for partner notification of sexually transmitted diseases—Los Angeles County, California, 2003. *Morbidity and Mortality Weekly Report*. 2004;53:129–131.

127. Rietmeijer CA, Bull SS, McFarlane M, Patnaik JL, Douglas J. Risks and benefits of the internet for populations at risk for sexually transmitted infections. *Sexually Transmitted Diseases*. 2003;30:15–19.

128. McFarlene M, Bull SS, Rietmeijer CA. The internet as a newly emerging risk environment for sexually transmitted diseases. *Journal of the American Medical Association*. 2000;284:443–446.

129. Klausner JD, Wolf W, Fischer-Ponce L, Zolt I, Katz MH. Tracing a syphilis outbreak through cyberspace. *JAMA*. 2000;284:447–449.

130. Tomnay JE, Pitts MK, Fairley CK. New technology and partner notification—why aren't we using them? *International Journal of STD & AIDS*. 2005;16:19–22.

131. Bovi AM. Ethical guidelines for use of electronic mail between patients and physicians. *American Journal of Bioethics*. 2003;3:1–6.

132. Anderton JP, Valdiserri RO. Combating syphilis and HIV among users of internet chatrooms. *Journal of Health Communication*. 2005;10:665–671.

133. Binik YM, Mah K, Kiesler S. Ethical Issues in conducting sex research on the internet. *The Journal of Sex Research*. 1999;36:82–90.

134. Brooks RG, Menachemi N. Physicians' use of email with patients: factors influencing electronic communication and adherence to best practices. *Journal of Medical Internet Research*. 2006;8(1):e2.

135. Centers for Disease Control and Prevention. Internet use and early syphilis among men who have sex with men—San Francisco, California, 1999–2003. *Morbidity and Mortality Weekly Report*. 2003;52:1229–1232.

136. Centers for Disease Control and Prevention. *Sexually Transmitted Disease Surveillance, 2003*. Atlanta, GA: Department of Health and Human Services; 2004.

137. Seal DW. HIV-related issues and concerns for imprisoned persons throughout the world. *Current Opinion in Psychiatry*. 2005;18:530–535.

138. Berkman A. Prison health: the breaking point. *American Journal of Public Health*. 1995;85:1616–1618.

139. Schady FF, Miller MA, Klein SJ. Developing practical "tips" for HIV/AIDS service delivery in local jails. *Journal of Public Health Management Practice*. 2005;11:554–558.

140. Hogben M, St. Lawrence J. HIV/STD risk reduction interventions in priosn settings: observations from the CDC. *Journal of Women's Health and Gender-based Medicine*. 2000;9:587–592.

141. Kansas department of corrections. Programs and services: consent to or refusal of medical treatment. http://docnet.dc.state.ks.us/IMPPs/Chapter10/10127.pdf 2006. Accessed April 26, 2006.

142. State of Tennessee Department of Correction. Consent/refusal of treatment. http://www.state.tn.us/correction/pdf/113-51.pdf 2006. Accessed April 26, 2006.

143. Vogt RP. When an inmate refuses medical care. *Correctcare*. 2005.

144. Newman S, Girasek D, Friedman H. Using qualitative methods to design an epidemiologic study on sexually transmitted diseases in female prisoners. Letter to the editor. *Sexually Transmitted Diseases*. 2003;30:531–532.

145. Brindis CD, Loo VS, Adler NE, Bolan GA, Wasserheit JN. Service integration and teen friendliness in practice: a program assessment of sexual and reproductive health services for adolescents. *Journal of Adolescent Health*. 2005;37:155–162.

146. VanDevanter N, Messeri P, Middlestadt S, et al. A community-based intervention designed to increase preventive health care seeking among adolescents: the gonorrhea action project. *American Journal of Public Health*. 2005;95:331–337.

147. Crosby R, St. Lawrence J. Adolescents' use of school-based health clinics for reproductive health services: data from the National Longitudinal Study of Adolescent Health. *Journal of School Health*. 2000;70:22–27.

148. Reddy DM, Fleming R, Swain C. Effect of mandatory parental notification on adolescent girls' use of sexual health care services. *JAMA*. 2002;288:710–714.

149. Franzini L, Marks E, Cromwell PF, et al. Projected economic costs due to health consequences of teenagers' loss of confidentiality in obtaining reproductive health care services in Texas. *Archives of Pediatric Adolescent Medicine*. 2004;158:1140–1146.

150. Santelli J, Ott MA, Lyon M, Rogers J, Summers D. Abstinence-only education policies and programs: a position paper of the Society for Adolescent Medicine. *Journal of Adolescent Health*. 2006;38:83–87.
151. Santelli J, Ott MA, Lyon M, Rogers J, Summers D, Schleifer R. Abstinence and abstinence-only education: a review of U.S. policies and programs. *Journal of Adolescent Health*. 2006;38:72–81.
152. Suarez-Al-Adam M, Raffealli M, O'Leary A. Influence of abuse and partner hyper-masculinity on the sexual behavior of Latinas. *AIDS Education and Prevention*. 2000;12:263–274.
153. Wingood GM, DiClemente RJ. The effects of an abusive primary partner on the condom use and sexual notification practices of African-American women. *American Journal of Public Health*. 1997;87:1016–1018.
154. Semaan S, Lauby J, O'Connell A, Cohen A. Factors associated with perceptions of, and decisional balance for, condom use with main partner among women at risk for HIV infection. *Women and Health*. 2003;37:53–69.
155. Adimora AA, Schoenbach VJ. Social context, sexual networks, and racial disparities in rates of sexually transmitted infections. *Journal of Infectious Diseases*. 2005;191:S115–S122.
156. Latka M. Drug-using women need comprehensive sexual risk reduction interventions. *Clinical Infectious Diseases*. 2003;37:S445–S450.
157. Amaro H. Love, sex and power. *American Psychologist*. 1995;50:437–446.
158. Harrison AE, Silenzio VM. Comprehensive care of lesbian and gay patients and families. *Primary Care*. 1996;23:41–46.
159. Jillson IA. Opening closed doors: improving access to quality health services for LGBT populations. *Clinical Research and Regulatory Affairs*. 2002;19:153–190.
160. Young RM, Meyer IH. The trouble with "MSM" and "WSW": erasure of the sexual-minority person in public health discourse. *American Journal of Public Health*. 2005;95:1144–1149.
161. Des Jarlais DC, Semaan S. Interventions to reduce the sexual risk behavior of injecting drug users. *International Journal of Drug Policy*. 2005;16S:S58–S66.
162. Quan VM, Steketee RW, Valleroy L, Weinstock H, Karon J, Janssen R. HIV incidence in the United States, 1978–1999. *JAIDS*. 2002;31:188–201.
163. Cami J, Farre M. Drug addiction. *New England Journal of Medicine*. 2003;349:975–986.
164. Griffiths. A "components" model of addiction within a biopsychosocial framework. *Journal of Substance Use*. 2005;10:191–197.
165. Roy DJ. Injection drug use and HIV/AIDS: an ethics commentary on priority issues. *Health Canada*. 2000.
166. Friedman SR, Cooper HLF, Tempalski B, et al. Relationships of deterrence and law enforcement to drug-related harms among drug injectors in U.S. metropolitan areas. *AIDS*. 2006;20:93–99.
167. Edlin BR, Kresina TF, Raymond DB, et al. Overcoming barriers to prevention, care, and treatment of hepatitis C in illicit drug users. *Clinical Infectious Diseases*. 2005;40:S276–S285.
168. Edlin BR. Hepatitis C prevention and treatment for substance users in the United States: acknowledging the elephant in the living room. *International Journal of Drug Policy*. 2004;15:81–91.
169. Des Jarlais DC. Research, politics and needle exchange. *American Journal of Public Health*. 2000;90:1392–1394.
170. Wodak A, Cooney A. Effectiveness of sterile needle and syringe programs. *International Journal of Drug Policy*. 2005;16:S31–S44.
171. Lurie P, Drucker E. An opportunity lost: HIV infections associated with lack of a national needle-exchange programme in the USA. *Lancet*. 1997;349:604–608.

172. Wodak A, Lurie P. A tale of two countries: attempts to control HIV among inject-ing drug users in Australia and the United States. *Journal of Drug Issues.* 1996;27:117–134.

173. Coutinho RA. Needle exchange, pragmatism, and moralism. *American Journal of Public Health.* 2000;90:1387–1388.

174. Des Jarlais DC, Perlis T, Arasteh K, et al. HIV incidence among injection drug users in New York City, 1990 to 2002: Use of serologic test algorithm to assess expansion of HIV prevention services. *American Journal of Public Health.* 2005;95:1439–1444.

175. Vlahov D. The role of epidemiology in needle exchange programs. *American Journal of Public Health.* 2000;90:1390–1392.

176. Des Jarlais DC. Research, politics and needle exchange. *American Journal of Public Health.* 2000;90:1392–1394.

177. Vlahov D, Des Jarlais DC, Goosby E, et al. Needle exchange programs for the pre-vention of human immunodeficiency virus infection: epidemiology and policy. *American Journal of Epidemiology.* 2001;154:S70–S77.

178. National Commission on AIDS. The Twin Epidemics of Substance Use and HIV: Full Report. Washington, DC: U.S. National Commission on AIDS; 1991.

179. National Institutes of Health. Interventions to prevent HIV risk behaviors. Washington, DC: National Institutes of Health; 1997. Report No.: 15 (2).

180. *Preventing HIV Transmission: The Role of Sterile Needles and Bleach.* Washington, D.C.: National Academy Press; 1995.

181. The Cochrane Collaborative Review Group on HIV Infection and AIDS. Evidence Assessment: Strategies for HIV/AIDS Prevention, Treatment and Care. University of California, San Francisco, Institute for Global Health; 2004. Accessed August 5, 2005.

182. Vlahov D, Junge B. The role of needle exchange programs in HIV prevention. *Public Health Reports.* 1998;113:75–80.

183. Hagan H, McGough JP, Thiede H, Hopkins S, Duchin J, Alexander ER. Reduced injection frequency and increased entry and retention in drug treatment associated with needle-exchange participation in Seattle drug injectors. *Journal of Substance Abuse Treatment.* 2000;19:247–252.

184. Ksobiech K. A meta-analysis of needle sharing, lending, and borrowing behaviors of needle exchange program attenders. *AIDS Education and Prevention.* 2003;15:257–268.

185. Broadhead RS, van Julst Y, Heckathorn DD. The impact of a needle exchange's closure. *Public Health Reports.* 1999;114:439–447.

186. Cross JE, Saunders CM, Bartelli D. The effectiveness of educational and needle exchange programs: a meta-analysis of HIV prevention strategies for injecting drug users. *Quality and Quantity.* 1998;32:165–180.

24

Policy and Behavioral Interventions for STDs

Jonathan M. Zenilman, M.D.

Policy making in public health is a multidisciplinary activity that has a major impact on how public health problems are addressed. While most assume that relevant science should form the basic foundation for development of public health policy, the way that connection is bridged and how the science is interpreted are frequently influenced by the political arena within which they exist. STD prevention and reproductive health are not immune to this reality.

This chapter will first describe and define the core functions of public health, which provide a critical context for policy making. The basis and specific domains of policy making and how they relate to preventing STDs will be explored, using case study examples to highlight specific points. The interface of science and policy making and the political arena within which they function will also be woven into the discussion.

Core Public Health Functions

The Institute of Medicine (IOM) defined public health as consisting of three core functions—*assessment, assurance,* and *policy development* (1–3). Policy development will be discussed here in the context of the other two major components. In addition, many authorities also propose *communication* as a fourth function.

Assessment is the collection, analysis, and dissemination of health status information in a systematic manner. For STD control, assessment includes the collection of morbidity data, the collection of behavioral surveillance data(4), as well as outbreak investigations. These activities include support of surveillance systems at local, state, and federal levels, and publication of documents such as CDC's annual STD Surveillance Report and MMWR articles.

Assurance is the provision of access to necessary community-wide health services. In many settings, especially care settings where clinical care has a direct impact on disease transmission, assurance may involve a public health agency directly providing care (5). Although clinical care provision is often perceived by the public as a major function of public health, this endeavor can be treacherous to public health agencies, because uncompensated clinical care in an environment without universal health care coverage is expensive. Besides clinical care and counseling activities, the assurance function is the basis for many regulatory activities, such as quality regulation of drugs and laboratories, and licensing of providers.

Behavioral Interventions for Prevention and Control of Sexually Transmitted Diseases.
Aral SO, Douglas JM Jr, eds. Lipshutz JA, assoc ed. New York: Springer Science+
Business Media, LLC; 2007.

Policy development (1) is the process through which decisions about problems are made, followed by the establishment of goals and a means to reach them. According to the Institute of Medicine, public health policy decisions should have a sound scientific knowledge base (1). In classical political theory, as outlined by Lasswell, the outcome of this process (i.e., the policy) is a commitment to a particular course of action with broad implications for society (6). While policies can be developed by the private sector and government, only those established by government are binding. In an ideal world, policies are developed with objective data along with logical conclusions and recommendations. However, consensus about conclusions and resulting recommendations is typically difficult to achieve. In turn, politics almost always play a role in policy development. It is thus important to distinguish policy from politics. *Politics* is a process of bargaining, negotiation, and compromise that determines "who gets what, when, and how" (7) and frequently influences policy development. Furthermore, politics are necessarily linked to values and not uniformly linked to science. A *policy* perspective of an issue is intended to "elucidate and expand the range of alternatives" for a resolution to a problem while a *political* perspective by nature aims to decrease the range of alternatives based on a particular set of values (8). A good example of an STD *policy* document is the Institute of Medicine report in 1997—*The Hidden Epidemic* (9)—which identified four major policy objectives to address the epidemic of STDs in the United States:

1. Overcome barriers to adoption of healthy sexual behaviors.
2. Develop strong leadership, strengthen investment, and improve information systems for STD prevention.
3. Design and implement essential STD services in innovative ways for adolescents and under served populations.
4. Ensure access to quality clinical STD services.

Communication (10,11) includes provision of health promotion messages and realistic risk assessment. Besides delivering messages to the general population, a major communication objective is to insure that public health officials have appropriate training and tools to adequately address public health needs, especially in times of crisis. Communication is also audience-dependent, a nuance that is often overlooked. Communication skills for a medical audience would differ substantially from those required for policymakers or special interest groups.

Process for Policy Development and Implementation

Public health policy is developed and implemented through legislation, regulation, and guidance.

Legislation

Legislation provides the legal framework for defining and establishing public health policy as well as the vehicle that provides funding to implement such policy. One of the prime examples of how legislation has impacted public health policy for STD control was the passage of federal venereal disease control legislation during the 1930s, which provided justification and federal authorization of spending for public health services related to STD control. The justification for federal involvement was the potential for the transmission of STDs across state lines.

Authorizing legislation (12) provides support for surveillance; public health control functions, such as partner notification; and laboratory testing, which is typically part of large initiatives. Initiatives can be either through specific authorizations, such as the Ryan White Care Act, which began in 1991 (13) or as part of an overall budgetary process, such as the national gonorrhea screening program which began in 1972 (14) and the Infertility Prevention Program (focused on chlamydia screening), which became a part of the STD prevention budget in the late 1980s (15–17). Delineating specific federal and local roles is important. For example, federal funds under the STD public health acts cannot be used for the provision of clinical care, which is primarily seen as a local function.

Legislation invariably has to adapt to specific political needs. One of the major issues facing STD controllers is that a large number of individuals at particularly high-risk for STIs are marginalized, may be incarcerated, do not or cannot vote, and therefore have poor political representation. Stigmatization of persons with STDs has been historically problematic. Effective development of public health programs requires developing and building a constituency, partnering with impacted groups, enlisting the support of the provider community and finally, convincing legislators that there is potential for the public good.

Regulation

Regulation is one expression of policy and can take a number of forms. Since this is a very broad topic, discussion will be limited to regulatory frameworks that are relevant for STD control. Regulation usually requires underlying legislation to provide a legal framework, which is critical for enforcement.

Regulation of Professionals
All states require credentialing and licensing for professionals involved in the care of patients, including physicians, nurses, social workers, pharmacists, and laboratory technologists. Such practice is intended to assure competency, and often is required for reimbursement. Currently, there are no credentialing requirements for public health professionals who are not direct care providers, such as epidemiologists or program managers.

Laboratory Regulation
Clinical laboratories are regulated by state and federal governments, with a major focus on quality assurance and tracking of specimens. The Clinical Laboratory Improvement Act of 1988 (CLIA) is the major federal laboratory regulatory legislation which has impacted STD care providers. Quality assurance is especially important in STD care because of the implications of clinical results. Regulation can also include reporting requirements by laboratories for communicable diseases. Before new diagnostic tests can be used in patient care, they have to be approved, usually by the FDA (see below).

Drug, Vaccine, and Diagnostic Test Regulation

This function is performed by the Food and Drug Administration, whose mandate is to assure that drugs used are effective and safe. The manufacturer must meet stringent criteria and present results of carefully conducted clinical trials.

Case Studies: Regulation

Over-the-Counter Acyclovir

Acyclovir is a highly effective antiviral medication that is indicated for the treatment and suppression of genital herpes. The drug has minimal side effects, and most experts consider it safe to use even in pregnancy (18). In the mid-1990s, advocacy groups and the manufacturer proposed to the FDA that the drug be licensed for over the counter (OTC) sale (19). The major supporting argument was that acyclovir is most effective when taken early in the course of a herpes outbreak. Since patients often have to wait several days before being able to see a health care provider, and since the drug is safe, OTC status would facilitate rapid treatment. Arguments against licensure included concern over self-diagnosis and misdiagnosis of other genital ulcer diseases as well as concerns over development of antiviral resistance due to potential overuse (20,21). After active debate in the literature as well as at regulatory hearings. Nevertheless, the FDA elected not to approve acyclovir as an OTC drug. This debate was largely informed by scientific considerations.

Plan B (Over-the-Counter Emergency Contraceptive)

Plan B (emergency contraception) was proposed as an OTC drug in 2003. Plan B is most effective when taken within 48 hours after unprotected intercourse (22). The arguments in favor of approval were based on scientific evidence and implementation practicalities (23,24). Similar to those presented for the acyclovir debate, the drug's safety record was impeccable, and women often had to wait more than 48 hours to see a physician or health care provider, especially on weekends and holidays. Furthermore, experience with OTC use in both Western Europe and a number of states was highly favorable (25). In contrast, the arguments against Plan B were politically rather than scientifically driven. Contrary to scientific evidence (26), antiabortion activists claimed that Plan B was an abortifacient. Other groups contended that OTC licensure would lead to behavioral disinhibition and increased high-risk sexual behaviors (27) though scientific evidence counters this concern (28). The FDA Advisory Committee voted overwhelmingly to approve Plan B as an OTC. In an unprecedented move, however, the Commissioner overruled the committee. Because of the perception that the Commissioner's decision was influenced by conservative political pressure and not guided by the recommendations of the scientific advisory committee, Dr. Susan Wood, the FDA official in charge of women's health, resigned. Women's health groups felt that this impasse was a critical issue and used it as a tool to address what they felt to be governmental disregard for the scientific basis for reproductive health policies and the FDA regulatory policy in particular (29). In 2006, the issue was mostly resolved when the FDA approved OTC Plan B for women over 18 years old. This decision was based on the science indicating a likely high level of benefit with minimal harm.

Partner-Delivered Therapy

Treatment of exposed partners is a cornerstone of control policy for bacterial STDs. However, partner notification (PN) and treatment is not widely implemented for gonorrhea and chlamydia. This occurs for three reasons. First, PN is labor intensive and in an era of limited budgets, many health departments have either reduced these resources or redirected them to HIV and syphilis control. Second, index cases often refuse to name exposed partners. Third, there are no data to demonstrate that PN provided by health department personnel is cost-effective (30,31).

Partner-delivered therapy (PDT) has been proposed as an alternative to traditional partner services (32–34). PDT has been shown to reduce re-infection rates in persons with gonorrhea and chlamydia. However, implementing PDT faces a number of regulatory challenges (35), including;

1. Physician issues: In prescribing PDT, does a third party (the unnamed partner) become a patient by proxy, and does the physician incur liability, especially for prescribing drugs without seeing the patient?
2. Can a pharmacy dispense drugs to an individual without a prescription?
3. Do these issues result in violations of the Medical Practice Acts and Pharmacy laws, which may subject the practitioners to disciplinary action?

Because the drugs commonly used are safe, STD programs have lobbied in a number of states to establish PDT as a recognized standard of care, including changing the appropriate regulations. In California, this was done through lobbying, advocating, and ultimately enacting changes in the laws and regulations. Under current law, California physicians are allowed to provide medication to sexual partners of individuals diagnosed with chlamydia without fear of regulatory action by state medical boards. In Washington State, another approach has been for the Health Department to act as agent. Partners of individuals diagnosed with gonorrhea or chlamydia are directed to designated pharmacies where they can confidentially obtain medications, subsidized by the Health Department. In this setting, the Health Department received a regulatory interpretation which allowed pharmacies to dispense the medication without a direct prescription.

Guidance

Guidance is developed by government agencies to help responsible parties adhere to laws, regulations or recommendations promulgated by the government. From the clinical perspective, the CDC's *Sexually Transmitted Diseases Treatment Guidelines* (18) is a widely disseminated document that provides clinicians with current clinical practice recommendations. Although the document clearly states that they are "only guidelines," they are widely adopted and recognized as "clinical standard of care" by STD programs and other provider communities. CDC's guidelines for HIV counseling and testing, which were first released in 1986, targeted a wide audience, including clinicians, public health program managers, and the larger private health community (36). These guidelines were instrumental in the rapid dissemination of HIV testing resources throughout the country, and in ascertaining quality assurance for lab performance and behavioral counseling. Other examples are CDC's recent recommendations by the Advisory Committee on Immunization Practice (ACIP) for use of quadrivalent HPV vaccine (37), which provides guidance on the use of newly licensed vaccines, and CDC recommendations on HIV testing in health care settings, which encourages routine HIV testing in a variety of health care settings (38).

Relationship of Core Public Health Functions to Policy: Assessment and Assurance in the STD Context

Development of STD policy and programs requires a clear understanding of morbidity and other assessment measures, underscoring the need for effective disease and behavioral surveillance. Surveillance should proactively guide policy that results in the development of interventions. For example, the focus of the syphilis elimination program on African-American populations was a direct response to increases in syphilis in that population during the early 1990s, which was in part related to drug abuse (39). The chlamydia intervention screening programs developed during the 1980s were a response to increased recognition that chlamydia was an important cause of pelvic inflammatory disease (40) as well as technological innovation which made chlamydia testing possible in the typical clinical setting (41).

The STD control issues which face policy makers in the United States include an expanding and diverse population, persistence of high rates of STDs especially in minority and poor populations, a fragmented health care system, and dynamic epidemics. Allocation of resources between clinical services, screening, public health outreach, and surveillance is a continual challenge. Furthermore, emerging public health threats, such as bioterrorism and pandemic influenza, pose challenges to more established programs for ongoing public health issues such as STD control. These challenges not only include competition for funding but also competition for experienced staff.

Differential Government Roles in Developing and Implementing STD Policy

The programs and implications of STD prevention policy are different at various levels of government. At the local level, the major focus is on local assessment and service provision. Local governments, such as municipal and county governments in the United States, generally provide access to free or low-cost STD services (5). In addition to STD services, they may also provide additional reproductive health care services, such as family planning and adjunctive services like partner notification. Often, these services are provided with local health care dollars, supplemented by state funding. In addition, a critical component of local government is implementation of reproductive health education in public school systems.

At the state level, there are a variety of additional STD prevention functions. State governments are often involved in providing assurance of service delivery, both for clinical services and general public health services. In some states, county health department employees are actually part of the state civil service systems. Besides providing access to care, state governments provide overall education guidelines to school systems, including development of curricula as part of health and science education. State governments also have a growing role in funding of clinical care services. In some states, Medicaid and other publicly funded care programs can provide funding to public health services. An example of this is Minnesota, where a state-wide managed health care system provides support for public health clinics to offer reproductive health services (42). In addition, states are responsible for professional regulation of providers such as nurse practitioners and physicians.

The federal government also has substantial impact on development of STD and reproductive health policy. The federal government expresses STD policy largely through the Centers for Disease Control and Prevention and Prevention (CDC) and, to a lesser degree, through the National Institutes of Health (NIH) and other federal agencies. The CDC supports the development of STD treatment guidelines (18), which are widely used for both clinical care and quality assurance, not only in the United States but also throughout the world. The CDC also provides support for national surveillance programs for a variety of sexually transmitted infections. Most of public health surveillance for STDs is passive. However, large periodic national surveys, such as the National Health and Nutrition Evaluation Survey (NHANES) (43) and the National Survey of Family Growth (NSFG) (44), provide opportunities for periodic assessment of broad parts of the population on a cross-sectional basis. The federal government also supports STD research through a variety of different sources. NIH supports research in basic science of STD, STD vaccine development, as well as targeted STD intervention research programs. NIH research is largely hypothesis-driven. In contrast, CDC research support is often operationally driven, focusing on quality improvement indicators, development of surveillance methods and systems, and health process indicators. The federal government also has the capability of instituting large national initiatives, such as the syphilis elimination and the chlamydia screening/infertility prevention programs described above. Implementation of federal program initiatives is usually accomplished through appropriation of funding.

Policy Development, Public Health, and the Public Arena

Balancing Individual Liberties and the Public Good

Critical to policy development in public health is understanding the inherent challenge of balancing the overall health needs of the population with individual choice and liberty. At its extreme, public health authority is based in police powers. Practices to prevent infectious disease transmission may conflict with societal privacy norms, notions of personal autonomy or even civil rights. For example, public health entities have the authority to incarcerate an individual who is noncompliant with antituberculosis therapy, or to notify individuals that they have been exposed to a sexually transmitted or other communicable disease. Use of such authority is essentially abrogating privacy and intruding on personal autonomy. In a democratic society, a cost-benefit calculation would determine that the public good often outweighs privacy and freedom liberties.

Community Influence

Community support is essential for the development of public health policies. Thus, another way of looking at policy development is informing, educating, and empowering communities, processes that are dependent on both the assessment and communication public health functions. Mobilization of community partnerships is integral to policy development because such partners are the basis for political support. Political support is dependant essentially on the electoral process. If policy makers recognize community support and consensus for a public health initiative, political will to support those initiatives is greatly increased.

Potential advocates for STD policy can result in coalitions of grass-roots organizations and political organizations that may not be intuitively obvious. For example, women's groups have traditionally coalesced around issues of specific interest, such as infertility prevention, maternal-fetal health, and reproductive health. These issues can catalyze a natural alliance between the women's caucus in the congressional leadership and STD prevention interests. Grass-roots community organizing, following the models of nongovernmental organizations seen in international settings and developing countries, have been effective in influencing legislators when addressing the needs of particular populations. Probably the best example of community organizing has been in the area of HIV treatment and prevention. Early in the epidemic, community groups, especially those in the gay community, were especially effective in humanizing those affected by the disease. They also focused on legislative action, resulting in a treatment programs such as those funded by the Ryan White Care Act, and prevention and research programs.

Advocacy partnerships vary widely, depending on the specific objective. For example, two of the major advocacy groups for STD control are the American Social Health Association (ASHA) and the National Coalition of STD Directors (NCSD). Each has a different audience. ASHA largely focuses on consumers (patients) and provides resources and information, especially on chronic viral infections such as genital herpes and genital HPV infection. ASHA also advocates in the general public sector on the overall medical and economic impact of STDs. NCSD represents State public health programs and has typically collaborated with traditional public health advocates, such as the American Public Health Association and associations of county health officials. NCSD educates policy makers about a variety of issues related to STD prevention and control including funding for surveillance, public health infrastructure, and STD core support services.

One of the best partnership examples was the syphilis elimination program initiated in the late 1990s (45–49). This effort was fueled by substantial concern, in both the African American community and the public health community, over the increased rates of syphilis in heterosexual African Americans. Previous syphilis control programs were hampered by poor access to marginalized populations. In the African-American community, these problems were complicated by the historical legacy of discrimination and the Tuskegee syphilis study. Partnership with the affected community was seen as critical to success.

The *National Plan to Eliminate Syphilis from the United States* was released in 1999 (50). A key feature of this program was recognizing the need to interact with community partners. These partners included public health advocacy groups, health providers, grass-roots community organizations and supportive churches. The program start-up had many trust-building initiatives, including open discussion of past discrimination and of the Tuskegee study. One overall objective, which was achieved, was to provide support to enable and empower community members to deal with syphilis as a health problem and not as a stigmatizing issue. Achievement would not have been possible without developing successful partnerships. Tools for developing partnerships, which are translatable to multiple settings are available at the CDC Syphilis Elimination web site (51).

Communicating Policy with Senior Officials

Policy messages need to be effectively communicated to politicians in order to effect change. At times, these communications can be based on cost effectiveness arguments and savings for the health care system. At other times, policy communication may be emergently necessary due to political embarrassment. For example, in 1997–1998, a syphilis epidemic in Baltimore (52,53) embarrassed local political leaders, which in turn resulted in the rapid provision of resources (54). Effective utilization of these resources by health care personnel resulted in an extremely positive relationship between health department staff and the political process, which in turn enhanced future funding levels.

A common error made by many scientists and public health officials is overlooking the political realm. Political decision making is an art form. A briefing for policy makers should be concise and is typically provided in the form of a briefing paper, a talking points memo, and a very short presentation. Talking points memos are short, one-page documents that present the policy question, the stakeholder constituencies, and the pros and cons of policy options, closing with a recommendation and justification.

Economic Influences on Policy Making: Cost-Effectiveness

The cost and cost-effectiveness of public health programs is an area of increasing interest, and there is a growing amount of cost-effectiveness data for many STD diagnostic and therapeutic interventions, especially chlamydia screening (55–57). Such analyses are critically important when addressing policy makers, because effective prevention often requires investment of financial resources. STD interventions are usually less expensive than interventions typically used in general medical practice. For example, the annual costs of medical interventions for conditions such as end-stage renal disease, advanced coronary artery disease, and HIV treatment are between $30,000 and $60,000 per year.

Cost-effectiveness data need to be carefully evaluated. For example, cost effectiveness should be used as a tool only when the savings are seen as prevention of subsequent medical costs, Quality-Adjusted Life-Years (QALY), or Disability-Adjusted Life Years (DALY), all of which are internationally recognized normalization approaches. Some authorities recommend using full cost analyses, including indirect costs (e.g., lost income, overall societal benefit). See Chapter 21 in this book for more discussion about cost effectiveness analysis.

Managed care organizations (MCOs) have historically looked closely at cost-effectiveness of care and can be another potential source of support for STD advocacy. Vertically integrated MCOs, where the organization provides *and* pays for all medical and prevention services, are natural test beds for evaluating public health prevention interventions that result in later cost savings. In these systems, a single payer, which is also the provider, is responsible for the prevention services, medical services, hospital care, and all associated services. Therefore, cost savings realized by prevention result in increased revenue at the bottom line for the provider through decreased complication rates and a decreased need for treatment services. For example, large, vertically-integrated MCOs such as the Kaiser Permanente groups and Group Health of Puget Sound have been especially active in developing cost-effectiveness models for many diseases, including STD prevention initiatives (42,58–61). This model contrasts with the typical care reimbursement system in the United States, where investment in prevention services by either a hospital or health department results in savings not for the provider of these services but rather for the organization that pays for care (e.g., Medicare, Medicaid, other insurers). In this latter system, there is no feedback loop to compensate or reward for increased prevention.

Public Health Policy and the Prevention Cost Paradox

One of the most important issues facing prevention analysts is the cost paradox. The United States is largely structured for health care on a payment scheme. Therefore, payment is provided for clinical services rendered, not for morbidity that is prevented or population-level health promotion. This results in a clinical paradox (62). For example, it is often difficult to garner adequate funding for prevention initiatives; however, practitioners are well aware of the large sums of money spent on complications of preventable diseases, resulting in both practical and ethical dilemmas. The practical issues are that prevention programs are very difficult to tangibly assess, especially for the layperson and the policy maker. Furthermore, it is very difficult—medically, ethically, and politically—to refuse to provide care to sick individuals, even at the terminal phase of illness. Solutions to this problem have been evasive. One solution is a vertically integrated managed care system, such as Kaiser Permanente, in which clinical care and preventive care are all funded through the same financial source, as described above. In such a situation, there is a direct incentive to reduce overall costs, not just costs on the prevention side.

Case Study: Effective Intervention without Implementation—The Failure of Translational Follow-Through

Although there has been substantial research on behavioral interventions, there has been little investment in implementation. One of the best examples in this area is Project RESPECT. Project RESPECT was a large multi-center behavioral intervention project which was conducted by CDC from1992 to 1995 in five STD clinics (63,64). Project RESPECT conclusively showed that behavioral intervention in an STD clinic (high risk) setting can yield benefits, both in terms of behaviors such as increased condom use and decreased STD rates. Despite this demonstrated effectiveness, the Project RESPECT intervention was never implemented in the vast majority of STD clinics. This occurred for a number of reasons. First, the demonstration project clearly indicated the need for increased support and training of staff and improved infrastructure. Second, in underfunded programs, if managers are presented a choice between allocating funds for treating symptomatic STDs or investing in behavioral counseling, treating symptomatic patients is always prioritized. Finally, the savings from preventing HIV and other STDs primarily accrue to the health insurers, not to the prevention agencies.

Case Study: Chlamydia and Infertility Prevention—Successful Screening Intervention for Women, but Not for Men

An example of both the advantages and disadvantages of the legislative process is the development of the chlamydia control and prevention initiatives. The major morbidity of chlamydia was well-appreciated to be the development of pelvic inflammatory disease and subsequent infertility. Therefore, as chlamydia screening initiatives were developed, it became very clear that women should be their initial targets, primarily to prevent development of these subsequent complications. Chlamydia prevention was marketed to legislators in the 1980s as an infertility and neonatal infection prevention program.

Although this approach resulted in broad-based political support, it was limited by its failure to support screening of men or partner management. Although a number of venues have begun to implement chlamydia screening of men (e.g., correctional centers, job core centers, adolescent clinics, STD clinic) (65), no federal programs currently support male screening.

Using Science to Instruct Policy

Framing the Issue for Success

Case Study from the United Kingdom

How an issue is framed can significantly impact its ability to be successfully addressed through policy. One of the best examples of using data to successfully inform policy and effective advocacy was development of the National Strategy for Sexual Health and HIV in the United Kingdom in 2001 (66). Concern over increased pregnancy and STD rates in the United Kingdom prompted a Parliamentary Commission of Inquiry in 2002 (67). The Commission recommended greater investment in STD services, increased support of National Health Service (NHS) STD interventions, and implementation of a national chlamydia screening program.

This initiative has had broad-based support (68,69). The Commission's report to Parliament largely focused on improving *sexual health* rather than on *sexual disease* or consequences. From a clinical care perspective, the goals included improving health care and social care for people living with HIV, and reducing the stigma associated with HIV and *sexually transmitted infections* (STIs). The linking of STI care to HIV care resulted in substantial support from the HIV advocacy community for improved care services. The sexual health plan included specific clinical provision issues, such as providing more patient-friendly services at the NHS facilities. The plan also addressed social issues, including improved sex education, prevention initiatives, overall reduction of social inequality, and specific outreach to vulnerable groups such as homosexual men, injecting drug users, and immigrants. The Commission was able to assess the problems with input from stakeholders and based on that assessment, develop an acceptable strategy that promoted sexual health and expanded clinical services.

Policy Controversies in the United States

The United States has the highest rate of teenage pregnancy among other developed countries, and nearly one million of these are terminated annually through therapeutic abortion (70). Although the abortion rate has dropped significantly over the past decade, it is still much higher than that seen in other developed countries.

Despite the large number of unwanted pregnancies and high STD rates, one of the most contentious policy issues in the United States has been sex education for adolescents. The foci of the two primary competing programs are *abstinence-only* and *comprehensive sex* education (71). Both approaches include the biology of reproduction. However, abstinence-only education programs place great emphasis on the adverse impacts of sexual intercourse prior to marriage (72–74), and contraception and condom use as prevention strategies are not included. In contrast, comprehensive sex education includes all forms of disease prevention, such as delayed onset of sexual intercourse, abstinence, health promotion, and appropriate use and benefits of contraception and condoms (75).

In addition, service delivery access, in general, presents real and substantive problems. Over 45 million persons in the United States currently lack health insurance. Although there have been significant advances in providing access to services for children and young adults, there are still important gaps, especially for adolescents, older males, and women who are not pregnant or do not have dependents. When teens and young adults do choose to seek reproductive health services, they face substantial structural barriers. Without parental consent, they frequently cannot access insurance for which they are eligible, payment, and/or transportation. For those covered under a parent's insurance plan, confidentiality may be an important barrier to seeking care because the service delivery and payment notifications that are typically mailed out to the subscriber.

Case Study: The Efficacy of Condoms—Interpretation of Empirical Data

An important intersection of policy and science revolves around the issue of condom promotion as a major form of STD prevention. Despite a long history of being recommended and used both for contraception and STD control, condoms actually lack formally and rigorously obtained clinical data demonstrating effectiveness (76,77). The absence of such studies is largely related to the fact that condom efficacy is difficult to study, especially since study designs would require that all individuals at a minimum be counseled about standard public health practice, which includes condom use. Thus, it is unethical to conduct a trial where individuals are exposed to sexually transmitted infections without recommending use of a condom. Therefore, indirect methodologies have to be used, resulting in problems with selection and reporting bias. Even under these constraints, however, there are increasing data that condoms are effective in reducing risk of transmission of HIV, gonorrhea, herpes, and chlamydia (77). In addition, there are ecological data from large country-level programs as in Thailand, where national campaigns to increase condom use resulted concurrently in structural interventions (i.e., 100% condom use regulations in brothels, development of alternative recreational activities for army personnel), destigmatization of HIV in public discourse, and substantial (over 90%) decreases in STDs (78,79). The 100% condom campaign has been promoted extensively by the Thai Ministry of Health, and more recently, by other countries in Southeast Asia, such as Cambodia and Vietnam (80,81).

In 2000, the NIH held a consensus conference to assess the data on condom efficacy (76). The motivations for this conference were largely driven by an emerging political debate in the late 1990s which argued that, since there were no data from randomized clinical trials on condom efficacy, they should not be promoted as an effective means to prevent STDs (76). Based on review of the published literature, the conference concluded that apart from HIV and gonorrhea, there was little efficacy data to demonstrate condom effectiveness for most STDs. Some organizations focused on the absence of data as justification for discouraging the recommendation of condom use in high-risk situations (82). The dearth of data also provided justification for Congress to enact subsequent legislation that directed the FDA (83) to mandate labeling on condom packaging that indicated both the "overall effectiveness" *and* the "lack of effectiveness" in preventing STDs, including condom efficacy for specific STDs. This mandate represented a changed emphasis from the FDA regulations in place since 1987 which required that condom packages include language emphasizing the *effectiveness* of condoms against STDs when used properly. The explicit goal of the new mandate was to inform consumers about the *limitations* of the device (84).

In response, there was a large surge in research to evaluate condom efficacy using more methodologically sound designs (73). Innovative clinical trial designs evaluated data seen in patients from sexual partnerships (85, 86). Other studies used sophisticated retrospective analyses of previous data sets, like those collected for such purposes as STD vaccine trials (87). A recent prospective study showed that condom use reduces male to female transmission of human papillomavirus (HPV) (88), an area of great interest to policy makers. The growing body of scientific evidence showing that condoms reduce the transmission risk of most STDs, including human papillomavirus (89), more firmly supports recommendations regarding the importance of condoms in STD/HIV prevention among individuals who choose to be sexually active (18). See Chapter 10 in this book for more extensive discussion of the latest studies on male condoms.

Case Study: Abstinence-Only Sex Education

Abstinence-only education has been the primary sex education policy of the federal government in the United States since the mid-1990s (90). Funded through the 1996 Social Security Act, Title V, Section 510 (88) as well as Special Projects of Regional and National Significance (SPRANS) as part of block grants starting in 2005 (91), abstinence-only education programs must adhere to the following guidance:

A. Have as its exclusive purpose teaching the social, psychological, and health gains to be realized by abstaining from sexual activity
B. Teach abstinence from sexual activity outside marriage as the expected standard for all school-age children
C. Teach that abstinence from sexual activity is the only certain way to avoid out-of-wedlock pregnancy, STDs, and other associated health problems
D. Teach that a mutually faithful, monogamous relationship in the context of marriage is the expected standard of sexual activity
E. Teach that sexual activity outside the context of marriage is likely to have harmful psychological and physical effects
F. Teach that bearing children out-of-wedlock is likely to have harmful consequences for the child, the child's parents, and society
G. Teach young people how to reject sexual advances and how alcohol and drug use increases vulnerability to sexual advances

H. Teach the importance of attaining self-sufficiency before engaging in sexual activity

Abstinence–only sex education is by definition not comprehensive. Yet, it is important to note that national surveys have shown that over 88% of American adults have had vaginal sexual intercourse prior to marriage (92). Though almost all adults (94%) and teens (92%) believe it is important that society give a strong message that teens delay sex until after high school (93), most believe that the abstinence-only approach will not prevent STDs or unwanted pregnancies (94). Most also think teens who are sexually active should have access to birth control (94).

Study results from abstinence-only approaches must be carefully examined before conclusions are drawn. For example, data from large nationally based prospective surveys of adolescents have shown that abstinence-only programs and the use of virginity pledges delayed the onset of coital debut by six months (95). However, although these programs delayed the onset of coitus, when it did occur, the virginity pledgers were less likely to use contraception and condoms than others, resulting in increased risk for pregnancy and STDs. When analyzed over time, the cumulative STD and pregnancy rates in the virginity pledge groups were similar to those of the nonabstinent group, and in some subsets, were actually higher. Findings were stable across both socioeconomic and ethnic lines. These data suggest that lack of comprehensive sex education, which affords the young individual the tools to use for protection in case sexual intercourse occurs unexpectedly or in an unplanned fashion, reduces the STD and pregnancy prevention benefits of abstinence programs. The few studies to date that have reported positive results from abstinence-only programs have had significant methodological limitations (e.g., measuring short-term behaviors, small sample sizes, use of nonstandard statistical data, use of self-reported vs. laboratory-confirmed STIs) (73,75).

Therefore, in this case, the emphasis of the national public health policy on abstinence-only education for youth is discordant with the practices and attitudes of the vast majority of the American population as well as the existing science. In contrast to this approach, peer-reviewed research on abstinence-only education and comprehensive sex education (72,73) has led many prestigious organizations to recommend a different policy direction. For example, the Institute of Medicine (96), the American Academy of Pediatrics (97), and the American Psychological Association (98) have all concluded that sex education for adolescents needs to offer comprehensive approaches to optimize prevention (including abstinence), and that abstinence-only programs leave adolescents vulnerable and unarmed with the tools they need to prevent harmful outcomes.

Science, Policy Making, and Politics in STD Prevention and Reproductive Health: Tensions and Promise

The Institute of Medicine concluded that health policy making should be driven by public health concerns and based on scientific knowledge (1). Yet, politics clearly influences the way science, policy making and public health practice converge, especially in the field of reproductive health. The controversies in the United States about emergency contraception, condoms, and abstinence education exemplify the influence of politics on how public health problems are addressed. Similar observations can be made in the field of global warming where environmental scientists have recently argued the importance of distinguishing policy from politics as a way to ensure that science instructs policy without political bias. Science, they would argue, cannot resolve political differences since scientific results can be interpreted to support different political agendas (8,99). Rather, scientists might more usefully and more objectively link their results to policy. In other words, scientific inquiry should not only show results but should also offer policy options based on those results. Using science to justify a political agenda after that agenda has been defined removes the objectivity of the science (99).

Policy making as a core function of public health plays a critical role in effective STD prevention. If policy options are not informed by science, political agendas may weaken the effectiveness of STD prevention efforts. At the same time, one cannot ignore the influence of politics on policy makers. Partnerships between the public and private sectors can constructively fuel the political arena within which policy is developed. To maximize STD prevention efforts, STD prevention scientists, public health practitioners, health care providers and the general public must recognize the complementary but different roles of science, policy and politics in formulating effective public health programs.

Acknowledgments: The author acknowledges support from NIH grant K13-AI01633. Ms. Lin Rucker provided invaluable assistance in preparing the manuscript. I also acknowledge the review and constructive comments from Dr. Stephen Teret of Johns Hopkins Bloomberg School of Public Health and an anonymous reviewer.

References

1. Institute of Medicine. *The Future of Public Health.* Washington, DC: National Academy Press; 1988:1–18,35–55.
2. Institute of Medicine. *Healthy Communities: New Partnerships for the Future of Public Health.* Washington, DC: National Academy Press; 1996:33–50.
3. Scutchfield FD, Keck CW. *Principles of Public Health Practice.* Albany, NY: Delmar Publishers; 1997:111–212.
4. McGarrigle CA, Fenton KA, Gill ON, Hughes G, Morgan D, Evans B. Behavioural surveillance: the value of national coordination. *Sex Transm Infect.* 2002;78:398–405.
5. Suen J, Magruder C. National profile: overview of capabilities and core functions of local public health jurisdictions in 47 states, the District of Columbia, and 3 U.S. territories, 2000-2002. *J Public Health Manag Pract.* 2004;10:2–12.
6. Lasswell HD, Kaplan A. *Power and Society: A Framework for Political Inquiry.* New Haven, CT: Yale University Press; 1950:55–102.
7. Lasswell HD. *Politics: Who Gets What, When, How, with Postscript.* New Haven, CT: Yale University Press; 1958:13–27.
8. Pielke RA Jr. When scientists politicize science: making sense of controversy over The Skeptical Environmentalist. *Environmental Science & Policy.* 2004;7: 405–417.
9. Institute of Medicine. *The Hidden Epidemic: Confronting Sexually Transmitted Diseases.* Washington, DC: National Academy Press; 1997:1–17.
10. Haider M. *Global Public Health Communication: Challenges, Perspectives, and Strategies.* Sudbury, MA: Jones and Bartlett Publishers; 2005:1–150.
11. Institute of Medicine. *Public Health Risks of Disasters: Communication, Infrastructure, and Preparedness—Workshop Summary.* Washington, DC: National Academies Press; 2005:7–18.

12. Code of Federal Regulations. Part 51b_Project Grants for Preventive Health Services. Available at: http://a257.g.akamaitech.net/7/257/ 2422/12feb20041500/ edocket.access.gpo. gov/cfr_2004/octqtr/42cfr51b.406.htm. Accessed September 13, 2006.

13. Health Resources and Services Administration. Ryan White CARE Act, 1990. Available at: http://hab.hrsa.gov/history.htm. Accessed September 13, 2006.

14. Brown ST, Wiesner PJ. Problems and approaches to the control and surveillance of sexually transmitted agents associated with pelvic inflammatory disease in the United States. *Am J Obstet Gynecol.* 1980;138(7 Pt 2):1096–1100.

15. Stamm WE, Holmes KK. Measures to control chlamydia trachomatis infections: an assessment of new national policy guidelines. *JAMA.* 1986;256:1178–1179.

16. Centers for Disease Control and Prevention. Recommendations for the prevention and management of chlamydia trachomatis infections, 1993. *MMWR.* 1993;42(RR-12):1–39.

17. Cates W Jr, Rolfs RT Jr, Aral SO. Sexually transmitted diseases, pelvic inflammatory disease, and infertility: an epidemiologic update. *Epidemiol Rev.* 1990;12:199–220.

18. Centers for Disease Control and Prevention. Sexually transmitted diseases treatment guidelines, 2006. *MMWR.* 2006;55(No. RR-11):1–94.

19. Fife K. Over-the-counter Acyclovir: an idea whose time has come. *Sex Transm Dis.* 1996;23:174–176.

20. Handsfield HH. Acyclovir should not be approved for marketing without prescription. *Sex Transm Dis.* 1996;23:171–173.

21. Sande MA, Armstrong D, Corey L, Drew WL, Gilbert D, Moellering RC Jr, Smith LG. Perspectives on switching oral acyclovir from prescription to over-the-counter status: report of a consensus panel. *Clin Infect Dis.* 1998;26:659–663.

22. Piaggio G, von Hertzen H, Grimes DA, Van Look PF. Timing of emergency contraception with levonorgestrel or the Yuzpe regimen. Task Force on Postovulatory Methods of Fertility Regulation. *Lancet.* 1999;353:721.

23. Food and Drug Administration. Nonprescription Drugs Advisory Committee and the Advisory Committee for Reproductive Health Drugs. December 16, 2003. Available at http://www.fda.gov/ohrms/dockets/ac/ 03/slides/4015s1.htm,

24. Grimes DA, Raymond EG. Emergency contraception. *Ann Intern Med.* 2002;137:180–189.

25. Davis D. Safety Review for Plan B. Presentation to Food and Drug Administration, December 16, 2003. Available at: http://www.fda.gov/ ohrms/dockets/ac/03/slides/4015S1_03_FDA-Davis.ppt.

26. Pruitt SL, Mullen PD. Contraception or abortion? Inaccurate descriptions of emergency contraception in newspaper articles, 1992-2002. *Contraception.* 2005;71:14–21.

27. Couzin J. Drug Regulation—Plan B: a collision of science and politics. *Science.* 2005;310:38–39.

28. Raine TR, Harper CC, Rocca CH, et al. Direct access to emergency contraception through pharmacies and effect on unintended pregnancy and STIs: a randomized controlled trial. *JAMA.* 2005;293:54–62.

29. Wood SF. Women's health and the FDA. *N Engl J Med.* 2005;353:1650–1651.

30. Mathews C, Coetzee N, Zwarenstein M, Guttmacher S. Partner notification. *Clin Evid.* 2004;(11):2113–2120.

31. Low N, McCarthy A, Roberts TE, et al. Partner notification of chlamydia infection in primary care: randomised controlled trial and analysis of resource use. *BMJ.* 2006;332:14–19.

32. Kissinger P, Mohammed H, Richardson-Alston G, et al. Patient-delivered partner treatment for male urethritis: a randomized, controlled trial. *Clin Infect Dis.* 2005;41:623–629.

33. Golden MR. Expedited partner therapy for sexually transmitted diseases. *Clin Infect Dis.* 2005;41:630–633.

34. Golden MR, Whittington WL, Handsfield HH, et al. Effect of expedited treatment of sex partners on recurrent or persistent gonorrhea or chlamydial infection. *N Engl J Med.* 2005;352:676–685.

35. Golden MR, Anukam U, Williams DH, Handsfield HH. The legal status of patient-delivered partner therapy for sexually transmitted infections in the United States: a national survey of state medical and pharmacy boards. *Sex Transm Dis.* 2005;32:112–114.

36. Centers for Disease Control and Prevention. Public health service guidelines for counseling and antibody testing to prevent HIV infection and AIDS. *MMWR.* 1987;36:509–515.

37. Centers for Disease Control and Prevention. ACIP Provisional Recommendations for the Use of Quadrivalent HPV Vaccine. (date of vote: June 29, 2006) Available at: http://www.cdc.gov/nip/recs/provisional_recs/hpv.pdf. Accessed September 12, 2006.

38. Centers for Disease Control and Prevention. Revised recommendations for HIV testing of adults, adolescents, and pregnant women in health care settings. *MMWR.* 2006;55(RR-14):1–17.

39. Williams LA, Klausner JD, Whittington WLH, Handsfield HH, Celum C, Holmes KK. Elimination and reintroduction of primary and secondary syphilis. *American Journal of Public Health.* 1999;89:1093–1097.

40. Svensson L, Mardh PA, Westrom L. Infertility after acute salpingitis with special reference to chlamydia trachomatis. *Fertil Steril.* 1983/;40:322–329.

41. Centers for Disease Control and Prevention. Screening tests to Detect *Chlamydia trachomatis* and *Neisseria gonorrhoeae* infections—2002. MMWR 2002;51(No. RR-15).

42. Magid DJ, Stiffman M, Anderson LA, Irwin K, Lyons EE. Adherence to CDC STD guideline recommendations for the treatment of *Chlamydia trachomatis* infection in two managed care organizations. *Sex Transm Dis.* 2003;30:30–32.

43. Schillinger JA, Xu F, Sternberg MR, et al. National seroprevalence and trends in herpes simplex virus type 1 in the United States, 1976–1994. *Sex Transm Dis.* 2004;31:753–60.

44. Mosher WD, Chandra A, Jones J. Sexual behavior and selected health measures: men and women 15-44 years of age, United States, 2002. *Adv Data.* 2005;362:1–55.

45. Hook EW, 3rd. Is elimination of endemic syphilis transmission a realistic goal for the USA? *Lancet.* 1998;351(Suppl 3):19–21.

46. Hook EW 3rd. Elimination of syphilis transmission in the United States: historic perspectives and practical considerations. *Trans Am Clin Climatol Assoc.* 1999;110:195–203;110:195,203; discussion 203–204.

47. Satcher D. From the CDC: syphilis elimination: history in the making—closing remarks. *Sex Transm Dis.* 2000;27:66–67.

48. St Louis ME, Wasserheit JN. Elimination of syphilis in the United States. *Science.* 1998;281:353–354.

49. Thomas RJ, MacDonald MR, Lenart M, Calvert WB, Morrow R. Moving toward the eradication of syphilis. *Mil Med.* 2002;167:489–495.

50. Centers for Disease Control and Prevention. The National Plan to Eliminate Syphilis from the United States. Atlanta, GA: U.S. Department of Health and Human Services, CDC, National Center for HIV, STD, and TB Prevention; 1999;1–84.

51. Centers for Disease Control and Prevention. Syphilis Elimination Effort Toolkit. Available at: http://www.cdc.gov/std/see/. Accessed September 13, 2006.

52. Centers for Disease Control and Prevention (CDC). Outbreak of primary and secondary syphilis—Baltimore City, Maryland, 1995. *MMWR.* 1996;45:166–169.

53. Schumacher CM, Bernstein KT, Zenilman JM, Rompalo AM. Reassessing a large-scale syphilis epidemic using an estimated infection date. *Sex Transm Dis.* 2005;32:659–664.

54. No author listed. Baltimore loses number one spot. *AIDS Patient Care STDS.* 2000;14:676.

55. Jackson B. Relative Cost-effectiveness of different tests for *Chlamydia trachomatis. Ann Intern Med.* 2005;142:308; author reply 308–309.

56. Honey E, Augood C, Templeton A, et al. Cost effectiveness of screening for *Chlamydia trachomatis*: a review of published studies. *Sex Transm Infect.* 2002;78:406–412.

57. Pozniak AL. Screening for chlamydia: what is the cost? *Curr Opin Infect Dis.* 2005;18:35–36.

58. Burstein G, Snyder M, Conley D, et al. Screening females for *Chlamydia trachomatis* (CT) in a large managed care organization (MCO). A New HEDIS Measure. *J Pediatr Adolesc Gynecol.* 2000;13:91.

59. Burstein GR, Snyder MH, Conley D, Boekeloo BO, Quinn TC, Zenilman JM. Adolescent chlamydia testing practices and diagnosed infections in a large managed care organization. *Sex Transm Dis.* 2001;28:477–483.

60. Scholes D, Anderson LA, Operskalski BH, BlueSpruce J, Irwin K, Magid DJ. STD prevention and treatment guidelines: a review from a managed care perspective. *Am J Manag Care.* 2003;9:181–189; quiz 190–191.

61. Scholes D, Stergachis A, Heidrich FE, Andrilla H, Holmes KK, Stamm WE. Prevention of pelvic inflammatory disease by screening for cervical chlamydial infection. *N Engl J Med.* 1996;334:1362–1366.

62. Chaulk CP, Zenilman J. Sexually transmitted disease control in the era of managed care: "magic bullet" or "shadow on the land"? *J Public Health Manag Pract.* 1997;3:61–70.

63. Kamb ML, Fishbein M, Douglas JM Jr, et al. Efficacy of risk-reduction counseling to prevent human immunodeficiency virus and sexually transmitted diseases: a randomized controlled trial. Project RESPECT Study Group. *JAMA.* 1998;280:1161–1167.

64. Fishbein M, Hennessy M, Kamb M, et al. Project Respect Study Group. Using intervention theory to model factors influencing behavior change. Project RESPECT. *Eval Health Prof.* 2001;24:363–384.

65. Schillinger JA, Dunne EF, Chapin JB, et al. Prevalence of *Chlamydia trachomatis* infection among men screened in 4 U.S. cities. *Sex Transm Dis.* 2005;32:74–77.

66. Department of Health (United Kingdom). The National Strategy for Sexual Health and HIV. London: Department of Health; 2001. Available at: http://www.dh.gov.uk/assetRoot/04/05/89/45/04058945.pdf

67. Adler MW. Sexual health—health of the nation. *Sex Transm Infect.* 2003;79:85–87.

68. Sherrard J, Robinson AJ. The MSSVD, the National Sexual Health and HIV Strategy for England and Genitourinary Medicine Education. *Sex Transm Infect.* 2003;79:166–167.

69. Rogstad KE, Henton L. General practitioners and the national strategy on sexual health and HIV. *Int J STD AIDS.* 2004;15:169–172.

70. Strauss LT, Herndon J, Chang J, Parker WY, Bowens SV, Berg CJ. Abortion surveillance—United States, 2002. *MMWR Surveill Summ.* 2005;54:1–31.

71. Kirby D. *Emerging Answers—Research Findings on Programs to Reduce Teen Pregnancy* (Summary). Washington, DC: National Campaign to Prevent Teen Pregnancy; 2001; p7.

72. Fortenberry JD. The limits of abstinence-only in preventing sexually transmitted infections. *J Adolesc Health.* 2005;36:269–270.

73. Santelli J, Ott MA, Lyon M, Rogers J, Summers D, Schleifer R. Abstinence and abstinence-only education: a review of U.S. policies and programs. *J Adolesc Health*. 2006;38:72–81.

74. Santelli J, Ott MA, Lyon M, Rogers J, Summers D. Abstinence-only education policies and programs: a position paper of the society for adolescent medicine. *J Adolesc Health*. 2006;38:83–87.

75. Kirby D. Reflections on two decades of research on teen sexual behavior and pregnancy. *J Sch Health*. 1999;69:89–94.

76. National Institute of Allergy and Infectious Diseases. Workshop Summary: Scientific Evidence on Condom Effectiveness for Sexually Transmitted Disease prevention, June 12-13, 2000. Bethesda, MD: National Institutes of Health; 2001. Available at: http://www3.niaid.nih.gov/research/topics/STI/pdf/condomreport.pdf

77. Holmes KK, Levine R, Weaver M. Effectiveness of condoms in preventing sexually transmitted infections. *Bull World Health Organ*. 2004;82:454–461.

78. Ainsworth M, Beyrer C, Soucat A. AIDS and public policy: the lessons and challenges of "success" in Thailand. *Health Policy*. 2003;64:13–37.

79. Celentano DD, Bond KC, Lyles CM, et al. Preventive intervention to reduce sexually transmitted infections: a field trial in the Royal Thai Army. *Arch Intern Med*. 2000;160:535–540.

80. World Health Organization. WHO's current programmes in Viet Nam. Available at: http://www.un.org.vn/who/programme.htm. Accessed September 20, 2006.

81. Wong ML, Lubek I, Dy BC, Pen S, Dros S, Chhit M. Social and behavioural factors associated with condom use among direct sex workers in Siem Reap, Cambodia. *Sex Transm Infect*. 2003;79:163–165.

82. Boonstra H. Public Health Advocates Say Campaign to Disparage Condoms Threatens STD Prevention Efforts. Guttmacher Report on Public Policy. March 2003.

83. Public Law 106–554—Dec. 21, 2000. Available at: http://www.ewg.org/issues_content/mercury/20031222/DataQualityAct.pdf. Accessed September 20, 2006.

84. Statement before Subcommittee on Criminal Justice, Drug Policy, and Human Resources Committee on Government Reform before the US House of Representatives, March 11, 2004. Available at: http://www.fda.gov/ola/2004/condom0311.html. Accessed September 20, 2006.

85. Warner L, Newman DR, Austin HD, et al. Condom effectiveness for reducing transmission of gonorrhea and chlamydia: the importance of assessing partner infection status. *Am J Epidemiol*. 2004;159:242–251.

86. Warner L, Stone KM, Macaluso M, Buehler JW, Austin HD. Condom use and risk of g6norrhea and chlamydia: a systematic review of design and measurement factors assessed in epidemiologic studies. *Sex Transm Dis*. 2006;33:36–51.

87. Wald A, Langenberg AG, Link K, et al. Effect of condoms on reducing the transmission of herpes simplex virus type 2 from men to women. *JAMA*. 2001;285:3100–3106.

88. Winer RL, Hughes JP, Feng Q, et al. Condom use and the risk of genital human papillomavirus infection in young women. *N Engl J Med*. 2006;354: 2645–2654.

89. Steiner MJ, Cates W Jr. Condoms and sexually transmitted infections. *N Engl J Med*. 2006;354:2642–2643.

90. Social Security Administration. Separate Program for Abstinence Education. Available at: http://www.ssa.gov/OP_Home/ssact/title05/0510.htm. Accessed September 13, 2006.

91. Health Resources and Services Administration. Abstinence Education. Available at: http://mchb.hrsa.gov/programs/adolescents/abstinence.htm. Accessed September 13, 2006.

92. Laumann, EO, Gagnon JH, Michael RT, Michaels S. *The Social Organization of Sexuality: Sexual Practices in the United States*. Chicago: University of Chicago; 1994:203–213.

93. National Campaign to Prevent Teen Pregnancy. America's Adults and Teens Sound off about Teen Pregnancy—An Annual National Survey. December 2003. Available at: http://www.teenpregnancy.org/resources/data/pdf/wov2003.pdf

94. American Public Health Association. APHA National Survey, 2004. Harris Interactive for Research!America. Available at: http://www.researchamerica.org/polldata/2004/apha2004.pdf

95. Bruckner H, Bearman P. After the Promise: the STD consequences of adolescent virginity pledges. *J Adolesc Health*. 2005;36:271–278.

96. Institute of Medicine *No Time to Lose: Getting More from HIV Prevention*. Washington, DC: National Academy Press; 2001:116–120.

97. Klein JD, AAP Committee on Adolescence. adolescent pregnancy: current trends and issues. *Pediatrics*. 2005;116:281–286.

98. American Psychological Association. Resolution in Support of Empirically Supported Sex Education and HIV Prevention Programs for Adolescents. Available at: http://www.apa.org/releases/sexed_resolution.pdf. Accessed September 15, 2006.

99. Sarewitz D. Liberating science from politics. *American Scientist*. 2006;35:104.

Index

Printed in the United States
97155LV00004BB